Healthy China

Healthy China: Deepening Health Reform in China

Building High-Quality and Value-Based Service Delivery

A copublication of the World Bank and the World Health Organization

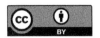

Contents

Boxes

Figures

Tables

Preface

During the past three decades, China has achieved a momentous social transformation, pulling 600 million people out of poverty. At the same time, it has made impressive strides in health. Since the launch of a new round of reforms in 2009, China has invested substantially in expanding health infrastructure, achieved nearly universal health insurance coverage, promoted more equal access to public health services, and established a national essential medicine system.

These measures have significantly improved the accessibility of health services, greatly reduced child and maternal mortality, cut the incidence of infectious disease, and considerably improved the health outcomes and life expectancy of the Chinese population: average life expectancy reached 76.34 years in 2015, 1.51 years longer than in 2010. And the country's overall health level has reached the average of other middle- and high-income countries, achieving better health outcomes with less input. These achievements have been well recognized internationally.

China has now reached a turning point. It is starting to face many of the same challenges and pressures that high-income countries face. The Chinese population over the age of 65 is approximately 140 million, and that cohort is expected to grow to 230 million by 2030. High-risk behaviors like smoking, sedentary lifestyles, and alcohol consumption as well as environmental factors such as air pollution take a huge toll on health, and noncommunicable diseases account for more than 80 percent of the 10.3 million deaths every year. At the same time, with higher economic growth, increased personal incomes, and fast-changing in consumption patterns, people are demanding more and better health care. As a result of all these factors, expenditures on health care have increased continuously in recent years. For China, this rapid growth in health expenditure may be difficult to sustain amid the country's economic slowdown.

The Chinese government fully recognizes the need to make strategic shifts in the health sector to adapt to these new challenges. President Xi Jinping and Premier Li Keqiang have placed great importance on health care reform. As President Xi has pointed out, it would not be possible to build a well-off society without universal health coverage. He also indicated that China should shift its focus and resources toward the lower levels of care, aiming to provide its citizens with public health and basic health services that are safe, effective, accessible, and affordable. Premier Li has held several State Council executive meetings to set priorities in health care reform and asked for the development of a basic health care system covering all urban and rural residents. The State Council has set up a Leading Group for Deepening Health Care Reform to strengthen multisector coordination, which provides a strong institutional guarantee for the reforms.

In July 2014 in Beijing, the Chinese government, the World Bank, and the World Health Organization committed to working together on a joint health reform study to further improve the policy formulation and to deepen the health reform. This report, *Healthy China: Deepening Health Reform in China*, is the outcome of this joint study. Following the successful model of previous flagship reports such as *China 2030* and *Urban China*, this report offers a blueprint for further reforms in China's health sector.

In July 2016, Minister of Finance Lou Jiwei, Minister of the National Health and Family Planning Commission Li Bin, and Deputy Minister of Human Resources and Social Security You Jun, joined by World Bank Group President Jim Yong Kim and Bernhard Schwartländer, the World Health Organization representative to China, jointly launched the Policy Summary of this report at the Diaoyutai Guesthouse in Beijing. The Policy Summary has received wide praise from the media and academia, has been disseminated to the health policy makers in all the provinces in China, and has served as an important instrument for policy making.

The report's main theme is the need for China to transition its health care delivery system toward people-centered, high-quality, integrated care built on the foundation of a strong primary health care system. Such a system offers both better health care for its citizens and better value for its economy.

To that end, the report offers a comprehensive set of eight interlinked recommendations that can prepare the Chinese health system for the demographic and health challenges it faces. It focuses not only on the top-level design for reform but also on the important question of how to make reform work on the ground. It builds on extensive analysis of literature and case studies from high- and middle-income countries as well as on ongoing innovations in China that offer lessons and experiences for bringing about desired change. The report draws upon cutting-edge thinking about the science of delivery that can help in the scaling up of health reforms—from prefecture to province and, ultimately, nationwide.

Our hope is that this report will provide the research, analysis, and insight to help central and local authorities plan and execute major restructuring of the health care delivery system in China during the 13th Five-Year Plan period of 2016–20. Getting this reform right is crucial to China's social and economic success in the coming decades. We believe that China's experience with health service delivery reform carries many lessons for other countries, and we hope this report can also contribute to a global knowledge base on health reform.

Acknowledgments

This study was organized jointly by China's Ministry of Finance (MoF), National Health and Family Planning Commission (NHFPC), and Ministry of Human Resources and Social Security (MoHRSS); the World Health Organization (WHO); and the World Bank. The study was proposed by Premier Li Keqiang, Vice Premier Liu Yandong, Minister Lou Jiwei of MoF, Minister Li Bin of NHFPC, Minister Yin Weimin of MoHRSS, and World Bank Group President Jim Yong Kim. WHO Director-General Margaret Chan provided valuable leadership and guidance at the initiation as well as at the critical junctions of the study. In particular, Vice Premier Liu hosted two special hearings on the progress and main findings for the study in March of 2015 and 2016.

Under the overall leadership of Minister Lou (MoF) and World Bank Managing Director and Chief Operating Officer Sri Mulyani Indrawati, the report was overseen by a joint team from the five participating organizations, led by the following: MoF vice ministers Yaobin Shi and Weiping Yu; NHFPC vice ministers Zhigang Sun and Xiaowei Ma; MoHRSS Vice Minister Jun You and former vice minister Xiaoyi Hu; WHO Regional Director for the Western Pacific Shin Young-soo; WHO representative to China Bernhard Schwartländer; Vivian Lin, director, Division of Health Sector Development, WHO Western Pacific Regional Office; Axel van Trotsenburg,

World Bank vice president, East Asia and Pacific Region; Timothy Grant Evans, senior director of the World Bank's Health, Nutrition & Population (HNP) Global Practice (GP); Olusoji Adeyi, director of the Bank's HNP GP; Bert Hofman, World Bank country director for China, the Republic of Korea, and Mongolia; Mara Warwick, World Bank operations manager for China, Korea, and Mongolia; and Toomas Palu, global practice manager for the Bank's HNP GP in the East Asia and Pacific Region.

Valuable advice was provided by the members of the team's external advisory panel: Michael Porter, Bishop William Lawrence University Professor at the Institute for Strategy and Competitiveness, Harvard Business School; Donald Berwick, president emeritus, senior fellow, and former president and chief executive officer of the Institute for Healthcare Improvement and former administrator of the Centers for Medicare and Medicaid Services; Winnie Yip, professor of health policy and economics at the Blavatnik School of Government, University of Oxford; Ellen Nolte, coordinator of the European Observatory at the London School of Economics and Political Science and the London School of Hygiene & Tropical Medicine; Yanfeng Ge, director-general, Department of Social Development Research, Development Research Center of the State Council, China; and Shangxi Liu, director-general, Chinese Academy of Fiscal Sciences.

A technical working group (TWG), consisting of technical leads from each of the government agencies as well as the World Bank and WHO, was formed at the beginning of the study. The TWG has led technical communications, provided important comments, and facilitated research data from different departments of the Ministries. Its members included Yao Licheng, Peng Xiang, Wang Lei, and Wang Min (MoF); Jiao Yahui, Zhao Shuli, Zhuang Ning, Liu Yue, Qin Kun, and Chen Kai (NHFPC); Wang Guodong, Zhao Zhihong, and Song Chengjin (MoHRSS); Gerard La Forgia, Shuo Zhang, and Rui Liu (World Bank); and Martin Taylor, Wen Chunmei, and Stephanie Dunn (WHO).

Within the World Bank, task team leaders Gerard La Forgia and Mukesh Chawla received significant on-the-ground support from Shuo Zhang as well as from Elena Glinskaya, Daixin Li, and Rui Liu in the World Bank's Beijing office. Martin Taylor was the core team member from WHO, with support from Clive Tan, Ding Wang, and Tuo Hong Zhang of WHO and from Edward Hsu and Jiadi Yu of the World Bank Group's International Finance Corporation (IFC). Mickey Chopra, Jeremy Veillard, Enis Baris, and Patrick Osewe served as the World Bank's internal peer reviewers of the study reports. Valuable inputs were received from Simon Andrews (IFC) and Hong Wang (Bill and Melinda Gates Foundation). The joint study team also acknowledges media coordination work from Li Li; translation and proofreading work from Shuo Zhang, Rui Liu, and Tianshu Chen; editing work from Rui Liu and Tao Su; and the tremendous administrative support from Tao Su, Sabrina Terry, Xuan Peng, Lidan Shen, Shunuo Chen, and Xin Feng.

The report was prepared and coordinated under the technical leadership of Gerard La Forgia. The chapter authors comprised Tania Dmytraczenko, Magnus Lindelow, Ye Xu, and Hui Sin Teo (chapter 1); Asaf Bitton, Madeline Pesec, Emily Benotti, Hannah Ratcliffe, Todd Lewis, Lisa Hirschhorn, and Gerard La Forgia (chapter 2); Ye Xu, Gerard La Forgia, Todd Lewis, Hannah Ratcliffe, and Asaf Bitton (chapter 3); Rabia Ali, Todd Lewis, Hannah Ratcliffe, Asaf Bitton, and Gerard La Forgia (chapter 4); Gerard La Forgia, Antonio Duran, Jin Ma, Weiping Li, and Stephen Wright (chapter 5); Mukesh Chawla and Mingshan Lu (chapter 6); Shuo Zhang and Edson Araújo (chapter 7); Karen Eggleston, Barbara O'Hanlon, and Mirja Sjoblom (chapter 8); James Cercone and Mukesh Chawla (chapter 9); and Kedar S. Mate, Derek Feeley, Donald M. Berwick, and Gerard La Forgia (chapter 10). Mukesh Chawla, Joy De Beyer, Aakanksha Pande, Rachel Weaver, and Ramesh Govindaraj did the technical and content editing of the final report.

Case studies and background studies were drawn from 21 provinces, autonomous regions, and municipalities in China: Beijing, Shanghai, Tianjin, Chongqing, Sichuan, Yunnan, Guizhou, Ningxia, Qinghai, Anhui, Shandong, Guangdong, Jiangsu, Jiangxi, Henan, Zhejiang, Hubei, Hunan, Fujian, Xiamen, and Shenzhen. Other case and background studies were drawn internationally from Brazil, Denmark, Germany, the Netherlands, New Zealand, Norway, Portugal, Singapore, Turkey, the United Kingdom, and the United States.

Many international and China experts contributed through these studies. By chapter, the contributors comprised Hui Sin Teo, Rui Liu, Daixin Li, Yuhui Zhang, Tiemin Zhai, Jingjing Li, Peipei Chai, Ling Xu, Yaoguang Zhang, David Morgan, Luca Lorenzoni, Yuki Murakami, Chris James, Qin Jiang, Xiemin Ma, Karen Eggleston, and John Goss (chapter 1); Zlatan Sabic, Rong Li, Rui Liu, Qingyue Meng, Jin Ma, Fei Yan, Sema Safir Sumer, Robert Murray, Ting Shu, Dimitrious Kalageropoulous, Helmut Hildebrandt, and Hubertus Vrijhoef (chapter 2); Xiaolu Bi, Agnes Couffinhal, Layla McCay, and Ekinadose Uhunmwangho (chapter 3); Rabia Ali, Todd Lewis, Hannah Ratcliffe, Asaf Bitton, and Gerard La Forgia (chapter 4); Weiyan Jian, Gordon Guoen Liu, and Baorong Yu (chapter 5); Christoph Kurowski, Cheryl Cashin, Wen Chen, Soonman Kwon, Min Hu,

Lijie Wang, and Alex Leung (chapter 6); Guangpeng Zhang, Barbara McPake, Xiaoyun Liu, Gilles Dussalt, and James Buchan (chapter 7); Jiangnan Cai, Yingyao Chen, Qiulin Chen, Ian Jones, and Yi Chen (chapter 8); Dan Liu (chapter 9); and Aviva Chengcheng Liu (chapter 10). Chinese officials who provided significant support with the coordination of field studies and mobilization of research data included Licheng Yao, Xiang Peng, and Yan Ren (MoF); Ning Zhuang, Kun Qin, Rui Zhao, and Chen Ren (NHFPC); and officials in provinces.

During the study preparation, six technical workshops and several consultative roundtables were organized with active participation from the MoF, NHFPC, MoHRSS, and select provincial governments. These workshops served as platforms for reciprocal policy dialogue and for receiving timely and constructive feedback from the government partners and researchers on the preliminary study findings. The following leaders, officials, and experts made presentations and important contributions to the discussions: Shaolin Yang, Guifeng Lin, Shixin Chen, Yingming Yang, Qichao Song, Haijun Wu, Aiping Tong, Weihua Liu, Licheng Yao, Yuanjie Yang, Yu Jiang, Wenjun Wang, Lei Wang, Xuhua Sun, Fei Xie, Xiang Peng, Lei Zhang, Min Wang, Yi Jiang, Shaowen Zhou, Qi Zhang, and Chenchen Ye (MoF); Yan Hou, Wannian Liang, Minghui Ren, Chunlei Nie, Yuxun Wang, Wei Fu, Jinguo He, Feng Zhang, Shengguo Jin, Jianfeng Qi, Hongming Zhu, Yang Zhang, Ruirong Hu, Ning Zhuang, Changxing Jiang, Liqun Liu, Yilei Ding, Yue Liu, Ling Xu, Kun Qin, Ge Gan, Zhihong Zhang, Yongfeng Zhu, Kai Chen, Yi Wang, Jianli Han, Yan Chen, Xiaorong Ji,

Yujun Jin, Chen Ren, Rui Zhao, Liang Ye, Xiaoke Chen Meili Zhang, and Ru Yuhong (NHFPC); Qinghui Yan, Shuchun Li, Chengjin Song, Jun Chang, Yutong Liu, Guodong Wang, Zhengming Duan, Yongsheng Fu, Kaihong Xing, Wei Zhang, Jiayue Liu, and Chao Li (MoHRSS); Yanfeng Ge and Sen Gong (Development Research Center of the State Council); Shangxi Liu (MoF Academy of Fiscal Sciences); Hongwei Yang, Zhenzhong Zhang, and Weiping Li (NHFPC China National Health Development Research Center [CNHDRC]); Dezhi Yu, Junwen Gao, Lijun Cui, and Beihai Xia (Anhui Commission for Health and Family Planning [CHFP]); Dongbo Zhong and Haichao Lei (Beijing CHFP); Xiaochun Chen, Wuqi Zeng, and Xu Lin (Fujian CHFP); Xueshan Zhou and Shuangbao Xie (Henan CHFP); Patrick Leahy and Henrik Pederson (IFC); Xiaofang Han, Qingyue Meng, Gordon Liu, Jiangnan Cai, Asaf Bitton, Jin Ma, Wen Chen, James Cercone, Ian Forde, Barbara O'Hanlon, Karen Eggleston, Fei Yan, Guangpeng Zhang, Xiaoyun Liu, Qiulin Chen, Min Hu, Lijie Wang, Antonio Duran, and Dan Liu (World Bank consultants); and Bang Chen, Junming Xie, Roberta Lipson, Beelan Tan, Sabrinna Xing, Jane Zhang, Alex Ng, Yuanli Liu, Jianmin Gao, Baorong Yu, Mario Dal Poz, James Buchan, Ducksun Ahn, and Stephen Duckett.

The study team recognizes and appreciates additional funding support from the Bill & Melinda Gates Foundation via its Results for Development Institute and from the IFC. The joint study team is also grateful for all contributions and efforts from any individuals and teams not named above.

Abbreviations

ACC-AHA CVD	American College of Cardiology and American Heart Association cardiovascular disease
ADHC	Ageing, Disability, and Health Care
AEHG	Aier Eye Hospital Group
AHRQ	Agency for Healthcare Research and Quality (United States)
ARCH	Automated Record for Child Health (Boston, United States)
BHLC	Better Health at Lower Cost
BMIs	basic medical insurances
BoG	Board of Governors (foundation trusts, United Kingdom)
BoHRSS	Bureau of Human Resources and Social Security (China)
BRIICS	Brazil, Russian Federation, India, Indonesia, China, and South Africa
BSC	balanced scorecard
CAPEX	capital expenditure
CCGs	clinical commissioning groups (United Kingdom)
CDC	Center for Disease Control and Prevention (United States)
CDSS	computerized decision support systems
CEC	Clinical Excellence Commission (Australia)
CEO	chief executive officer
CHA	Chaoyang Hospital Alliance (Beijing, China)
CHC	community health center
China CDC	Chinese Center for Disease Control and Prevention
CHS	community health station
CHWs	community health workers
CIF	capital investment fund
CIP	capital investment planning
CME	continuing medical education
CMS	Centers for Medicare & Medicaid Services (United States)
CON	Certificate of Need

CONU	Certificate of Need Unit
COPD	chronic obstructive pulmonary disease
CPC	Communist Party of China
CQI	continuous quality improvement
CVA	cerebrovascular accident
DALY	disease-adjusted life year
DMC	district medical center
DRC	Development and Reform Commission (provincial)
DRGs	diagnosis-related groups
ECG	electrocardiogram
EDL	Essential Drug List
EHR	electronic health record
FACS	Family and Consumer Services
FCH	Foshan Chancheng Hospital
FDS	family doctor system
FHS	Family Health Strategy (Brazil)
FTs	foundation trusts (United Kingdom)
GDP	gross domestic product
GH	Great Health (Zhenjiang, Jiangsu Province)
GIS	geographic information system
GP	general practitioner
HAS	Haute Autorité de Santé (France)
HASU	hyperacute stroke unit (England, United Kingdom)
HCA	health care alliance
HFPC	Health and Family Planning Commission (provincial)
HHS	Department of Health and Human Services (United States)
HIRA	Health Insurance Review and Assessment Service (Republic of Korea)
HMC	hospital management council/center
HSR	health services research
ICT	information and communication technology
IFC	International Finance Corporation (World Bank)
IHI	Institute for Healthcare Improvement (United States)
IMAI	Integrated Management of Adolescent and Adult Illness
IOM	Institute of Medicine (United States)
IPCD	Insurance Program for Catastrophic Diseases
IQWiG	Institute for Quality and Efficiency in Health Care (Germany)
IT	information technology
JCUH	James Cook University Hospital (England, United Kingdom)
LG	leadership group
LLG	local leading group
M&E	monitoring and evaluation
MBS	Medicare Benefits Schedule (Australia)
MDT	multidisciplinary team

MFA	Medical Financial Assistance
MI	myocardial infarction
MoCA	Ministry of Civil Affairs
MoF	Ministry of Finance
MoH	Ministry of Health
MoHRSS	Ministry of Human Resources and Social Security
MoLSS	Ministry of Labor and Social Security
MQCCs	medical quality control committees
MSA	medical savings account
MSAC	Medical Services Advisory Committee (Australia)
MSMGC	Medical Service Management and Guidance Center (of NHFPC)
NCD	noncommunicable disease
NCMS	New Cooperative Medical Scheme
NCQA	National Committee for Quality Assurance
NDP	National Demonstration Project on Quality Improvement in Health Care (United States)
NDRC	National Development and Reform Commission
NGO	nongovernmental organization
NHFPC	National Health and Family Planning Commission
NHIA	National Health Insurance Administration (Taiwan, China)
NHIS	National Health Insurance Service (Republic of Korea)
NHS	National Health Service (United Kingdom)
NICE	National Institute for Health and Care Excellence (United Kingdom)
NPDT	National Primary Care Development Team (United Kingdom)
NPO	nonprofit organization
NQF	National Quality Forum (United States)
NRCMS	New Rural Cooperative Medical Scheme
NSW	New South Wales (Australia)
OECD	Organisation for Economic Co-operation and Development
OSS	social health organization (Brazil)
P4Q	pay-for-quality
PACE	Program of All-Inclusive Care for the Elderly (United States)
PACS	Community Health Agents Program (Programa de Agentes Comunitários de Saúde, Brazil)
PACS	picture archiving and communications system
PACT	Patient-Aligned Care Team (U.S. Veterans Health Administration)
PAD	peripheral artery disease
PCG	primary care group
PCIC	people-centered integrated care
PCMH	patient-centered medical home
PCT	primary care trust
PDCA	plan-do-check-act (cycle)
PDSA	plan-do-study-act
PFP	private-for-profit

PHC	primary health care
PHIFMC	Public Health Insurance Fund Management Centre (Sanming, China)
PLG	provincial leading group
PNFP	private-not-for-profit
PPP	public-private partnership
PPP	purchasing power parity
PSA	public service announcement
PSU	public service unit
QoC	quality of care
QOF	Quality and Outcomes Framework (United Kingdom)
RHS	Regional Health System (Singapore)
RMB	renminbi
SCHRO	State Council Health Reform Office
SES	Secretariat of Health, State Government of São Paulo
SHI	social health insurance
SHINe	Singapore Healthcare Improvement Network
SIKS	Integrated Effort for People Living with Chronic Diseases
SOE	state-owned enterprise
SPHCC	Strengthening Primary Health Care Capacity (Feixi County, Anhui Province)
SPSP	Scottish Patient Safety Programme
SRE	serious reportable event (NQF, United States)
SROS	Regional Strategic Health Plan (Schéma Régional d'Organisation Sanitaire, France)
SU	stroke unit (England, United Kingdom)
TCM	traditional Chinese medicine
TFY	Twelfth Five-Year Plan (Hangzhou, Zhejiang Province)
THC	township health center
THE	total health expenditure
TLC	Transformative Learning Collaborative
TQM	total quality management
UEBMI	Urban Employee Basic Medical Insurance
UHC	universal health coverage
ULS	unidades de saúde local (Portugal)
URBMI	Urban Resident Basic Medical Insurance
VAT	value added tax
VC	venture capital
VHA	Veterans Health Administration (United States)
WAHH	Wuhan Asia Heart Hospital
WHO	World Health Organization
WMS	World Management Survey
WOFI	wholly owned foreign investment

Note: All dollar amounts are U.S. dollars unless otherwise indicated.

Executive Summary

China's Health System

Following decades of double-digit growth that lifted more than 600 million people out of poverty, China's economy has slowed in recent years. The moderating growth adds a new sense of urgency to strengthening human capital and ensuring that the population remains healthy and productive, especially as the economy gradually rebalances toward services and the society experiences shifting demographics and disease burdens. An area that demands particular attention in this context is health care, which is critical not only to improving equity but also to ensuring that people live healthier as they live longer.

Furthermore, slower economic growth opens the door for much-needed reforms in the health sector, because continuing on the present path would be both costly and unaffordable: government expenditures on health (including health insurance) would increase threefold, to about 10 percent of China's gross domestic product (GDP) by 2060, in the absence of cost containment measures, but these expenditures would be kept to under 6 percent of GDP if adequate reforms are undertaken. China now faces an opportunity to rebalance its health care system by embarking on a high-value path to better health at an affordable cost.

Reform Initiatives and Benefits

China has already launched major reform initiatives to improve health sector performance and meet the expectations of its citizenry. In 2009, the government unveiled an ambitious national health care reform program, committing to significantly raise health spending to provide affordable, equitable, and effective health care for all by 2020. Building on an earlier wave of reforms that established a national health insurance system, the 2009 reforms, supported by an initial commitment of RMB 850 billion, reaffirmed the government's role in the financing of health care and provision of public goods.

After nearly six years of implementation, the 2009 reforms have made a number of noteworthy gains: they have achieved near-universal health insurance coverage at a speed with few precedents. Benefits have been gradually expanded, use of health services has increased, and out-of-pocket spending on health—a major cause of impoverishment for low-income populations—has fallen. Indeed, since 2009, the average life expectancy at birth today has increased by more than 30 years; it took rich countries twice that long to achieve the same gains.

Health Service Delivery Challenges

China now faces emerging challenges in meeting its citizens' health care needs associated with a rapidly aging society and the increasing burden of noncommunicable diseases (NCDs). The trends of reduced mortality and fertility have led to a rapidly aging society, while social and economic transformation have brought urbanization and lifestyle changes, in turn leading to emerging risk factors of obesity, sedentary lifestyles, stress, smoking, abuse of alcohol and other substances, and exposure to pollution.

NCDs are already China's number one health threat, accounting for more than 80 percent of the 10.3 million premature deaths annually and 77 percent of disability-adjusted life years (DALYs) lost in 2010, not far off the share in Organisation for Economic Co-operation and Development (OECD) countries of 83 percent. Importantly, 39.7 percent (males) and 31.9 percent (females) of all NCD deaths in China are "premature"—that is, under the age of 70—compared with 27.2 percent (males) and 14.7 percent (females) in Japan and 37.2 percent (males) and 25.1 percent (females) in the United States. For populations aged 30–70 years, the probability of dying from cardiovascular disease, cancer, diabetes, or chronic respiratory disease is 19.5 percent in China, compared with 9.3 percent in Japan and 14.3 percent in the United States.

These trends add to the complexity China is facing and to which the health system must respond by reducing the major risk factors for chronic disease; addressing those influences that drive exposure to these risk factors, including the environment; and ensuring the provision of services that meet the requirements of those with chronic health problems.

The 2009 reforms produced substantial positive results in expanded insurance coverage and better health infrastructure, but much still needs to be done to reform health care delivery in China. Since 2005, health care spending in China has been growing at a rate of about 5–10 percentage points higher than GDP growth. Affordability of health services remains a concern to both citizens and government. Although out-of-pocket expenditures have declined significantly in recent years, they remain high, at 29.9 percent of total spending, compared with an average of 21 percent in high-income countries. Social insurance funds are already under increasing pressure to not run into debt.

Although spending growth started from a comparatively low level, the trend is not likely to reverse in the near future because expenditure pressures will continue to grow. For example, addressing the health needs of millions of people with diabetes, hypertension, and other chronic diseases who are currently undiagnosed and not receiving any care will be costly.

However, China also needs to address the low-value and cost-escalating aspects of its delivery system. China faces major challenges in transforming its hospital-centric and volume-driven delivery system into one that delivers high-quality care at affordable costs at all levels and that meets peoples' demands and expectations. Motivated by profits and poorly governed, too many public hospitals are embodiments of both government and market failures. Health financing is fragmented, and insurance agencies have remained largely passive purchasers of health services.

As for the quality of care, information is limited, but available evidence suggests that there is significant room to improve. A shortage of qualified medical and health workers at the primary care level compromises the health system's ability to carry out the core functions of prevention, case detection, early treatment of common illnesses, referral, care integration, and gatekeeping.

China is transforming its capital investment planning from input-based parameters (which tend to focus on bed numbers and facility size) to parameters that are based on population served. The government has also opened the hospital sector to private investment, but the private sector's ability to improve access and quality care is constrained by China's weak regulatory and public purchasing environment.

The Health Expenditure Outlook

Although China is still a comparatively low spender on health care, it needs to avoid the trap observed in several OECD countries of rapidly increasing health spending combined with only marginal gains in health outcomes. A high-cost path will result in two or three times the per capita spending of the low-cost path and will not necessarily lead to significantly better outcomes.

Although factors other than health care and health spending contribute to health outcomes, it is instructive that the United States has a *poor-value* health care system, spending nearly $9,000 per capita (at purchasing power parity [PPP]). Singapore has a relatively *high-value* system, spending under $4,000 per capita and achieving better health outcomes and higher life expectancy than the United States (figure ES.1).

This does not mean that China should emulate one system over the other. The starting points and contexts are substantially different. As China continues to grow, an inconvenient truth is that health spending will increase. However, the rate of increase can be controlled by prudent choices as to the organization and production of health services and the efficient use of financial and human resources.

Doing nothing is not an option. A study commissioned by the World Bank and carried out with researchers from China concluded that business as usual will result in real health expenditure growth of 9.4 percent a year from 2015 to 2020, during which GDP was projected to grow by 6.5 percent a year.[1] In the period 2030–35, during which GDP is projected to slow down (this study uses 4.6 percent per year as the basis for projection), health expenditure will grow by 7.5 percent per year. In other words, without deepening the health reform, health expenditure in China will increase in real terms (2014 prices) from RMB 3,531 billion in 2015 to RMB

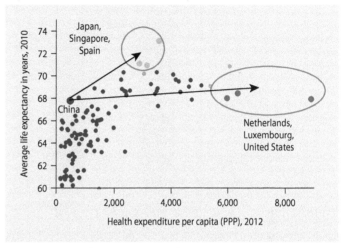

FIGURE ES.1 **Life expectancy relative to per capita health expenditure, selected countries, early 2010s**

Source: Economist Intelligence Unit 2014; WHO (various years).
Note: PPP = purchasing power parity.

15,805 billion in 2035—an average increase of 8.4 percent per year. This will increase health expenditure from 5.3 percent of GDP in 2015 to 9.1 percent of GDP in 2035.

Under the business-as-usual scenario, more than 60 percent of the growth in health expenditure is expected to be in inpatient services. Inpatient expenditure will grow by RMB 7,915 billion, compared with outpatient expenditure growth of RMB 3,328 billion, pharmaceutical expenditure growth of RMB 1,256 billion, and growth of other health expenditure of RMB 155 billion.

China could, however, achieve significant savings—equivalent to 3 percent of GDP—if it could slow down the main cost drivers (figure ES.2). To realize these savings, the growth in hospitalization needs to come down and use of outpatient care needs to go up. This implies strengthening the primary care system, raising people's confidence in the health system outside of the hospital setting, providing high quality people-centered care that is integrated across all levels, and enriching people's experience with the health care system. The potential for savings also allows for affordable fiscal space for needed investments into people-centered integrated care that would be well below the potential savings to be achieved.

FIGURE ES.2   Main drivers of projected health expenditure in China, 2015–35

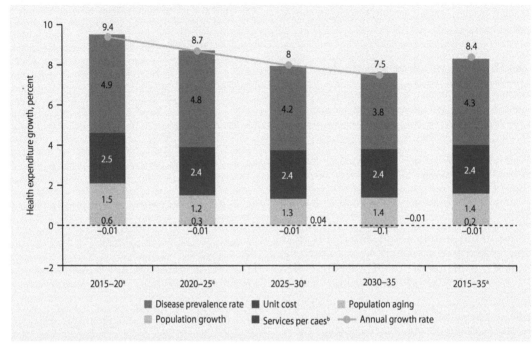

Source: World Bank estimations.
a. Growth rates of −0.01 percent pertain to population growth, which has been negative.
b. "Services per case" refers to the number of outpatient visits per disease episode—or hospital discharges, in the case of inpatient services—across 19 disease categories.

The Health System Reform Outlook

Recognizing these challenges, China's leaders have adopted far-reaching policies to put in place a reformed delivery system. On October 29, 2015, the 18th Session of the Central Committee of the Fifth Plenary Session of the Communist Party of China (CPC) endorsed a national strategy known as "Healthy China," which places population health improvement as the primary strategic goal of the health system. This strategy has guided the planning and implementation of health reforms under the 13th Five-Year Development Plan, 2016–20.

The government has also initiated enabling legislative actions. The Basic Health Care Law—which will define the essential elements of the health care sector, including financing, service delivery, pharmaceuticals, and private investment—has been included in the legislative plan of the National People's Congress of China and is being formulated by the congress.

These policy directives contain the fundamental components of service delivery reform and emphasize strengthening the three-tiered system (including primary care and community-based services), instituting human resources reform, optimizing use of social insurance, and encouraging private investment in health care. The policies also support "people first" principles such as

- Building harmonious relationships with patients;
- Promoting greater care integration between hospitals and primary care facilities through tiered service delivery and use of multidisciplinary teams and facility networks;
- Shifting resources toward the primary level;
- Linking curative and preventive care;
- Reforming public hospital governance; and
- Strengthening regional service planning.

However, although important progress has been observed, it is mostly limited to pilot projects, which suggests the need to strengthen implementation and emphasize scaling-up.

China already has a mixed health delivery system comprising both public and private providers, and this system requires strong government steering to deliver on government objectives. In this context, the role of the government at both the central and provincial levels needs to shift from top-down administrative management of services and functions through mandates and circulars (a remnant of the "legacy system") to indirect governance, whereby the government guides public and private providers to deliver health services and results aligned with government objectives.

Currently—and despite policy directives mandating separation of functions in the health sector—the government is still involved in multiple functions, including oversight, financing, regulation, management, and service provision. In contrast, many OECD countries are converging on a health delivery model in which the government plays a larger role in financing, oversight, and regulation and a relatively limited role in direct management and service provision.

What matters, however, are the policy instruments and accountability mechanisms used to align organizational objectives with public objectives. Tools include grants, contracts, regulations, public information and disclosure rules, independent audits, and tax policies, among others. Some are already in use in China. Other core government functions in a mixed delivery system include establishing public purchasing arrangements, guiding health service and capital investment planning, setting and enforcing quality standards and monitoring, regulating public and private hospitals, accrediting medical professionals and facilities, and creating a system of medical dispute resolution.

By using these tools, the government defines public and private roles, creates a level playing field for public and private providers, and develops a path for more formalized and transparent public and private

engagements that are aligned with public priorities. However, international experience suggests that these tools should be sufficiently strong and transparent—and that government should possess adequate enforcement and data monitoring capacity—to defend the public interest and avoid policy and regulatory capture by powerful private (and public) actors.

Report Background and Structure

This report was proposed by Chinese Premier Li Keqiang at a July 2014 meeting with the World Bank Group President Jim Yong Kim and World Health Organization (WHO) Director-General Margaret Chan. It is a product of joint initiatives of five institutions: China's Ministry of Finance, Health and Family Planning Commission, and Ministry of Human Resources and Social Security; the World Bank; and WHO. It has two objectives: (a) provide advice on core actions and implementation strategies in support of China's vision and policies on health reform, and (b) contribute technical inputs into the implementation of the 13th Five-Year Development Plan.

The report is based on 20 commissioned background studies; more than 30 case studies from China, middle-income countries, and OECD countries on various themes; visits to 21 provinces in China; six technical workshops; and inputs from a diversified team of policy makers, practitioners, academicians, researchers, and interested stakeholders who came together to dissect, analyze, and discuss the main sectoral reform areas in this intensive two-year effort.

The report consists of 10 chapters, the first summarizing the major health and health system challenges facing China and providing a rationale for the recommendations detailed in this report. The next eight chapters constitute the main body of the report as follows:

- "Lever 1: Shaping Tiered Health Care Delivery with People-Centered Integrated Care"

- "Lever 2: Improving Quality of Care"
- "Lever 3: Engaging Citizens in Support of the PCIC Model"
- "Lever 4: Reforming Public Hospital Governance and Management"
- "Lever 5: Realigning Purchasing and Provider Incentives"
- "Lever 6: Strengthening the Health Workforce"
- "Lever 7: Strengthening Private Sector Engagement in Health Service Delivery"
- "Lever 8: Modernizing Health Service Planning to Guide Investment"

The final chapter, "Strengthening Implementation of Health Service Delivery Reform," focuses on implementation and scaling-up. Based on the broader implementation literature, it describes an actionable implementation "system" framework and corresponding strategies relevant to the Chinese context to promote effective and scalable implementation.

The Recommendations

The report proposes eight sets of strategic reform directions, referred to as "levers,"

representing a comprehensive package of interventions to deepen health reform. Each lever contains a set of recommended core action areas and corresponding implementation strategies to guide the "what" and "how" of deepening service delivery reform; the action areas and strategies are meant to provide policy guidance at all governmental levels.

The levers are conceptualized to be interlinked and are not designed to be implemented as independent actions (figure ES.3). For example, actions taken by frontline health care providers will require strong institutional support combined with financial and human resource reforms to achieve the reform goals.

Service Delivery Levers

First, and at the core of the recommendations, is the full adoption of a reformed service delivery model—referred to as people-centered integrated care (PCIC)—to accelerate progress toward China's vision of health service delivery reform and improve value for money. PCIC refers to a care delivery model organized around the health needs

FIGURE ES.3   Eight interlinked levers to deepen health care reform in China

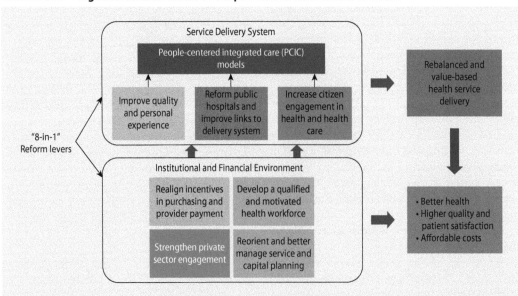

of individuals and families. The bedrock of a high-performing PCIC model is a strong primary care system that is integrated with secondary and tertiary care through formal links, good data, information sharing among providers and between providers and patients, and the active engagement of patients in their care. It uses multidisciplinary teams of providers who track patients with e-health tools, measures outcomes over the continuum of care, and relentlessly focuses on continually improving quality. Curative and preventive services are integrated to provide a comprehensive experience for patients and measurable targets for facilities. Large secondary and tertiary hospitals have new roles as providers of complex care and leaders in workforce development. Measurement, monitoring, and feedback are based on up-to-date, easily available, validated data on the care, outcomes, and behaviors of providers and patients.

Primary care is a central organizing paradigm for the production of key health system functions. International experience suggests that no country can provide high-quality, person-centered care at lower costs without a robust primary care system. In China, frontline village, township, and district health facilities need to continue to be strengthened and better staffed to provide an attractive PCIC model. Improved frontline facilities can provide a gatekeeping role for hospital and specialized services while providing better follow-up care for recently discharged patients. Empanelment can be used to identify reference populations (for example, diabetics) who will receive care by a team of providers who create registries of such patients to facilitate proactive management and a population-based approach to care.[2] In some areas, primary care providers are sufficiently strong to perform these functions. In others, some functions will need the support of county and district hospitals and can be gradually transferred to primary care once capacity is strengthened.

The "family doctor" system in Shanghai and other Chinese cities is already piloting empanelment, registries of patients with chronic diseases, and initial forms of gatekeeping. Families who contract with the system are assigned to a general practitioner who works with a team to manage care for 800–1,000 families. Empanelment is also an integral underlying feature of small-scale but successful delivery models in Germany (the Gesundes Kinzigtal integrated care system); Canterbury, New Zealand (the Health Services Plan); and the United States (Patient-Centered Medical Homes). As in Shanghai, empanelment is voluntary, and patients can opt out at any time.

In the PCIC approach, health services are integrated across provider levels and across space, time, and information through alliances or networks. The networks responsible for implementing PCIC function on a "3-in-1" principle: one system, one population, one pool of resources. In rural areas, the 3-in-1 principle can be applied to the tiered network consisting of village clinics, township health centers (THCs), and county hospitals, while in the cities the networks will consist of community health stations, community health centers (CHCs), and district hospitals. There can be multiple networks in cities and counties, which would allow for patient choice. In geographically dispersed areas, networks can be established virtually or through contracting arrangements.

In China, the current tiered delivery system was designed to operate as an integrated network. However, separate organization and management, loose definition of provider functions across tiers, constrained financial flows, and fragmented governance arrangements have limited the ability to integrate service provision and provide more continuous care. Nevertheless, well-organized, integrated networks of tiered service delivery—such as those emerging in Zhenjiang, Feixi (Anhui Province), and Huangzhong (Qinghai Province)—should be mainstreamed.

Within each network, the functions and responsibilities of each provider level need to be clearly defined. This will necessarily involve shifting low-complexity care out of hospitals. Initially, at least, networks need to avoid incorporating or being operated by tertiary hospitals, only because the tertiary hospitals might use the network to capture additional patients rather than to shift low-complexity care to lower levels. Avoiding "hospital capture" is also important to promote the strengthening of primary care and service integration.

However, secondary hospitals will be important network members in terms of providing technical support and training for the network. Initially, county and district hospitals will play a strong technical role in network operations and implementing PCIC, in part because these facilities already have good working relationships with primary care providers in many areas in China. A networkwide managerial unit will be responsible for selecting, deploying, and supervising resources in the most efficient way possible to achieve network objectives. Ideally, this management unit should be the executive arm of a governance structure and be separate from the government administrative apparatus.

Second, to improve the quality of care, the report recommends that a regulatory authority be established that provides a high level of technical oversight. PCIC requires strong government leadership and stewardship for building capacity to improve the quality of health care. A regulatory entity would promote scientific, evidence-based medicine by developing standardized clinical pathways and overseeing their implementation in clinical practice. It would also be a key resource for clinical practitioners to access a range of clinical, public health, and social care information, including safe practice guidelines, technology appraisals and guidance, quality standards, and implementation tools. Quality improvement is recognized as a continuous effort, which will require continuous monitoring and benchmarking of health care service delivery and building up the performance information infrastructure to monitor progress.

A coordinated institutional architecture committed to helping the nation improve health care quality and to overseeing related efforts is increasingly the path followed by many countries (such as the National Institute for Health and Care Excellence in the United Kingdom and the National Quality Forum in the United States). China could consider establishing a similar agency that, reporting to the central government, would be responsible for coordinating all efforts geared toward quality assurance and improvement and would actively engage all stakeholders in implementing quality assurance and improvement strategies. It would develop standardized clinical pathways and oversee their implementation in clinical practice, set quality standards, accredit and certify both public and private providers, measure and track performance, conduct research, and otherwise build capacity in advancing health care quality. The agency would ideally be co-led by representatives of relevant ministries and key professional and scientific bodies and would include other stakeholders such as community representatives.

Third, recognizing the key role of patient trust for the success of the PCIC model, the report recommends that patients be actively engaged and empowered in the process of seeking care through measures that increase their knowledge and understanding of the health system. Optimal use of scarce resources requires that patient preferences shape decisions about investment and disinvestment in services, which in turn requires a two-way communication between multidisciplinary clinical teams and their patients. Without this exchange, decisions are made with avoidable ignorance at the front lines of care delivery, services fall short of meeting needs while exceeding wants, and efficiency declines over time.

The report recommends strong patient engagement and self-management practices to help patients manage their conditions. Patient self-management refers to patients' active participation in their treatment and providers' consideration of patient treatment preferences. It offers a more collaborative approach in which providers and patients work together to identify problems, set priorities, establish goals, create treatment plans, and solve issues. Patient self-management involves systematically educating patients and their families about their conditions, how to monitor them, and how to incorporate healthy behaviors into their lifestyles. It also involves training of clinicians to communicate better with patients. By promoting systems for patient self-management, health systems can empower individuals to reduce their utilization of and make more informed decisions relating to office visits, medication, and procedures.

Several of the case studies commissioned for this report exemplify such patient engagement and self-management approaches, including the following:

- *In Shanghai,* the "family doctor" system encourages patients and families to jointly set treatment goals with their providers, and monthly patient satisfaction scores track progress.
- *In Germany,* Gesundes Kinzigtal (a health care management company whose name translates as "healthy Kinzig valley") emphasizes joint treatment goal setting and attainment. Shared decision-making tools augment this process along with case managers who support the patient through their conditions and behavior changes.
- *In the United States,* the Veterans Health Administration encourages self-management through disease-specific action planning and intensive education, especially around medication management.
- *In Denmark,* the SIKS (Integrated Effort for People Living with Chronic Diseases) project prioritizes patient involvement in developing their own treatment plans, setting goals through shared care plans, and providing feedback about whether these goals were met in partnership with the care team.

Fourth, the report suggests deep reforms in the governance and management of public hospitals to improve their performance in cost control, quality of care, and patient satisfaction. Reforming hospitals is part and parcel of reforming service delivery and adapting PCIC-like models.

Hospitals will continue to play an important role, but one that becomes less financially dominant and more focused on providing only the specialized services that are most needed. As the capacity of primary care is strengthened and the PCIC model is put in place, a wide range of care processes will be shifted out of hospitals to ambulatory units (such as surgical and chemotherapy units) and primary care facilities. Hospitals will become centers of excellence but with adequate volume to deliver high-quality care. They can perform important training and workforce development functions. They can also focus more on biomedical research and providing clinical support to lower-level providers.

Some of these functions are slowly rolling out in China. Existing "alliances" in China already show the potential benefits of these organizational forms; their use and further development should be considered. In Feixi, county hospitals and THCs share medical resources and personnel as well as coordinate services between local THCs and their associated village clinics. Similarly, Huangzhong built local alliances to use county hospital resources to strengthen and integrate THCs. Zhenjiang leveraged key county and academic hospital resources to set up more integrated rehabilitation care. Importantly, payment schemes need to be adjusted to support these functions.

The report suggests comprehensive governance arrangements to improve performance of public hospitals and promote their integration into the service delivery system. A number of countries where public hospitals historically were directly administered (including Brazil, the Netherlands, Norway, Spain, the United Kingdom, and others) have taken steps to grant them greater independence. These steps include the following:

- Granting hospitals full autonomy to manage all assets and personnel, including civil service or "quota" staff (for example, to hire, dismiss, and determine compensation)
- Developing independent hospital governance boards with government and

nongovernment participation to oversee hospital management and performance

- Appointing professional managers through a merit-based selection process (although sometimes subject to a consultative process with government)
- Enacting laws defining the nature of autonomy and specifying board selection, membership, and functions; definition of social function and obligations; separation of functions between board and management; financial arrangements; and reporting and other accountability requirements (such as an annual independent audit).

China may want to consider regulating public hospitals under a broader legal framework setting the attributes, accountabilities (discussed below), and requirements of non-profit (and for-profit) health care organizations. Such legislation could also address the issue of hospital-based "quota" employees and criteria to access social insurance. Evaluations have shown that public hospitals operating with this full range of decision rights frequently perform better than public hospitals that are managed hierarchically by government administration. International and Chinese experience provide good examples of road maps for improving autonomy. For example, China's Dongyang Hospital manifests many of these features. Other emerging but less autonomous hospital governance models are also evident in Zhenjiang, Shanghai, and other cities.

Institutional and Financial Environment Levers

Fifth, the report makes a strong case for realigning purchasing and provider incentives in the health system to motivate the establishment of PCIC, strengthen primary health care delivery, and integrate services across the entire spectrum of health care. Effectively leveraging the power of strategic purchasing, contracting, and paying providers could improve the value of the government's large investment in the health sector in China and achieve greater value for money.

China has taken many important steps in recent years to build the role of health purchasing agencies, develop their institutional capacities, and test innovative contracting and provider payment approaches. Hence it is well positioned to build on the experiences of the many successful pilots and experiments—both within and outside the country—to further leverage the power of strategic purchasing and put in place a set of incentives that motivates providers at all levels. Suggested core actions include adopting volume-controlled, value-driven approaches to effectively manage the growth of expenditures; making incentive mechanisms coherent and consistent across the system; rationalizing the distribution of services by facility level; and strengthening the capacity of purchasing agencies.

The report proposes a realignment of incentives within a single, uniform, network-wide design in support of population health, quality of care, and cost containment. Prospective payment is more effective than fee-for-service for improving efficiency and quality and incentivizing PCIC-based delivery. For these mechanisms to work, they must (a) be defined and applied consistently across the full continuum of health care production and delivery, from primary care to tertiary interventions; and (b) be aligned so that all providers, including hospitals, physicians, and health centers, fall within their purview.

Some of the different options for reorienting incentives are being tested in China. To move public hospitals away from being profit centers to being public-interest entities, the report suggests changing how physicians are paid in hospitals and linking their remuneration to a metric of public interest built around measures of quality, patient satisfaction, and serving vulnerable populations. These measures are consistent with the government's May 2015 policy directive requiring that public hospitals operate for the public good instead of seeking lucrative gains and that health services be accessible, equal, and efficient for the people.

Sixth, the report recommends strengthening the health workforce in China to enable the implementation of a PCIC service delivery model. Covering the domains of production, recruitment, compensation, management, regulation, and performance evaluation, the suggested core actions include raising the status of primary health care workers, paying them well, strengthening their composition and competencies, and building an effective framework for governance and regulation of the health workforce.

Building a strong enabling environment for the development of the primary health care (PHC) workforce is key to implementing the PCIC model. To raise the status of primary care, general practice must be established as a specialty with equivalent status to other medical specialties and with the same attributes of well-regulated standards of practice. This will require building a consensus and shared understanding among government, health providers, and the public of the centrally important role of primary care together with hospitals in providing the full continuum of care to the citizens.

China may like to consider introducing primary-care-specific career development prospects to develop and incentivize the primary care workforce. This strategy includes separate career pathways for general practitioners, nurses, mid-level workers, and community health workers that enable career progression within PHC practice. Current pilots of a separate accreditation for rural assistant physicians as well as a separate professional title promotion system for PHC workers are good examples of this approach.

The report also proposes reforming the compensation system to provide strong incentives for good performance. The compensation system needs to be revised to reduce reliance on service revenue-based bonuses and to increase base salaries and hardship allowances. Although a combination of fixed payment with variable performance-based payments is desirable, the latter should focus on quality improvements (for example, pay-for-quality schemes).

In addition, nonfinancial incentives should be introduced to attract and retain health workers in rural and remote areas. International experiences suggest that financial incentives alone cannot always provide sufficient motivation, and nonfinancial incentives have an important role in meeting special needs. Commonly used options including rotating housing, job opportunities for spouses, and opportunities for further training (scholarships for college-level studies, in-service training, and so on). Professional isolation can be avoided by using communication technologies that facilitate knowledge sharing with other providers.

Seventh, the report recognizes that although China has formulated several policies to encourage private sector engagement in the health system, much remains to be done to integrate the private entities into the national health system and motivate them to deliver good-quality health services that improve the lives and health of China's population. Measures suggested include (a) the enunciation and adoption of a shared vision of the private sector's potential contribution to national health system goals; (b) regulations that better align private sector health services with social goals; and (c) the establishment of a level playing field for the public and private sectors to better promote active private sector engagement. Through this approach, the incentives and conditions under which the whole health sector operates would move China toward a well-integrated world-class health system that yields better health outcomes and financial protection for the nation's investments in health.

The private sector can play many important roles in the production and delivery of health services, and it is important that China articulate a clear vision to steer the course of private engagement. If properly harnessed, the private sector can deliver value through business model innovation and a commitment to quality and transparency. The private sector can contribute most effectively in areas where the public sector is currently weakest and where market forces can play an important role—that is, where patients can make informed choices, as in the case of long-term care, home care, and so on.

In areas where patients are typically not able to make choices, the expansion of the private sector should be gradual and cautious as well as predicated upon the establishment of a strong purchasing function. In other words, China should leverage the potential gains that involvement of the private sector in health would bring but be careful not to get into a situation that would make it difficult to reverse course.

China should also adopt policies and regulatory measures to guide private sector engagement and minimize the risks associated with growth of poor-quality private providers. The private sector in China and abroad contains examples of business models that deliver high quality at low cost, as well as poor models that rely on overprescribing services, false advertising, and cherry-picking patients and thus fail to serve social interests. As China moves from a wholly public system to one of mixed delivery, it needs to have in place the right regulation and payment incentives to motivate all health providers to operate in the best medical and social interest, irrespective of whether they are publicly or privately owned. Indeed, China is at a critical point in private sector development and must avoid many of the pitfalls encountered in other countries as they opened up their health sectors. China will need to consider the full range of regulatory instruments—including legal prohibition, disclosure rules, industry self-regulation, and audits—to foster private engagement in the health sector in areas where it can best serve the social interest and to deter companies with vested interests from influencing hospital (and physician) behaviors, whether for-profit, nonprofit, or public. Through appropriate regulation and oversight, China can accelerate the shift in the private sector from low-quality to high-quality private providers.

Private and public providers of health services should be subject to the same set of rules and regulations. Licensing a private facility remains cumbersome, unpredictable, and costly compared with public facilities and to a large extent depends on the whims and will of local government officials.

Provincial governments should receive clearer guidance on private sector planning, entry requirements, surplus use, and other community service requirements, and enforcement should be strictly monitored. Likewise, the private sector should be assured that it will enjoy treatment similar to public institutions in such aspects as access to health professionals, land use, equipment purchasing, designated medical insurance, and professional title appraisal. A critical factor to leveling the playing field is ensuring that social insurance payments follow the patients to their chosen providers. As social insurers continue to strengthen their purchasing functions, the government could consider introducing equal contracting standards and payment principles ("pay for quality, not quantity") for both public and private providers for health services. This will encourage a virtuous circle, where both public and private providers spur each other toward achieving better value.

Eighth, the report recommends a fundamental change in how capital investment decisions are made in China's health sector by modernizing health service planning. More specifically, the report suggests moving away from traditional input-based planning toward capital investments based upon region-specific epidemiological and demographic profiles. Shifting from a strategy that is driven by macro standards to one that is determined by service planning based on real population needs will help China better align its huge capital investments—projected to reach $50 billion annually by 2020—with the demands of an affordable, equitable health care system and achieve value for money for its massive investments in the health sector.

Moving from capital investment planning to a people-centered service planning model will require prioritization of public investments according to burden of disease, where people live, and the kind of care people need on a daily basis. Service planning offers the opportunity to remake the health provider network—its design, culture, and practices—to better meet the needs of patients and families and the aspirations of those who provide their care. Within this service planning approach, capital investment planning (which is necessary to optimally use funding opportunities such as insurance and public reimbursements) can guide the development of facilities of the future, change the status quo of today, and ensure that excess capacity is not created to further exacerbate inefficiency and capital misallocation Allowing population needs to drive service and capital investment planning will make an important correction in the current system and will direct delivery of health services toward a people-centered model.

Countries that have strong planning traditions, such as France and the United Kingdom, follow a needs-based planning approach linked to specific health challenges. These countries incorporate demographic and epidemiological considerations in developing their service plans, and they factor in private sector capacity in planning for a balance between market demand and supply. This approach allows them to focus on integrated networks delivering services for defined catchment populations, allocate capital funds to provinces to acquire and upgrade physical assets such as property and equipment, and correct for equity and the level of population vulnerability.

Ensuring that available assets deliver the most cost-effective delivery solution requires the development of a regulatory framework that directs capital investment away from expansion and toward deepening of the existing infrastructure's capacity to better meet the population's health needs. This regulatory framework should encourage integrated capital planning and allocation across sectors of care to capture the potential cost and quality advantages of integration. In addition, capital planning needs to be integrated into a medium-term expenditure framework to bring together planning and budgeting, strengthen capital spending by facilitating multiyear funding programs, and incorporate the operation and maintenance costs of investments into expenditure projections. At the same time, planning standards should be tightened to close loopholes in the existing

guidelines and reduce excess capacity and duplication in the network.

Another practice to consider is periodic issuance of specific guidance on implementing standards and investment appraisals—a drill that OECD countries with advanced capital planning processes (such as Australia and the United Kingdom) routinely carry out by issuing "green papers" on various policies to support local authorities in interpreting those policies.

Finally, China should consider setting provincial caps on capital spending or "earmarked" allocations by level of care to promote new development of ambulatory solutions for surgery, chemotherapy, dialysis, imaging, and so on that would reduce the need for hospital beds and expensive infrastructure and bring services closer to the people.

Implementation of Health Care Reforms

The report's final chapter addresses the central challenge of how to implement the important changes suggested in the eight levers and recommends tools to operationalize and sustain the core actions and implementation strategies suggested. It presents an operational framework that focuses on four "implementation" systems: macro implementation and influence, coordination and support, service delivery and learning, and monitoring and evaluation. Recognizing the strong association between high-quality implementation and the probability of obtaining better program performance, it recommends establishing an enabling organizational environment as a precondition for effective implementation. Without it, progress may be elusive.

Transforming the commitment of central-level leadership to deepening health care reforms by operationalizing a value-based delivery system will require (a) defining central and local governmental roles within a policy implementation framework and (b) putting in place the right governance, organizational, and shared learning plat-forms. Despite a consensus that China's reform policies are sufficiently robust, most observers acknowledge that the country has had difficulty translating these policies into scalable and sustained actions. Current insti-tutional fragmentation and vested interests make it difficult to maintain or scale up even effective pilots. Appropriate governance, organizational, and shared learning plat-forms are key preconditions to effective implementation and represent the critical first steps in the prioritization and sequencing of interventions necessary to build a modern 21st-century health system. These platforms will need strong and persistent central gov-ernment support to make them work.

The central government must take the lead in guiding and overseeing implementation of the reforms, including the eight levers. China may like to consider assigning this mandate to the State Council, which would prepare a uniform policy implementation framework to orient reform planning and execution by local governments.

This framework would not be a one-size-fits-all blueprint but would need to be opera-tional in nature, specifying categorically *what* to do as well as what *not* to do. In turn, local governments would need to have full authority to decide on *how* to do what needs to be done, including developing, executing, and sequencing implementation plans based on local conditions but according to the pol-icy implementation framework specified by the State Council.

Strengthening accountability arrange-ments, particularly at the provincial and local levels, is another essential ingredient to facili-tate effective implementation. Any gover-nance arrangement should be sufficiently powerful to align institutional standpoints and to leverage government interests when dealing with providers and vested interests. One solution is to form empowered leader-ship groups or councils at the provincial or prefecture levels led by government leaders (governors and mayors). A few such councils already exist in China. At any level, the coun-cils will require strong leadership and

political support and be fully empowered (and accountable) to support reform imple-mentation within their jurisdictions.

The proposed councils should consist of representatives from the various government agencies involved in the health sector as well as representatives from providers, the private sector, and community leaders. The councils should be held accountable to the central gov-ernment through central-local intergovern-mental performance or "task" agreements that specify implementation benchmarks, anticipated results of the reforms, and, ulti-mately, population health indicators. These implementation performance measures should also be incorporated into the career promotion system for provincial and local leaders. Importantly, the councils will direct government agencies involved in human resource management, planning, and financ-ing to enact the changes required to create an enabling environment for the reforms.

China may also wish to create Transformation Learning Collaboratives (TLCs) at the network and facility levels as the fundamental building blocks to imple-ment, sustain, and scale up reforms on the front line. The shift in organizational goals from a treatment orientation to an outcome orientation will require fundamental changes in organizational culture. Health care organizations—whether networks, hospitals, CHCs, or THCs—must adopt continuous learning and problem-solving approaches to encourage innovation and a new culture of care. At the same time, pol-icy guidance from national and provincial officials will need to be customized and adapted at the front lines of service deliv-ery. The service delivery model envisioned for China includes several important changes at care sites, as specified under Lever 1 (shaping service delivery with PCIC). Although these changes can and should be driven by national, provincial, and local leadership, implementing them at local sites will require assistance for local learning, problem solving, and adaptation.

The driving vision behind the TLC con-cept is to assist and guide local care sites (such as village clinics, THCs, CHCs, and county and district hospitals) to implement and scale up the reformed service delivery model and close the gap between *knowing* and *doing*. A TLC is a structure for rapidly disseminating better practices for change to all facilities in a network, whether in a county or city. Each TLC can be organized as a short-term (12–15-month) learning system, which brings together teams from each participating facility, ideally within a specific network.

Before launching a TLC, for example, county network officials agree to the slate of interventions that will be implemented as well as a set of measures to track the implementation progress of all participating facilities (and institutions). The facility-level teams meet face-to-face in "learning sessions" every four to six months to discuss implementation successes, barriers, and challenges; share better practices; and describe lessons learned. In between these face-to-face meetings are "action periods" when facility teams test and implement interventions in their local settings—and collect and report data to measure the impact of these reforms. Teams submit regular progress reports for the entire TLC to review and are supported by site visits, conference calls, and other web-based discussions facilitated by implementation experts.

The most successful clinics and centers would become mentors and coaches to those that are struggling. Using both meetings and ongoing virtual exchanges, participating sites will help each other to overcome barriers and accelerate their progress. Such learning alliances have been successfully applied to support service delivery reform in England, Scotland, Singapore, Sweden, and the United States.

Implementing suitable reform pathways in an ordered manner has the potential to begin rebalancing China's health system toward people-centered integrated care. Done rigorously and with effective learning, measurement, and feedback loops, these reform pathways have the potential to improve the quality and efficiency of key services delivered across the entire system.

Notes

1. According to the latest World Bank growth estimates (issued June 2018), China grew by 6.9 percent in 2017 and is projected to grow by 6.5 percent in 2018, 6.3 percent in 2019, and 6.2 percent in 2020.
2. Empanelment is the process by which all patients in a given facility or geographic area are assigned to a primary care provider or care team.

Introduction

China's Road to Health Care Reform

Deepening health sector reform is arguably one of the major social undertakings facing China. In 2009, China unveiled an ambitious national health care reform program, committing to significantly raise health spending to provide affordable, equitable, and effective health care for all by 2020. Building on an earlier wave of reforms that established a national health insurance system, the 2009 reforms, supported by an initial financial commitment of RMB 1,380 billion, reaffirmed the government's role in the financing of health care and the provision of public goods.

After nearly six years of implementation, the 2009 reforms have made many noteworthy gains. Among them, China has achieved near universal health coverage (UHC) at a speed with few precedents globally or historically. Benefits have also been gradually expanded. For example, the New Rural Cooperative Medical Scheme (NRCMS), which targets rural populations, has become more comprehensive, incrementally adding outpatient benefits while including coverage for specific diseases. Treatment for many conditions no longer represents a poverty-inducing shock for rural residents.

Massive investments in health infrastructure and human resource formation at the grassroots level and significant expansion of access to basic public health services have fueled impressive gains. For example, health insurance coverage has stayed above 95 percent. Service capacity has increased, use of health services has risen, and out-of-pocket spending as share of total health expenditures has fallen, leading to more equitable access to care and greater affordability. For example, by 2014 the reimbursement rates were raised for inpatient services under the three main social insurance schemes (Urban Employee Basic Medical Insurance [UEBMI] scheme, Urban Resident Basic Medical Insurance [URBMI], and New Cooperative Medical Scheme [NCMS]); consequently, the differences between them significantly narrowed, reaching 80 percent, 70 percent, and 75 percent, respectively. Twelve categories of basic public services, including care for several chronic conditions, are now covered free of charge. The essential drug program is helping to reduce irrational drug use and improving access to effective drugs. The reforms, including subsequent regulations, have encouraged greater private sector participation, in part to reduce overcrowding in public facilities. The governments have spent huge sums on the construction of primary health care facilities. The capacity of primary health care services has been greatly strengthened.

Finally, the 2009 reforms also spearheaded hundreds of innovative pilots in health financing, public hospitals, and grassroots service delivery—several of which are examined in this report—and provided a strong foundation for the next stage of reform. China is progressing quickly to achieving UHC, and some of the reforms' achievements have attracted worldwide attention.

Challenges Ahead

China now faces emerging challenges in meeting the health care needs of its citizens, associated with a rapidly aging society, the increasing burden of noncommunicable diseases (NCDs), and the rising prevalence of risk factors. The trends of reduced mortality and fertility have led to a rapidly aging society, while social and economic transformation has brought urbanization and changed lifestyles, leading to the emerging risk factors of obesity, sedentary lifestyles, stress, smoking, abuse of alcohol and other substances, and exposure to pollution and traffic accidents. NCDs are already China's number one health threat.

These trends add to the complexity China is facing and to which the health system will have to respond by reducing the major risk factors for chronic disease; addressing those influences that drive exposure to these risk factors (such as the environment); and ensuring the provision of services that meet the requirements of those with chronic health problems. Rising incomes and levels of education contribute to population demands for more and better health services. China's health system will be judged on how well it handles these new challenges.

China needs to avoid the risks of developing a high-cost, low-value health system (box I.1). The health system is hospital-centric, fragmented, and volume-driven. Cost-inducing provider incentives and lack of attention to quality are major system shortcomings. The delivery system has a bias toward doing more treatment rather than improving population health outcomes and toward admitting patients to hospitals rather than treating them at the primary care level. Services are unintegrated (or uncoordinated) across provider tiers (tertiary, secondary, and primary) and between preventive and curative services.

BOX I.1   What is value in health care?

Value is defined as health outcomes for the money spent (Porter 2010). Others offer a more expanded definition involving a combination of better outcomes, quality and patient safety, and lower costs (Yong, Olsen, and McGinnis 2010). In terms of reform or change strategies to improve health services, value involves "shift[ing] the focus from the volume and profitability of services provided—physicians visits, hospitalizations, procedures, and [diagnostic] tests—to the patient outcomes achieved" (Porter 2010, 3). The concept involves making effective links between health care and health outcomes.

"Low-value care" refers to services that have little or no benefit in terms of health outcomes, are clinically ineffective or even harmful, and are cost-ineffective (compared with alternatives). The term encompasses multiple concepts (and terms) that contribute to excess costs, low-quality care, and poor health outcomes, including inappropriate care, unsafe care, unnecessary care, overutilization, misuse, overtreatment, overdiagnosis, missed prevention opportunities, and waste.

The high prevalence of NCDs suggests that care is suboptimal.

In addition, health financing is institutionally fragmented, and insurance agencies have remained passive purchasers of health services. Effective engagement with the private sector is in its infancy, and service planning has not been modernized. There is a shortage of qualified medical and health workers at the primary care level, which further compromises the system's ability to carry out the core functions of prevention, case detection, early treatment, and care integration.

The Next Stage: "Healthy China"

Recognizing these challenges, China's leaders have adopted far-reaching policies to put in place a reformed delivery system. On October 29, 2015, the 18th Session of the Central Committee of the Fifth Plenary Session of the Communist Party of China (CPC) endorsed a national strategy known as "Healthy China," which places population health improvement as the main system goal. This strategy guided the planning and implementation of health reforms under the 13th Five-Year Development Plan, 2016–20 (State Council 2016), as noted in box I.2.

The government has also initiated enabling legislative actions. The Basic Health Care Law—which will define the essential elements of the health care sector including financing, service delivery, pharmaceuticals, private investment, and so on—has been included in the legislative plan of the National People's Congress of China and is being formulated by the congress.

The CPC Central Committee Suggestions for the 13th Five-Year Development Plan and other recent policy directives (*Guo Wei Ji Ceng Fa* No. 93, 2015) contain the fundamental components of service delivery reform. For example, policies emphasize strengthening the three-tiered system (including primary care and community-based services), instituting human resources reform, optimizing use of social insurance, and encouraging private investment ("social capital") to support health care.

The government policies also support "people first" principles such as

- Building harmonious relationships with patients;
- Promoting greater care integration between hospitals and primary care facilities through tiered service delivery and use of multidisciplinary teams and facility networks;

BOX I.2   Communist Party of China's endorsement of "Healthy China" strategy

"China will deepen the reform of the medical and health systems, promote the interaction of medical services, health insurance, and pharmaceutical supply, implement the tiered delivery system, and establish primary care and modern health care systems that cover both urban rural areas.

"Efforts should be made to optimize the layout of medical institutions, improve the medical service system featuring the interaction and complementarity of higher and lower levels of institutions, improve the model of medical service at the grassroots level, develop distance medical service, promote the flow of medical resources to the grassroots level and rural areas, and promote work concerning general practitioners, family doctors, and the medical service capacity of highly needed areas, and electronic medical records.

"Efforts should be made to encourage social forces to develop the health service industry, promote the equal treatment of non-profit private hospitals and public hospitals, strengthen supervision and control of medical quality, improve mechanisms for dispute resolution, and build harmonious relations between doctors and patients."

Source: "Suggestions of the CPC Central Committee on the 13th Five-Year Plan for National Economic and Social Development on the Promotion of a 'Healthy China'" (English translation), 42–43.

- Shifting resources toward the primary level;
- Linking curative and preventive care;
- Reforming public hospital governance; and
- Strengthening regional service planning.

These are some of the essential features and supporting elements of a value-driven delivery system that incorporates a new service delivery model, the full adoption of which will facilitate achievement of China's vision of service delivery reform. However, although important progress has been observed, it is mostly limited to pilot projects, which suggests the need to strengthen implementation and emphasize scaling-up. Acknowledging the difficulty of implementing these reforms and the time required to achieve scale, they are collectively referred to as reforms of the emerging "deepwater" phase.

China also faces an unenviable conundrum: as its economy slows down, health spending is not likely to follow suit. Indeed, as the population ages and new technologies are further integrated into preferred treatment options, the upward pressures on health spending will become even more pronounced. In the face of these opposing trends, China will soon need to come up with a new model of health production, financing, and delivery, which responds to the needs and expectations of its population but at the same time is grounded in the economic reality of today, based on the economic new normal.

China has already decided that doing nothing is not an option: continuing to provide quality health services under the current arrangement will result in increasing health costs and a heavier burden on the state exchequer or households or both. In fact, because reforms take time to work their way through the complex health care system, the time to *implement* and *scale up* transformative measures is now, before it gets too late and even more expensive.

In moving forward with the delivery reforms, China should consider maintaining its focus on achieving more health rather than more treatment. This would suggest shifting the focus from rewarding volume and sales to rewarding health outcomes as well as achieving more value for the money spent. It would also suggest paying particular attention to providing affordable and equitable health care for all population groups, so that the poor and disadvantaged people do not face the risks of catastrophic medical spending and forgo medical care because of unaffordability.

Shifting from a health care delivery system focused on production of treatments to one focused on value and producing health suggests a strategic agenda that aligns all stakeholders and works toward three goals: attaining better health for the population, providing better quality and care experience for individuals and families, and achieving affordable costs.

Report Objectives and Audience

The objective of this report is to provide advice on core actions and implementation strategies in support of China's vision and policies on health reform, particularly in relation to service delivery. A more immediate objective is to contribute technical inputs for the implementation of the 13th Five-Year Development Plan.

There is much to learn from national and international innovations and experiences to successfully reform service delivery. In China, for example, many successful pilot initiatives have not yet been scaled up. These initiatives represent opportunities that China can build upon to shape a world-class service delivery system. At the same time, China can draw on the experience of Organisation for Economic Co-operation and Development (OECD) countries that are reshaping their health delivery systems to address similar challenges posed by chronic diseases, aging populations, and cost pressures. Drawing on commissioned case work and analysis as well as the broader literature, the report summarizes lessons learned from Chinese and international experiences and recommends actions to support policy implementation.

The report is intended for central- and provincial-level policy makers and regulators as well as planners and implementers at the local level, including insurers and providers. Policy makers may want to focus on the recommended levers and corresponding core actions. The strategies for central and provincial government proposed in the implementation model (described in chapter 10) would also be of interest to this group. Meanwhile, planners and implementers can center their attention on the core actions and corresponding specific implementation strategies. They would also benefit from the frontline elements of the proposed implementation model.

Before proceeding, a couple of caveats are in order: This study centers on reforms to improve health service delivery and the supporting financial and institutional environment in China. Resource and time constraints did not allow for analysis of other important reform themes that can be the subjects of future research. These include China's pharmaceutical industry, its tobacco industry, the education and licensing of medical professionals, traditional Chinese medicine (and its integration with Western medicine), and dissemination and use of medical technologies. Some of the links between aged care, health care, and social services in China will be taken up in a forthcoming World Bank study.

Report Structure

Chapter 1 summarizes the major health and health system challenges facing China and provides a rationale for the recommendations detailed in this report. More-specific challenges are highlighted in each of the subsequent chapters according to theme.

The next eight chapters (chapters 2–9) constitute the main body of the report (table I.1): each chapter concentrates on a single "lever" or strategic direction to support the planning and implementation of the government's vision of reform. The levers aim to provide policy implementation guidance to all governmental levels. Each lever contains a set of recommended core action areas and corresponding implementation strategies to guide the *what* and *how* of deepening service delivery reform.

These levers are interlinked and should not be considered or implemented as independent sets of actions. To be sure, actions taken by frontline providers will require strong institutional support combined with financial and human resource reforms to achieve the triple goals (attaining better population health, better quality of care, and affordable costs). In short, the eight levers represent a comprehensive package of interventions to deepen health reform.

TABLE I.1   *Deepening Health Reform in China* **report chapters**

Chapter no.	Chapter title
1	Impressive Gains, Looming Challenges
2	Lever 1: Shaping Tiered Health Care Delivery with People-Centered Integrated Care
3	Lever 2: Improving Quality of Care
4	Lever 3: Engaging Citizens in Support of the PCIC Model
5	Lever 4: Reforming Public Hospital Governance and Management
6	Lever 5: Realigning Incentives in Purchasing and Provider Payment
7	Lever 6: Strengthening the Health Workforce
8	Lever 7: Strengthening Private Sector Engagement in Health Service Delivery
9	Lever 8: Modernizing Health Service Planning to Guide Investment
10	Strengthening the Implementation of Health Service Delivery Reform

Service Delivery Levers

How health services are organized and delivered—and how providers relate to each other and to patients—matters. "People-centered integrated care" (PCIC) is the term used to refer to a health care delivery model organized around the health needs of individuals and families. PCIC—also discussed in the World Health Organization's (WHO) recently proposed "WHO Global Strategy of People-Centered and Integrated Health Services" (WHO 2015a, 2015b)—comprises characteristics that seek to achieve better health and better quality at affordable costs, or in other words, *more value for the money spent.* It is not a one-size-fits-all model. How PCIC is implemented in practice depends on local conditions.

Based on the WHO strategy and the broader literature, PCIC involves several strategic directions, referred to as "levers," at the service delivery level (covered in chapters 2–5):

1. Reorienting the model of care, particularly in terms of strengthening primary health care, changing the roles of hospitals, and integrating providers across care levels and among types of services
2. Continuously improving the quality of care
3. Engaging people to make better decisions about their health and health-seeking behaviors
4. Improving the governance and management of hospitals.

Broadly, the bedrock of a high-performing PCIC model is a strong primary care system that is integrated with secondary and tertiary care through formal links, good data, and information sharing among providers and between providers and patients, and active engagement of patients in their care. It uses multidisciplinary teams of providers who track patients with e-health tools, measures outcomes over the continuum of care, and relentlessly focuses on improving quality. Feedback and audit mechanisms ensure continuous learning and quality improvement. Curative and preventive services are integrated to provide a comprehensive experience for patients and measurable targets for facilities. Hospitals have new roles as providers of complex care and leaders in workforce development. They also adopt more robust governance arrangements and management practices. Measurement, monitoring, and feedback are based on up-to-date, easily available, and validated data on the care, outcomes, and behaviors of providers and patients.

Internationally, many countries are implementing PCIC-like models to address challenges similar to those facing China: cost escalation, questionable quality of care, and stagnant gains in health outcomes. Australia, Brazil, Canada, Denmark, Germany, New Zealand, Singapore, the United Kingdom, and the United States are some of the countries testing reformed service delivery models that incorporate features of PCIC. Though expanding rapidly, PCIC-like approaches remain local or regional in most of these countries. Preliminary results suggest that gains can be made in outcomes, quality, and cost containment, but results vary considerably within and across countries. Implementing these reforms at scale would make China a world leader in reform service delivery and place it at the vanguard in health system innovation and development with insightful lessons for many countries.

Financial and Institutional Environment Levers

Establishing an enabling institutional environment together with strengthening incentives and accountabilities are underlying but recognized drivers of successful PCIC implementation and improved service delivery globally (WHO 2015b). China is no different. Implementation and sustained development of service delivery reform in China will require fundamental shifts in incentives, capabilities, and accountabilities, especially in the ways that services are purchased, providers are paid, people are reimbursed, and providers report on performance and are held accountable for better care and alignment with public priorities.

These shifts will require strong governance arrangements and sustained high-level government support. The success of PCIC, for example, will depend on improving the primary care workforce, raising compensation and competencies of primary care clinicians, and reforming human resource management practices. The implementation of service delivery reform will also be enhanced through developing more effective forms of public-private engagement. Finally, new approaches to service and capital investment planning will be required to align investment planning with the new service delivery model. Realigning incentives, developing a qualified and motivated workforce, strengthening private sector engagement, and improving capital and service planning are the levers taken up in chapters 6–9.

China already has a mixed health delivery system consisting of both public and private providers, and this system requires strong government steering to deliver on public objectives. In this context, the role of the government, at both the central and provincial levels, needs to shift from top-down administrative management of services and functions through mandates and circulars (a remnant of the "legacy system") to indirect governance whereby government guides public and private providers to deliver health services and results aligned with government objectives. Currently—and despite policy directives mandating separation of functions in the health sector—the government is still involved in multiple functions, including oversight, financing, regulation, management, and service provision. By comparison, many OECD countries are converging on a health delivery model in which the government plays a large role in financing, oversight, and regulation and a relatively limited role in direct management and service provision.

What matters, however, are the policy instruments and accountability mechanisms used to align organizational objectives with public objectives. Tools include grants, contracts, regulations, public information and disclosure rules, independent audits, and tax policies, among others. Some are already in use in China. Other core government functions in a mixed delivery system include establishment of public purchasing arrangements, guidance of health service and capital investment planning, setting and enforcement of quality standards and monitoring, regulation of public and private hospitals, accreditation of medical professionals and facilities, and creation of a system of medical dispute resolution.

By using these tools, the government defines public and private roles, creates a level playing field for public and private providers, and develops a path for more formalized and transparent public and private engagements that are aligned with public priorities. However, international experience suggests that these tools should be sufficiently strong and transparent—and that government should possess adequate enforcement and data monitoring capacity—to defend the public interest and avoid policy and regulatory capture by powerful private (and public) actors.

Moving Forward with Implementation

The final chapter concludes with recommended strategies, coordination arrangements, and organizational platforms to facilitate sustained implementation and full scaling-up of reforms. Based on the broader implementation literature, it describes an actionable implementation "system" framework and corresponding strategies relevant to the Chinese context to promote effective and scalable implementation. Recommendations on the sequencing and timing of rollout to reach full scale are also provided.

Supporting Case Studies and Appendixes

Finally, case studies commissioned for this study are referenced throughout the report. For details about each of the case studies, see chapter 2, annex 2B. In addition, at the end of the volume, appendix A presents the following supplementary tables:

- *Table A.1:* Eight Levers and Recommended Core Actions
- *Table A.2:* Government Policies in Support of the Eight Levers
- *Table A.3:* New Policy Guidelines on Tiered Service Delivery and Recommended Core Actions

References

Guo Wei Ji Ceng Fa. 2015. "NHFPC Opinions on Further Standardizing the Management of Community Health Services and Improving the Quality of Service." *Guo Wei Ji Ceng Fa,* No. 93.

Porter, Michael E. 2010. "What Is Value in Health Care?" *New England Journal of Medicine* 363 (26): 2477–81.

State Council. 2016. "The 13th Five-Year Plan for Economic and Social Development of the People's Republic of China (2016–2020)." Translated by the Compilation and Translation Bureau, Central Committee of the Communist Party of China. Beijing: Central Compilation & Translation Press. http://en.ndrc.gov.cn /policyrelease/201612/P0201612076457 66966662.pdf.

WHO (World Health Organization). 2015a. "People-Centered and Integrated Health Services: An Overview of the Evidence. Interim Report." Report WHO/HIS/SDS/2015.7, WHO, Geneva.

———. 2015b. "WHO Global Strategy on People-Centered and Integrated Health Services: Interim Report." Report WHO/HIS/SDS /2015.6, WHO, Geneva.

Yong, P. L., L. A. Olsen, and J. M. McGinnis, eds. 2010. *Value in Health Care: Accounting for Cost, Quality, Safety, Outcomes, and Innovation.* Washington, DC: National Academies Press.

Impressive Gains, Looming Challenges

Introduction

China has been a pioneer in primary care and public health, and, more recently, in universal insurance coverage. The introduction of bare-foot doctors,[1] community or workplace health insurance, and ambitious public health campaigns drove improvements—combined with higher incomes, lower poverty, and better living standards (sanitation and water quality, education, nutrition, and housing)—that significantly reduced mortality rates and brought an unprecedented increase in life expectancy (Caldwell 1986; Yang and others 2008).

The health sector in China has undergone a series of wide-ranging reforms aimed at providing affordable, equitable, and effective health care. Social health insurance was introduced in phases beginning in 1998, first covering formal sector workers, then expanding to the rural population in 2003, and finally extending to informal sector workers, children, and the elderly in urban areas in 2007. Health spending rose significantly in 2009, when the government injected RMB 850 billion into the financing of health care. As a result, China has achieved near-universal health insurance coverage at a speed that has few precedents, reaching over 95 percent in both urban and rural areas since 2011. At the same time, the increase in government subsidies to social insurance schemes has increased the utilization of health services and reduced the share of out-of-pocket spending in total health expenditures.

Notwithstanding recent accomplishments, however, the health care system in China is experiencing major challenges that are contributing to cost escalation, increasing citizen discontent, and threatening future health system gains:

- *Emerging demographic and epidemiological trends,* including a rapidly aging population and the onslaught of noncommunicable diseases (NCDs) and corresponding risk factors
- *Quality of care issues,* including insufficient attention to measuring and improving the quality of health care service delivery
- *Internal systemic factors,* such as the top-heavy structure of the delivery system and unreasonable provider incentives, that all contribute to rising costs

This chapter first reviews these three challenges and then examines the resulting inefficiencies and their potential spending implications.

China's Changing Health Care Needs

Driven by improvements in disease prevention and access to medical care—as well as by higher incomes, lower poverty, and better living standards (stemming from progress in sanitation and water quality, education, nutrition, and housing), China has achieved a rapid decline in mortality and an unprecedented increase in life expectancy (Blumenthal and Hsiao 2005; Caldwell 1986; Yang and others 2008). A child born in China today can expect to live more than 30 years longer than his forebears half a century ago; it took rich countries twice that long to achieve the same gains (Deaton 2013).

In addition, fertility has declined sharply, declining from 6.0 children per woman of reproductive age in 1950 to 2.9 children per woman in 1979 (Hesketh, Lu, and Xing 2005; Smith, Strauss, and Zhao 2014). Fertility continued to fall, albeit more gradually, after China's introduction in 1979 of the one-child policy, and it has stabilized at approximately 1.7, well below the replacement rate of 2.1.

An Aging Population

Although reductions in mortality and fertility represent progress, these demographic changes are creating a rapidly aging population. The "graying" of the population has profound implications for China's economic and social policies and places new demands on the health system to deliver care that ensures that people live healthy longer lives. In 2013, China had 202 million people aged 60 years or older, who made up 15 percent of its total population.[2] Their number is expected to double by 2030 and grow to more than a third of the population by 2050 (UN DESA 2013, 2015).

China will have far less time than the Organisation for Economic Co-operation and Development (OECD) countries to adjust to the challenges imposed by an aging population (figure 1.1). For example, at the current rate of demographic change, it will experience in 26 years the degree of population aging that took 115 years to occur in France (Kinsella and Phillips 2005).

The share of working-age people in China's population peaked in 2010 at 74 percent and has now started to decline. In 2015, at the current retirement age of 60, there were 4.1 workers for each retiree; this ratio will fall to 1.4 workers per retiree by 2050. According to some estimates, if China is to avoid postponing the retirement age, this shift in the dependency ratio will require a doubling of the tax rate to finance elderly people's income benefits (Smith, Strauss, and Zhao 2014).

The graying of China's population also has profound implications for the country's mortality and morbidity profile. A mere quarter century ago, 41 percent of the burden of disease in China came from injuries; communicable diseases; and newborn, nutritional, and maternal conditions—a profile little different from that of the average low- to middle-income country today (figure 1.2). Now NCDs are responsible for 77 percent of the loss of healthy life and for 85 percent of all deaths, giving China a profile similar to that of most OECD countries (IHME 2010).

Cardiovascular diseases and cancers alone account for more than two-thirds of China's total mortality (WHO 2014). Strokes, ischemic heart disease, chronic obstructive pulmonary disease, and lung cancer top the list

FIGURE 1.1   Aging of the population in China compared with selected countries, 1950–2050

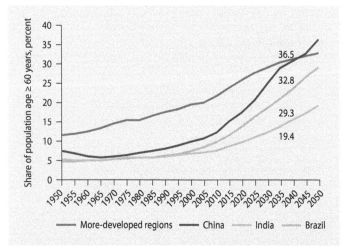

Source: UN DESA 2015.
Note: "More-developed" countries are defined according to World Health Organization (WHO) criteria.

FIGURE 1.2   Prominence of NCDs in the burden of disease and causes of mortality

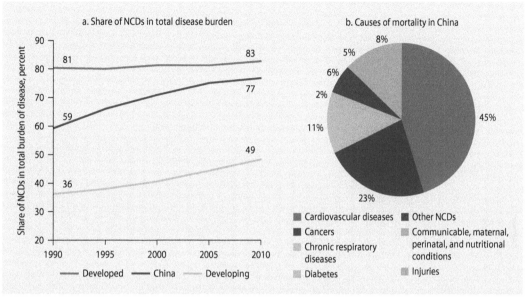

a. Share of NCDs in total disease burden

b. Causes of mortality in China

Sources: IHME 2010; WHO 2014.
Note: NCDs = noncommunicable diseases. Groups of "developed" and "developing" countries are defined according to the World Health Organization (WHO) criteria.

of causes of premature mortality, while diabetes, along with musculoskeletal disorders and major depressive disorders, has emerged as a principal cause of years lived with disability (IHME 2010; Yang and others 2013).

NCDs and Changing Risk Factors

The NCD epidemic will continue to grow. By some estimates, the number of NCD cases among Chinese people older than 40 years of age is predicted to double or even triple over the next two decades; diabetes will be the most prevalent disease, and lung cancer cases are likely to increase fivefold (Wang, Marquez, and Langenbrunner 2011).

Even more than the aging of the population, other powerful forces behind the growth of chronic illnesses in China are high-risk behaviors such as smoking, poor diets, sedentary lifestyles, and alcohol consumption, as well as environmental factors such as air pollution (Batis and others 2014; Gordon-Larsen, Wang, and Popkin 2014; Ng and others 2014; Yang and others 2008). Adult overweight prevalence nearly tripled between 1991 (11.8 percent) and 2009 (29.2 percent), with

the stronger increase taking place among men. An alarming 49 percent of Chinese men are daily smokers—a proportion more than twice the OECD average (figure 1.3, panel a). And alcohol consumption per capita nearly doubled between 2000 and 2010, to 5.8 liters of pure alcohol per capita per year—a steeper increase than in Brazil and India and quickly catching up to the OECD average of 9 liters (figure 1.3, panel b).

These risk factors are strongly associated with the major causes of morbidity and mortality in China. Causality has been established between smoking and lung, liver, stomach, esophageal, and colorectal cancers, which together contribute close to a fifth of all premature mortality in the Chinese population (HHS 2014; IHME 2012). Cardiovascular diseases, China's leading cause of mortality, are also attributable to smoking as well as to air pollution, poor diet, and high blood pressure. In 2005, 2.33 million cardiovascular deaths among Chinese adults aged 40 years and older were due to high blood pressure (He and others 2009).

This hypertension problem is worsening. According to the China Nutrition and Health

FIGURE 1.3   Smoking and alcohol consumption, international comparisons

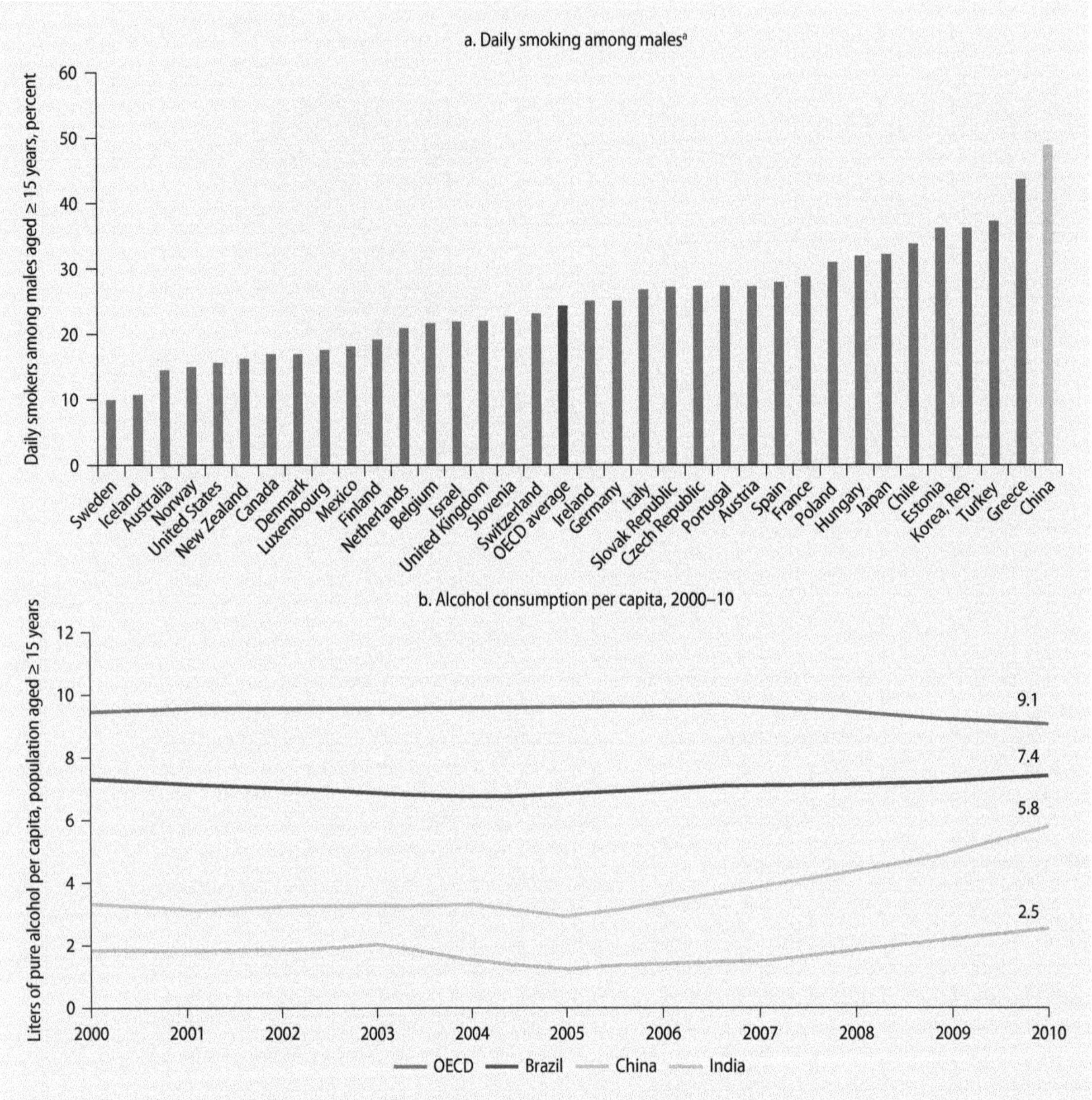

a. Daily smoking among males[a]

b. Alcohol consumption per capita, 2000–10

Source: OECD 2015.
Note: OECD = Organisation for Economic Co-operation and Development.
a. Data on smoking are for 2013 or nearest year.

Survey, the crude prevalence of hypertension in the population aged 15 years and older increased from 5.1 percent in 1959 to 18.8 percent in 2002. By 2012, the estimated prevalence of hypertension among middle-aged adults reached 40 percent (Chow and others 2013; Feng, Pang, and Beard 2014)— which translates into more than 200 million people living with hypertension and a prevalence higher than in many middle- and high-income countries (figure 1.4, panel a).

Likewise, the prevalence of diabetes—a cause of premature mortality and a contributing factor to cardiovascular disease—is high and rising (figure 1.4, panel b). The diabetes prevalence rate rose from

2.5 percent in the early 1990s to between 9.7 percent and 11.6 percent of the adult population two decades later (depending on the estimates) and is projected to reach 13 percent by 2035 (Guariguata and others 2014; Xu and others 2013; Yang and others 2010). Using data from the nationally representative China National Diabetes and Metabolic Disorders Study (2007–08), Yang and others (2011) found that 30 percent of the sample studied had three or more cardiovascular risk factors; applied to the Chinese population, this translates into more than 300 million people—equivalent to roughly the entire population of the United States— being at high risk for cardiovascular disease.

Chronic disease can have disastrous outcomes for individuals and society. If not effectively managed, diabetes, hypertension, and other chronic conditions tend to result in complications, which in turn may lead to disability, suffering, or premature death. The economic costs of chronic disease— associated with health care, lost productivity, caregiving, and loss of healthy life—can be enormous. At the system level, the direct medical costs of NCDs in China were $210 billion in 2005 and are estimated to reach more than $500 billion by 2015 (Bloom and others 2013). Considering the impact of NCDs on labor supply and capital accumulation, the total economic impact of the five major NCDs on China is projected to be $27.8 trillion for the period 2012–30.

NCDs also pose a threat to the financial health of households because they are expensive to treat and often require care over an extended period. In 2009, the average out-of-pocket spending per hospital admission due to NCDs had already mounted to 50 percent of the disposable annual income of an urban resident ($750 per capita per year) and 1.3 times that of a rural resident ($291 per capita per year), while a coronary artery bypass operation cost 1.2 times and 6.4 times the annual disposable income of an urban and rural resident, respectively (Chen and Zhao 2012). A 2011 study found that 37.6 percent of low-income patients reported not being hospitalized despite being advised to do so, because most of them (89.1 percent)

faced financial constraints (Wang, Marquez, and Langenbrunner 2011).

The rising burden of NCDs and their associated costs poses a significant challenge for China's health system. There is no quick, simple way to meet the challenge of chronic illnesses, but there is much that the health system can do to improve outcomes and reduce these costs—by preventing the onset of disease; providing early diagnosis and effective management through regular monitoring; supporting changes in behavior; and encouraging appropriate use of pharmaceuticals and other therapies. Dealing effectively

FIGURE 1.4   Prevalence of hypertension and diabetes in China and selected other countries, early 2010s

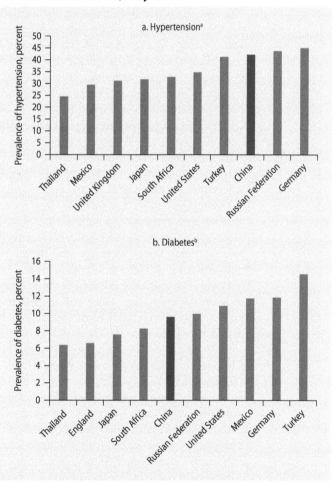

Sources: Chow and others 2013; Guariguata and others 2014; Ikeda and others 2014.
Note: The figures show the percentage of the population diagnosed with hypertension or diabetes in specific age groups.
a. The hypertension age group is 35–84 years, except for China and Germany, for which the upper age limit is 70 and 74, respectively.
b. The diabetes age group is 20–79 years.

with chronic medical conditions requires both continuity and coordination of care because, unlike episodic acute medical conditions, NCDs often call for interventions from multiple providers over long periods. Over the past decade, many OECD countries have introduced reforms to strengthen public health programs and primary health care and improve the coordination of care. A growing body of evidence shows that such reforms can have important benefits not only in improving outcomes but also in controlling cost escalation.

Health System Reform in China: A Brief Overview

The collapse of the planned economy during the 1980s, and the massive unemployment and layoffs associated with the reform of state-owned enterprises during the 1990s, resulted in a drastic reduction in health protection in both urban and rural areas, and by 2001 households were paying 60 percent of all health care costs out-of-pocket (Feng, Lou, and Yu 2015). Alongside the economic transition from the planned economy to a market economy since the 1970s, the Chinese government took a series of policy measures to reform the health care facilities. The focus of these measures was to enhance hospitals' financial and operational autonomy as well as to improve their efficiency and effectiveness. Because of these policy measures, the hospitals became more and more financially independent, though they still remained under the jurisdiction of the health departments.

Over the past three decades, hospitals in Chinese cities have improved dramatically, and difficulties in seeking health services, receiving surgeries, and getting admitted for inpatient care have been greatly reduced. However, the regulatory role of governments was not strong enough during the autonomy enhancement process. As a result, chaotic competition occurred in the market, and the hospital sector became more profit-driven. Health facilities were given full financial autonomy and allowed to generate revenues

in the form of markups for drugs and some services. This created incentives for drug prescribing and overservicing that remain a feature of China's health system today. Disparities between urban and rural areas and among regions widened drastically, and health care expenditure grew rapidly as a result of pervasive overservicing and waste (Chen 2009; Ma, Lu, and Quan 2008).

Expansion of Health Care Coverage and Utilization

In the late 1990s, concerns about the affordability of health care led the state to begin a major expansion of health insurance coverage. Initially, the expansion focused on reestablishing insurance for formal sector workers with the introduction of the Urban Employee Basic Medical Insurance (UEBMI) scheme in 1998. This was followed by the introduction of the New Cooperative Medical Scheme (NCMS) in 2003, offering subsidized health insurance for China's rural population, and the Urban Resident Basic Medical Insurance (URBMI) for the urban poor and informal sector workers in 2007.

Insurance coverage expanded at a remarkable pace, reaching more than 90 percent of the population in urban areas and 97 percent of those in rural areas by 2013 (figure 1.5).[3] By design, the *depth* of insurance coverage expanded more gradually. When they were first launched, the NCMS and URBMI covered only inpatient services. Reimbursements were later extended to outpatient services, and reduced copayments were permitted for public health priorities such as hospital deliveries and the identification and treatment of chronic diseases (Yip and others 2012). Although these changes have helped to reduce disparities across the fragmented insurance schemes over time, the UEBMI continues to be better funded and to offer more generous benefits than the other two schemes (Liang and Langenbrunner 2013; Meng and Tang 2010; Yip and others 2012).

China's achievement of almost universal health insurance coverage has coincided with

FIGURE 1.5   Coverage of social health insurance in China, 2003–13

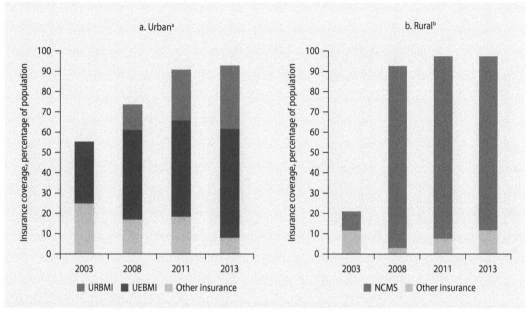

Sources: Center for Statistics and Information data, National Health and Family Planning Commission; Meng and others 2012.
a. UEBMI = Urban Employee Basic Medical Insurance. URBMI = Urban Resident Basic Medical Insurance.
b. NCMS = New Cooperative Medical Scheme (2003 data include the predecessor to NCMS, the Cooperative Medical Scheme). "Other" insurance comprises the government insurance scheme, the labor insurance scheme, and other commercial and noncommercial schemes.

an equally remarkable increase in the use of some health services (figure 1.6). Hospital admissions, for instance, increased more than twofold between 2003 and 2013 (Meng and others 2012). Insurance has significantly raised the use of inpatient services (Babiarz and others 2012; Liu and Zhao 2014; Yu and others 2010; Zhang, Yi, and Rozelle 2010). Insurance uptake has also been associated with a rise in specific services such as annual medical checkups and services for other public health priorities that are either free or almost free of charge to patients (Lei and Lin 2009; Meng and others 2012; Yip and others 2012).

Reforms to Address Coverage Shortcomings

Several studies point to shortcomings in the design of the insurance schemes that make it difficult to achieve better results. Providers face pressure to generate revenue to cover operational costs and a bonus system that ties staff remuneration to facility revenues.

Together these features create incentives for increasing patients' average length of stay and service volume, particularly for items with high price–cost margins, such as drugs and high-technology services. They inflate the charges to patients (including, in some cases, postreimbursement charges) and drive up health care costs overall (Li and others 2012; Liu, Wu, and Liu 2014; Meng and others 2012; Yang and Wu 2014).

The government recognizes these shortcomings and has attempted to address them through national policies that reduce outpatient copayments for priority chronic conditions, establish zero markup on sales of drugs in primary care facilities and (more recently) in some hospitals, and separate revenues from expenditures in lower-level facilities (table 1.1).[4] Additionally, in July 2015 the government launched insurance to cover catastrophic illnesses, extending financial protection for families at risk of being impoverished by health expenditures.

These policies may be having the desired effects,[5] but they are stopgap measures that

FIGURE 1.6   Trends in health service use in China, by visit type, 2003–13

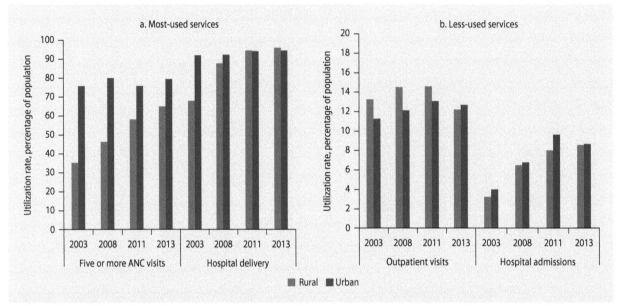

Sources: Center for Statistics and Information data, National Health and Family Planning Commission (NHFPC); Meng and others 2012.
Note: ANC = antenatal care.

address the symptoms rather than the structural deficiencies in financing and service delivery that prevent China from having a world-class health system.

Reforms to Strengthen Prevention, Primary Care, and Integration of Services

Chinese policy makers have increasingly seen that the health system suffers from hospital-centrism and fragmentation. As part of a reform of the rural health system that was launched in the early 2000s, policies envisaged that township health centers and village clinics would play important roles, with effective coordination and collaboration across the tiers of the system.[6] The importance of primary care was reinforced in subsequent years, including a growing emphasis on developing community health services and their associated workforces as well as on adjusting the coverage and reimbursement arrangements of the NCMS and URBMI to promote the use of services at the community level.[7]

The 2009 "Opinions of the [Communist Party of China] Central Committee and the State Council on Deepening the Health Care System Reform" further emphasized the importance of primary care and promoted regional health planning and coordinated management of the health system across levels of government. Since 2009, more-specific reforms have been introduced to strengthen primary care and promote integration. As discussed further in chapter 2, these have included proposed increases in salary levels, and the introduction of performance-based pay, in community-level institutions.[8] The concept of "general practice" was subsequently introduced, identifying primary care as the first point of contact and emphasizing continuity in the relationship between general practitioners and the population.[9] Policies also call for large-scale investments to construct and equip community-level health institutions and to train health workers at the village and township levels.[10]

The government made further commitments in 2013 and 2014 to enhance integration between hospitals and primary care facilities[11] and in 2015 to shift resources toward the primary level. In 2013, the central government invested in a program to improve

TABLE 1.1   Major reforms to extend financial protection and contain health care costs in China, 2009–15

Year	Reform document	Issuing agencies (document number)	Key content
2009	Opinion on Establishing the National Essential Medicines System	Ministry of Health (*Weiyaozheng fa* 2009, No. 78)	Establishes an essential medicines list and suggests that community health centers and country hospitals pilot zero markup for medicines on the list
2009	Opinion on Improving Government Health Subsidy	Ministry of Finance, National Development and Reform Commission, Ministry of Civil Affairs, Ministry of Human Resources and Social Security, and Ministry of Health (*Caishe* 2009, No. 66)	Suggests that local government pilot the retention of all revenue from health facilities, including from the sale of medicines (as opposed to allowing facilities to retain such revenues)
2011	Opinions on Further Improving the Reform of Health Insurance Payments	Ministry of Human Resources and Social Security (*Renshenbu fa* 2011, No. 63)	Implements payment reforms in the UEBMI scheme (for example, DRGs, capitation, and global budget) to control the increase of medical expenditures
2012	Notification on Health Sector Development in the 12th Five-Year Plan[a]	State Council (*Guo fa* 2012, No. 57)	For NCMS and URBMI: • Gradually increases government subsidy to RMB 360 per capita by 2015 • Increases reimbursement ceiling • Increases reimbursement rates for inpatient care to 75 percent; outpatient care to 50 percent; specific treatments for select chronic conditions (such as diabetes and mental health) and NCDs (such as cancer and Parkinson's disease) to 100 percent • Stipulates that basic outpatient care should be covered broadly by 2015
2012	Opinions on Promoting Rural Residents' Catastrophic Insurance	Ministry of Health (*Weizhengfa fa* 2012, No. 74)	Supplements insurance coverage for 20 high-expense priority conditions (such as childhood leukemia, congenital heart disease, uremia, and lung cancer)
2012	Notification on Implementing the Catastrophic Insurance for Urban and Rural Residents	National Development and Reform Commission, Ministry of Health, Ministry of Finance, Ministry of Civil Affairs, and China Insurance Regulatory Commission (*Guoyigaiban fa* 2012, No. 2605)	Stipulates that a portion of the URBMI and NCMS funds be used to finance catastrophic expenditures of beneficiaries of the respective schemes (the exact portion to be determined by local government)
2012	Opinion on Implementing the Control of Total Medical Insurance Payment	Ministry of Human Resources and Social Security, Ministry of Finance, and Ministry of Health (*Renshebu fa* 2012, No. 70)	Suggests implementation of payment reforms across all schemes (for example, DRGs, capitation, and global budget) to control the increase of medical expenditures
2012	Guidance on Promoting Reform of the NCMS Payment System	Ministry of Health, Ministry of Finance, and National Development and Reform Commission (*Weinongwei fa* 2012, No. 28)	Implements payment reforms (for example, for DRGs, capitation, and global budget) to control the increase of medical expenditures
2013	Opinion on Consolidating and Improving the Essential Medicine System and New Operating Mechanism	General Office of the State Council (*Guoban fa* 2013, No. 14)	Establishes zero markup policy for medicines on the essential list at the grassroots level
2013	Opinion on Establishing an Emergency Medical Assistance System	General Office of the State Council (*Guoban fa* 2013, No. 15)	Reimburses medical expenses for emergency room admission for patients without capacity to pay

(Table continued next page)

TABLE 1.1   Major reforms to extend financial protection and contain health care costs in China, 2009–15   *Continued*

Year	Reform document	Issuing agencies (document number)	Key content
2014	Guidance on Further Implementation of Basic Health Insurance Reimbursement Across Pooling Regions	Ministry of Human Resources and Social Security, Ministry of Finance, and National Health and Family Planning Commission (*Renshebu fa* 2014, No. 93)	Suggests that local government pilot the portability of insurance across pooled funds
2015	Opinion on Comprehensively Scaling Up Reform of County-Level Public Hospitals	General Office of the State Council (*Guoban fa* 2015, No. 33)	Extends the zero markup policy to all county hospitals
2015	Main Tasks of Deepening Medical Reform[a]	General Office of the State Council (*Guoban fa* 2015, No. 34)	• Increases government subsidy to NCMS and URBMI to RMB 380 per capita • Increases reimbursement rate for outpatients to 50 percent and inpatient services to 75 percent
2015	Opinion on Pilot Comprehensive Reform of Urban Public Hospitals	General Office of the State Council (*Guoban fa* 2015, No. 38)	Extends the zero markup policy to all pilot cities
2015	Notification of the Opinion to Comprehensively Scale Up Urban and Rural Residents' Catastrophic Medical Insurance	General Office of the State Council (*Guoban fa* 2015, No. 57)	• Extends supplemental coverage for catastrophic medical expenditures to 700 million patients (with reinsurance with commercial companies) • Increases reimbursement for eligible patients by 10–15 percent
2015	Notification of Measures for Administration of National Essential Medicine Directory	National Health and Family Planning Commission (*Guoweiyaozheng fa* 2015, No. 52)	Creates a database of essential drug prices for all schemes
2015	Guidance on Promoting Tiered Care Service Delivery System	General Office of the State Council (*Guoban fa* 2015, No. 70)	Promotes health insurance payment reform and improves health service pricing mechanism to support the tiered care system
2015	Several Opinions on the Control of Unreasonable Growth of Medical Expenses in Public Hospitals	National Health and Family Planning Commission, National Development and Reform Commission, Ministry of Finance, Ministry of Human Resources and Social Security, and State Administration of Traditional Chinese Medicine (*Guoweitigai fa* 2015, No. 89)	Eight cost-containment measures and a list of 21 monitoring indicators, including the following: • Reduces the percentage of drug revenue to 30 percent of overall revenue (excl. TCM) • Reduces the revenue of consumables below RMB 20 per RMB 100 of revenue generated (excl. revenue from medicines) in pilot public hospitals by 2017 • Promotes provider payment reform, ensures application of clinical pathway management to 30 percent of hospitalization patients, and implements DRG system on at least 100 disease types

Note: DRG = diagnosis-related group; NCDs = noncommunicable diseases; NCMS = New Cooperative Medical Scheme; TCM = traditional Chinese medicine; UEBMI = Urban Employee Basic Medical Insurance; URBMI = Urban Resident Basic Medical Insurance.
a. Umbrella reforms that are implemented through subsequent more specific policy documents.

the capacity and service provision of traditional Chinese medicine as a way to further augment frontline service delivery capacity. In 2015, the central government enacted a series of policies and supported investments to promote a more patient-focused delivery system with multiple tiers.[12]

Policies in support of community-level health care have also been backed by investments. Between 2009 and 2012, the central

government invested $19 billion in building, renovating, and equipping thousands of village clinics, community health centers, and township health centers. New training programs for primary health care providers have spread across the country, and thousands of new workers have been trained to provide frontline primary health care. A number of technical cooperation relationships between hospitals and village clinics have begun to improve the skills of frontline health workers and to encourage coordination across levels of the health system. China has also made large investments in information systems in community-level health institutions, as well as in piloting the general-practice model, vertical integration, and gatekeeping with patient-referral systems.

Notwithstanding the impressive expansion and improvement of community-level health facilities, the overall impact of the reforms to promote primary care and integration has been limited for several reasons:

- *Difficulty in attracting and retaining qualified health professionals at the community level.* Despite a policy push to improve conditions, salaries and incentives for work at this level have not been adequate considering the professional and financial opportunities that are available in higher-level institutions.
- *Contradictions in policy.* Cross-government policies on personnel and budgeting restrict the scope for raising compensation for work in the health sector and for expanding the health workforce.
- *Lack of incentives for local governments and providers to restructure the health system and pursue integration.* Indeed, rather than promoting coordination and cooperation, current financing arrangements have stimulated expansion of the volume and complexity of care as well as competition among providers.

In addition to broader financing and service delivery reforms, the government has introduced various initiatives to improve the care of chronic diseases. Some local governments started experimenting with community-based disease management programs in the early 2000s. Building on their experiences, the central government defined the management of chronic diseases as a priority public health service area in 2009, highlighting the important role of community-level providers.[13] The National Health and Family Planning Commission's 2012–15 "Work Plan for Prevention and Treatment of Chronic Diseases" sets ambitious goals, including coverage of key interventions and reduction of chronic-disease prevalence and related mortality.[14]

In parallel, the central government has developed protocols for chronic-disease management and has promoted the introduction and expansion of disease management programs by the local governments. Some parts of China have achieved significant progress in implementing these policy commitments.

Meeting China's Health Care Needs: Key Challenges

Recalibrating the health system has become more urgent as China's changing demographic and epidemiological profiles—as well as its rising health care costs and slowing economy—exert growing pressures. The rapidly evolving needs pose important challenges for policy makers in the drive to create an equitable system that uses resources efficiently to produce good health outcomes.

These challenges, discussed below, include excessive use of hospitals for care that could be provided effectively and much more cheaply in primary care facilities; uneven and inadequate quality of care; strong incentives to provide medically unnecessary services; rising costs and poor value for money; and disappointing health outcomes.

Hospital-Centrism and Weakness in Primary Care

China's health system remains hospital-centric and fragmented. The number of hospital beds doubled between 1980 and 2000 (from 1.2 million to 2.17 million) and doubled again in 13 years (to 4.58 million in 2013). The number of hospital beds per 1,000 population has more than doubled from 2000 to 2015 (figure 1.7). Although starting from a lower base, the expansion of hospital capacity in China runs counter to international trends. Most OECD countries, with the notable exception of the Republic of Korea, significantly reduced the number of hospital beds per 1,000 population

FIGURE 1.7   Hospital beds in China and selected OECD countries, 2000 and 2013

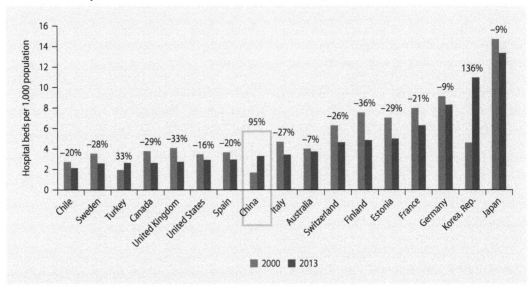

Source: OECD 2015.
Note: OECD = Organisation for Economic Co-operation and Development. Percentages shown above the bars for each country represent the change between 2000 and 2013.

over the past decade, in many cases by as much as 30 percent (OECD 2015), as shown in figure 1.7. China today has more hospital beds per 1,000 population than Canada, Spain, the United Kingdom, or the United States.

China's hospitalization rate reached 14.1 percent in 2013, up from 4.7 percent in 2003, an annual growth rate of 11.5 percent. The volume of hospitalization in both secondary and tertiary hospitals tripled in roughly the same period (Xu and Meng 2015).

The expansion and use of China's hospital capacity has been shifting toward higher-level facilities. Between 2002 and 2013, the numbers of tertiary and secondary hospitals rose by 82 percent and 29 percent, respectively, while the number of primary care providers declined by 6 percent (figure 1.8, panel a). Health workers, especially those with formal medical education (a measure of health service quality), have been moving to high-level facilities and have become particularly concentrated in hospitals (Meng and others 2009; Xu and Meng 2015).

Moreover, China's technology boom—fueled by an increasing reliance on patient examination (to generate revenue to compensate for the tighter regulation of

medicine sales profits)—has disproportionately favored the hospital sector (figure 1.8, panel b). The gap between the value of high-priced medical devices in hospitals versus those in township health centers and below widened by a factor of three, from RMB 157 billion to RMB 473 billion (Xu and Meng 2015).

This trend is significant in view of the experience in high-income economies, where technology has been a major driver of the increase in health care expenditures (de la Maisonneuve and Oliveira Martins 2013; Smith, Newhouse, and Freeland 2009). Appropriate use of medical technologies can improve the quality of care, but if providers' incentives are not well aligned, there is a danger that the mere availability of equipment can induce its overuse.

Although secondary hospitals still provide the largest volume of inpatient services, hospitalizations are growing by 18.3 percent per year at the tertiary level compared with annual growth of 14.1 percent at the secondary level (Xu and Meng 2015). Further, county hospitals are replacing township health centers as the principal providers of inpatient services in rural areas.

FIGURE 1.8 **Trends in the number and use of health care facilities in China, by level**

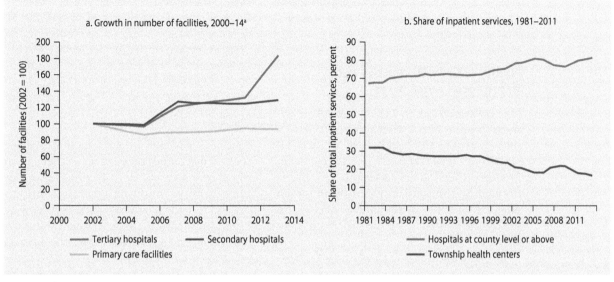

a. Growth in number of facilities, 2000–14[a]

b. Share of inpatient services, 1981–2011

Tertiary hospitals — Secondary hospitals
Primary care facilities

Hospitals at county level or above
Township health centers

Source: Xu and Meng 2015.
a. "Primary care facilities" refers to village clinics and township health centers in rural areas and to community health centers and stations in urban areas.

As for outpatient visits, all types of providers have experienced rapid growth since 2004. However, hospitals are playing a greater role in such services. From 2010 to 2014, the share of all health care facility outpatient services that occurred in hospitals increased from 34.9 percent to 39.1 percent, while the proportion in primary care facilities dropped from 61.9 percent to 57.4 percent.

As described earlier, China's initiatives aimed at strengthening tiered service provision include (a) capital investments and capacity building at the primary care level; (b) national policies that promote gatekeeping, referral systems, and vertically integrated networks (such as medical groups); and (c) payment reforms to improve financing and provider incentives at lower levels of care.

Little systematic information is available by which to gauge the success of these initiatives. On the coordination of care across different providers, the results from localized experiments have thus far been limited and uneven (Meng 2015). In Fuzhou, McCollum and others (2014) found that coordination across levels of health providers was unsatisfactory. In Qingdao, case studies of the community health center (CHC) gatekeeping

pilot show indications of success: the proportion of inpatients in hospitals who had been referred there by CHCs increased rapidly, from 2.7 percent in 2007 to 57 percent in 2010, and average medical expenditure per hospital admission was 6 percent lower for patients referred by CHCs than for those who had sought care directly at hospitals. Similarly, the Shenzhen pilot achieved a 40 percent increase in the share of insured patients who used CHCs as their first point of contact. In Chongqing, by contrast, studies of the two-way referral policy found no evidence of improvement in two-way referral after the reforms; fewer than a quarter of all acute outpatient visits were the result of referral services, and the vast majority of those were upward referrals. In the vertically integrated networks in Beijing, upward referrals were also more frequent than downward referrals.

Hospitals are full-service facilities and have little financial incentive to turn away patients and the associated revenues. With their enhanced infrastructure and human resource capacity, which draw patients to them, hospitals are in the driver's seat. Any attempt to create an effective integrated tiered delivery system will require fundamental changes—at both the hospital and the primary care levels—in a system that has significant room for marked improvement in quality, whether perceived or real.

Quality of Care: Disparities and Inappropriate Incentives

The quality of health care services is often understood as the degree to which the services increase the likelihood of desired health outcomes and are consistent with current professional knowledge. Quality is affected by the availability of basic inputs (adequate supplies of equipment, drugs, and personnel) as well as by the process of care delivery.

In assessing quality, fundamental questions concern whether the nurse or physician asks the right questions, performs the appropriate tests and exams, reaches the correct diagnosis, communicates effectively with the patient, prescribes the appropriate treatment, and provides comfort to the patient. These questions are fundamental both from an individual patient's perspective and at the system level: systematic underuse, overuse, and inappropriate use of drugs and procedures results in wasted resources and subpar health outcomes.

Although systematic evidence is hard to come by, quality is known to be a significant issue in China's health system. Concerns about quality are the main reason why it is difficult to redirect patients to primary care facilities: patients perceive huge disparities in the quality of care among different levels of providers (Bhattacharyya and others 2011; Jing and others 2015; Yang and others 2014).

Available evidence shows that many health professionals lack the basic skills needed to diagnose and treat common conditions effectively. A doctor's qualifications are a strong correlate of technical quality, yet large variations persist between rural and urban areas in doctor training and qualification standards. In one study using simulated patients, village doctors asked on average just 18 percent of the questions that were recommended

to make a proper diagnosis and only slightly more than a third of the questions that were deemed essential (Sylvia and others 2015). When presented with an unstable-angina case, village doctors performed only 15 percent of the recommended examinations, and only 26 percent of their clinical diagnoses were correct. Overall, treatment was considered correct or partially correct in only about half of the interactions. In addition, in 75 percent of the interactions, village doctors dispensed medication, 64 percent of which was determined to be unnecessary or harmful by an auditing physician. Efforts have been made to address these problems by expanding training and the use of clinical protocols and guidelines, but the impact needs to be further improved.

Arguably, the most salient quality issue in China is that of overservicing. Excessive prescription of drugs and procedures not only increases the risk of medical harm to patients and undermines trust in the system, but also wastes scarce resources that, if used appropriately, could improve population health outcomes and reduce health inequalities.

China's health care facilities derive significant incomes from the sale of medicines and certain services. Over time, this feature has translated into financial incentives for individual providers to prescribe drugs and perform diagnostic and other procedures, while at the same time shaping patients' expectations of what constitutes "good" health care.

Numerous studies have shown that overprescription is now pervasive in China. A prescription audit study on village clinics in Shandong found that the average number of drugs per prescription (three) and the rates of use of antibiotics (60 percent), intravenous injection drugs (53 percent), and steroids (20 percent) all exceeded the reference levels in the World Health Organization (WHO) index system of rational drug prescription (Yin and others 2015). A series of experiments to test the underlying motives for overprescription in China concluded that financial incentive is the major driver (Currie, Lin, and Meng 2014; Currie, Lin, and Zhang 2011).

Rising Costs Amid Room for Efficiency Improvement

Health expenditures in China have been rising steadily at a faster rate than income. Over the past two decades, total spending on health increased fourteenfold from about RMB 220 billion (1985) to RMB 3,170 billion (2013) in real terms.[15] In 2015, China spent 5.98 percent on health as a share of gross domestic product (GDP), close to the average of 6.1 percent in middle- to high-income countries. This gap has been narrowing, spurred mostly by growth in public spending—including for social health insurance, which is heavily subsidized by the government.

China's tax-financed government budget for health nearly doubled its share of national health spending between 2001 and 2013 (from 16 percent to 30 percent). Most of the budget increase was used to increase public subsidies for social health insurance.[16] Since 2001, the share of China's total health spending paid by social health insurance has grown from a quarter to more than one-third, while that of households' out-of-pocket payments has dropped from 60 percent to less than one-third (figure 1.9).

There is no single correct or best level of government spending on health, but the rapid rise in China raises concerns about affordability, particularly considering the country's relatively small government revenue base (11.3 percent of GDP), which is below the average for upper-middle-income, and even low-income, countries (14.4 percent and 13.4 percent, respectively. Even during China's period of record-breaking growth in GDP and increases in central government subsidies resulting from reform policies, local governments in the country's less-developed regions were feeling the fiscal constraints of meeting centrally mandated levels of funding to support social programs, including health care (Long and others 2013).[17] Concerns about affordability have prompted an increased focus on cost containment, with measures ranging from direct price controls or budget caps (through supply-side measures to control the volume and unit prices of services) to increased cost-sharing and demand-side measures designed to affect usage patterns.

Experience from other countries has shown that cost-control measures differ in how well they contain costs and that they can sometimes adversely affect broader health system goals such as quality and responsiveness. Hence, in many OECD countries, instead of simply attempting to control costs, the focus of health system reform has increasingly shifted to promoting value for money.

FIGURE 1.9   Composition of health spending in China, 1997–2013

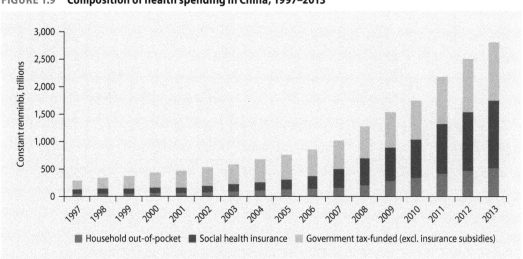

Source: Global Health Expenditure Database, World Health Organization, http://apps.who.int/nha/database.

There are ample opportunities to improve value for money in China's health care system. The most obvious is to curb waste and inefficiency. Chisholm and Evans (2010) estimated that, globally, 20–40 percent of total health spending was wasted, mainly because of technical inefficiencies related to human resource management, inappropriate use of medicines, medical errors and other types of suboptimal quality, and corruption and fraud. In China, despite scant systematic data on these issues, there is plenty of scope both to control costs and to improve outcomes by reducing unnecessary use of medicines and procedures.

Pharmaceutical spending per capita, for example, has increased more than threefold over the past decade (figure 1.10, panel a). Although spending on medicines has declined as a share of total health expenditure, it still accounts for more than 40 percent (figure 1.10, panel b). This share is large compared with those of other countries in East Asia and the Pacific and with the OECD average of 16 percent.[18] As noted above, concerns have been rising about irrational use of medicines in China, and in particular about excessive use of antibiotics (Currie, Lin, and Zhang 2011; Yin and others 2013; Yin and others 2015). A key driver of this practice is the financial incentive to prescribe antibiotics (Currie, Lin, and Meng 2014), which results in antibiotic abuse, unnecessary health expenditure, and the public health threat of antimicrobial resistance. Yip and others (2014) show that reforms of provider payment arrangements—in particular, capitation with pay for performance—have been effective in curtailing overprescribing and inappropriate prescribing as well as in reducing per-visit costs in parts of China.

Another indicator of the efficiency of health expenditure is the share of health spending that is incurred in hospital settings. Hospital-based care often entails intensive use of resources, including advanced medical technology and procedures, resulting in a

FIGURE 1.10 Pharmaceutical spending in China and international comparisons

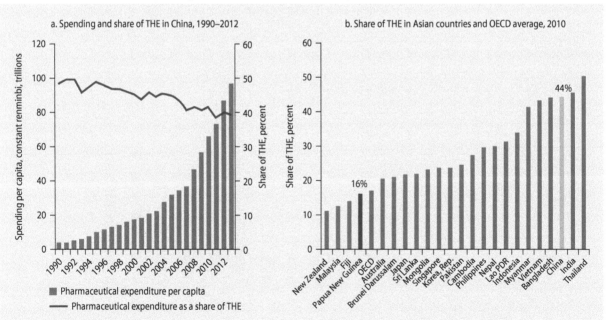

Sources: 2014 China National Health Accounts Report data, China National Health Development Research Center (CNHDRC); OECD and WHO 2014.
Note: THE = total health expenditure. OECD = Organisation for Economic Co-operation and Development. The data vary slightly depending on the source: according to the CNHDRC, pharmaceutical expenditure as a share of GDP in China in 2010 was 42 percent, whereas the OECD and WHO estimate is 44 percent.

FIGURE 1.11   Composition of health spending in China, by provider type, 1990 and 2013

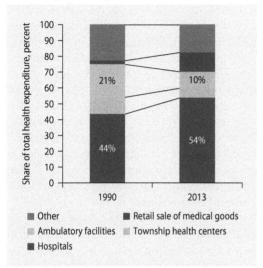

Source: 2014 China National Health Accounts Report data, China National Health Development Research Center (CNHDRC).

FIGURE 1.12   Percentage of outpatient visits in hospitals, China and selected countries, 2013

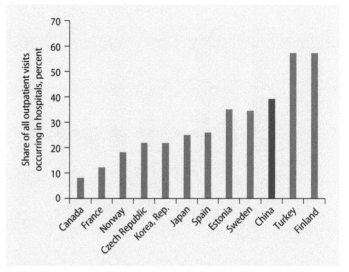

Sources: 2014 China National Health Accounts Report data, China National Health Development Research Center (CNHDRC); OECD 2015.
Note: Data for Spain are for 2011.

high cost per episode of treatment. Hospitals account for 54 percent of China's total health expenditure (figure 1.11), compared with the OECD average of 38 percent (OECD 2015). And the average length of stay for inpatient services—a key driver of higher costs—is longer in China (9.8 days) than in OECD countries (7.3 days).

Good tertiary care is essential in a health system, but in many instances, care can be more appropriately and less expensively provided in a community facility or in an outpatient setting. A large share of outpatient consultations in China (nearly 40 percent) take place in hospitals (figure 1.12).

Many studies point to the inefficiencies that arise when patients bypass lower-level facilities to seek care in hospitals, particularly the better-equipped and better-staffed tertiary hospitals, where provider-induced overuse of medical technologies and of procedures with high profit margins is well documented (Eggleston and others 2008; He and Meng 2015; Sun, Wang, and Barnes 2015). These inefficiencies have been attributed to specific features of the financing and delivery system such as reliance on the fee-for-service payment method, lack of effective referral or tiered

copayment, distorted price schedules that favor drugs and high-technology procedures over other health care services, concentration of health workers and other resources in urban areas, and medical staff remuneration tied to volume- and revenue-based bonus payments (Li and others 2012; Liu, Wu, and Liu 2014).

China will need to adopt a more comprehensive approach to reform that corrects dysfunctions across levels of care if it is to achieve appropriate care-seeking behavior by patients and to increase the use of affordable, quality primary care services (He and Meng 2015). Current inefficiencies are costly not only for the health system but also for patients who face congestion in high-level hospitals and incur expenditures associated with sometimes unnecessary procedures.

Out-of-pocket payments have been rising in real terms as a whole, although the trend may vary for specific health insurance schemes (figure 1.13). This is to be expected: as incomes rise, households are better able to afford goods and services, and health care is no exception. But the important question is whether households are having to pay catastrophically high costs for health services or are being pushed into poverty by health care costs.

FIGURE 1.13   Trends in out-of-pocket health care payments in China, by insurance type, 2003–13

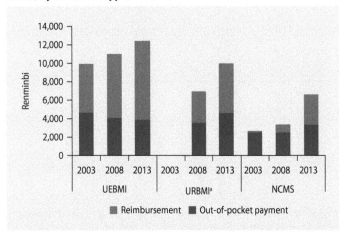

Source: Tang 2014.
Note: NCMS = New Cooperative Medical Scheme; UEBMI = Urban Employee Basic Medical Insurance; URBMI = New Urban Resident Basic Medical Insurance.
a. No 2003 data are available for URBMI, which was not launched until 2007.

As noted earlier in this chapter, evidence of the effects of China's reforms in extending financial protection to patients is mixed. By some estimates, the ratio of out-of-pocket expenditures to disposable personal income may be rising (Zhang and Liu 2014). At the household level, there is some evidence that health insurance has had positive impacts. For instance, the rate of self-discharge from hospital for financial reasons has declined steadily since 2003 (Meng and others 2012). But the incidence of catastrophic levels of health care spending has remained stable: Liu, Wu, and Liu (2014) found that reimbursements through insurance mechanisms were more than offset by increases in spending associated with patients' use of higher-level facilities, longer lengths of stay, and use of more expensive treatment items.

Though the share of out-of-pocket payments in total health expenditures in China has declined impressively—from 60 percent to 30 percent in little more than a decade—it remains high relative to the OECD average of 21 percent. Moreover, the decline has not benefited urban and rural populations evenly. For the rural population, out-of-pocket payments still account for 50 percent of total per capita health spending, and rural households

continue to spend a considerable share of their income on health: 8.4–10 percent of their annual household income, depending on the measure used (Liang and Langenbrunner 2013; Long and others 2013).

Cost pressures in China's health sector are likely to worsen in coming decades. As in many other countries, the aging of the population; the growing prevalence of chronic disease; and the introduction and expanded use of new drugs, procedures, and other medical technology are all putting upward pressure on spending. Expenditure pressures will also come from addressing coverage gaps and disparities in the health system.

China's health insurance coverage is now nearly universal, but it is still shallow and there are important exclusions. An analysis of reimbursement data shows that the effective reimbursement rate under both URBMI and the New Rural Cooperative Medical Scheme (NRCMS) is about 50 percent (considering deductibles, exclusions, and so on), even though the reimbursement rates of the schemes are 70–75 percent (Liang and Langenbrunner 2013). The shortfall is largely due to insufficient funds, especially in the NCMS.

In practice, insurance beneficiaries continue to pay significant health costs out of pocket and to incur catastrophic expenditures despite having insurance coverage; this is particularly true for rural residents, the poor, and households with members suffering from chronic disease, and it is an important cause of citizen discontent (Yang 2015; Zhang, Yi, and Rozelle 2010). Further, several studies find that insurance coverage is positively associated with prereimbursement charges because insured patients are more likely than the uninsured to receive more types of treatment, seek care in higher-level facilities, and stay longer in the hospital, all of which contribute to higher costs (Liu, Wu, and Liu 2014; Wang, Liu, and Liu 2014; Yang and Wu 2014). The resulting trend is an increase in prereimbursement costs with no significant difference in out-of-pocket or postreimbursement payments, except for patients insured under UEBMI.

Extending financial protection and reducing rural–urban disparities are important policy objectives, but they entail significant fiscal costs. Additionally, as detailed in the following section of this chapter, millions of people with diabetes, hypertension, and other chronic diseases are currently undiagnosed and not receiving the care they need. Any effort to deepen coverage, improve the quality of care, and reduce the large gaps in entitlements under China's different health insurance schemes will require substantial increases in government spending.

Poor Outcomes

Life expectancy: After a period of rapid improvements in health, during which China recorded impressive progress in reducing maternal and infant mortality, recent investments are not translating into greater longevity for the population (figure 1.14). Although China still performs well relative to other countries—having a higher life expectancy at birth than would be expected at its level of income and health spending—its global comparative position of advantage has deteriorated (figure 1.15).

Hypertension: For chronic conditions associated with the principal causes of loss of healthy life, large gaps in health care coverage remain despite steady increases in diagnosis, awareness, and treatment. Hypertension statistics provide an example. Between 1991 and 2002, China's hypertension awareness rate increased from 26.3 percent to 30.2 percent, the treatment rate increased from 12.1 percent to 24.7 percent, and the control rate increased from 2.8 percent to 6.1 percent. This translates into about 30 million hypertensive patients who received treatment and about 6 million whose symptoms were under control (Liu 2011).

However, 130 million hypertensive patients (65 percent) are still unaware of their condition. Most live in rural areas, where mortality from the major complication of hypertension—stroke—exceeds that in urban areas. Among people with hypertension who are aware of their condition, 30 million (43 percent) have not received treatment, and among those who are receiving treatment, 75 percent do not have their blood pressure under control.

In their analysis of the 2011–12 China Health and Retirement Longitudinal Study of people aged 45 years or older, Feng, Pang, and Beard (2014) find further improvements in diagnosis, treatment, and

FIGURE 1.14   Life expectancy trends in China relative to total spending on health, 1995–2013

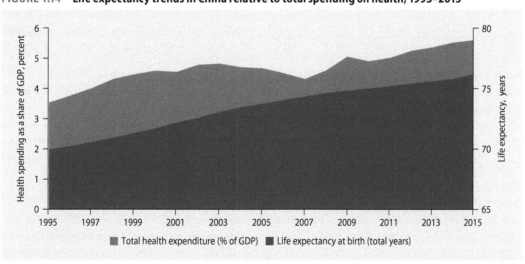

Source: World Bank 2015; China Health Statistics.

FIGURE 1.15   Performance (life expectancy) relative to health spending and income, international comparisons

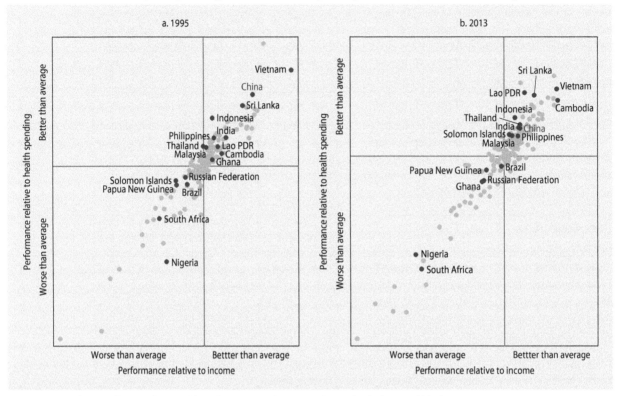

Sources: Global Health Expenditure Database, World Health Organization, http://apps.who.int/nha/database; World Bank 2015.
Note: Performance is measured by life expectancy at birth. Both axes are log scale.

control (to 56.2 percent, 48.5 percent, and 19.2 percent of the sample, respectively). Nonetheless, 33 percent of the randomly selected sample had hypertension that was not well controlled (figure 1.16). In short, there is still much room for improvement in hypertension prevention and management.

The proportions of hypertensive people who are aware, treated, and controlling their high blood pressure are lower in China than the averages in middle-income countries—whose overall management of hypertension is, in turn, worse than that of high-income countries (table 1.2). In the United States, 85.3 percent of people aged 35–84 years who have hypertension are aware of their health condition, 80.5 percent are on medication, and 59.1 percent have their blood pressure controlled (Chow and others 2013; Ikeda and others 2014).

Diabetes: Better prevention and management of diabetes is another enormous opportunity and challenge for public health policy in the next few decades. Low awareness of diabetes is a major obstacle for treatment and control of blood glucose, and 60–70 percent of China's diabetic population are unaware of their condition (Xu and others 2013; Yang and others 2010). Between 1979 and 2012, no obvious improvement took place in awareness of diabetes.

Treatment and control of diabetes increased among those who were aware of their condition. But only 25–40 percent of patients with diabetes received treatment, and only 20–40 percent of those treated achieved adequate glycemic control (defined as HbA1c<7 percent) (Li and others 2013; Xu and others 2013). By comparison, 50 percent of diabetic patients in the United States were adequately controlled (Selvin and others 2014).

TABLE 1.2   **Hypertension diagnosis, treatment, and control in selected countries, 2013**

Adults aged 35–84 years, percent

Country	Diagnosed	Treated	Controlled
China	41.6	34.4	8.2
Thailand	46.0	38.4	17.7
Turkey	49.7	29.0	6.5
South Africa	52.8	37.6	21.0
Germany	53.1	39.2	7.4
Mexico	55.8	49.5	28.0
United Kingdom	62.5	53.5	32.3
Bangladesh	62.7	54.6	30.2
Jordan	73.9	71.0	38.2
Russian Federation	74.9	59.9	14.2
United States	85.3	80.5	59.1
Japan	—	48.9	22.9

Sources: Chow and others 2013; Ikeda and others 2014.
Note: — = not available.

FIGURE 1.16   **Management of hypertension and diabetes in China, circa 2010**

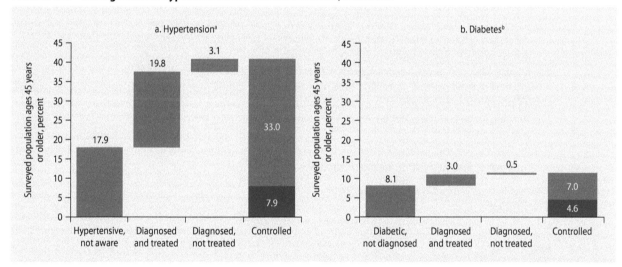

Sources: Feng, Pang, and Beard 2014; Xu and others 2013; Yang and others 2010.
a. Hypertension figures are for 2011–12.
b. Diabetes figures are for 2007 and 2010, using a mid-range of estimates from Xu and others (2013) and Yang and others (2010).

Impact of Selected Policy Changes on Health Expenditures

As noted earlier, China spends less on health as a share of GDP than most OECD countries—but its rate of growth of spending on health, especially public spending, is higher than that of all OECD countries. An OECD study projects that, at this rate, public spending on health in China will triple by 2060 to approximately 8 percent of GDP (de la Maisonneuve and Oliveira Martins 2013). There is no doubt that with further declines in poverty and increases in prosperity, the demand for health care will increase. But it does not have to increase threefold. Indeed, the same OECD study also concluded that China could limit its public expenditures on health to reasonable levels under 5 percent of GDP if adequate reforms are undertaken.

The salience and nature of these reforms is the focus of this book.

A study commissioned by the World Bank, conducted together with researchers from China (the China National Health Development Research Center) and Australia (the University of Canberra), projects that if the health spending between 1993 and 2012 is any indication (as analyzed and decomposed by Zhai and others 2015),[19] current health spending in China will increase in real terms (2014 prices) from RMB 3,591 billion in 2015 to RMB 18,039 billion in 2035, equivalent to an average increase of 8.4 percent per year. This would increase China's health expenditure from 6 percent of GDP in 2016 to 9.1 percent of GDP in 2035.[20]

The most important driver of the increase in health expenditures (accounting for about 55 percent) is the rising number of services per case of disease.[21] Excess health price inflation (the increase in prices of medical goods and services relative to prices of other goods and services) accounts for a further 26 percent, while demographic factors, such as population aging and population growth, make up the balance (19 percent), as shown in figure 1.17.

An important question to consider here is how much further China needs to increase its inpatient and outpatient service provision to bring it to world best practice. To answer this question, consider the rate of hospital discharge in high-income economies (figure 1.18). France had a discharge rate of 166 per 1,000 persons in 2013, compared with 179 per 1,000 in Australia. The median hospital discharge rate in OECD countries in 2013 was 162 per 1,000. In East Asia, discharge rates vary, from 111 per 1,000 in Japan in 2011; 138 per 1,000 in Taiwan, China; and 147 per 1,000 in the Republic of Korea in 2011. (Zhai and others 2015).

In OECD countries, the median discharge rate rose from 159 discharges per 1,000 persons in 2003 to 162 per 1,000 in 2013. Over the same period—10 short years—the discharge rates in China jumped from 47 per 1,000 (30 percent of the OECD median) to 134 per 1,000 (83 percent). At this rate, discharge rates will increase to 201 per 1,000 by 2020 and to 241 per 1,000 by 2030. In comparison, discharge rates in Taiwan, China, will increase to 152 per 1,000 in 2020 and to 182 per 1,000 in 2030.

Likewise, outpatient services per case of disease in China are currently growing at an annual rate of 5.2 percent. By 2035, outpatient services in China will be 62 percent of the outpatient service levels in Taiwan, China.

The World Bank study shows that if China were to reduce inpatient use growth and keep it growing at levels comparable to Taiwan, China, hospital spending would be reduced to RMB 3,566 billion in 2035, or 1.8 percent of GDP, compared with RMB 9,562 billion, or 4.8 percent of GDP, under the business-as-usual scenario of no spending reduction. In other words, health system reforms that lower the utilization of inpatient services will result in significant savings, equivalent to 3 percent of GDP, and bring health spending down to 6 percent of GDP by 2035. This finding is supported by the considerable evidence from pilot health reforms in China, which have succeeded in reducing the use of health inputs without compromising the quality of care and in curbing expenditures and out-of-pocket outlays (Cheng 2013; Gao,

FIGURE 1.17   Main drivers of projected health expenditure increases in China, 2015–35

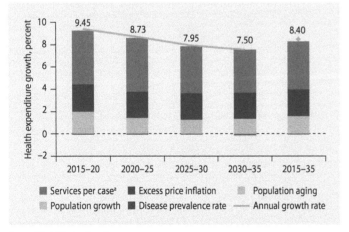

Source: World Bank estimations.
a. "Services per case" refers to the number of outpatient visits per disease episode—or hospital discharges, in the case of inpatient services—across 19 disease categories.

FIGURE 1.18 **Hospital discharge rates, selected countries and economies, 2000–14**

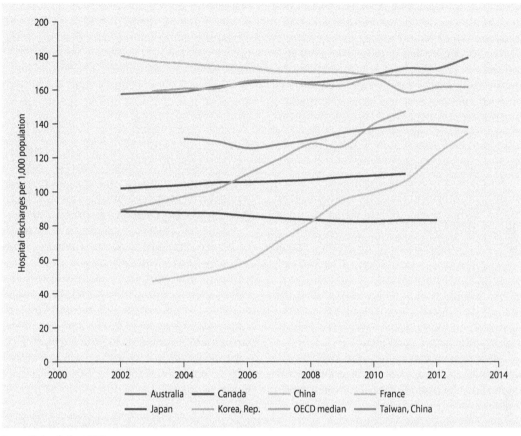

Source: Zhai and others 2015.
Note: OECD = Organisation for Economic Co-operation and Development.

Xu, and Liu 2014; Yip and others 2014). Most importantly, this finding highlights the significant impact that health system reforms can have on health spending in the medium to long term.

We note that though health policy decisions can noticeably affect trends in health spending, rising expenditures on health also reflect improvements in medical technologies, rising incomes, and demographic and epidemiological factors. Societies invest in health because these investments have the potential to generate significant value. This value comes from longer life and absence of disability, which, although not reflected in GDP, increase individual well-being and tend to be highly valued by society.

Value also comes from reducing the direct economic costs of poor health—which are reflected in the use of health services, reduced labor supply and productivity, and possible impacts on savings and investment associated with illness and premature death (Bloom and others 2013). Of course, the extent to which savings are realized depends on how well the health system performs in improving health outcomes.[22]

Conclusion

Weaknesses in primary care, hospital-centrism, lack of integration, and uneven quality impede China's achievement of better health outcomes and higher returns to investments in health. Shifting spending from hospitals to primary care facilities and improving the quality and coordination of care would improve outcomes and enhance the efficiency of spending. These gains would come from strengthened primary and secondary health care, reductions in medical complications and hospital admissions, and fewer years of disability and poor health in old age. Savings in the short term are likely to be outweighed by the cost of expanding the coverage of interventions and improving quality, but the returns over the longer term—from slower growth in health spending and reduced economic costs of ill health—are likely to be significant.

As China's economy continues to grow, health spending will inevitably rise. But how fast it rises can be controlled by prudent choices about the organization and production of health services and the more efficient use of resources. Continuing along the current high-cost path to improved health outcomes would result in two or three times the per capita spending associated with a low-cost path and would not necessarily lead to significantly better outcomes.

Although factors other than health care and health spending contribute to health outcomes, it is instructive that the United States

has a poor-value health care system, spending $9,146 per capita (2013, at purchasing power parity [PPP]), whereas Japan and Singapore get much higher value, spending only a little over $3,500 per capita (2013) and achieving much better health outcomes and higher life expectancy than the United States (figure 1.19). A large part of Japan's success in ensuring value for money, for instance, is its management of expenditures by encouraging the use of more cost-effective services, such as emphasizing primary care in the insurance benefits package and promoting investment in facilities that provide high-priority services (Maeda and others 2014).

China will need to implement a new model of health care production, financing, and delivery that responds to the needs and expectations of the population but at the same time is grounded in today's economic reality. Doing nothing is not an option: continuing to provide health services in the current environment using the current delivery model will raise health costs and impose heavier burdens on the government or households, or both.

FIGURE 1.19   Life expectancy relative to per capita health expenditure, selected countries, early 2010s

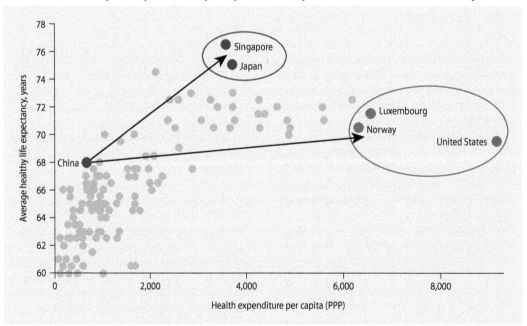

Source: Global Health Observatory data repository, World Health Organization, http://apps.who.int/gho/data.
Note: PPP = purchasing power parity.

Notes

1. Barefoot doctors are "farmers who received a short medical and paramedical training, to offer primary medical services in their rural villages" (Yang and Wang 2017).
2. Demographic data, by age group, from National Bureau of Statistics of China, *2014 China Statistical Yearbook*. Beijing: China Statistics Press.
3. The urban/rural classification is according to hukou (residence registration). Migrant workers are captured as rural residents and typically have NCMS coverage. Not being insured in the cities where they spend most of their time hinders their access to health care because NCMS copayments are higher for providers outside rural areas (Peng and others 2010; Yip and others 2012).
4. In addition, a number of subnational governments have experimented with provider payment reforms, including capitation and prospective payments, to lessen the incentives to drive up service volume.
5. Analysis of the 2013 China Health and Nutrition Survey, which would shed light on the impact on these policies on health service use and out-of-pocket payments, was not publicly available at the time of this publication.
6. Sources of the rural health system reform policies include the 2002 "Decision on Further Strengthening Rural Health Work" issued by the Central Committee of Communist Party of China and State Council and the Ministry of Health's 2002 "Opinion on Reform and Management of Rural Health Facilities."
7. Government guidance on development of primary care and community health services included the State Council's 2006 "Guidance on Development of Community Health Services in the Cities"; the 2007 "Guiding Opinions of the State Council about the Pilot Urban Resident Basic Medical Insurance"; and the 2007 "Guiding Opinions Regarding Perfecting Measures of Pooling and Reimbursement of the New Rural Cooperative Medical Scheme" issued by the Ministry of Health, Ministry of Finance, and State Administration of Traditional Chinese Medicine.
8. "Guiding Opinions Regarding Implementing Performance-Based Salary in Public Institutions on Public Health and Primary Care," Ministry of Human Resources and Social Security (2009).
9. "Guidance on the Establishment of a General Practitioner System," State Council (2011).
10. "Planning and Implementation Plan of Deepening Health System Reform during the Twelfth Five-Year Plan," State Council (2012).
11. "Announcement on Publishing 2013 National Health Work Conference Document," Ministry of Health (2013); "Announcement on carrying out some key work in the New Rural Cooperative Medical Scheme," Ministry of Health (2014).
12. The 2015 State Council documents include the following: "Guidance on Comprehensive Pilot Reform of Urban Public Hospitals," NHFPC (*Guoban fa* 2015, No. 38); "Guidance on Comprehensively Scaling-Up Reform of County-Level Public Hospitals" (*Guoban fa* 2015, No. 33); "Guidance of the General Office of the State Council on Promoting Multi-Level Diagnosis and Treatment System" (No. 70); and "Guidance on Promoting Tiered Care Service Delivery System" (No. 93).
13. "Opinions on Promoting the Gradual Equalization of Basic Public Health Services," Ministry of Health and Ministry of Finance (2009).
14. Specific goals include ensuring that 40 percent of the hypertensive and diabetic patients receive standardized disease control interventions, limiting the increase in stroke incidence to 5 percent, reducing stroke mortality by 5 percent, and reducing prevalence of chronic obstructive pulmonary disease (COPD) to below 8 percent. The policy calls for further specific targets to be set at the local level.
15. Health spending data from the 2014 China National Health Accounts Report, China National Health Development Research Center (CNHDRC), Beijing.
16. According to China's system of health accounts (2011 edition), social health insurance is classified as part of general government health expenditures, and this category includes tax-financed subsidies to social health insurance. For international comparability, we present data according to this classification in the charts of this report. Disaggregated data on tax-financed insurance subsidies were provided by the China National Health Development Research Center (CNHDRC).
17. Public subsidies mainly benefited the least-developed Western provinces.

18. The data vary slightly depending on the source. According to the China National Health Development Research Center's (CNHDRC) 2014 National Health Accounts Report, pharmaceutical expenditure as a share of GDP in China in 2010 was 42 percent, whereas the OECD and WHO 2010 estimate is 44 percent. The CNHDRC estimates that the share was 40 percent in 2013.

19. Zhai and others (2015) found that the growth in total health expenditure from 1993 to 2012 was driven mainly by rapid increases in real expenditure per case, which contributed 8.2 percentage points to the 11.6 percent total growth in health expenditures. Excess health price inflation and population aging contributed 1.3 and 1.2 percentage points, respectively. Reduction in disease prevalence led to modest savings, and population growth was a small contributor to the growth in expenditures.

20. Figures differ slightly from the China National Health Accounts data presented earlier because projections were done for current expenditures only, excluding capital formation, which is lumpy and difficult to predict. Projections also differ from those produced for OECD countries and the BRIICS countries (Brazil, Russian Federation, India, Indonesia, China, and South Africa) by de la Maisionneuve and Oliveira Martins (2013) and for China by Lorenzoni and others (2015), which used a component-based model that considers the age and sex structure of the population; population growth and aging (adjusted for longevity to account for savings in health costs due to additional years of good health); income; health-relative prices; and other unexplained factors.

21. The number of "services per case" is the number of outpatient visits (or hospital discharges, in the case of inpatient services) per disease episode by age group across 19 disease categories and 17 age groups.

22. In the United Kingdom, this consideration led the Treasury-appointed Wanless Commission to recommend increases in government spending on health both to improve health and to control health care costs (Wanless and others 2007).

References

Babiarz, Kimberly S., Grant Miller, Hongmei Yi, Linxiu Zhang, and Scott Rozelle. 2012. "China's New Cooperative Medical Scheme Improved Finances of Township Health Centers but Not the Number of Patients Served." *Health Affairs* 31 (5): 1065–74. doi:10.1377/hlthaff.2010.1311.

Batis, Carolina, Daniela Sotres-Alvarez, Penny Gordon-Larsen, Michelle A. Mendez, Linda Adair, and Barry Popkin. 2014. "Longitudinal Analysis of Dietary Patterns in Chinese Adults from 1991 to 2009." *British Journal of Nutrition* 111 (8): 1441–51. doi:10.1017/S0007114513003917.

Bhattacharyya, Onil, Yin Delu, Sabrina T. Wong, and Chen Bowen. 2011. "Evolution of Primary Care in China 1997–2009." *Health Policy* 100 (2–3): 174–80. doi:10.1016/j.healthpol.2010.11.005.

Bloom, David E., Elizabeth T. Cafiero, Mark E. McGovern, Klaus Prettner, Anderson Stanciole, Jonathan Weiss, Samuel Bakkila, and Larry Rosenberg. 2013. "The Economic Impact of Noncommunicable Disease in China and India: Estimates, Projections, and Comparisons." NBER Working Paper No. 19335, National Bureau of Economic Research, Cambridge, MA.

Blumenthal, David, and William Hsiao. 2005. "Privatization and Its Discontents—The Evolving Chinese Health Care System." *New England Journal of Medicine* 353 (11): 1165–70.

Caldwell, John C. 1986. "Routes to Low Mortality in Poor Countries." *Population and Development Review* 12 (2): 171–220. doi:10.2307/1973108.

Chen, Junshi, and Wenhua Zhao. 2012. "Diet, Nutrition, and Chronic Disease in Mainland China." *Journal of Food and Drug Analysis* 20: 222–25.

Chen, Zhu. 2009. "Launch of the Health-Care Reform Plan in China." *The Lancet* 373 (9672): 1322–24.

Cheng, Tsung-Mei. 2013. "A Pilot Project Using Evidence-Based Clinical Pathways and Payment Reform in China's Rural Hospitals Shows Early Success." *Health Affairs* 32 (5): 963–73. doi: 10.1377/hlthaff.2012.0640.

Chisholm, Dan, and David B. Evans. 2010. "Improving Health System Efficiency as a Means of Moving towards Universal Coverage." *World Health Report (2010)* Background Paper 28, World Health Organization, Geneva.

Chow, Clara K., Koon K. Teo, Sumathy Rangarajan, Shofiqul Islam, Rajeev Gupta,

Alvaro Avezum, Ahmad Bahonar, Jephat Chifamba, Gilles Dagenais, and Rafael Diaz. 2013. "Prevalence, Awareness, Treatment, and Control of Hypertension in Rural and Urban Communities in High-, Middle-, and Low-Income Countries." *Journal of the American Medical Association* 310 (9): 959–68.

Currie, Janet, Wanchuan Lin, and Juanjuan Meng. 2014. "Addressing Antibiotic Abuse in China: An Experimental Audit Study." *Journal of Development Economics* 110: 39–51. doi:10.1016/j.jdeveco.2014.05.006.

Currie, Janet, Wanchuan Lin, and Wei Zhang. 2011. "Patient Knowledge and Antibiotic Abuse: Evidence from an Audit Study in China." *Journal of Health Economics* 30 (5): 933–49. doi:10.1016/j.jhealeco.2011.05.009.

de la Maisonneuve, Christine, and Joaquim Oliveira Martins. 2013. "A Projection Method for Public Health and Long-Term Care Expenditures." OECD Economics Department Working Paper No. 1048, Organisation for Economic Co-operation and Development, Paris.

Deaton, Angus. 2013. *The Great Escape: Health, Wealth, and the Origins of Inequality.* Princeton, NJ: Princeton University Press.

Eggleston, Karen, Li Ling, Meng Qingyue, Magnus Lindelow, and Adam Wagstaff. 2008. "Health Service Delivery in China: A Literature Review." *Health Economics* 17 (2): 149–65. doi: 10.1002/hec.1306.

Feng, Jin, Pingyi Lou, and Yangyang Yu. 2015. "Health Care Expenditure over Life Cycle in the People's Republic of China." *Asian Development Review* 32 (1): 167–95.

Feng, Xing Lin, Mingfan Pang, and John Beard. 2014. "Health System Strengthening and Hypertension Awareness, Treatment and Control: Data from the China Health and Retirement Longitudinal Study." *Bulletin of the World Health Organization* 92 (1): 29–41.

Gao, Chen, Fei Xu, and Gordon G. Liu. 2014. "Payment Reform and Changes in Health Care in China." *Social Science and Medicine* 111: 10–16. doi:10.1016/j.socscimed.2014.03.035.

Gordon-Larsen, P., H. Wang, and B. M. Popkin. 2014. "Overweight Dynamics in Chinese Children and Adults." *Obesity Reviews* 15: 37–48. doi: 10.1111/obr.12121.

Guariguata, L., D. R. Whiting, I. Hambleton, J. Beagley, U. Linnenkamp, and J. E. Shaw. 2014. "Global Estimates of Diabetes Prevalence for 2013 and Projections for 2035." *Diabetes Research and Clinical Practice* 103 (2): 137–49.

He, Alex Jingwei, and Qingyue Meng. 2015. "An Interim Interdisciplinary Evaluation of China's National Health Care Reform: Emerging Evidence and New Perspectives." *Journal of Asian Public Policy* 8 (1): 1–18. doi:10.1080/17516234.2015.1014299.

He, Jiang, Dongfeng Gu, Jing Chen, Xigui Wu, Tanika N. Kelly, Jian-feng Huang, Ji-chun Chen, Chung-Shiuan Chen, Lydia A. Bazzano, and Kristi Reynolds. 2009. "Premature Deaths Attributable to Blood Pressure in China: A Prospective Cohort Study." *The Lancet* 374 (9703): 1765–72.

Hesketh, Therese, Li Lu, and Zhu Wei Xing. 2005. "The Effect of China's One-Child Family Policy after 25 Years." *New England Journal of Medicine* 353 (11): 1171–76. doi: doi:10.1056/NEJMhpr051833.

HHS (U.S. Department of Health and Human Services). 2014. *The Health Consequences of Smoking—50 Years of Progress: A Report of the Surgeon General.* Atlanta: Centers for Disease Control and Prevention.

IHME (Institute for Health Metrics and Evaluation). 2010. "Global Burden of Diseases Study: China Profile." IHME, University of Washington, Seattle.

———. 2012. "Global Burden of Diseases Study: China Profile." IHME, University of Washington, Seattle.

Ikeda, Nayu, David Sapienza, Ramiro Guerrero, Wichai Aekplakorn, Mohsen Naghavi, Ali H. Mokdad, Rafael Lozano, Christopher J. L. Murray, and Stephen S. Lim. 2014. "Control of Hypertension with Medication: A Comparative Analysis of National Surveys in 20 Countries." *Bulletin of the World Health Organization* 92 (1): 10–19C.

Jing, Limei, Zhiqun Shu, Xiaoming Sun, John F. Chiu, Jiquan Lou, and Chunyan Xie. 2015. "Factors Influencing Patients' Contract Choice with General Practitioners in Shanghai: A Preliminary Study." *Asia-Pacific Journal of Public Health* 27 (2 Suppl): 77S–85S. doi:10.1177/1010539514561654.

Kinsella, Kevin, and David R. Phillips. 2005. "Global Aging: The Challenge of Success." *Population Bulletin* 60 (1): 5–42.

Lei, Xiaoyan, and Wanchuan Lin. 2009. "The New Cooperative Medical Scheme in Rural China: Does More Coverage Mean More

Service and Better Health?" *Health Economics* 18 (S2): S25–S46. doi: 10.1002/hec.1501.

Li, Min-zhi, Li Su, Bao-yun Liang, Jin-jing Tan, Qing Chen, Jian-xiong Long, Juan-juan Xie, and others. 2013. "Trends in Prevalence, Awareness, Treatment, and Control of Diabetes Mellitus in Mainland China from 1979 to 2012." *International Journal of Endocrinology* 2013: Article ID 753150. doi:10.1155/2013/753150

Li, Ye, Qunhong Wu, Ling Xu, David Legge, Yanhua Hao, Lijun Gao, Ning Ning, and Gang Wan. 2012. "Factors Affecting Catastrophic Health Expenditure and Impoverishment from Medical Expenses in China: Policy Implications of Universal Health Insurance." *Bulletin of the World Health Organization* 90: 664–71.

Liang, Lilin, and John C. Langenbrunner. 2013. "The Long March to Universal Coverage: Lessons from China." Universal Health Coverage (UNICO) Study Series 9, World Bank, Washington, DC.

Liu, Hong, and Zhong Zhao. 2014. "Does Health Insurance Matter? Evidence from China's Urban Resident Basic Medical Insurance." *Journal of Comparative Economics* 42 (4): 1007–20. doi:10.1016/j.jce.2014.02.003.

Liu, Kai, Qiaobing Wu, and Junqiang Liu. 2014. "Examining the Association between Social Health Insurance Participation and Patients' Out-of-Pocket Payments in China: The Role of Institutional Arrangements." *Social Science and Medicine* 113: 95–103. doi:10.1016/j.socscimed.2014.05.011.

Liu, L. S. 2011. "2010 Chinese Guidelines for the Management of Hypertension." *Zhonghua xin xue guan bing za zhi* 39 (7): 579–615.

Long, Qian, Ling Xu, Henk Bekedam, and Shenglan Tang. 2013. "Changes in Health Expenditures in China in the 2000s: Has the Health System Reform Improved Affordability?" *International Journal for Equity in Health* 12: 8.

Lorenzoni, Luca, David Morgan, Yuki Murakami, and Chris James. 2015. "The OECD Health and Long-Term Care Expenditure Projection Model and Its Application to China." Background report, Organisation for Economic Co-operation and Development (OECD), Paris.

Ma, Jin, Mingshan Lu, and Hude Quan. 2008. "From a National, Centrally Planned Health System to a System Based on the Market: Lessons from China." *Health Affairs* 27 (4): 937–48.

Maeda, Akiko, Edson Araujo, Cheryl Cashin, Joseph Harris, Naoki Ikegami, and Michael R. Reich. 2014. *Universal Health Coverage for Inclusive and Sustainable Development: A Synthesis of 11 Country Case Studies.* Directions in Development Series. Washington, DC: The World Bank.

McCollum, Rosalind, Lieping Chen, Tang Chen Xiang, Xiaoyun Liu, Barbara Starfield, Zheng Jinhuan, and Rachel Tolhurst. 2014. "Experiences with Primary Health Care in Fuzhou, Urban China, in the Context of Health Sector Reform: A Mixed Methods Study." *The International Journal of Health Planning and Management* 29 (2): e107–e126. doi:10.1002/hpm.2165.

Meng, Qingyue. 2015. "Overview of Efforts to Improve Primary Health Care and Enhance Integration in China." World Bank, Washington, DC.

Meng, Qingyue, and Shenglan Tang. 2010. "Universal Coverage of Health Care in China: Challenges and Opportunities." *World Health Report (2010)* Background Paper, 7, World Health Organization, Geneva.

Meng, Qingyue, Jing Yuan, Limei Jing, and Junhua Zhang. 2009. "Mobility of Primary Health Care Workers in China." *Human Resources for Health* 7 (24): 5.

Meng, Qun, Ling Xu, Yaoguang Zhang, Juncheng Qian, Min Cai, Ying Xin, Jun Gao, Ke Xu, J. Ties Boerma, and Sarah L. Barber. 2012. "Trends in Access to Health Services and Financial Protection in China between 2003 and 2011: A Cross-Sectional Study." *The Lancet* 379 (9818): 805–14. doi: http://dx.doi.org/10.1016/S0140-6736(12)60278-5.

Ng, S. W., A. G. Howard, H. J. Wang, C. Su, and B. Zhang. 2014. "The Physical Activity Transition among Adults in China: 1991–2011." *Obesity Reviews* 15: 27–36. doi:10.1111/obr.12127.

OECD (Organisation for Economic Co-operation and Development). 2015. "OECD Health Statistics 2015." Database, OECD, Paris. http://www.oecd.org/els/health-systems/oecd-health-statistics-2015-country-notes.htm.

OECD and WHO (Organisation for Economic Co-operation and Development and World Health Organization). 2014. *Health at a Glance: Asia/Pacific 2014.* Paris: OECD.

Peng, Yingchun, Wenhu Chang, Haiqing Zhou, Hongpu Hu, and Wannian Liang. 2010. "Factors Associated with Health-Seeking

Behavior among Migrant Workers in Beijing, China." *BMC Health Services Research* 10: 10.

Selvin, Elizabeth, Christina M. Parrinello, David B. Sacks, and Josef Coresh. 2014. "Trends in Prevalence and Control of Diabetes in the United States, 1988–1994 and 1999–2010." *Annals of Internal Medicine* 160 (8): 517–25.

Smith, James P., John Strauss, and Yaohui Zhao. 2014. "Healthy Aging in China." *Journal of the Economics of Ageing* 4: 37–43. doi:10.1016/j.jeoa.2014.08.006.

Smith, Sheila, Joseph P. Newhouse, and Mark S. Freeland. 2009. "Income, Insurance, and Technology: Why Does Health Spending Outpace Economic Growth?" *Health Affairs* 28 (5): 1276–84. doi:10.1377/hlthaff.28.5.1276.

Sun, Zesheng, Shuhong Wang, and Stephen R. Barnes. 2015. "Understanding Congestion in China's Medical Market: An Incentive Structure Perspective." *Health Policy and Planning.* doi:10.1093/heapol/czv062.

Sylvia, Sean, Yaojiang Shi, Hao Xue, Xin Tian, Huan Wang, Qingmei Liu, Alexis Medina, and Scott Rozelle. 2015. "Survey Using Incognito Standardized Patients Shows Poor Quality Care in China's Rural Clinics." *Health Policy and Planning* 30 (3): 322–33. doi:10.1093/heapol/czu014.

Tang, Shenglan. 2014. "Developing More Equitable and Efficient Health Insurance in China." Paulson Policy Memorandum, Paulson Institute, Chicago.

UN DESA (United Nations Department of Economic and Social Affairs). 2013. "World Population Aging 2013." Report ST/ESA/SER.A/348, UN DESA Population Division, United Nations, New York.

————. 2015. "World Population Prospects: The 2015 Revision, Key Findings and Advance Tables." Working Paper No. ESA/P/WP.241, UN DESA Population Division, United Nations, New York.

Wang, Shan, Lihua Liu, and Jianchao Liu. 2014. "Comparison of Chinese Inpatients with Different Types of Medical Insurance before and after the 2009 Health Reform." *BMC Health Services Research* 14 (443): 8.

Wang, Shiyong, Patricio Marquez, and John Langenbrunner. 2011. "Toward a Healthy and Harmonious Life in China: Stemming the Rising Tide of Non-Communicable Diseases." Report 62318-CN, World Bank, Washington, DC.

Wanless, Derek, John Appleby, Anthony Harrison, and Darshan Patel. 2007. *Our Future Health Secured? A Review of NHS Funding and Performance.* London: King's Fund.

WHO (World Health Organization). 2014. "Noncommunicable Diseases (NCD) Country Profiles: China." Factsheet, WHO, Geneva. http://www.who.int/nmh/countries/chn_en.pdf.

World Bank. 2015. *World Development Indicators 2015.* Washington, DC: World Bank.

Xu, Jin, and Qingyue Meng. 2015. "People-Centered Health Care: Towards a New Structure of Health Service Delivery in China." World Bank, Washington, DC.

Xu, Y., L. Wang, J. He, Y. Bi, M. Li, T. Wang, L. Wang, Y. Jiang, M. Dai, and J. Lu. 2013. "Prevalence and Control of Diabetes in Chinese Adults." *Journal of the American Medical Association* 310 (9): 948.

Yang, Gonghuan, Lingzhi Kong, Wenhua Zhao, Xia Wan, Yi Zhai, Lincoln C. Chen, and Jeffrey P. Koplan. 2008. "Emergence of Chronic Noncommunicable Diseases in China." *The Lancet* 372 (9650): 1697–1705. doi:10.1016/S0140-6736(08)61366-5.

Yang, Gonghuan, Yu Wang, Yixin Zeng, George F. Gao, Xiaofeng Liang, Maigeng Zhou, Xia Wan, Shicheng Yu, Yuhong Jiang, and Mohsen Naghavi. 2013. "Rapid Health Transition in China, 1990–2010: Findings from the Global Burden of Disease Study 2010." *The Lancet* 381 (9882): 1987–2015.

Yang, Huajie, Xiang Huang, Zhiheng Zhou, Harry H. X. Wang, Xinyue Tong, Zhihong Wang, Jiaji Wang, and Zuxun Lu. 2014. "Determinants of Initial Utilization of Community Health Care Services among Patients with Major Noncommunicable Chronic Diseases in South China." *PLoS ONE* 9 (12): e116051. doi:10.1371/journal.pone.0116051.

Yang, Wei. 2015. "Catastrophic Outpatient Health Payments and Health Payment-Induced Poverty under China's New Rural Cooperative Medical Scheme." *Applied Economic Perspectives and Policy* 37 (1): 64–85. doi:10.1093/aepp/ppu017.

Yang, Wei, and Xun Wu. 2014. "Paying for Outpatient Care in Rural China: Cost Escalation under China's New Co-operative Medical Scheme." *Health Policy and Planning.* doi:10.1093/heapol/czt111.

Yang, Wenying, Juming Lu, Jianping Weng, Weiping Jia, Linong Ji, Jianzhong Xiao, Zhongyan Shan, Jie Liu, Haoming Tian, and Qiuhe Ji. 2010. "Prevalence of Diabetes among Men and Women in China." *New England Journal of Medicine* 362 (12): 1090–1101.

Yang, Zhao-Jun, Jie Liu, Jia-Pu Ge, Li Chen, Zhi-Gang Zhao, and Wen-Ying Yang. 2011. "Prevalence of Cardiovascular Disease Risk Factors in the Chinese Population: The 2007–08 China National Diabetes and Metabolic Disorders Study." *European Heart Journal* 33: 213–20. doi: 10.1093/eurheartj/ehr205.

Yin, Wen-qiang, Zhong-ming Chen, Hui Guan, Xue-dan Cui, Qian-qian Yu, Hai-ping Fan, Xin Ma, and Yan Wei. 2015. "Using Entropy Weight RSR to Evaluate Village Doctors' Prescription in Shandong Province under the Essential Medicine System." *Modern Preventive Medicine* 42 (3): 2.

Yin, Xiaoxv, Fujian Song, Yanhong Gong, Xiaochen Tu, Yunxia Wang, Shiyi Cao, Junan Liu, and Zuxun Lu. 2013. "A Systematic Review of Antibiotic Utilization in China." *Journal of Antimicrobial Chemotherapy* 68 (11): 2445–52. doi:10.1093/jac/dkt223.

Yip, Winnie, Timothy Powell-Jackson, Wen Chen, Min Hu, Eduardo Fe, Mu Hu, Weiyan Jian, Ming Lu, Wei Han, and William C. Hsiao. 2014. "Capitation Combined with Pay-for-Performance Improves Antibiotic Prescribing Practices in Rural China." *Health Affairs* 33 (3): 502–10. doi:10.1377/hlthaff.2013.0702.

Yip, Winnie, Chi-Man Yip, William C. Hsiao, Wen Chen, Shanlian Hu, Jin Ma, and Alan Maynard. 2012. "Early Appraisal of China's Huge and Complex Health-Care Reforms." *The Lancet* 379: 10. doi:10.1016/S0140-6736(11)61880-1.

Yu, Baorong, Qingyue Meng, Charles Collins, Rachel Tolhurst, Shenglan Tang, Fei Yan, Lennart Bogg, and Xiaoyun Liu. 2010. "How Does the New Cooperative Medical Scheme Influence Health Service Utilization? A Study in Two Provinces in Rural China." *BMC Health Services Research* 10: 9.

Zhai, Tiemin, John Goss, Jinjing Li, Rachel Davey, and Yohannes Kinfu. 2015. "Main Drivers of Recent Health Expenditure Growth in China: A Decomposition Analysis." *The Lancet* 386, Suppl 1: S46. doi:10.1016/S0140-6736(15)00627-3

Zhang, Linxiu, Hongmei Yi, and Scott Rozelle. 2010. "Good and Bad News from China's New Cooperative Medical Scheme." *IDS Bulletin* 41 (4): 10.

Zhang, Lufa, and Nan Liu. 2014. "Health Reform and Out-of-Pocket Payments: Lessons from China." *Health Policy and Planning* 29 (2): 217–26.

2

Lever 1: Shaping Tiered Health Care Delivery with People-Centered Integrated Care

The People-Centered Integrated Care (PCIC) Model

A country's health care service delivery system should ensure that patients receive appropriate, high-quality care in the best setting for their needs in a timely, equitable, and affordable fashion. This report uses "people-centered integrated care" (PCIC) to refer to a flexible model that is organized around the health needs of individuals and their families. The term is shortened, for easier translation, from the World Health Organization's (WHO) global strategy on "people-centered and integrated health services" (WHO 2015a). Box 2.1 defines PCIC, drawing on the WHO strategy.

The goal of PCIC is to provide the right service at the right place and the right time. In addition to responding to patient needs and perspectives, this approach prioritizes integration and coordination of services across the spectrum of care, from promotion and prevention to curative and palliative needs to reduce fragmentation and wasteful use of resources across a health system.

The foundation of PCIC is primary health care. Without a robust primary health care system, no country can provide high-quality,

effective PCIC while also keeping costs low. Effective PCIC promotes primary care as the patients' first point of contact for most of their health care needs, coordinating care with other providers, such as hospitals, at different levels of the health care system and across the spectrum of health needs. Ultimately, adopting PCIC implies a process of rebalancing and structuring China's delivery system into functional and accountable networks of tiered and interconnected providers.

In China, a paradigm shift toward a PCIC-like model is already under way from a policy perspective, as chapter 1 discussed. Of particular relevance are recent State Council guidelines that outline the roles and responsibilities of different levels of a tiered delivery system.[1] These guidelines establish the essential tenets and features of the PCIC delivery model in China and set the stage for the core actions outlined later in this chapter.

The new guidelines include the following important features:

- Strengthening grassroots providers
- Promoting first contact at the grassroots level
- Establishing two-way referrals

BOX 2.1   People-centered integrated care (PCIC) defined

People-centered care is "an approach to care that consciously adopts the perspectives of individuals, families and communities, and sees them as participants as well as beneficiaries of trusted health systems that respond to their needs and preferences in humane and holistic ways."

Integrated care consists of "health services that are managed and delivered in a way that ensures people receive a continuum of health promotion, disease prevention, diagnosis, treatment, disease management, rehabilitation and palliative care services, at the different levels and sites of care within the health system and according to their needs throughout their life course."

Source: WHO 2015a, 10–11.

- Defining provider roles while fostering the integration of providers across a tiered delivery system
- Emphasizing special care arrangements to treat and manage chronic diseases
- Expanding the supply of general practice physicians ("general practitioners") to staff primary care facilities
- Organizing provider networks
- Advancing the use of information and communications technology for electronic health systems

Across the globe, PCIC initiatives that prioritize primary health care are gaining traction as central parts of health care reform. Their core features—strengthened primary care, a focus on patient needs, and care integration across provider levels—are ubiquitous. In the United States, the patient-centered medical home (PCMH) model has become an important form of primary care improvement. Across highly functioning health systems such as those in Australia, Canada, Denmark, the Netherlands, and the United Kingdom, PCIC-like reforms are taking shape. Even middle-income countries such as Brazil, Costa Rica, Singapore, and Turkey show a marked orientation toward reshaping service delivery toward PCIC. Though they are expanding rapidly, PCIC-like approaches remain local or regional in many countries.

Based on a review of international experience—including a range of Chinese initiatives for establishing PCIC—this chapter assesses the benefits of a shift to PCIC as well as the challenges China is likely to face in broadening the reliance of its health care system on PCIC. It then discusses actions in eight core areas that will help guide the decisions of Chinese authorities as they seek to broaden the implementation of PCIC. The chapter concludes by summarizing the outlook in China on the PCIC core action areas. The focus of the discussion is on organizing the delivery system around the needs of patients and achieving integration between the different components of the system.

Benefits of Adopting PCIC

Although results are often context-specific and most of the available evidence comes from PCIC initiatives in high-income countries, preliminary findings suggest that adopting PCIC can improve health outcomes, quality, and patient experience. Annex 2A reviews the evidence on effects of PCIC-like models on health outcomes, quality, and costs, drawing on findings from more than 300 studies, including 10 Chinese case studies that were commissioned for this report. In summary, PCIC adoption has had the following results:

- *Reduced hospitalizations and use of emergency care.* Reviews of a wide variety of PCIC approaches—including those of the U.S. Program of All-Inclusive Care for the

Elderly (PACE) and the U.S. Veterans Health Administration's Patient Aligned Care Teams (PACT)—highlight reductions in patients' visits to emergency departments, unscheduled readmissions, and lengths of hospital stays (Ali 2015; Ali and Li 2015b). Hospital admission rates for conditions that can be treated with ambulatory care have often declined.

- *Improved clinical care processes.* PCIC interventions improved pain assessment and treatment, adequacy of medicine dosages, patients' adherence to prescriptions, use of care plans, and patient education. For example, of the 48 clinical processes studied in the PACT case study, 41 improved (Ali and Li 2015b).

- *Improved outcomes and patient satisfaction.* PCIC interventions decreased patients' pain, improved the quality of life, and reduced the severity of depression. Other benefits included better glycemic control and lipid profiles and improvements in physical function, nutritional status, and physical balance. When measured, patient satisfaction almost always increased.

- *Mixed impacts on costs.* Nearly all the studies examined short-term impacts on costs, and their findings varied considerably within and across countries. Some PCIC interventions in Europe and the United States have generated savings, but the clear majority of studies show limited or inconclusive evidence on cost stabilization or curtailment, and a handful even report cost increases (Hebert et al. 2014). Further research is needed to determine whether better quality and outcomes will bring about cost savings in the long term. In China, with its current bias toward specialty services over primary care services, there is probably greater potential for cost savings.

- *Improved balance of health system resources and needs.* At the health system level, adopting PCIC enables a shift in the balance of care so that resources are allocated to better respond to needs. This shift can reduce the duplication of health investments and services, unnecessary use of health care facilities, and waiting times for care. PCIC can also improve patient safety by reducing medical errors, increasing the uptake of screening and prevention programs, improving diagnostic accuracy, increasing the appropriateness and timeliness of referrals, and improving equity across the care system.

An exhaustive review of the literature on PCIC initiatives globally (WHO 2015a, 2015b) identified an array of potential benefits to individuals, communities, health workers, and health systems (as listed in box 2.2).

International experience shows that better outcomes at potentially lower costs are produced by systems that prioritize the critical primary health care functions: accessibility, comprehensive capacities for most general nonemergent clinical needs, continuity of care and information, continual quality improvement, and integration of care (Friedberg, Hussey, and Schneider 2010; Macinko, Starfield, and Erinosho 2009). It also suggests that, though there is no one model for providing PCIC, at the service delivery level PCIC should encompass at least the following four strategic goals:[2]

- Organizing the model of care around the health needs of patients, which in China is likely to entail strengthening primary health care and changing the roles of hospitals
- Integrating providers across care levels and among types of services
- Continuously improving the quality of care
- Engaging people to make better decisions about their health and health-seeking behaviors.

Challenges to PCIC Implementation in China

The 22 case studies commissioned by the World Bank for this report yield insights into the challenges China is likely to face in implementing PCIC-based reforms in service delivery. Ten of the studies were of PCIC

BOX 2.2   **Potential benefits of people-centered integrated care**

Benefits to individuals and their families
- Increased satisfaction with care and better relationships with care providers
- Improved access to and timeliness of care
- Improved health literacy and decision-making skills that promote patient independence
- Shared decision making with professionals along with increased patient and family involvement in care planning
- Increased ability to self-manage and control long-term health conditions
- Better coordination of care across different care settings.

Benefits to health professionals and community health workers
- Improved job satisfaction
- Decreased workloads and reduced burnout
- Role enhancement that expands workforce skills, so workers can assume a wider range of responsibilities
- Education and training opportunities to learn new skills, such as working in team-based health care environments.

Benefits to communities
- Improved access to care, particularly for marginalized groups
- Improved health outcomes and healthier communities, including greater levels of health-seeking behaviors
- Better ability for communities to manage and control infectious diseases and respond to crises

- Greater influence and better relationships with care providers that build community awareness of, and trust in, care services
- Greater engagement and participatory representation in decision making about the use of health resources
- Clarification of citizens' health care rights and responsibilities
- Care that is more responsive to community needs.

Benefits to health systems
- Better balance of care so that resources are allocated closer to needs
- Improved equity and enhanced access to care for all
- Improved patient safety through reduced medical errors and adverse events
- Increased uptake of screening and preventive programs
- Improved diagnostic accuracy and appropriateness and timeliness of referrals
- Reduced hospitalizations and lengths of stay through stronger primary and community care services and better management and coordination of care
- Reduced unnecessary use of health care facilities and waiting times for care
- Reduced duplication of health investments and services
- Reduced overall costs of care per capita
- Reduced mortality and morbidity from both infectious and noncommunicable diseases.

Source: WHO 2015a, 12.

---

improvement initiatives in China, and 12 were of initiatives in other middle- and high-income countries (table 2.1; for more details, see annex 2B).

Through interviews with planners and personnel in hospitals and primary care centers in China and other countries, these case studies highlighted the typical issues that arise when improving primary care and better integrating care across the tiers of the health care system. Importantly, as

highlighted in this and other chapters, innovative initiatives are under way in China to address these challenges.

First among these challenges, the case studies found that, at the primary care level, systems need to be established for registering or empaneling patients[3] *and stratifying them by their conditions and risks.* Experience with gatekeeping in China is limited, and referral systems need improvement to support the goal of having patients' first contact be at the

TABLE 2.1   Summary list of commissioned case studies on PCIC-based health care reforms in China and other selected countries

In-text reference	Case study	Location
Chinese case studies		
Beijing, CHA	Beijing Chaoyang Hospital Alliance (CHA), four cases	Beijing
Beijing, PKU IDS	Peking University Renmin Hospital Integrated Delivery System (PKU IDS), four cases	Beijing
Feixi, SPHCC	Strengthening Primary Health Care Capacity (SPHCC)	Feixi (Anhui province)
Hangzhou, TFY	Twelfth Five-Year Plan (TFY)	Hangzhou (Zhejiang province)
Huangzhong, HCA	Health Care Alliance (HCA)	Huangzhong (Qinghai province)
Shanghai, FDS	Family Doctor System (FDS)	Shanghai
Shanghai, RLG	Shanghai Ruijin-Luwan Hospital Group (RLG), four cases	Shanghai
Xi, IC	Integrated Care (IC)	Xi (Henan province)
Zhenjiang, GH	Great Health (GH)	Zhenjiang (Jiangsu Province)
Zhenjiang, ZKG	Jiangsu Zhenjiang Kangfu Hospital Groups (ZKG), four cases	Zhenjiang (Jiangsu Province)
International case studies		
Canterbury, HSP	Health Services Plan (HSP)	Canterbury, New Zealand
Denmark, SIKS	Integrated Effort for People Living with Chronic Diseases (SIKS)	Denmark
Fosen, DMC	District Medical Center (DMC)	Fosen, Norway
JCUH, AEC	James Cook University Hospital (JCUH), Ambulatory Emergency Care (AEC)	England
Kinzigtal, GK	Gesundes Kinzigtal (GK)	Kinzigtal, Germany
Maryland, CareFirst	CareFirst Patient-Centered Medical Home	Maryland, United States
Netherlands, DTC	Maastricht Diabetes Care (DTC)	Netherlands
Portugal, ULS	Local Health Unit (ULS)	Portugal
Singapore, RHS	Regional Health Systems (RHS)	Singapore
Turkey, HTP	Health Transition Plan (HTP)	Turkey
United States, PACE	Program of All-Inclusive Care for the Elderly (PACE)	United States
VHA, PACT	Veterans Health Administration (VHA), Patient Aligned Care Teams (PACT)	United States

Note: For more detailed descriptions of each of the case studies, see annex 2B (table 2B.1).

primary care level rather than at a hospital. Downward referral systems—that is, from hospital to primary care—function irregularly. Although there is a clear movement toward forming multidisciplinary teams, in much of China the health care workforce lacks the knowledge, skills, and culture needed to work collaboratively. Despite the government's calls to integrate preventive and curative care at the primary level, integration remains insufficient throughout the country. Unattractive compensation levels discourage qualified professionals and health workers from seeking and retaining positions at the grassroots level.

Second, hospitals in China have strong financial incentives to capture both inpatients and outpatients and not to shift or integrate care provision to lower levels, because of their high dependency on fee-for-service revenues. Hospitals' willingness to shift care to facilities at lower levels of the health system will usually favor those patients for whom the revenue receipts do not cover costs (such as geriatric patients with long stays). Each facility is paid separately for the care it provides, and except in the Xi County (Henan province) experiment (Ali and Li 2015a), few facilities have attempted to share earnings or savings from improved coordination. Though China is experimenting with the formation of integrated facility networks, known as hospital alliances, some of these alliances are dominated by large hospitals and become channels to capture patients at higher levels of care.

Third, providers and facilities are not compensated—or not fully compensated— for the provision of integrated care. For example, Beijing Chaoyang Hospital provides a small yearly stipend to physicians who rotate to community health centers on a part-time basis, but at a rate too low to cover the "lost income" they could have made by providing hospital-based care (Jian and Yip 2015). Primary care physicians rarely receive additional income for activities related to care coordination, and primary care facilities cannot retain savings they may earn if they coordinate care and increase efficiency.

Fourth, patients in China have few incentives to use primary care as a first point of entry. Government policy allows patients direct access to hospitals for all care. Relative to hospitals, primary care facilities have limited drug formularies and fewer well-qualified professionals—which limits the demand from patients with complex conditions. Because the copayments charged at hospital outpatient departments are little higher than those at primary care facilities, out-of-pocket cost differences do not deter patients from preferring hospitals.

Fifth, integration requires administrative coordination beyond what currently exists in China. Networks that consist of facilities in different political-administrative jurisdictions (such as municipality, district, and county) have difficulty coordinating decision making and staff behavior regarding patient flows,

overlapping services, financing arrangements, human resources, and logistics. The formation of health maintenance organizations has not overcome this difficulty. Two cases with arguably the best examples of care coordination, Xi County and Zhenjiang-Kangfu, operate within a single administrative jurisdiction (Ali and Li 2015a; Li and Jiang 2015).

Finally, though China has adopted many innovations in health information and communication systems, these initiatives often lack interoperability. Many of them center on supporting hospitals rather than grassroots providers.

The case studies suggest that China should consider unified, standardized local and national systems to measure and improve the quality of primary health care service delivery, chronic disease management, and patient satisfaction. Such measurement systems should be linked to improvement efforts.

China is not alone in facing challenges to the reform of health services. Many Organisation for Economic Co-operation and Development (OECD) countries have begun adopting PCIC as part of broader reform efforts to invest more in health systems (rather than in individual health programs and facilities)—reforms that are designed to address the needs of aging populations, the high and increasing incidence of noncommunicable diseases (NCDs), and escalating costs. The challenges they have faced in doing so include transforming the acute care and "illness treatment" orientation of traditional care models; reversing the often top-heavy, pyramidal structures of their service delivery systems; and reducing fragmentation of management and services between facilities and service levels (Cercone and O'Brien 2010; Porter 2010; WHO 2008).

Some of the OECD reforms have also aimed to alter traditional relationships between providers and patients away from the current model, which has tended to be limited to the moment of the consultation, centered on discrete interventions, limited to a single medical professional's advice to an individual patient during the consultation, and conceiving of the patient's responsibility as merely following the provider's advice.

Core Action Areas and Implementation Strategies

Based on the commissioned case studies and, where appropriate, the broader case literature, this section outlines eight core action areas identified as fundamental to the establishment of effective PCIC systems (table 2.2). For each, we outline strategies that China's authorities may wish to adopt to guide implementation.

All the improvement initiatives featured in the case studies have used multiple strategies in pursuit of PCIC (figure 2.1). All initiatives included work to strengthen vertical integration and information and communication systems (core areas 3 and 5, respectively)—reflecting a need to improve coordination and

continuity to ensure the right care is given at the right place. Almost all of them sought to strengthen horizontal integration as well as performance measurement and feedback (core areas 4 and 7, respectively).

The least frequent area of focus was certification and accreditation (core area 8), which was seen in about one-quarter of the cases; none of the initiatives in China used this as an improvement strategy. Other approaches used for improving accountability and the standardization of care (core areas 1 and 2) include linking payment to quality, implementing clinical pathways and other standards of care (core area 6), and measuring patient satisfaction.

Within each action area, the PCIC initiatives used a range of strategies, chosen to match their identified priorities, the scope of the targeted areas for improvement, existing challenges, the health care system's strengths

TABLE 2.2   Eight core PCIC action areas and corresponding implementation strategies

Core action area	Implementation strategies
1: Primary health care as the first point of contact	• Use empanelment to facilitate population health management • Stratify empaneled population based on risk • Strengthen gatekeeping • Ensure accessibility
2: Multidisciplinary teams	• Define team goals, composition, roles, and leadership • Form individualized care plans between care teams and patients
3: Vertical integration, including new roles for hospitals	• Redefine the roles of facilities within a vertically integrated network • Establish provider-to-provider relationships • Develop formalized facility networks
4: Horizontal integration	• Promote the integration of different types of health care facilities • Provide integrated care around the individual user to promote more patient-centered care
5: Advanced information and communication technology (e-health)	• Establish standardized electronic health records systems accessible to providers and patients • Establish communication and care management functions • Ensure interconnectivity and interoperability
6: Integrated clinical pathways and functional dual referral systems	• Craft integrated pathways to facilitate care integration and decision support for providers • Promote dual referrals within integrated facility networks
7: Measurement, standards, and feedback	• Use standard performance measurement indicators • Create continuous feedback loops linked to action plans to drive quality improvement
8: Accreditation and certification	• Develop nationally and locally relevant accreditation criteria • Set indicator targets for certification

Note: PCIC = people-centered integrated care.

FIGURE 2.1   Frequency of PCIC interventions in commissioned case studies, by core action area

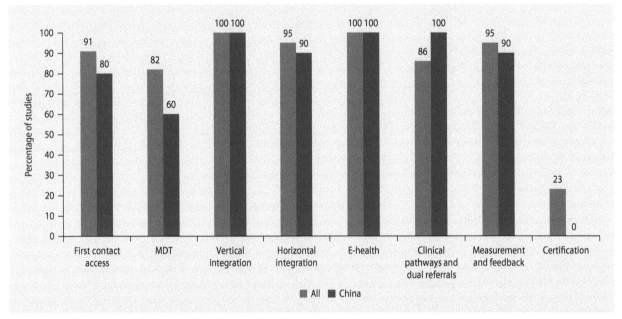

Note: PCIC = patient-centered integrated care; MDT = multidisciplinary team. For descriptions of all 22 case studies commissioned for this report, see annex 2B (table 2B.1).

and structure, the system's history of reform, and local traditions and culture.

Core Action Area 1: Primary Health Care as the First Point of Contact

Primary health care is the focal point of PCIC, addressing both individual and community health. One of the basic characteristics of a strong primary health care system is that it establishes primary health care as the first point of contact for most patients' needs. When patients consistently use trusted and competent primary health care providers as their entryway into a tiered health system, they can receive care that is continuous and coordinated across the range of health care delivery levels (hospital, primary care provider, and specialist). They thus receive the needed care at the right place and avoid unnecessary hospital admissions, procedures, risks, and medical expenses.

Based on the findings from the case studies, four strategies were identified for ensuring that primary health care is the first point of contact for patients for most of their health care needs: empanelment, risk stratification, gatekeeping, and accessibility.

Strategy 1: Use empanelment to facilitate population health management
Empanelment is the process by which all patients in a given facility or geographic area are assigned to a primary care provider or care team. It was considered a fundamental component in 10 of the 22 initiatives studied, including three of those in China. Empanelment is the mainstay of service delivery systems in a number of European countries, including Denmark; England, U.K.; Finland; the Netherlands; Scotland, U.K.; and Turkey. In China, adopting empanelment is likely to be an important step in improving patient-provider relationships and trust, in ensuring responsibility is taken at the primary care level for a population's health, and in shifting health-seeking behavior away from hospitals.

There are two main ways to approach empanelment: allowing patients an element of choice or assigning patients by geographic region—which is typically done using preexisting community demarcations. For example, the success of the Shanghai "family doctor" system (FDS) largely hinged on contracts between residents and primary health care providers (Ma 2015a). The FDS empaneled populations by neighborhood in all of its districts. It focused on building strong relationships between patients and primary care providers, which furthered community trust in the family doctors as the first point of contact in the health system.

China also used empanelment as a tool in shifting from fee-for-service care to providing more accessible, high-quality care in lower-level health facilities through integrated chronic disease management programs and improved e-health tools. Empanelment in Hangzhou (through implementation of its Twelfth Five-Year Plan [TFY]) was conducted by geographically restricted patient choice: residents were able to choose any primary health care provider in a community health center (CHC) within a specific area designated by their district health insurance. Each resident was contracted for a full year and could only choose one primary care provider at a time (Yan 2015a). Similarly, in Kinzigtal, Germany, health care management company Gesundes Kinzigtal (whose name translates as "healthy Kinzig Valley") empaneled its population by region to make sure that all the covered patients were linked to a primary health care team, but it allowed the patients to choose any primary care team within their region (Hildebrandt and others 2015; Nolte and others 2015).

Though simple, geographic empanelment can limit patients' choice of physician and thereby decrease their acceptance of the system. Empanelment by patient choice is an alternative approach that was used in other initiatives. In Turkey, the Health Transformation Plan of 2003 sought to establish family medicine centers in every district of the country, each with a defined reference population (Sumer 2015). The Turkish government initially decided to assign patients geographically to family medicine doctors, creating "patients' registries," while allowing patients to request to leave the original registry and join the panel of a different family physician even if the physician was outside their geographic area. This freedom of choice proved to be a challenge for continuity of care, particularly when patients moved between panels without effective communication between physicians. Further, transferring patient records could take significant time. If China were to implement a similar choice-based empanelment system, it would need to be supported by an effective, real-time information management system, to ensure that patient information is transferred efficiently whenever patients change providers.

In the United States, the private health insurance company CareFirst prioritized patient preference in the state of Maryland but also worked to ensure that all patients were assigned a regular source of primary health care as part of its PCMH payment model (Murray 2015). The company devised a complex process of "aligning" or attributing patients who did not have a chosen primary health care provider to a provider. It developed an algorithm to assign a primary care provider based on which physician the patient had last seen and how many times they had seen him or her. Importantly, CareFirst prioritized patient choice and reached out to the patients to confirm and update their empanelment assignment. At any point, a patient could contact CareFirst to switch to another primary health care provider. While labor-intensive, this alignment process allowed for patient empanelment in a country where there are no established empanelment practices.

A core component of empanelment is maintaining workable panel sizes (the number of patients assigned to a specific provider or team). Limiting this panel size is critical to achieve the goals of empanelment, allowing the primary care provider and team to deliver effective PCIC by focusing on the patient's needs. Overly large panel sizes can discourage the formation and maintenance of strong patient-provider relationships and inhibit the provision of coordinated quality care by limiting the time available for individual patients. Large panel sizes are often the result of fee-for-service based payment systems, which can lead providers and practices to prioritize the number of visits and patients seen over the quality of their interactions, care provided, and health outcomes.

Strategy 2: Stratify the risks of the empaneled population

One of the first tasks that PCIC planners must consider is defining the health needs of the target population. Risk stratification is the proactive identification of individuals within an empaneled reference population who are at higher risk of developing poor outcomes or who have, or risk having, high rates of service utilization, particularly hospitalization. The individuals thus identified can be proactively targeted for interventions designed to provide the needed higher-intensity, coordinated care within the primary health care setting. At the same time, these high utilizers can be engaged to understand and address their needs, as well as to reduce their preventable use of higher-cost, higher-intensity services. Risk stratification was featured in 10 of the 22 initiatives studied, including only one of the Chinese initiatives.

Risk stratification can be done at an individual patient level or based on disease burden. At the individual level, risk can be assessed based on clinical guidelines, on the presence of particular target conditions, or on a recent history of high utilization. Clinical staff can also use a summative process of their clinical intuition to create lists of patients whom they believe will need a higher level of attention from the team. The Xi Integrated Care initiative used the staff's summary clinical judgment to stratify patients by risk and to target the higher-risk patients for integrated clinical pathways to increase the delivery of appropriate

care and improve health outcomes (Ali and Li 2015a).

Other means to identify high-risk patients include a patient's past use of care facilities or current illness burden. In the United States, CareFirst's PCMH model in Maryland found that risk stratification based on history of use was highly effective without being overly burdensome to the provider (Murray 2015). The program uses an illness burden score to quantify patients' risk. Illness burden scores are calculated using the past 12 months of health insurance claims data and diagnoses (figure 2.2).

In Germany, physicians in Gesundes Kinzigtal complete a risk status questionnaire for each new patient as a part of the enrollment procedure. They use this information to compute risk for poor outcomes, which helps tailor a specialized care plan and goal-setting process for each patient (Hildebrandt and others 2015; Nolte and others 2015). This process ensures that higher-intensity services target those patients who are at higher risk for poor outcomes.

The Netherlands' Maastricht Diabetes Care and Denmark's Integrated Effort for People Living with Chronic Diseases (SIKS) initiatives both applied risk stratification by identifying specific diseases that were associated with high costs, required complicated management, or were associated with high risk for poor outcomes (Nolte and others 2015; Runz-Jørgensen and Frølich 2015; Vrijhoef and Schulpen 2015). SIKS created rehabilitation centers for people with four diseases: chronic obstructive pulmonary disease, diabetes, heart failure, and hip fracture, specifying clearly defined clinical entry criteria for each. Disease-based risk stratification allowed SIKS to reduce hospital admissions by 18 percent and outpatient visits by 24 percent (Runz-Jørgensen and Frølich 2015). Based on the success of the SIKS centers in Copenhagen, Denmark has scaled the approach into a national disease management program, which provides integrated comprehensive care for people with chronic diseases.

FIGURE 2.2   **Illness burden scorecard for patient risk stratification**

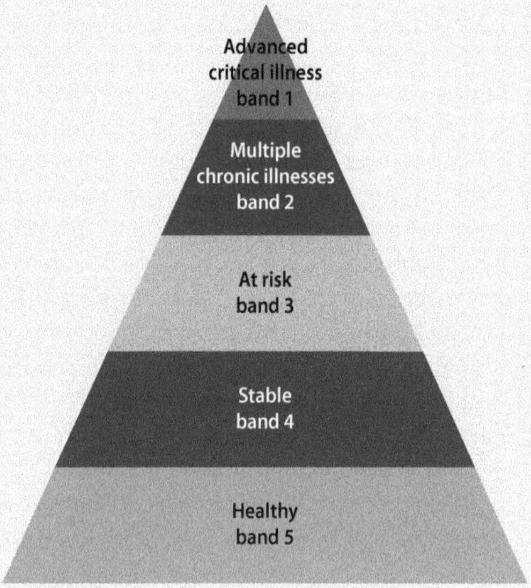

	Percent of population	Percent of cost	Cost PMPM
Advanced critical illness band 1 — **Illness burden (5.00 and above)** Extremely heavy health care users with significant advanced / critical illness.	3%	29%	$4,436
Multiple chronic illnesses band 2 — **Illness burden (2.00–4.99)** Heavy users of health care systems, mostly for more than one chronic disease.	8%	23%	$1,160
At risk band 3 — **Illness burden (1.00–1.99)** Fairly heavy users of health care system who are at risk of becoming more ill.	12%	21%	$578
Stable band 4 — **Illness burden (0.25–0.99)** Generally healthy, with light use of health care services.	27%	20%	$218
Healthy band 5 — **Illness burden (0–0.24)** Generally healthy, often not using health system.	50%	7%	$49

Source: O'Brien 2014.
Note: Graphic depicts the risk stratification used by insurance provider CareFirst in the state of Maryland, United States. PMPM = per member per month.

Strategy 3: Strengthen and target gatekeeping
Gatekeeping is an important mechanism for ensuring that patients receive the right care at the right place at the right time. Because patients may perceive gatekeeping as limiting their choice and imposing undue restrictions, gatekeeping systems must be designed with both patient autonomy and overall utilization controls in mind. Having primary health care providers as the gatekeepers is a way to manage patients' access to specialty care and can help to reduce overuse of inappropriate care. Gatekeeping arrangements must include a strong referral system so that those patients who need a higher level of care have access to it.

Gatekeeping can be done explicitly or implicitly. In *explicit gatekeeping*, patients cannot receive secondary or tertiary care without first seeing and getting approval from their primary health care provider, the "gatekeeper." This mechanism is often enforced by imposing financial or regulatory penalties on noncompliant patients or their providers. Hangzhou's TFY initiative used explicit gatekeeping for patients with hypertension or diabetes (Yan 2015a). These patients had to access the health care system through their primary care providers, who could then refer them to more-advanced care at the CHC.

In *implicit gatekeeping* systems, patients are strongly encouraged to see their primary health care provider before they visit a specialist, but they are not formally required to do so. This arrangement may be preferable to explicit gatekeeping because it allows greater patient choice. Turkey's Health Transformation Plan chose not to adopt a formal gatekeeping program. Instead, it gave patients a financial incentive to use family medicine practices as their first contact for problems by waiving the hospital copayment for patients who come to the hospital with a referral from their family physicians (Sumer 2015). This initiative decreased the number of patients coming to hospitals, but it also made family medicine physicians feel that they are sometimes used only for referrals to hospitals.

Strategy 4: Expand accessibility
Providing options for patients to see or speak to their providers when they perceive the need is a vital function of primary health care. Primary health care must be even more accessible and convenient than hospitals. After-hours care options and same-day visit opportunities strengthen the ability of primary health care to avoid unnecessary upstream utilization of more expensive care options. Increasing accessibility for patients was addressed in 14 (64 percent) of the 22 PCIC initiatives.

Financial incentives for providers can be used to improve patient access. In Maryland, the CareFirst insurance company paid each of its primary health care providers a monthly non-visit-based payment with quality bonuses that are partly determined by the providers' accessibility to patients (Murray 2015). Obtaining high scores on measures such as accessibility (on weekends, evening hours, and by telephone) and by giving patients access to their own medical records made providers eligible to receive bonuses. The financial incentives gave physicians the impetus to increase patients' access, including after-hours and electronic access, to their own electronic health records (EHRs).

Access standards can also be legislated. Before the district medical center (DMC) initiative began in Fosen, Norway, many districts did not have their own emergency care beds. Patients had to travel long distances to reach emergency care in tertiary medical centers. After the success of the DMC model, the national government mandated that every district establish emergency care beds, although it allowed the districts to choose where to do so, based on their infrastructure and their populations' needs (Forde, Auraasen, and Moreira 2015). By dictating the goal but allowing the districts choice in implementation, Norway ensured increased access to 24/7 emergency care for its citizens.

Other ways to increase access to primary health care include mobile clinics and home-based care. In a rural part of northwest China, Huangzhong in Qinghai Province implemented a health care alliance system in 2013 with the goal of fully integrating county, township, and village health centers (Meng, Luyu, and others 2015). For eldercare follow-up visits, primary health care facilities were supplemented with mobile clinics that were extended out from the county hospitals. The mobile clinics were capable of screening patients, transporting the critically ill to larger hospitals, and moving specimens to and from the primary health care facilities and the laboratory. In Zhenjiang, in China's eastern Jiangsu Province—Great Health's "3+X" teams were required to spend three days per week providing home visits to community members (Yan 2015b). Additional services they provided included appointment booking and online communication. These services were most often used by the elderly.

Under Turkey's Health Transformation Plan, family medicine physicians were required to conduct home visits and mobile clinics for patients who could not attend traditional clinics (Sumer 2015). These options were especially important in rural areas. The provision of home-based care, mobile health services, and mobile pharmacies are written into the contracts that family medicine practices make with the Ministry of Health. However, there have been some complaints that the time spent away from the office may create a gap in the continuity of care. Seven years after the start of the initiative, in 2010, Turkey also began to require that family medicine physicians serve nursing homes, prisons, and childcare centers by conducting community visits.

Core Action Area 2: Functioning Multidisciplinary Teams

Multidisciplinary teams are a building block for most successful PCIC initiatives. In principle, these teams are nonhierarchical groups of clinical and nonclinical staff whose goal is to provide comprehensive and integrated care for patients. Teams composed of clinical and nonclinical members with a variety of training backgrounds can provide a fuller range of services than individual health care providers.

Multidisciplinary teams were implemented by 17 (77 percent) of the 22 initiatives studied, and most were viewed as facilitators to PCIC. The initiatives used various approaches to make the multidisciplinary teams successful, including ensuring appropriate team composition and leadership and providing comprehensive, coordinated patient care.

Strategy 1: Define team goals, composition, roles, culture, and leadership

The starting point for defining an effective team is to define the health needs of the population and the role that primary care teams will play in responding to those needs. Aligning the goals of population health within a community to the composition and tasks of the team is a key initial planning step.

The personnel on a multidisciplinary team can vary, but clearly defining their roles and responsibilities is critical for success. Typically, the team leader is an experienced primary health clinician. For example, in the U.S. Veterans Health Administration's (VHA) PACT, the leader of each team was a physician, and the teams consisted of a nurse, medical assistant, pharmacist, care coordinator, and community social worker. The program required each care team to clearly define the role of each team member (figure 2.3) but allowed each team to adapt the roles of its members to its individual needs and context.

Multidisciplinary teams can designate a care coordinator to relieve stress on other team members, counsel patients on improving their health, and help patients navigate the delivery system. Because a large proportion of VHA patients had complicated chronic conditions that required well-coordinated care, each PACT team included a designated care coordinator who managed patients' appointments, follow-ups, referrals, test data, and discharge from the hospital. The care coordinator was a critical position on the care team, explicitly responsible for coordinating the clinical staff and the range of provided services (Ali and Li 2015b).

The multidisciplinary family doctor teams within Shanghai's FDS included a primary care physician as the core leader, along with a nurse, a public health physician, an assistant, and sometimes other professionals such as nutritionists and pharmacists (Ma 2015a). Similarly in Zhenjiang, Great Health's 3+X

FIGURE 2.3   Responsibilities of PACT members, U.S. Veterans Health Administration

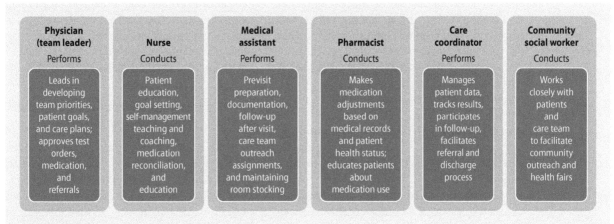

Physician (team leader)	Nurse	Medical assistant	Pharmacist	Care coordinator	Community social worker
Performs	Conducts	Performs	Conducts	Performs	Conducts
Leads in developing team priorities, patient goals, and care plans; approves test orders, medication, and referrals	Patient education, goal setting, self-management teaching and coaching, medication reconciliation, and education	Previsit preparation, documentation, follow-up after visit, care team outreach assignments, and maintaining room stocking	Makes medication adjustments based on medical records and patient health status; educates patients about medication use	Manages patient data, tracks results, participates in follow-up, facilitates referral and discharge process	Works closely with patients and care team to facilitate community outreach and health fairs

Source: Stout and others 2015.
Note: PACT = Patient Aligned Care Team.

teams comprised three members from a community health center and a varying number of volunteers from hospitals; generally, the three members were a primary care physician, a nurse, and one other preventive care staff member, while the hospital representatives (the "X") included other physicians, nurses, and administrative staff (Yan 2015b).

Multidisciplinary teams function best in a collaborative culture where providers communicate openly, trust one another, and are treated as equals. Teams must meet regularly and engage in frequent training and improvement efforts as a team. A comparison between the Norwegian and Portuguese PCIC improvement initiatives is illustrative. In the Norwegian case, a long history of cooperation and team mentality facilitated the development of multidisciplinary teams. Though they faced few requirements or mandates to work in teams, the DMC staff quickly developed a team spirit as the model was implemented (Forde, Auraasen, and Moreira 2015). Even the public health department and community psychiatric care service used the team approach, though their counterparts elsewhere in the world use hierarchical management models.

The Portuguese PCIC initiative also recognized the importance of multidisciplinary teams, and the reform explicitly called for the newly developed local health units (unidades de saúde local, or ULS) to work in multidisciplinary teams to provide primary, inpatient, and public health services. Unfortunately, the providers did not fully accept the concept of teamwork, and they reported that the process of creating functional multidisciplinary teams was a major barrier to care integration. Although on paper their multidisciplinary teams appeared similar to those elsewhere, a culture of teamwork and collaboration was generally missing. Fifteen years after the beginning of the ULS initiative, the teams still struggle to function (Forde, Auraasen, and Moreira 2015).

Importantly, collaborative cultures can be cultivated, as shown by the Health Services Plan in Canterbury, New Zealand. To foster a culture of collaboration, the architects of the plan clearly defined the targets and used emotional appeals to ensure that everyone understood the importance of working in multidisciplinary teams—rather than just mandating that they do so, as in the Portuguese case. To foster a collaborative culture from the start, the Canterbury leadership committees signed charters outlining the culture they agreed to uphold (Love 2015).

Strategy 2: Form individualized care plans between care teams and patients

A care plan provides a road map for all the providers who care for a patient. Care plans are generally used for high-risk patients but can be applied to all patients. They can also be used by patients themselves to manage their conditions at home. Successful care plans act as a contract of mutual commitments and contingency plans between the physician or nurse practitioner and the patient.

For example, in the Maryland case, CareFirst developed care plans for particularly high-risk and high-utilizing patients. Although CareFirst's local care coordinator played a role in initiating and maintaining the care plan, the key to a successful plan was the involvement of both the primary health care provider or nurse practitioner and the patients themselves. When care plans are subject to patient consent and can be accessed online by both the patient and the provider, they can also promote patient empowerment. To encourage providers to contribute the necessary time and effort to develop and maintain a care plan, CareFirst offered payments to primary care providers for established and maintained plans (Murray 2015).

Core Action Area 3: Vertical Integration Including New Roles for Hospitals

Vertical integration is a key element of tiered service delivery and involves communication and coordination among the primary, secondary, and tertiary health facilities delivering care. For China, achieving vertical integration will involve redefining the roles of, and interactions among, the facilities in all three tiers, especially hospitals, so that they work together toward the "3-in-1 principle: one system, one population, one pot of resources."

China's State Council guidance on tiered health care delivery recently outlined roles and responsibilities of facilities at different levels of the system,[4] and it is a good basis to build upon. As seen in some of the Chinese initiatives featured in the case studies, vertical integration can also link providers across the tiers of the system to provide support and technical assistance and to strengthen the quality of care.

Of the 22 PCIC initiatives studied for this report, 15 sought to strengthen vertical integration. Their strategies were of three broad types: (a) redefining facility roles within a vertically integrated network; (b) strengthening relationships among providers through technical assistance and skill building; and (c) developing formal networks of facilities based on the 3-in-1 principle.

Strategy 1: Redefine the role of facilities, especially hospitals, within a vertically integrated network

To ensure coordination and continuity, vertical integration requires cooperation among health facilities at different levels of the health care system, many of which may not have traditionally collaborated. It is necessary to define the roles of facilities so that they function within a robust vertically integrated network; to determine what range of services specific health facilities will provide; and to decide how higher-level facilities will support lower-level facilities through supervision, technical assistance, and partnership.

Internationally, the role of hospitals is changing. They are no longer stand-alone facilities at the center of the delivery system, nor are they the point of entry to care or "one-stop shops" for all services. Rather, they are becoming a part of networks of facilities that include other providers such as primary care facilities, diagnostic units, and social services (Porignon and others 2011). Within these networks, hospitals can become centers of excellence—concentrating

technology and expertise, focusing highly complex care, and providing valuable rescue services for life-threatening conditions. They can also share their personnel to provide technical assistance and training to facilities at lower levels of the system.

In China, the recent policy reform plans and policy directives of the central government emphasize the integration of health care across a tiered delivery system, with close collaboration between hospitals and primary care providers (State Council 2012, 2015).[5] Integrating county hospitals, township health centers (THCs), CHCs, and village clinics is not a particularly new concept in China but is one that continues to be difficult to implement. As in other reforms, the government aims to draw lessons from pilots. Several mostly hospital-led, small-scale initiatives seek to coordinate care or at least link hospitals with other providers. Most of these initiatives are linked to other reforms, with the integration of care being one of multiple goals for improving service delivery.

The experience of six of the Chinese initiatives highlights some of the issues associated with greater hospital integration into the delivery system. (For details of these initiatives, see annex 2C.) Except for Xi County's Integrated Care delivery model in Henan Province, the initiatives took place in large cities and involved tertiary hospitals, usually as the lead facility. Four were managed by hospital management groups or councils (HMCs),[6] one by a county health bureau, and another by a lead hospital.

Though their objectives were varied, all six initiatives sought to improve the capacity of affiliated primary care providers: that is, CHCs in urban areas and THCs in rural areas. They used rotating specialists who provided training and technical support; they improved referral systems; and they established a "green channel" to facilitate upward referrals from affiliated lower-level facilities. Only a few of the initiatives also designed payment systems to incentivize the coordination of care. Two initiatives—the Shanghai Rujin-Luwan Group and the Zhenjiang

Kangfu Hospital Group—each horizontally integrated a subset of diagnostic services in a single location. Both involved some degree of e-health innovation, such as introducing electronic consultations among providers for diagnostics and teleconferencing for training and clinical guidance (Jian and Yip 2015; Li and Jiang 2015; Ma 2015b). Programs in Xi County and Hangzhou established e-consultations so that patients attending primary care facilities could interact with hospital specialists (Ali and Li 2015a; Yan 2015a), while their provinces (Henan and Zhenjiang, respectively) implemented electronic record systems that their affiliated providers could access.

Often, integration can force health facilities into new roles that they find unfamiliar and uncomfortable. In these circumstances, clarifying roles from the outside can provide needed direction and guidance. A prime example of this is the Xi County case. In June 2014, four of the county's hospitals and 19 of its THCs were contracting with each other for inpatient care. The county established these contracts and clearly laid out roles and responsibilities for each level of facility. By linking payment and reimbursement to performance, the authorities incentivized the facilities to fulfill their responsibilities.

Findings from these case studies show some good results. Zhenjiang reports improvements in the number of patients under management for NCDs, while Xi County reports a significant increase in follow-up care of hypertensive patients, as well as in flows of two-way referrals. Further, the Zhenjiang Kangfu Hospital Group established multidisciplinary family health teams consisting of personnel from hospitals, CHCs, and public health teams to support integrated management of NCDs and maternal and child care. The same program established rehabilitation wards in four community health centers for patients who were discharged from geriatric and neurology departments and also implemented a payment system to incentivize chronic-care management in CHCs.

At the same time, challenges remain. Key features of integrated systems—gatekeeping, use of multidisciplinary teams, use of individual care plans coordinated by primary care facilities, patient tracking, and postdischarge care—and the associated policy measures still need to be improved and implemented. In Xi County, the flow of upward referrals continues to dwarf that of downward referrals, and the "green channel" (upward referral) admissions represent only a fraction of total admissions to hospitals.[7] Care shifting from hospitals to lower levels has also not been fully achieved.

Strategy 2: Establish provider-to-provider relationships through technical assistance and skill building

Links between providers across the vertical levels of care can be established and strengthened through hospitals helping to improve quality and competency at the lower levels of care facilities. Most of the Chinese initiatives used technical assistance provided by hospitals to primary health care facilities to establish the interfacility relationships and communication required for effective vertical integration.

Two such examples are Feixi County's Strengthening Primary Health Care Capacity (SPHCC) and Huangzhong County's health care alliance (HCA) initiatives, both of which established technical assistance programs between village clinics, THCs, and county hospitals (Meng, Luyu, and others 2015; Meng, Yinzi, and others 2015). The upper-level facilities were responsible for providing clinical technical assistance through training, education, and joint consultations to physicians in lower-level facilities. This interaction strengthened coordination between the levels and was further supported by an e-health system that allowed health facilities to communicate with one another.

In Hangzhou, the TFY health care reform created 46 "joint centers" in communities (Yan 2015a). The joint centers were staffed by hospital specialists (from four municipal hospitals) and primary care physicians to manage patients with diabetes and hypertension.

Features included tracking and coordinating care across the delivery chain, using integrated care pathways, crafting individual care plans for patients, and fostering the active involvement of hospital specialists in the postdischarge care delivered in CHCs. The joint centers also established a peer-to-peer mentoring program that paired CHC physicians with hospital endocrinologists and cardiologists to improve the CHCs' management of chronic diseases.

Zhenjiang's Great Health initiative required hospital specialists to work at least five half-days per week at community health centers to provide outpatient services, inpatient rounds, case discussion, and lectures (Yan 2015b). The CHCs also provided training opportunities for their employees at the core hospital. For example, the Liming Community Health Center in the Rehabilitation Health Care Group sent one doctor per year for training at the neurology department in the First People's Hospital. Further, three or four specialists in traditional Chinese medicine, internal medicine, and pediatrics were placed in CHCs for a year to provide intensive training for staff there. Unique to Zhenjiang's Great Health initiative, the integrated health care groups addressed multisite licensed physicians and could effectively use them and their skills when it came to providing technical assistance. Zhenjiang also created a special fund for downward mobilization of resources, such as for technical assistance; from this fund the government reimburses a tertiary hospital RMB 80,000 for each specialist that it sends to support a CHC.

In Shanghai, the Ruijin-Luwan Hospital Group implemented a "specialist–general practitioner joint outpatient" service in CHCs and then developed a training plan for primary health care providers in these centers (Jian and Yip 2015; Ma 2015b). The training covered basic theories of general practice; basic knowledge of internal medicine, surgery, and diagnosis; treatment of frequently occurring diseases; provision of people-centered community health services; computer skills; and community health service management.

Strategy 3: Develop formalized facility networks

In many health systems, vertical integration has been driven by the creation of provider networks. At their most developed, these networks offer a broad continuum of care across all possible service lines, connected seamlessly through e-health tools, and often take on financial risk for the health outcomes of the populations they serve. Looser, including "virtual," networks also exist for vertical integration. These virtual networks often form out of proximity or with the goal to negotiate favorable contracts with payers. Because they often lack strong governance structures and shared e-health tools, such as unified patient records, looser networks are often less successful at curbing costs while integrating care.

There are many ways in which China can create networks that achieve PCIC goals without fostering control by hospitals. In Xi County, the integration of care between the county hospital, THCs, and village clinics was one goal of an externally financed project that broadly aimed to improve the accessibility, affordability, and quality of rural health care. The Xi Integrated Care initiative created a more formalized network of health facilities that jointly cared for patients (Ali and Li 2015a). It also used a financial incentive scheme to reinforce the integration across facilities and encouraged providers to recognize the connectedness of their system.

The initiative greatly emphasized the importance of following guidelines for clinical and integrated care. These guidelines explicitly advised how and at what facility level to care for a patient with a given condition, and also specified the criteria for referrals and postdischarge care for more than 100 conditions at each provider level. Liaison officers were hired at the THCs to manage care coordination and referrals and to oversee the use of customized care plans for follow-up by village clinics. The project developed metrics to assess the application of the integrated pathways and introduced EHRs that were accessible countywide.

Service agreements among county hospitals, THCs, and village clinics reflected the above features. Although no penalties were imposed for noncompliance with the service agreements, Xi County introduced a payment mechanism in which insurance payments for inpatient care were shared between the county hospital and the THCs, encouraging providers to shift care out of the hospital to ensure postdischarge care and hospital–THC coordination.

However, networks should not be solely operated by hospitals. In Singapore, the movement to integrate public health services, secondary hospital care, and contract with primary health care providers through regional health systems (RHSs) aimed to move away from the concept of the hospital as the anchor of the system. Instead, the Singapore RHSs aimed to center the system on the patient's needs (Teo 2015).

Hospital capture can occur when hospitals "capture" patients who could be treated in primary care and pull them up into the hospital system. To avoid hospital capture, the management of the RHS was separate from hospital management, and the chairperson of the private corporation that oversees all RHSs was a government-appointed employee. These actions signaled an important shift away from the hospital-centric model and toward a PCIC system.

Core Action Area 4: Horizontal Integration

Horizontal integration aims to provide more complete and comprehensive services— including promotional, preventive, curative, rehabilitative, and palliative care— coordinated by the providers at the frontline facility. Such service integration allows for more effective management of health care delivery and better-coordinated care within a cohesive health system centered on the needs of the patient rather than the convenience of the delivery system. Horizontal integration can also contribute to more efficient use of resources by reducing wasteful service duplication. Half of the 22 cases reported horizontally integrating care.

Strategy 1: Promote horizontal integration through service colocation
At the systems level, horizontal integration may take the form of colocation of services within a single facility. For example, the DMC initiative in Fosen, Norway, integrated public health, primary health care, and emergency care into one facility, thus allowing the population to access public health and primary care services—from vaccinations to emergency medical care—within one location (Forde, Auraasen, and Moreira 2015).

Hangzhou's TFY created joint centers for NCDs in CHCs. The centers integrated public health, specialty care, and primary care for NCDs, successfully transforming previously fragmented care delivery and making it easier for patients to receive a broader array of services within a single visit to a frontline facility (Yan 2015a).

Horizontal integration can also help to achieve greater economies of scale. The Zhenjiang Great Health initiative consolidated clinical diagnosis facilities and laboratories across hospitals and CHCs into single units, reducing service overlap and allowing for the more efficient use of resources (Yan 2015b).

Strategy 2: Provide integrated care around the individual user to promote more patient-centered care
Horizontal integration enables the provision of holistic and comprehensive care for the individual patient, bringing together preventive and curative treatments and looking beyond specific diseases to the person as a whole. At the patient level, a holistic approach to care goes beyond the traditionally defined medical components and addresses psychosocial and contextual contributors to disease. In the United States, for example, the Program of All-Inclusive Care for the Elderly (PACE) case study highlighted how the program sought to provide both comprehensive medical care and holistic care by integrating services across disciplines (Ali 2015). PACE achieved holistic care through home-based care services, meal delivery, intensive social work, and a nuanced understanding of frail

elders' challenges to maintaining their home-based independence.

As part of the primary health care initiative in Hangzhou's TFY implementation, contracts between physicians and area residents covered integrated home-based services, living support, and community day care or nursing centers for the elderly (Yan 2015a). The services were based on residents' needs and included medical care and social activities.

Feixi County's SPHCC initiative emphasized the importance of integrating holistic care into modern medical services and created a partnership between a traditional medicine center and a THC in Zipeng (Meng, Yinzi, and others 2015). As a result, the Zipeng branch of the Feixi Hospital of Traditional Chinese Medicine fully integrated health care organizations of varying levels and types, including both traditional and modern Chinese medicine. Because traditional Chinese medicine is important to many of the country's citizens, combining it with modern care better accounted for patients' desires and belief systems and encouraged their overall engagement in their treatment plans.

Core Action Area 5: Advanced ICT (e-Health)

Within an advancing technological environment, a robust e-health platform is the backbone of an interconnected health care system that puts patients at the center of their care (Bates and Bitton 2010). Use of information and communication technology (ICT) lays the foundation for successful communication between facilities and also provides health workers and patients with the opportunity to participate in the improved service process, care management, and decision making.

With ICT, patients have the tools to more fully engage with their care. Such an e-health platform can greatly enhance the functionality and effectiveness of a primary health care system by connecting providers to achieve horizontal and vertical integration, coordination, and continuity of information over time.

This coordination has been shown to result in more effective care and to decrease the unnecessary costs related to duplication of testing, inappropriate medication, and avoidable complications due to gaps in follow-up. Use of ICT also helps enable PCIC by facilitating new forms of interaction beyond short in-person visits—including, for instance, multifaceted shared EHRs with registries, telephone or web consultations, and online appointment scheduling systems.

The time, effort, and resources needed to achieve the putative savings from adopting e-health systems are substantial. E-health strategies were used by 21 (95 percent) of the 22 PCIC improvement initiatives, which clearly shows the importance and core function of the Core Action Area 5 strategies in strengthening the health service system. Three main e-health strategies emerged from the cases: applying EHRs, establishing electronic communication and management functions, and ensuring interoperability.

Strategy 1: Establish EHR systems that are accessible to providers and patients

At the center of an effective e-health system is the EHR, which has been shown to improve clinical decision support, registries, team care, care transitions, personal health records, telehealth technologies, and measurement (Bates and Bitton 2010). When these key factors function smoothly in a health care setting, both providers and patients experience a more coordinated care pathway. Providers across different levels can communicate in real time and easily access patients' current and updated health information in one place.

For example, Xi County's integrated care initiative implemented a new clinical management system using EHRs, including key information such as how the dual referral system operates (Ali and Li 2015a). This system links inpatient and outpatient care, enabling THCs to monitor the clinical services provided by village clinics. Physicians at the THCs could also view the outcome of follow-up appointments as well as the clinical pathways and the individualized care plans developed by the upper-level facility doctors. Xi's new system also captured patient referrals.

Hangzhou's TFY reform provided area residents with a citizen card and a database of "intelligent services" that held all patients' lifetime health information and allowed it to be shared between providers (Yan 2015a). The database housed information such as records of antenatal care and delivery, child care, health screenings, NCD management, diagnosis and treatment, hospitalization, and laboratory testing.

EHR systems that allow patients access to their own health records can also increase patients' empowerment and engagement in their care. For example, the U.S. VHA developed a patient portal called My HealtheVet to support patients' self-management of their health needs (Ali and Li 2015b). A patient portal is a website where patients can view their personal health record, refill prescriptions, view lab results, send secure messages to their physician, and review their physician's notes. The portal was reported to have been helpful in coordinating and integrating care for veterans. Recent studies show it has improved patients' experiences of care and connections with their personal health teams.

Strategy 2: Establish communication and care management functions

ICT can help expand access through online appointment scheduling, video conferencing, and mobile workstations; it can also help improve patient safety. Online appointment scheduling is one method to improve patient access to health services. Turkey's Health Transformation Plan created a central physician appointment system that schedules appointments for primary, secondary, and tertiary facilities over the telephone and online (Sumer 2015). This system allowed patients to request an appointment with a specific physician, at a specific office location, or in a specialty area and reduced the long waiting times at clinics.

In China, both Shanghai's FDS and Xi County's Integrated Care initiative aimed to

reach a younger generation by using WeChat, a Chinese messaging app. This proved to be a quick and easy way to get health information to patients, who could use it to check physician information, make appointments, and update their registration and payment forms.

Telemedicine and video conferencing played a particularly important role in Norway at the rural Fosen DMC. Video conferencing expanded access in two ways: (a) primary health care providers could consult with secondary and tertiary care providers, and (b) patients could see secondary care providers (Forde, Auraasen, and Moreira 2015). When the center was first established, six videoconference units were purchased and connected to the secondary hospital, St. Olav's (a three-hour drive from Fosen). The primary health care providers at the DMC all participated in a daily morning video meeting with St. Olav's. In these meetings, physicians discussed current DMC patients and could seek consultations from specialists as needed. As providers became comfortable with the video conferencing software and developed relationships with each other, they expanded the videoconferences to include patient consultations. This capability was used especially during night visits to the acute care center.

The primary care providers' workstations in Huangzhong's health care alliance provide another example of how to expand access to quality care through e-health. These mobile workstations, which were piloted in 2013 in 30 districts, could be carried by village doctors to more-remote locations (Meng, Luyu, and others 2015). Doctors could use them to conduct a number of medical exams (including elderly checkups and health assessments, hypertension management, diabetes management, electrocardiogram monitoring, and pulse oximetry testing) and to upload data and results to the system's health information services. The workstations gave clinicians better mobility when it came to follow-up care, and local residents trusted the results of the high-tech device more than the unaided diagnoses made by the village doctors.

The use of e-health tools has effectively improved patient safety. For example, Feixi County's SPHCC initiative used ICT to reduce overprescription and to promote more accurate and careful administration of medications to patients in THCs and village clinics (Meng, Yinzi, and others 2015). Medical information technology systems, using clinical decision-support tools, stored recommended lists of drugs for 50 outpatient diseases that were cared for in primary health care facilities. Once a diagnosis was put into the system, a set list of possible medications appeared, and the physician could only choose a drug from that list.

Similarly, in Xi County, the EHR system improved patient safety by linking the tiers of the health system, allowing clinical pathways to be put in place with guidelines about how to care for a patient with a particular illness (Ali and Li 2015a). If a physician deviated from the pathway, the change was recorded; approved deviations were monitored by a quality control officer, and any changes in care had to be made in consultation with the hospital unit director.

Strategy 3: Ensure interoperability of e-health tools across facilities and services
E-health tools carry great potential to improve the quality and safety of care, but they must be interoperable between facilities; that is, they must be capable of being accessed by different providers in different facilities. Where multiple e-health systems function, a major challenge exists in getting them to "talk to each other."

Interoperability (when the records can be lawfully used across institutions) needs to be built into an e-health system from the start. In Norway, Fosen's DMC achieved interoperability between its records and those of the secondary hospital with which it partnered (St. Olav's). Because the DMC was developed with this partnership in mind, it adopted the same EHR system as St. Olav's rather than create its own information system. Thus, the physicians at the DMC could view any patient record they needed at any time of day,

simultaneously with the providers at St. Olav's (Forde, Auraasen, and Moreira 2015).

Core Action Area 6: Integrated Clinical Pathways and Functional Dual Referral Systems

Integrated clinical pathways attempt to standardize the treatment and referral pathways that providers use in at least two levels of a health system to address particular conditions. They also clarify relationships and responsibilities between the different providers in the system. Because these pathways may finally lead to referrals to another level of care, they are most effective in the context of strong vertical integration. Dual referrals include referrals from primary to secondary care and also referrals back to primary from secondary care. Integrated pathways and strong dual referral systems are important to facilitate providing the right care at the right time.

Of the 22 case studies, 15 (68 percent) applied integrated care pathways, and 13 (59 percent) used dual referrals. Two main strategies were applied: (a) crafting integrated pathways to facilitate care integration and decision support for providers, and (b) promoting dual referrals within integrated facility networks.

Strategy 1: Craft integrated care pathways to facilitate care integration and decision support for providers
Clinical pathways help integrate care across providers and provide valuable decision support. As a part of the Canterbury Health Services Plan in New Zealand, clinicians developed a program called Health Pathways, which created 570 clinical pathways for referral (figure 2.4). The pathways made secondary-care referral decisions explicit to reduce variation in referral patterns and avoid unnecessary or duplicate referrals. Measures used to maximize their effectiveness included biannual reviews for quality by a group of clinicians; periodic clinical audits; and updating through a formal modification process.

FIGURE 2.4   Sample health pathway for COPD, Canterbury Health Services Plan, New Zealand

Assessment	Management	Request

• Make a diagnosis of COPD
  • Consider COPD in current and ex-smokers who are symptomatic
  • Consider COPD for any current or ex-smoker who had an emergency treatment for a respiratory condition
  • In patients who have never smoked, consider diagnosis other than COPD
  • Differentiate between asthma and COPD
• Arrange spirometry with bronchodilator
  • Mandatory for accurate diagnosis
  • Peak flow testing is inadequate
• Other investigations
  • Chest x-ray: only arrange if suspicious of other conditions
  • Blood tests: CBC and BMP if possible coexisting heart failure
  • Pulse oximetry: if < 92% on two occasions when resting, refer for arterial gas testing
• Look for comorbidities
• Determine COPD classification (A, B, C, or D)
	• Record confirmed case in Disease Register
	• Nonpharmacological interventions are as important as drug treatments for all patients with COPD, particularly
	  • Smoking cessation: This is the single most important intervention. Provide advice at every opportunity.
	  • Exercise: Encourage exercise and consider pulmonary rehabilitation for all, especially groups B and D, as it improves quality of life, reduces dyspnea, and improves exercise tolerance.
	  • Identification and management of commonly associated comorbidities: Patients in groups B and D have high rates of cardiovascular comorbidity.
	• Important interventions for all patients include
	  • Annual influenza immunization
	  • Advice on occupational factors
	  • Acute exacerbation management
	  • COPD action plan
	  • Adequate home heating or subsidy for heating
	• Consider other interventions, especially for group D patients
	• Specific management depends on the severity group
		• Request respiratory physician assessment if
		  • Diagnostic uncertainty
		  • Age > 40 years
		  • Severe disease group (group D) and age > 55 years
		  • Frequent exacerbations
		  • Difficult to control symptoms
		  • Uncommon sputum pathogens
		  • Sleep-disordered breathing
		  • Home oxygen required
		• If appropriate, consider community respiratory services
		• Your patient may also wish to consider private respiratory sociality assessment.

Source: Adapted from Love 2015.
Note: COPD = chronic obstructive pulmonary disease; CBC = complete blood count; BMP = basic metabolic panel.

Based on international best practices, the pathways were tailored to the needs and interests of the local population. Because of the high degree of clinical rigor used to develop and evaluate these pathways, physicians placed high trust in them and used them intensely: more than 80 percent of physicians viewed the Health Pathways website at least six times per week. Physicians reported feeling that their referral decisions were more rational and that care was more tailored to patient needs (Love 2015).

The health care initiative in Xi County also emphasized the importance of adhering to clinical pathways, which were established for 188 diseases in county hospitals and 104 diseases within THCs at an inpatient level

(Ali and Li 2015a). The pathways defined the scope of responsibility for hospitals and THCs, clarified when patients should be transferred to a THC for continued inpatient care, and provided guidelines for discharge and follow-up care at village clinics (figure 2.5).

All the county hospitals and THCs had full-time liaison officers who were responsible for soliciting feedback from patients and staff, coordinating dual referrals, making appointments, and transferring patient records when a referral was necessary. At the village clinic level, 21 disease-specific pathways were created and implemented to support decision making and strengthen a dual referral system between the clinics and THCs.

FIGURE 2.5 Sample responsibilities for dual referrals in Xi County

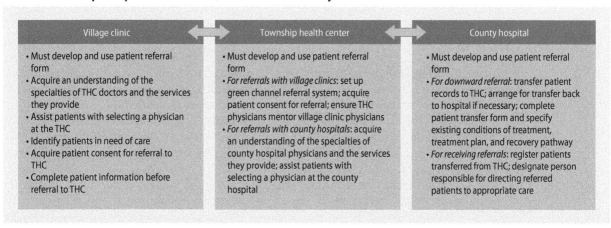

Village clinic	Township health center	County hospital
• Must develop and use patient referral form • Acquire an understanding of the specialties of THC doctors and the services they provide • Assist patients with selecting a physician at the THC • Identify patients in need of care • Acquire patient consent for referral to THC • Complete patient information before referral to THC	• Must develop and use patient referral form • *For referrals with village clinics*: set up green channel referral system; acquire patient consent for referral; ensure THC physicians mentor village clinic physicians • *For referrals with county hospitals*: acquire an understanding of the specialties of county hospital physicians and the services they provide; assist patients with selecting a physician at the county hospital	• Must develop and use patient referral form • *For downward referral*: transfer patient records to THC; arrange for transfer back to hospital if necessary; complete patient transfer form and specify existing conditions of treatment, treatment plan, and recovery pathway • *For receiving referrals*: register patients transferred from THC; designate person responsible for directing referred patients to appropriate care

Source: Ali and Li 2015a. ©World Bank. Permission required for reuse.
Note: THC = township health center.

Strategy 2: Promote dual referrals within integrated facility networks

All the Chinese PCIC initiatives that were studied employed upward referrals using the "green channel." As described in the case studies, patients who were referred upward through the green channel from participating facilities in their system were expected to receive expedited care at hospitals. In practice, however, green channels functioned irregularly. Downward referrals from hospitals to CHCs were rare, and some patients resisted them.

Notably, the dual referral system in Xi County's Integrated Care initiative was incentivized by cost sharing and reimbursement. Under this scheme, upper-level facilities were reimbursed for the entire cost of a referred case and shared the payment they received with the lower-level facility, depending on a previously determined price and the care workload. The reimbursement depended on whether the patient care pathway had been satisfactorily fulfilled in both health facilities (Ali and Li 2015a). This system encouraged hospitals to refer patients to lower-level health facilities to save costs and bed space.

Core Action Area 7: Measurement Standards and Feedback

Establishing a performance measurement system is critical to ensuring the quality and performance of a PCIC-based system. The performance measurement indicators need to reflect the national standards, which in turn should reflect the core functions and goals of the PCIC-based service delivery system, including coordination, comprehensiveness, integration, and technical and experiential quality. However, collecting only the indicator information would not improve the system's performance; formation of a feedback cycle is required to ensure that the performance results are communicated to stakeholders at all levels, ranging from the community and providers through to management and policy makers

Performance measurement can also identify early positive outliers that can teach others and point to effective intervention components for broader implementation. Of the 22 initiatives studied, 20 (91 percent) used measurement and evaluation to strengthen their performance.[8] Two common strategies for promoting measurement and feedback emerged: (a) development and use of standardized performance metrics; and (b) creation of feedback loops to drive continuous quality improvement.

Strategy 1: Use standardized indicators for performance measurement

Performance measurement should be standardized through the use of common, verifiable, and meaningful performance indicators. For example, the Gesundes Kinzigtal initiative in Germany used standardized reports based on a core set of measurement standards for care providers, the management team, and other stakeholders (Hildebrandt and others 2015; Nolte and others 2015). The measurement covered the system, technical quality, and service-experience quality (the patients' experiences), and it included the dimensions of structure, process, outcomes, quality, integration, patient experience, and efficiency. The use of performance measurement facilitated communication related to progress and enabled comparisons across facilities.

The outcomes and processes chosen for measurement should reflect the priorities of the system. The leaders and managers of the Huangzhong health care alliance developed a quality and safety evaluation system that could measure a set of core components broader than medical services, including management (financial management and village clinic management), disease and prevention control, patient satisfaction, and Chinese traditional medicine services (Meng, Luyu, and others 2015). The metrics used for primary health care reflected the priority goal of improvement within the primary health care workforce—focusing on provider availability, motivation, and performance; patient satisfaction; the number and quality (enthusiasm, skills, and ability) of the workforce; and some system measures, including indicators of coordination within the health service network.

Many OECD countries have established and implemented patient-reported outcome measures and patient-reported experience measures as part of their health system performance assessment systems (Klazinga 2014).

Strategy 2: Create continuous feedback loops linked to action plans to drive quality improvement

To drive improvement, standardized performance measures must be fed back to the appropriate stakeholders so that results can be used to improve quality. A commitment to identifying, learning from, celebrating, and spreading identified effective practices is important at all levels of the system. These processes will accelerate change, motivate providers and managers, and further increase the value and use of performance-measurement data.

Measurement information needs to be communicated to all levels of the PCIC system—starting with patients and communities, who can become active partners in strengthening primary health care by publicly sharing data on facility performance and community health and by building their capacity to understand results and engage in improvement and advocacy. Such engagement allows communities and providers to hold health systems accountable for the quality, responsiveness, and outcomes of the care provided. Care teams and managers at the facility and subnational level are other vital users of measurement information. They may need support and encouragement to use feedback to understand and improve their performance within the context of the facility, network, and broader care system.

To transform performance data into action and improvement requires regular feedback loops that enable the identification of gaps in services and that drive and support continuous learning and correction. A strong focus on feedback, linked to action at all levels of the system, is critical. To ensure ongoing learning requires a resilient system with the following main elements: performance measurement, feedback and review of the data, identification of gaps, and design and implementation of interventions. Each of these elements needs to be underpinned by support and training of staff in improvement methods. The cycle continues with remeasurement to assess whether gaps have been closed and whether new gaps have been identified.

For example, the PACE case outlines how the program's charter provided for continual feedback (figure 2.6) through a Quality Assessment and Performance Improvement program that is data-driven, community-led, and iterative (Ali 2015). Providers received the performance measurement results regularly so they could review their personal performance and identify problem areas across the practice. Many PACE centers instituted monthly, biweekly, or even daily feedback processes, combining required, optional, and facility-initiated performance measurement.

All PACE centers followed the Health Plan Management System of the Centers for Medicare and Medicaid Services (CMS) and were required to report basic information on core performance measures every quarter to CMS (figure 2.7). Following a recommendation by the National PACE Association, individual institutions within PACE have recognized the value in continual quality improvement efforts and have begun collecting additional measures focused on local priorities.

In Feixi's SPHCC initiative, the county's THCs used a nine-dimensional evaluation tool to measure and improve their performance (Meng, Yinzi, and others 2015). This tool was used twice per year and became a basis for budget allocation and performance-based financing. THC directors' salaries were tied to evaluation results; negative reviews resulted in penalties for the directors and also affected governmental funding. Some health facilities found evaluation to be helpful because it pushed them to provide high-quality care, and top-performing facilities received praise and recognition from the government.

Core Action Area 8: Accreditation and Certification

Accreditation is a formal process by which an independent body conducts an external assessment of a health care organization's performance in relation to previously defined metrics and published standards. At its core, accreditation is a defined mechanism for externally assuring accountability for minimal standards to be met across the

FIGURE 2.6   **PACE continual feedback loop**

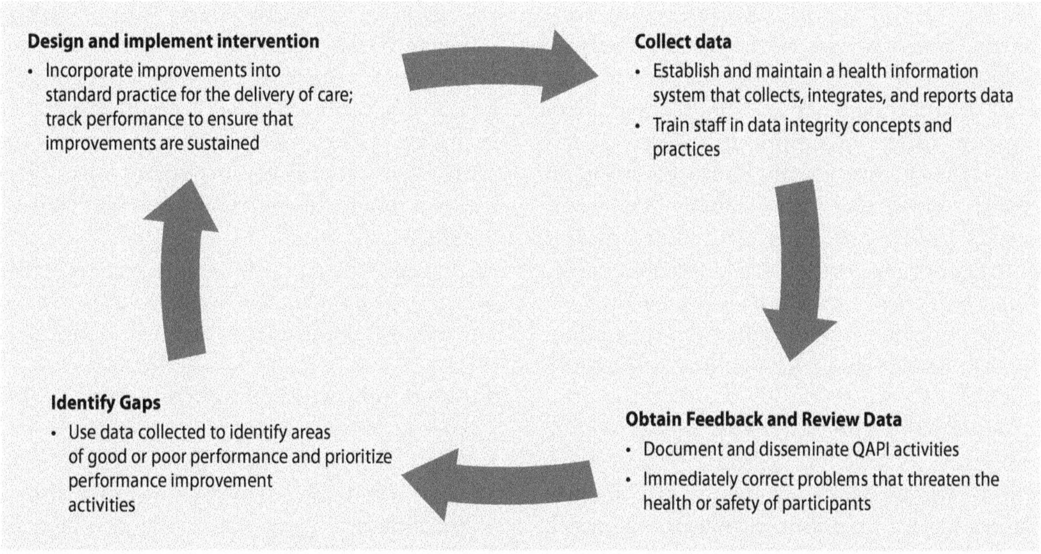

Design and implement intervention
- Incorporate improvements into standard practice for the delivery of care; track performance to ensure that improvements are sustained

Collect data
- Establish and maintain a health information system that collects, integrates, and reports data
- Train staff in data integrity concepts and practices

Identify Gaps
- Use data collected to identify areas of good or poor performance and prioritize performance improvement activities

Obtain Feedback and Review Data
- Document and disseminate QAPI activities
- Immediately correct problems that threaten the health or safety of participants

Source: Ali 2015. ©World Bank. Permission required for reuse.
Note: PACE = Program of All-Inclusive Care for the Elderly; QAPI = Quality Assessment and Performance Improvement.

FIGURE 2.7   **Types of data collected by PACE centers**

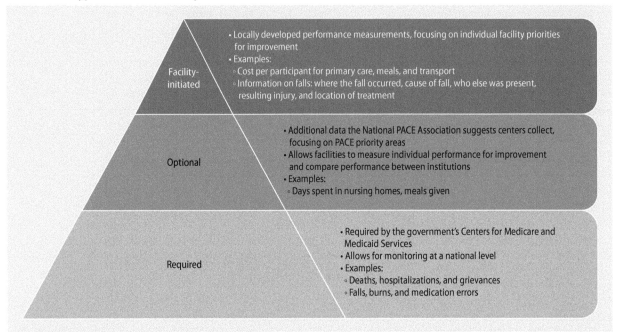

Source: Ali 2015. ©World Bank. Permission required for reuse.
Note: PACE = Program of All-Inclusive Care for the Elderly.

health care delivery system. Accreditation differs from licensure, which is generally considered a government regulatory responsibility and is designed to set minimum standards to protect public health and safety. Accreditation sets standards that are considered optimal and achievable but are more rigorous than the minimum standards used for licensure, and it has the stated intent to foster a culture of improvement (Mate and others 2014). The terms accreditation and certification are often used interchangeably, but accreditation usually applies only to organizations, while certification may apply to individuals as well (Salmon and others 2003).

In 2005, the Chinese government reformed its hospital accreditation system, moving away from a focus on infrastructure and equipment and toward a broader range of criteria including scientific management, patient safety, and service quality.

Although the changes are in the right direction, the guidelines leave considerable discretion to local government in operationalizing and implementing the system (Wagstaff and others 2009). As a result, the accreditation process does not cover many key health care delivery organizations, including THCs, village clinics, and private sector health delivery organizations. This limits comparability of performance across localities.

A recent review of 44 health care accreditation programs in 38 countries reported six key features (Braithwaite and others 2012):

• Development or adoption of a set of health care standards
• Enrollment of members who assess their own performance against those standards
• Recruitment, education, and management of a workforce of industry surveyors

- Deployment of teams of surveyors to health care organizations to assess progress against the standards
- Evaluation of survey teams' reports
- Award of accreditation status (if eligible) for a period of three to five years.

External organizational and clinical certification (or accreditation) standards are critical to ensuring high-quality, reliable, and safe care organizations (Greenfield and others 2012). However, accreditation featured in only 5 of the 22 PCIC performance improvement initiatives studied for this report. Their strategies to launch accreditation include developing criteria and setting targets.

Strategy 1: Develop certification criteria that are nationally and locally relevant

Criteria for accrediting primary care facilities need to reflect the priorities and structure of a PCIC-based delivery system. They should define model standards in areas ranging from infrastructure (resources, information technology, and human resources); systems organization (integration and hospital and primary health care roles); and care delivery characteristics (people-centeredness, comprehensiveness, continuity, and coordination) to facilitate desired health outcomes.

For example, for a facility to be recognized as a PCMH—a form of PCIC facility recently launched in the United States—it must meet the following criteria established by the National Committee for Quality Assurance (NCQA): team-based care, care coordination, patient self-management, enhanced access and continuity, care management, and quality improvement. Performance metrics based on these standards can be used to assess the quality of care being provided and to compare performance across providers and facilities in a standardized way.

Looking ahead, China may wish to draw on a wide array of easily available and scientifically proven protocols and guidelines for care that are available on websites sponsored by the NCQA and other organizations. When setting criteria, it will be important to consider the reporting burden and to streamline the number of measures adopted. For example, the Aarogyasri Health Care Trust, which insures more than 65 million people in the Indian state of Andhra Pradesh, recently began identifying standards that will be required of all hospitals that are empaneled to provide care to the Trust's beneficiaries. The Trust is working closely with India's National Accreditation Board of Hospitals, as well as with insurers from several states, to develop a shared set of standards that will encourage other hospitals to also achieve accreditation and thus improve their quality of care (Smits, Supachutikul, and Mate 2014).

Strategy 2: Set targets and use them to accredit facilities

Once the accreditation criteria have been developed, the next steps are to set targets and apply the criteria through a transparent and reliable mechanism. Under the VHA's PACT model (Ali and Li 2015a), a primary health care facility must meet certain criteria to be recognized as a PCMH by the NCQA. The NCQA uses a point-based system with three levels of classification, and it also requires a facility to score higher than 50 percent on each of six "must-pass" elements to receive accreditation (table 2.3). Many primary care facilities publicize their attainment of these recognition levels to attract patients (Bitton, Martin, and Landon 2010).

New accreditation programs benefit from setting relatively achievable standards based on the current status of local health care facilities and making a commitment to upgrade their standards over time. Malaysia and Thailand have each adopted this approach. Malaysia has issued four versions of its hospital standards since starting its accreditation program in 1999. Thailand's progressive changes include introducing a stepwise recognition program in 2004, followed by patient safety goals in 2006 (Smits, Supachutikul, and Mate 2014).

TABLE 2.3 NCQA certification guidelines for patient-centered medical homes

Standards	Elements	Possible points
Patient-centered access	Patient-centered appointment access	4.5
	24/7 access to clinical advice	3.5
	Electronic access	2.0
	Total	10.0
Team-based care	Continuity	3.0
	Medical home responsibilities	2.5
	Culturally and linguistically appropriate services	2.5
	Practice team	4.0
	Total	12.0
Population health management	Patient information	3.0
	Clinical data	4.0
	Comprehensive health assessment	4.0
	Use data for population management	5.0
	Implement evidence-based decision support	4.0
	Total	20.0
Care management and support	Identify patients for care management	4.0
	Care planning and self-care support	4.0
	Medication management	4.0
	Use electronic prescribing	3.0
	Support self-care and shared decision making	5.0
	Total	20.0
Care coordination and care transitions	Test tracking and follow-up	6.0
	Referral tracking and follow-up	6.0
	Coordinate care transitions	6.0
	Total	18.0
Performance measurement and quality improvement	Measure clinical quality performance	3.0
	Measure resource use and care coordination	3.0
	Measure patient and family experience	4.0
	Implement continuous quality improvement	4.0
	Demonstrate continuous quality improvement	3.0
	Report performance	3.0
	Use certified e-health record system technology	Not scored
	Total	20.0
	Overall total	100.0

Source: NCQA 2014.
Note: NCQA = National Committee for Quality Assurance. Patient-centered medical homes are a primary care model for providing comprehensive, coordinated care across all elements of the broader health care system in ways centered on individual patients' needs, accessibility of services, high quality of care, safety, and accountability ("Defining the PCMH," Patient Centered Medical Home Resource Center, U.S. Department of Health and Human Services [accessed June 13, 2018], https://pcmh.ahrq.gov/page/defining-pcmh).

Moving Forward on the PCIC Core Action Areas

China has already begun reforms in some of the eight core action areas for achieving PCIC, including introducing nearly universal health insurance coverage, reducing markups on sales of medication, and strengthening inputs, including health facility infrastructure and training of health care workers. Although recent reforms have led to improvements, developing a high-quality PCIC system that can rein in costs, increase value for money, and improve population health outcomes will require further reforms.

These reforms must be shaped by current circumstances and by lessons from improvement initiatives in China and in other countries. It is not feasible to address all eight action areas at the same time, and within each action area, strategies will need to be prioritized. Thus, it will be crucial for Chinese authorities to develop clear implementation guides or toolkits on what to implement and how, with indications on where and how local adaptations are needed. These guidelines will need to be supported with measurement and feedback systems to monitor the implementation of improvement efforts and troubleshoot problems as needed.[9]

China will also need to address provider payment mechanisms and ensure they are aligned with and actively support the chosen improvement interventions for PCIC. Achieving integration will require joint accountability for costs and quality through networks of care, strong dual referrals, and a health information system that helps patients receive coordinated care across providers and facilities.

Effective use of ICT to create e-health systems has been a key to success in almost all the cases studied. These e-health systems are structured and implemented in varying ways, but at their core is an EHR that is accessible across providers, and by patients, in a given region or locality. China needs to implement e-health systems that not only facilitate and document interactions between providers and patients, but also serve as coordination mechanisms for dual referrals and promote comprehensive, team-based care. Importantly, e-health systems must allow providers and facilities at different levels of the network to communicate with each other so that patients' care can be transferred seamlessly across them. In addition, an effective e-health system that can detect patients who need more-intensive services (for example, patients with recurrent hospitalizations, poor control of NCDs, or frequent primary health clinic visits) will be needed, while to respond effectively to the needs of these patients will require individualized care plans and multidisciplinary teams.

The case studies highlight the role played by stable and consistent management. Attention to building the necessary skills and capacities within a cadre able to support the goals of the improvement is essential. Important management functions will be to support performance measurement to identify gaps, drive improvement through supportive supervision, and ensure accountability. One-third of the case studies noted that flexibility and "opportunistic" implementation were major factors in success. Allowing the managers of facilities some degree of autonomy to address unexpected challenges and local opportunities for innovation—and encouraging them to share the lessons they have learned—will be important, regardless of the pathway taken.

Finally, effective measurement and feedback loops need to be designed and implemented to monitor and strengthen initiatives as they are started and scaled up. And meaningful patient engagement will be crucial throughout the change process.

Annex 2A   Summary of PCIC Impact Findings by Case Studies

TABLE 2A.1   Impact frequency of studies on PCIC initiatives, by PCIC model and impact area
Number of studies

Model	Impact	Hospitalizations and ED use	Processes of care	Intermediate health outcomes and mortality	Patient experience	Costs	Citations
General PCIC (52 studies)	Improvement	17	7	21	9	22	Guanais and Macinko (2009); Hildebrandt and others (2015); Macinko and others (2011); Nolte and Pitchforth (2014); RAND (2012); Schulte and others (2014); World Bank (2015)
	No change or worsened	5	4	10	1	2	
	Insufficient or inconclusive evidence, or not measured	30	41	21	42	28	
PCMH (14 studies)	Improvement	12	7	4	2	6	Bitton (2015); DeVries and others (2012); Fifield and others (2013); Friedberg and others (2014); Friedberg and others (2015); Gilfillan, Tomcavage, and Rosenthal (2010); Hebert and others (2014); Nelson and others (2014); Reid and others (2010); Reid and others (2013); Rosenthal and others (2013); van Hasselt and others (2015); Wang and others (2014); Werner and others (2014); World Bank (2015)
	No change or worsened	2	1	1	0	2	
	Insufficient or inconclusive evidence, or not measured	0	6	9	12		
PACE (16 studies)	Improvement	9	0	7	1	0	Beauchamp and others (2008); Chatterji and others (1998); DHCFP (2005); Kane, Homyak, and Bershadsky (2002); Kane and others (2006a, 2006b); Mancuso, Yamashiro, and Felver (2005); Meret-Hanke (2011); Mukamel, Bajorska, and Temkin-Greener (2002); Mukamel and others (2006); Mukamel and others (2007); Mukamel, Temkin-Greener, and Clark (1998); Temkin-Greener, Bajorska, and Mukamel (2008); Weaver and others (2008); Wieland and others (2000); Wieland and others (2010)
	No change or worsened	1	0	1	3	0	
	Insufficient or inconclusive evidence, or not measured	6	16	8	12	16	
Disease or case management (257 studies)	Improvement	82	22	64	28	34	Elissen and others (2012); Elissen and others (2015); Frølich, Jacobsen, and Knai (2015); Nolte and Pitchforth (2014); Runz-Jørgensen and Frølich (2015); Struijs, de Jong-van Til, and others (2012); Struijs, Mohnen, and others 2012); Vadstrup and others (2011)
	No change or worsened	29	6	25	8	37	
	Insufficient or inconclusive evidence	17	0	14	10	9	
	Not measured	129	229	154	211	178	
China (6 studies)	Improvement	1	6	1	1	2	World Bank (2015)
	No change or worsened	0	0	0	0	0	
	Insufficient or inconclusive evidence	5	0	5	5	4	

Note: ED = emergency department; PACE = Program of All-Inclusive Care for the Elderly; PCIC = patient-centered integrated care; PCMH = patient centered medical home.

Annex 2B   Methodology and Summaries of 22 PCIC Performance Improvement Initiatives Described in the Case Studies

Case study research consisted of three stages:

1. In the first stage, each author completed a rapid mapping of the county or country's performance improvement initiative, the progress to date, and important contextual factors (policy, institutional, and financial environments).
2. In the second stage, the details of the initiative were further analyzed, focusing on key components of PCIC, implementation readiness, implementation strategies, and initial and intermediate outcomes of the initiative.
3. The third stage examined critical contextual factors influencing the initiative design, implementation approach, and successes and challenges. Researchers used a mixed-methods approach that consisted of both quantitative secondary research and qualitative work, including focus group discussions and key-informant interviews.

Because no applicable tool was identified from the existing literature, the authors developed a tool designed to capture the following information from the case studies:

- Challenges prompting the design and implementation of the PCIC performance improvement initiative
- Core initiative elements
- Strategies for initiative implementation
- Facilitators and barriers to implementation
- Lessons learned
- Adaptability of the initiative to the Chinese health care system
- Potential sustainability.

TABLE 2B.1   Nomenclature and summaries of 22 PCIC performance improvement initiatives

PCIC performance improvement initiative	Description	Citations
Chinese case studies		
Zhenjiang, Jiangsu province: Great Health	Zhenjiang city, on the Yangtze River in eastern China, implemented the Great Health initiative in 2011 to service its two main districts. Through this initiative, two health care groups, Rehabilitation Health Care Group and Jiangbin Health Care Group, were created that focused on vertical and horizontal integration with new "3+X" family health teams managing the care of all contracted residents.	Yan (2015b)
Shanghai: Family Doctor System	Huangpu and Pudong, two neighboring districts within coastal Shanghai, China, implemented the family doctor system (FDS) in April 2011. This case study focused on five community health centers within these districts. The FDS centered on strengthening the relationship between the general practitioner and contracted resident by using empanelment and improved frontline service delivery to establish a continuous health care relationship with a particular focus on the management of chronic diseases.	Ma (2015a)
Huangzhong, Qinghai province: Health Care Alliance	In northwest China, Huangzhong County implemented a health care alliance system in 2013 to vertically integrate county, township, and village health centers. By focusing on the creation of a unified administration, the integration of human resources, a tight dual referral arrangement, the interconnection of health information systems, and shared medical resources, an integrated "county-township-village" health system emerged.	Meng, Luyu, and others (2015)
Hangzhou, Zhejiang province: Twelfth Five-Year Plan	Hangzhou, capital of China's Zhejiang province, is home to more than 8 million individuals and has traditionally struggled to provide equal and sufficient health care to its citizens. To curb such obstacles, the Twelfth Five-Year Plan was implemented in 2011, and key aspects included integrated e-consultation services, noncommunicable disease joint centers, and collaborative services for medical and living support and nursing care.	Yan (2015a)

(Table continued next page)

TABLE 2B.1 Nomenclature and summaries of 22 PCIC performance improvement initiatives *Continued*

PCIC performance improvement initiative	Description	Citations
Feixi, Anhui province: Strengthening Primary Health Care Capacity	Feixi County, of Anhui province in eastern China, has a population of roughly 850,000 citizens. In 2009, Feixi became the pilot site for the government's Strengthening Primary Health Care Capacity initiative, which focused on strengthening four sectors: human resources, network building, organization and management, and working conditions.	Meng, Yinzi, and others (2015)
Xi, Henan province: Integrated Care Reform	In Xi County, China, the integrated care (IC) reform in 2012 addressed the low quality of care for noncommunicable diseases and disjointed health systems by implementing contracts between county hospitals, township health centers, and village clinics. The initiative focused on building a strong referral mechanism, providing technical assistance to lower-level facilities, and altering the payment system to support cost sharing, all of which have had considerable success, even in their early stages.	Ali and Li (2015a)
Beijing: Beijing Chaoyang Hospital Alliance (four cases)	The Beijing Chaoyang Hospital Alliance (CHA), started in late 2012, aimed to attract patients to use community health centers more frequently for minor ailments and to strengthen the collaboration between upper- and lower-level facilities. The CHA comprised a core hospital, a second tertiary hospital, a secondary hospital, and a number of community health centers, which coordinated care for patients. As a result of this structure, the growth rate of participating facilities rose from 2012 to 2013.	Jian and Yip (2015)
Beijing: Peking University-Renmin Hospital Integrated Delivery System (four cases)	Started in 2007, the Peking University (PKU)–Renmin Hospital Integrated Delivery System (IDS) in Beijing increased technical assistance between health facilities and improved communication between providers through an information technology system. Through this system, providers were able to engage in telediscussions and specialist education and training, thus supplementing available continuing education for all providers in the IDS.	Jian and Yip (2015)
Shanghai: Shanghai Ruijin-Luwan Hospital Group (RLG) (four cases)	In 2011, the Shanghai Ruijin-Luwan Group was established, consisting of Shanghai Jiaotong University as the core hospital, two secondary hospitals, and four community health centers, which serviced people in the immediate area. This health care group created a shared imaging and testing center that increased access for residents, provided "specialist–general practitioner joint outpatient" visits for patients in community health centers, and strengthened its previously existing primary care provider training base.	Jian and Yip (2015); Ma (2015b)
Zhenjiang, Jiangsu province: Jiangsu Zhenjiang Kangfu Hospital Group (ZKG) (four cases)	The Jiangsu Zhenjiang Kangfu Hospital Group began in late 2009 in Zhenjiang, China. This initiative integrated imaging, chemical laboratory, and pathology test departments and required primary health care facilities to take more responsibility for chronic-disease outpatient services. Additionally, the hospital group established "3+X" health teams and supported more frequent information exchange.	Li and Jiang (2015)
International case studies		
Denmark: Integrated Effort for People Living with Chronic Diseases (SIKS)	Denmark piloted its chronic disease rehabilitation programs in Copenhagen with four centers, called SIKS rehabilitation centers. Owing to the success of the centers, Denmark embarked on a national disease management program, which provides integrated comprehensive chronic disease care.	Nolte and others (2015); Runz-Jørgensen and Frølich (2015)
England, U.K.: James Cook University Hospital Ambulatory Emergency Care	The James Cook University Hospital (JCUH) is in northern England, where hospitals are public but semiautonomous. In the early 2000s, JCUH developed an Ambulatory Emergency Care Center where patients could receive same-day care using predetermined clinical guidelines for certain conditions instead of being hospitalized. Simultaneously, it developed patient care pathways and explicitly strengthened the interface between primary care physicians and the hospital.	Forde, Auraasen, and Moreira (2015)
Kinzigtal, Germany: Gesundes Kinzigtal (GK)	Gesundes Kinzigtal, a health care management company in the Black Forest area of Germany, launched in 2005 a unification of a nonprofit, physician-run organization (MQNK) and a health-science management and investment company (OptiMedis). The integrated organizational model focused on improving the health of the population as well as patient experience while considering a fair business plan that appropriately incentivized patients and providers to join.	Hildebrandt and others (2015); Nolte and others (2015)

(Table continued next page)

TABLE 2B.1 Nomenclature and summaries of 22 PCIC performance improvement initiatives *Continued*

PCIC performance improvement initiative	Description	Citations
Netherlands: Maastricht Diabetes Care (DTC) (In-text reference: Netherlands, DTC)	The Maastricht region in the south of the Netherlands developed an integrated framework for diabetes care whereby the insurers negotiate with the primary care physicians a price for a complete package of care for a specific disease. Based on the care package's success, the Netherlands expanded this program nationwide in 2010.	Vrijhoef and Schulpen (2015); Nolte and others (2015)
Canterbury, New Zealand: Health Services Plan	Canterbury, a district in central New Zealand, developed its Health Services Plan in 2007. The plan included initiatives like the Acute Demand Management Services, Health Pathways standardization of care for hundreds of conditions, and the Community Rehabilitation and Enablement Support Team. Concurrent enabling initiatives, including an electronic medical record system, an electronic referral system, clinical continuing education programs, and a formal alliance between health care facilities, supported the mission of developing people-centered, coordinated, and integrated health care.	Love (2015)
Fosen, Norway: District Medical Center	Fosen, Norway, a municipality in the fjords of northern Norway, developed a comprehensive district medical center (DMC) model. The Fosen DMC provides integrated, coordinated acute medical care to people in the community to help them avoid hospital stays. In 2012, Norway modeled its national health care initiative on Fosen's successful DMC model.	Forde, Auraasen, and Moreira (2015)
Portugal: Local Health Unit	In 1999, a small province in northwest Portugal created a local health unit (unidad de saúde local, or ULS) that provides integrated primary and secondary care to a defined geographic area (Matosinhos) with centralized management and coordinated services. Starting in 2007, seven more ULSs have been established and now serve 10 percent of the Portuguese population.	Forde, Auraasen, and Moreira (2015)
Singapore: Regional Health Systems	Singapore reorganized its health care system by developing six regional health systems (RHSs), which aim to provide horizontally and vertically integrated health care ecosystems. Each RHS developed interventions to provide integrated coordinated care. Examples of these interventions include Aged Care Transition, Aging in Place, Post-Acute Care at Home, Community Health Assist Schemes, Family Medicine Centers, and Integrated Care Pathways.	Teo (2015)
Turkey: Health Transformation Plan	Turkey's 2003 national Health Transformation Plan focused on the establishment of high-quality family medicine centers accountable for individual and population health in every district of the country. Restructuring of hospitals, physician payment, data management, and national health insurance facilitated this transformation.	Sumer (2015)
Maryland, United States: CareFirst Patient-Centered Medical Home	This case study describes the patient centered medical home payment model created by the health insurance company CareFirst of Maryland. Support from the insurance company and a new financial incentive structure supported improvement of frontline delivery services across the state, resulting in improved quality and lower utilization of hospital and specialty care services.	Murray (2015)
United States: Program of All-Inclusive Care for the Elderly (PACE)	PACE centers across the country provide coordinated, integrated, holistic care for frail, nursing-home-eligible patients in their own homes. Funded by capitation payments from Medicare and Medicaid, each PACE center cares for around 300 patients. The PACE model originated in California and has now spread to 30 states in the United States.	Ali (2015)
Veterans Health Administration, United States: Patient Aligned Care Teams	Across the United States, the patient-centered medical home (PCMH) model has been used to integrate and improve primary care. The Veterans Health Administration (VHA) drew on the PCMH model and created the Patient Aligned Care Team (PACT) model to reorganize the way it provides primary care and to be integrated into the rest of the system. VHA primary care is now based entirely on the PACT model, with early evidence of success.	Ali and Li (2015b)

Note: PCIC = patient-centered integrated care.

Annex 2C   Characteristics of Care Integration Initiatives Involving Hospitals

TABLE 2C.1   **Characteristics of six health care integration initiatives at Chinese hospitals**

Characteristic type	Beijing: Chaoyang Hospital Alliance	Beijing: Renmin Hospital Integrated Care Delivery System	Shanghai: Ruijin-Luwan Hospital Group	Zhenjiang: Kangfu Network	Hangzhou: NCD joint centers	Henan: Xi County Integrated Care
Basic features						
Administrative level	Municipal and district	Municipal but with significant national reach	Municipal and district	Mainly district	Municipal and district	County, township, and village
Initiation date	2012	2007	2011	2009	2013	2012
Participating facilities	Tertiary and secondary hospitals and CHCs	Mainly tertiary and secondary hospitals and CHCs	Tertiary and secondary hospitals and CHCs	Tertiary and secondary hospitals and CHCs	Tertiary hospitals and CHCs	County hospitals, THCs, and VCs
Lead facility	Tertiary hospital	Tertiary hospital	Tertiary hospital	Tertiary hospital	Tertiary hospital	County hospital
Lead organization to oversee and manage coordination	Hospital alliance "council"	Lead hospital	Hospital Group Council	Hospital management council	Informal municipal "leading team"	County health bureau
Payment system to support care integration	Subsidy to hospital physicians to consult in CHCs	No	No	Payment to CHCs for NCD management	No	Yes
Main innovation	Formation of a "Hospital Alliance" to improve care at CHCs	Academic seminars, clinical research exchanges, and technical training (teleconferencing)	Horizontal integration of lab, imaging, and radiotherapy services	Rehabilitation and recovery wards in CHCs; horizontal integration of lab, imaging, and pathology services	Joint outpatient centers in CHCs for hypertension and diabetes	Integrated care pathways, "service agreements," and liaison officers to coordinate care
Elements of integrated care						
Tracking patient contacts with delivery system	Referrals only	No	Referrals and subset of diagnostic tests	Referrals and tests	Yes	Yes
Gatekeeping	No	No	No	For NCMS and URBMI	No	No
PHC-based care coordination across providers	No	No	No	No	For diabetes and hypertension management at CHCs	Partial: THC physician monitors; VC provides care
Use of integrated care pathways and/or individual care plans	No	No	No	No	Care plans for hypertension and diabetes	Yes
Use of metrics to measure care coordination	No	No	Limited to referrals and diagnostic tests	Limited to referrals and diagnostic tests	Limited to referrals and diagnostic rates	Compliance with integrated pathways; referral tracking

(Table continued next page)

TABLE 2C.1   Characteristics of six health care integration initiatives at Chinese hospitals   *Continued*

Characteristic type	Beijing: Chaoyang Hospital Alliance	Beijing: Renmin Hospital Integrated Care Delivery System	Shanghai: Ruijin-Luwan Hospital Group	Zhenjiang: Kangfu Network	Hangzhou: NCD joint centers	Henan: Xi County Integrated Care
Hospital-related activities and roles						
Use of multidisciplinary care teams with participation of hospital professionals	No	No	No	Yes	Hospital specialists only	No
Hospital involvement in postdischarge follow-up care	No	No	No	Information provided to lower levels	Inpatients with diabetes and hypertension	Yes
Two-way referral system	Limited	Limited	Yes	Yes	Yes	Yes
Hospital "green" channel[a]	Yes	Very limited	Yes, but limited	Yes, but limited	Yes	Yes
Care shifted out of hospitals to appropriate levels	Limited: subset of patients requiring rehabilitation	No	Some shifting of tests from tertiary to secondary hospitals	Limited to one hospital department	No	No
Technical support, training, or supervision provided by hospitals to lower levels	Yes	Yes	Yes	Yes	Yes	Yes
E-health	E-consultations for imaging services	Remote laboratory testing and imaging; teleconferencing for training and technical support	Teleconferencing for training and technical support	EHRs accessed by providers at different levels	E-consultations with hospital specialists	EHRs accessed countywide; e-consultations with hospital specialists

Note: CHC = community health center; EHR = electronic health record; NCD = noncommunicable disease; NCMS = New Cooperative Medical Scheme; PHC = primary health care; THC = township health center; URBMI = Urban Resident Basic Medical Insurance; VC = village center.

a. A hospital "green" channel refers to facilitation of upward referrals from affiliated lower-level facilities, with the intent of expediting the care of the patients so referred.

Notes

1. For example, "Guidance of the General Office of the State Council on Promoting Multi-level Diagnosis and Treatment System," State Council (2015, No. 70).

2. The strategic service delivery goals for PCIC are developed from the following sources: Barr and others (2003); Berwick, Nolan, and Whittington (2008); Craig, Eby, and Whittington (2011); Curry and Ham (2010); Curtis and Hodin (2009); Ham and Walsh (2013); Hofmarcher, Oxley, and Rusticelli (2007); Øvretveit (2011); Shortell and others (2014); Wenzel and Rohrer (1994); and WHO (2007, 2015a, 2015b).

3. Empanelment is the process by which all patients in a given facility or geographic area are assigned to a primary care provider or care team.

4. "Guidance of the General Office of the State Council on Promoting Multi-level Diagnosis and Treatment System," State Council (2015, No. 70).

5. In addition, see "Supervision of Comprehensive Reform of County-Level Public Hospitals," State Council (2015).

6. Hospital management groups or councils are described further in chapter 5.

7. For example, "green channel" admissions accounted for less than 1 percent of total admissions in the Beijing Renmin Hospital system.

8. Implementation of improvement initiatives with feedback loops is further examined in chapter 10.

9. Chapter 10 outlines an implementation plan that starts with the replication of effective practices at a provincial level in a targeted selection of counties or municipalities within the province. As learning is integrated into the process, change will be accelerated as the reforms spread.

References

Ali, Rabia. 2015. "Programs of All-Inclusive Care for the Elderly (PACE) in the U.S.: Background and Rationale." Case study commissioned by the World Bank, Washington, DC.

Ali, Rabia, and Rong Li. 2015a. "Integrated Care Services in Xi County, Henan Province." Case study commissioned by the World Bank, Washington, DC.

———. 2015b. "Patient-Centered Medical Home (PCMH) Model of U.S. Veterans Health Administration." Case study commissioned by the World Bank, Washington, DC.

Barr, Victoria J., Sylvia Robinson, Brenda Marin-Link, and Lisa Underhill. 2003. "The Expanded Chronic Care Model: An Integration of Concepts and Strategies from Population Health Promotion and the Chronic Care Model." *Hospital Quarterly* 7 (1): 73–82.

Bates, D. W., and A. Bitton. 2010. "The Future of Health Information Technology in the Patient-Centered Medical Home." *Health Affairs (Millwood)* 29 (4): 614–21.

Beauchamp, Jody, Valerie Cheh, Robert Schmitz, Peter Kemper, and John Hall. 2008. "The Effect of the Program of All-Inclusive Care for the Elderly (PACE) on Quality." Mathematica Policy Research report for the Centers for Medicare & Medicaid Services, Princeton, NJ.

Berwick, Donald M., Thomas W. Nolan, and John Whittington. 2008. "The Triple Aim: Care, Health, and Cost." *Health Affairs* 27 (3): 759–69.

Bitton, A. 2015. "Taking the Pulse of PCMH Transformation Nationwide." Lecture presented at World Bank, Washington, DC, May 29.

Bitton, A., C. Martin, and B. E. Landon. 2010. "A Nationwide Survey of Patient-Centered Medical Home Demonstration Projects." *Journal of General Internal Medicine* 25 (6): 584–92.

Braithwaite, J., C. D. Shaw, M. Moldovan, D. Greenfield, R. Hinchcliff, V. Mumford, M. B. Kristensen, and others. 2012. "Comparison of Health Service Accreditation Programs in Low- and Middle-Income Countries with Those in Higher-Income Countries: A Cross-Sectional Study." *International Journal for Quality in Health Care* 24 (6): 568–77.

Cercone, James, and Lisa O'Brien. 2010. "Benchmarking Hospital Performance in Health." White paper, Sanigest International San Jose, Costa Rica.

Chatterji, Pinka, Nancy R. Burstein, David Kidder, and Alan White. 1998. "Evaluation of the Program of All-Inclusive Care for the Elderly (PACE) Demonstration: The Impact of PACE on Participant Outcomes." Report submitted to the Health Care Financing Administration by Abt Associates, Cambridge, MA.

Craig, Catherine, Doug Eby, and John Whittington. 2011. "Care Coordination Model: Better Care at Lower Cost for People with Multiple Health and Social Needs." IHI Innovation Series white paper, Institute for Healthcare Improvement, Cambridge, MA.

Curry, Natasha, and Chris Ham. 2010. *Clinical and Service Integration: The Route to Improved Outcomes.* London: King's Fund.

Curtis, Jessica, and Renée Markus Hodin. 2009. "Special Delivery: How Coordinated Care Programs Can Improve Quality and Save Costs." Paper, Community Catalyst, Boston.

DeVries, Andrea, C. H. Li, Gayathri Sridhar, Jill Rubin Hummel, Scott Breidbart, and John J. Barron. 2012. "Impact of Medical Homes on Quality, Health Care Utilization, and Costs." *American Journal of Managed Care* 18 (9): 534–44.

DHCFP (Division of Health Care Finance and Policy). 2005. "PACE Evaluation Summary." Unpublished manuscript, DHCFP, Commonwealth of Massachusetts, Boston.

Elissen, A. M., I. G. Duimel-Peeters, C. Spreeuwenberg, M. Spreeuwenberg, and H. J.

Vrijhoef. 2012. "Toward Tailored Disease Management for Type 2 Diabetes." *American Journal of Managed Care* 18: 619–30.

Elissen A. M. J., I. G. P. Duimel-Peeters, C. Spreeuwenberg, H. J. M. Vrijhoef, and E. Nolte. 2015. "The Netherlands." In *Assessing Chronic Disease Management in European Health Systems. Country reports,"* edited by Ellen Nolte, Cécile Knai, and Richard B. Saltman, 99–110. Copenhagen: World Health Organization Regional Office for Europe (acting as the host organization for, and secretariat of, the European Observatory on Health Systems and Policies).

Fifield, Judith, Deborah Dauser Forrest, Melanie Martin-Peele, Joseph A. Burleson, Jeanette Goyzueta, Marco Fujimoto, and William Gillespie. 2013. "A Randomized, Controlled Trial of Implementing the Patient-Centered Medical Home Model in Solo and Small Practices." *Journal of General Internal Medicine* 28 (6): 770–77.

Forde, Ian, Ane Auraasen, and Liliane Moreira. 2015. "Delivering Person-Centered Integrated Care: Three Case Studies from OECD Health Systems." Case studies commissioned by the World Bank, Organisation for Economic Co-operation and Development, Paris.

Friedberg, M. W., P. S. Hussey, and E. C. Schneider. 2010. "Primary Care: A Critical Review of the Evidence on Quality and Costs of Health Care." *Health Affairs (Millwood)* 29 (5): 766–72.

Friedberg, Mark W., Meredith B. Rosenthal, Rachel M. Werner, Kevin G. Volpp, and Eric C. Schneider. 2015. "Effects of a Medical Home and Shared Savings Intervention on Quality and Utilization of Care." *JAMA Internal Medicine* 175 (8): 1362–68.

Friedberg, Mark W., Eric C. Schneider, Meredith B. Rosenthal, Kevin G. Volpp, and Rachel M. Werner. 2014. "Association between Participation in a Multipayer Medical Home Intervention and Changes in Quality, Utilization, and Costs of Care." *Journal of the American Medical Association* 311 (8): 815–25.

Frølich, A, R. Jacobsen, C. Knai. 2015. "Denmark." In *Assessing Chronic Disease Management in European Health Systems. Country Reports,"* edited by E. Nolte and C. Knai, 17–26. Copenhagen: World Health Organization (acting as host for, and secretariat of, the European Observatory on Health Systems and Policies).

Gilfillan, R. J., J. Tomcavage, and M. B. Rosenthal. 2010. "Geisinger Medical Home Pilot Demonstrates Success." *Managed Care* 16: 607–14.

Greenfield, D., M. Pawsey, R. Hinchcliff, M. Moldovan, and J. Braithwaite. 2012. "The Standard of Health Care Accreditation Standards: A Review of Empirical Research Underpinning Their Development and Impact." *BMC Health Services Research* 12: 329.

Guanais, Frederico C., and James Macinko. 2009. "The Health Effects of Decentralizing Primary Care in Brazil." *Health Affairs* 28 (4): 1127–35.

Ham, Chris, and Nicola Walsh. 2013. "Making Integrated Care Happen at Scale and Pace." Briefing paper, Lessons from Experience Series, The King's Fund, London.

Hebert, Paul L., Chuan-Fen Liu, Edwin S. Wong, Susan E. Hernandez, Adam Batten, Sophie Lo, and Jaclyn M. Lemon. 2014. "Patient-Centered Medical Home Initiative Produced Modest Economic Results for Veterans Health Administration, 2010–12." *Health Affairs* 33 (6): 980–87.

Hildebrandt, Helmut, Alexander Pimperl, Oliver Gröne, Monika Roth, Christian Melle, Timo Schulte, Martin Wetzel, and Alf Trojan. 2015. "Gesundes Kinzigtal: A Case Study on People-Centered/Integrated Health Care in Germany." Case study commissioned by the World Bank, Washington, DC.

Hofmarcher, Maria M., Howard Oxley, and Elena Rusticelli. 2007. "Improved Health System Performance through Better Care Coordination." OECD Working Paper No. 3. Organisation for Economic Co-operation and Development, Paris.

Jian, Weiyan, and Winnie Yip. 2015. "Integrated Care in China: Case Study: PKU-Renmin Hospital IDS, Beijing Chaoyang Hospital Alliance, Shanghai Ruijin-Luwan Hospital Groups, Zhenjiang Kangfu Hospital Groups." School of Public Heath, Peking University. Case study commissioned by the World Bank, Washington, DC.

Kane, Robert L., Patty Homyak, and Boris Bershadsky. 2002. "Consumer Reactions to the Wisconsin Partnership Program and Its Parent, the Program for All-Inclusive Care of the Elderly (PACE)." *The Gerontologist* 42 (3): 314–320.

Kane, Robert L., Patricia Homyak, Boris Bershadsky, and Shannon Flood. 2006a.

"The Effects of a Variant of the Program for All-Inclusive Care of the Elderly on Hospital Utilization and Outcomes." *Journal of the American Geriatrics Society* 54: 276–83.

———. 2006b. "Variations on a Theme Called PACE." *Journal of Gerontology* 61a (7): 689–93.

Klazinga, Niek. 2014. "Update on OECD's Health Care Quality Indicator Project: Measurement, Information Systems, Policies and Governance in OECD Countries." Presentation to the European Commission's Patient Safety and Quality of Care Working Group, Brussels, March 13.

Li, Weiping and Mengxi Jiang. 2015. "China's Public Hospital Governance Reform: Case Study of Zhenjiang." China National Health Development Research Center, Beijing. Case study commissioned by the World Bank, Washington, DC.

Love, Tom. 2015. "People-Centered Health Care in Canterbury, New Zealand." Sapere Research Group. Case study commissioned by the World Bank, Washington, DC.

Ma, Jin. 2015a. "Primary Care–Centered Care in Two Districts in Shanghai." Shanghai Jiao Tong University. Case study commissioned by the World Bank, Washington, DC.

———. 2015b. "China's Public Hospital Governance Reform: Case Study of Shanghai." Shanghai Jiao Tong University. Case study commissioned by the World Bank, Washington, DC.

Macinko, J., V. B. D. Oliveira, M. A. Turci, F. C. Guanais, P. D. F. Bonolo, and M. F. L. Costa. 2011. "The Influence of Primary Care and Hospital Supply on Ambulatory Care–Sensitive Hospitalizations among Adults in Brazil, 1999–2007." *American Journal of Public Health* 101 (10): 1963–70.

Macinko, J., B. Starfield, and T. Erinosho. 2009. "The Impact of Primary Health Care on Population Health in Low- and Middle-Income Countries." *Journal of Ambulatory Care Management* 32 (2):150–71.

Mancuso, David, Greg Yamashiro, and Barbara Felver. 2005. "PACE: An Evaluation. 2005." Report No. 8.26, Washington State Department of Social and Health Services Research and Data Analysis Division, Olympia.

Mate, K. S., A. L. Rooney, A. Supachutikul, and G. Gyani. 2014. "Accreditation as a Path to Achieving Universal Quality Health Coverage." *Globalization and Health* 10: 68.

Meng, Qingyue, Zhang Luyu, Zhu Weiming, and Ma Huifen. 2015. "People-Centered Health Care: A Case Study from Huangzhong County, Qinghai Province." China Center for Health Development Studies, Peking University. Case study commissioned by the World Bank, Washington, DC.

Meng, Qingyue, Jin Yinzi, Yue Dahai, and He Li. 2015. "People-Centered Health Care: A Case Study from Feixi County, Anhui Province." China Center for Health Development Studies, Peking University. Case study commissioned by the World Bank, Washington, DC.

Meret-Hanke, Louise. 2011. "Effects of the Program of All-Inclusive Care for the Elderly on Hospital Use." *The Gerontologist* 51 (6): 774–85.

Mukamel, Dana B., Alina Bajorska, and Helena Temkin-Greener. 2002. "Health Care Services Utilization at the End of Life in a Managed Care Program Integrating Acute and Long-Term Care." *Medical Care* 40 (12): 1136–48.

Mukamel, Dana B., Derick R. Peterson, Helena Temkin-Greener, Rachel Delavan, Diane Gross, Stephen J. Kunitz, and T. Franklin Williams. 2007. "Program Characteristics and Enrollees' Outcomes in the Program of All-Inclusive Care for the Elderly (PACE)." *The Milbank Quarterly* 85 (3): 499–531.

Mukamel, Dana B., Helena Temkin-Greener, and Marleen L. Clark. 1998. "Stability of Disability among PACE Enrollees: Financial and Programmatic Implications." *Health Care Financing Review* 19 (3).

Mukamel, Dana B., Helena Temkin-Greener, Rachel Delavan, Derick R. Peterson, Diane Gross, Stephen Kunitz, and T. Franklin Williams. 2006. "Team Performance and Risk-Adjusted Health Outcomes in the Program of All-Inclusive Care for the Elderly (PACE)." *The Gerontologist* 46 (2): 227–37.

Murray, Robert. 2015. "The CareFirst Blue Cross–Blue Shield Patient-Centered Medical Home Model, Maryland, U.S.A." Case study commissioned by the World Bank, Washington, DC.

NCQA (National Committee for Quality Assurance). 2014. "PCMH 2014 Content and Scoring Summary." NCQA, Washington, DC.

Nelson, Karin M., Christian Helfrich, Haili Sun, Paul L. Hebert, Chuan-Fen Liu, Emily Dolan, and Leslie Taylor. 2014. "Implementation of the Patient-Centered Medical Home in the Veteran's Health Administration: Associations with Patient Satisfaction, Quality of Care,

Staff Burnout, and Hospital and Emergency Department Use." *JAMA Internal Medicine* 174 (8): 1350–58.

Nolte, Ellen, Anne Frølich, Helmut Hildebrandt, Alexander Pimperl, and Hubertus J. Vrijhoef. 2015. "Integrating Care: A Synthesis of Experiences in Three European Countries." European Observatory. Case studies commissioned by the World Bank, Washington, DC.

Nolte, Ellen, and Emma Pitchforth. 2014. "What Is the Evidence on the Economic Impacts of Integrated Care?" Policy Summary 11, World Health Organization Regional Office for Europe, Copenhagen (acting as the host organization for, and secretariat of, the European Observatory on Health Systems and Policies).

O'Brien, John Michael. 2014. "PCMH, TCCI & the CareFirst Model: 'Focus on Medication Management.'" PowerPoint presentation to event, "A Prescription for Savings: Medication Management and Improved Adherence," National Coalition on Health Care, Washington, DC, March 6.

Øvretveit, John. 2011. *Does Clinical Coordination Improve Quality and Save Money? Volume 1: A Summary Review of the Evidence.* London: The Health Foundation.

Porignon, Denis, Reynaldo Holder, Olga Maslovskaia, Tephany Griffith, Avril Ogrodnick, and Wim Van Lerberghe. 2011. "The Role of Hospitals within the Framework of the Renewed Primary Health Care Strategy." *World Hospital Health Service* 47 (3): 6–9.

Porter, Michael E. 2010. "What Is Value in Health Care?" *New England Journal of Medicine* 363: 2477–81.

RAND. 2012. "National Evaluation of the Department of Health's Integrated Care Pilots: Appendices." Technical report, RAND Corporation, Santa Monica, CA.

Reid, Robert J., Katie Coleman, Eric A. Johnson, Paul A. Fishman, Clarissa Hsu, Michael P. Soman, Claire E. Trescott, Michael Erikson, and Eric B. Larson. 2010. "The Group Health Medical Home at Year Two: Cost Savings, Higher Patient Satisfaction, and Less Burnout for Providers." *Health Affairs* 29 (5): 835–43.

Reid, Robert J., Eric A. Johnson, Clarissa Hsu, Kelly Ehrlich, Katie Coleman, Claire Trescott, and Michael Erikson. 2013. "Spreading a Medical Home Redesign: Effects on Emergency Department Use and Hospital Admissions." *Annals of Family Medicine* 11 (1): S1–S26.

Rosenthal, Meredith B., Mark W. Friedberg, Sara J. Singer, Diana Eastman, Zhonghe Li, and Eric C. Schneider. 2013. "Effect of a Multipayer Patient-Centered Medical Home on Health Care Utilization and Quality: The Rhode Island Chronic Care Sustainability Initiative Pilot Program." *JAMA Internal Medicine* 173 (20): 1907–13.

Runz-Jørgensen, Sidsel Marie, and Anne Frølich. 2015. "SIKS—The Integrated Effort for People Living with Chronic Diseases: A Case Study on People Centered/Integrated Health Care in Denmark." The Research Unit for Chronic Conditions, Bispebjerg Hospital, Denmark. Case study commissioned by the World Bank, Washington, DC.

Salmon, J. W., J. Heavens, C. Lombard, and Paula Tavrow, 2003. "The Impact of Accreditation on the Quality of Hospital Care: KwaZulu-Natal Province, Republic of South Africa." Operations Research Results Series report, published for the U.S. Agency for International Development (USAID) by the Quality Assurance Project, University Research Co., Bethesda, MD.

Schulte, T., A. Pimperl, A. Fischer, B. Dittmann, P. Wendel, and H. Hildebrandt. 2014. "Ergebnisqualität Gesundes Kinzigtal—quantifiziert durch Mortalitätskennzahlen. Eine quasi-experimentelle Kohortenstudie: Propensity-Score-Matching von Eingeschriebenen vs. Nicht-Eingeschriebenen des Integrierten Versorgungsmodells auf Basis von Sekundärdaten der Kinzigtal-Population." Health Data Analytics study for Gesundes Kinzigtal GmbH, Hausach, Germany.

Shortell, Stephen, Rachael Addicott, Nicola Walsh, and Chris Haim. 2014. "Accountable Care Organisations in the United States and England: Testing, Evaluation, and Learning What Works." Briefing paper, The King's Fund, London.

Smits, H., A. Supachutikul, and K. S. Mate. 2014. "Hospital Accreditation: Lessons from Low- and Middle-Income Countries." *Globalization and Health* 10: 65.

State Council. 2012. "The Twelfth Five-Year Plan for Health Sector Development." *Guo Fa* 2012, No. 57. http://www.wpro.who.int/health _services/china_nationalhealthplan.pdf.

———. 2015. "Evaluation Report on Urban Public Hospital Reform Pilots." State Council of the People's Republic of China, Beijing.

Stout, S., C. Klucznik, A. Chevalier, R. Wheeler, J. Azzara, L. Gray, D. Scannell, L. Sweeney, M. Saginario, and I. Lopes. 2015. "Cambridge Health Alliance Model of Team-Based Care: Implementation Guide and Toolkit." Cambridge Health Alliance, Cambridge MA.

Struijs, J., J. de Jong-van Til, L. Lemmens, H. W. Drewes, S. de Bruin, and C. Baan. 2012. "Three Years Bundled Payment System for Diabetes Care: Effects on Care Process and Quality of Care." National Institute for Public Health and the Environment, Bilthoven, Netherlands.

Struijs, J. N., S. M. Mohnen, C. C. M. Molema, J. T. de Jong-van Til, and C. Baan. 2012. "Effects of Bundled Payment on Curative Health Care Costs in the Netherlands: An Analysis for Diabetes Care and Vascular Risk Management based on Nationwide Claim Data, 2007–10." National Institute for Public Health and the Environment, Bilthoven, Netherlands.

Sumer, Safir. 2015. "Case Study for People-Centered Health Care in Turkey." Case study commissioned by the World Bank, Washington, DC.

Temkin-Greener, Helena, Alina Bajorska, and Dana B. Mukamel. 2008. "Variations in Service Use in the Program of All-Inclusive Care for the Elderly (PACE): Is More Better?" *Journal of Gerontology* 63A (7): 731–38.

Teo, Hui Sin. 2015. "Singapore's Experience with Care Integration." Case study commissioned by the World Bank, Washington, DC.

Vadstrup, E., A. Frølich, H. Perrild, E. Borg, and M. Røder. 2011. "Effect of a Group-Based Rehabilitation Programme on Glycaemic Control and Cardiovascular Risk Factors in Type 2 Diabetes Patients: The Copenhagen Type 2 Diabetes Rehabilitation Project." *Patient Education and Counseling* 84: 185–90.

Van Hasselt, M., N. McCall, V. Keyes, S. G. Wensky, and K. W. Smith. 2015. "Total Cost of Care Lower among Medicare Fee-for-Service Beneficiaries Receiving Care from Patient-Centered Medical Homes." *Health Services Research* 50 (1): 253–72.

Vrijhoef, J. M. Hubertus, and Guy Schulpen. 2015. "Care Group Zio: Integrated Health Care for People with Type 2 Diabetes: A Case Study on People Centered/Integrated Health Care in the Maastricht Region, the Netherlands." Maastricht University Medical Center. Case study commissioned by the World Bank, Washington, DC.

Wagstaff, A., M. Lindelow, S. Wang, and S. Zhang. 2009. *Reforming China's Rural Health System*. Directions in Development Series. Washington, DC: World Bank.

Wang, Qiuyan Cindy, Ravi Chawla, Christine M. Colombo, Richard L. Snyder, and Somesh Nigam. 2014. "Patient-Centered Medical Home Impact on Health Plan Members with Diabetes." *Journal of Public Health Management and Practice* 20 (5): E12–E20.

Weaver, Frances M., Elaine C. Hickey, Susan L. Hughes, Vicky Parker, Dawn Fortunato, Julia Rose, Steven Cohen, Laurence Robbins, Willie Orr, Beverly Priefer, Darryl Wieland, and Judith Baskins. 2008. "Providing All-Inclusive Care for Frail Elderly Veterans: Evaluation of Three Models of Care." *Journal of the American Geriatrics Society* 56: 345–53.

Wenzel, Richard P., and James E. Rohrer. 1994. "The Iron Triangle of Health Care Reform." *Clinical Performance and Quality Health Care* 2 (1): 7–9.

Werner, Rachel M., Anne Canamucio, Judy A. Shea, and Gala True. 2014. "The Medical Home Transformation in the Veterans Health Administration: An Evaluation of Early Changes in Primary Care Delivery." *Health Services Research* 49 (4): 1329–47.

WHO (World Health Organization). 2007. *People-Centered Health Care: A Policy Framework*. Geneva: WHO.

———. 2008. *The World Health Report 2008: Primary Health Care—Now More than Ever*. Geneva: WHO.

———. 2015a. "WHO Global Strategy on People-Centered and Integrated Health Services." WHO/HIS/SDS/2015.6, WHO, Geneva.

———. 2015b. "People-Centered and Integrated Health Services: An Overview of the Evidence." WHO/HIS/SDS/2015.7, WHO, Geneva.

Wieland, Darryl, Rebecca Boland, Judith Baskins, and Bruce Kinosian. 2010. "Five-Year Survival in a Program of All-Inclusive Care for Elderly Compared with Alternative Institutional and Home- and Community-Based Care." *Journal of Gerontology* 65 (7): 721–26.

Wieland, Darryl, Vicki L. Lamb, Shae R. Sutton, Rebecca Boland, Marleen Clark, Susan Friedman, Kenneth Brummel-Smith, and G. Paul Eleazer. 2000. "Hospitalization in the Program of All-Inclusive Care for the Elderly (PACE): Rates, Concomitants, and Predictors."

Journal of the American Geriatrics Society 48: 1373–80.

World Bank. 2015. *World Development Indicators 2015*. Washington, DC: World Bank.

Yan, Fei. 2015a. "Integrated Health Services Reform between Community Health Service Centers and Hospitals in Hangzhou, Zhejiang Province." School of Public Health, Fudan University. Case study commissioned by the World Bank, Washington, DC.

———. 2015b. "The Integrated Health Care System Based on Health Care Groups in Zhenjiang, Jiangsu Province, China." School of Public Health, Fudan University. Case study commissioned by the World Bank, Washington, DC.

3

Lever 2: Improving Quality of Care

Introduction

China's success in rebalancing service delivery toward people-centered integrated care (PCIC) will depend on the health system's ability to produce and deliver high-quality services. This means providing clinically safe, effective, and timely care—at all levels of peoples' interaction with the health system, but especially in primary care, which is the patient's first point of contact in an effective PCIC model. Indeed, efforts to improve the quality of care (QoC) to support PCIC will serve as a key lever to achieve China's reform aims of better population health, better patient experience, and more efficient health care.

"Quality" in health care—an abstract and complex concept (Dayal and Hort 2015; La Forgia and Couttolenc 2008)—was described in an Institute of Medicine (IOM) report as "the degree to which health services for individuals and populations increase the likelihood of desired health outcomes and are consistent with current professional knowledge" (Kohn, Corrigan, and Donaldson 1990). Drawing in part on the IOM report, Dlugacz, Restifo, and Greenwood (2004) define QoC as "care that is measurably safe, of the highest standard, evidence-based,

uniformly delivered, with the appropriate utilization of resources and services."

In the context of health systems, the term "quality" incorporates a range of positive features that contribute to the overall performance of health care systems, a view that underscores the "systems property" of quality rather than simply the duty of a physician, department or facility (IOM 2001). Indeed, evidence-based, high-quality, clinically appropriate care—delivered with high technical skills—is critical if China is to improve population health, patient experience, and efficiency of health care.

QoC matters because it is a determinant of health outcomes. Approximately 10–30 percent of the reduction in premature mortality over the past decade in Organisation for Economic Co-operation and Development (OECD) countries can be attributed to QoC improvements (Nolte and McKee 2011, 2012). Low QoC can lead to medical errors that harm rather than help patients: for example, the IOM documented up to 98,000 deaths per year because of medical errors in U.S. hospitals (Kohn, Corrigan, and Donaldson 1999). Potentially preventable hospitalization due to poor primary care accounted for 1 out of every 10 hospital stays in 2008 in the United States (Stranges and Stocks 2010). Low-quality care, as indicated by medical errors and adverse events, also drives up health spending. Medical errors alone cost the United States an estimated $19.5 billion in 2008 (Andel 2012; Stranges and Stocks 2010).

Better QoC is not only associated with better patient outcomes and experience, but is also vital to the efficiency and sustainability of the delivery system because of the close link between quality and costs. Research shows that high-quality care is not necessarily more expensive, but that low-quality care is associated with more hospitalizations, more intensive treatments and use of medicine, longer hospital stays, and unnecessary readmissions, resulting in wasted resources and poor outcomes (Baicker and Chandra 2004; Berwick, Nolan, and Wittington 2008).

Estimates of health care costs stemming from improper and unnecessary use of medicines exceeded $200 billion in 2012 in the United States (IMS Institute for Health Care Informatics 2013). Similarly, the United Kingdom's National Health Service was found to be wasting up to £2.3 billion a year on a range of unnecessary procedures and processes (Campbell 2014). Preventing medical errors could have saved US$3 billion annually in the Australian health system during 1995–96 (AHMAC 1996). In short, low-quality care can harm patients' health and compromise the efficiency of health systems.

In China, there is a need for information on QoC and the implications for spending. It is safe to assume that the quality-cost links observed elsewhere also exist in China, though more research would be needed to confirm this hypothesis. A dearth of reliable data and a weak institutional infrastructure for monitoring and evaluation of quality makes it difficult to assess how deficiencies in quality are affecting patient outcomes or driving up health spending (for example, by causing medical errors, adverse events, and unnecessary readmissions to hospitals). There is nonetheless a consensus that quality needs improvement, especially at primary health facilities (Yip and Hsiao 2015). Emerging evidence of variations in clinical quality suggests room for quality improvement in hospitals as well (Xu and others 2015).

Quality shortcomings have been associated with low utilization of primary care services (Bhattacharyya and others 2011; Zhang and others 2014) and an increasing number of patient-doctor disputes over medical practice, resulting in litigations and violence (Hesketh and others 2012). A well-documented quality problem is the overprescription of unnecessary services and drugs (Li and others 2012; Yin and others 2015; Yin and others 2013). Patients have expressed dissatisfaction about overprescription as well as poor attitude, lack of effort, and short consultation time with doctors and nurses (NCHS 2010).

In China, the National Health and Family Planning Commission (NHFPC) has launched initiatives to improve QoC through promoting clinical pathways, regulating market access, and developing clinical standards (NHFPC 2014). Implementation is just under way. However, some important quality improvement functions are not yet addressed, including developing, validating, and mandating the use of national standardized quality measures; managing the monitoring and evaluation of quality at the facility level; and coordinating efforts for quality improvement across various stakeholders.

In the past decade, most OECD countries have recognized continual quality improvement as a central goal of health sector development and have implemented systematic reforms to improve QoC. Governments increasingly act as stewards of the public and payers for health care, leading the changes in health care delivery to improve QoC. Drawing on their experience combined with relevant experience from China, this chapter is organized as follows:

- *"Conceptualizing, Assessing, and Improving the Quality of Care"* describes a conceptual framework for analyzing QoC.
- *"Challenges in the Quality of Care in China"* examines opportunities and challenges for quality improvement in the Chinese context.

- *"International Experience in Improving Health System Features for High Quality"* presents the experience of OECD countries in establishing the support infrastructure for quality improvement.
- *"Recommendations to China for Improving the Quality of Care"* proposes a set of core actions and implementation strategies China may wish to adopt for scaling up systematic quality improvement efforts.

Conceptualizing, Assessing, and Improving the Quality of Care

This section first examines what QoC means through a review of definitions and concepts used internationally. It then presents frameworks for assessing quality challenges and for improving quality in the broader policy and institutional environment. These frameworks are applied to the Chinese and OECD contexts in subsequent sections.

Conceptualizing the Quality of Care

Defining QoC, clarifying the goals of quality improvement, and measuring progress are not straightforward tasks. Most countries define it in terms of desirable features of care processes and outcomes that combine technical, patient experience, and affordability dimensions, as in the following examples:

- Safe, effective, efficient, timely, patient-centered, equitable (Institute of Medicine, United States)
- Clinically effective, safe, and good patient experience (National Health Service, United Kingdom)
- Doing the right thing for the right patient, at the right time, in the right way to achieve the best possible results (Agency for Health Care Research and Quality, U.S. Department of Health and Human Services; and a similar definition by the National Committee for Quality Assurance, United States)

- Improved individual experience of care; improved health of population; and reduced per capita costs of care for population (Institute of Health Care Improvement, United States)
- The degree of care given to the patient, with existing medical technology, resources, and capacity, and following professional ethics and clinical standards (National Health and Family Planning Commission, China) (NHFPC 2014).

Different stakeholders are likely to emphasize different aspects of quality. *Medical professionals* tend to emphasize the consistency of practice with current professional standards and evidence (IOM 2001). *Patients* value certain features such as infrastructure, provider communication, and waiting time (de Silva and Bamber 2014). *Policy makers and health managers* tend to focus on striking a balance between quality, cost, and equity. Moreover, quality is often a moving target, because new medical knowledge and technology tend to alter understanding of what is considered high-quality (or higher-quality) care, requiring a constant revisiting and updating of processes, standards, and metrics.

Quality can be considered to have two dimensions: technical and personal. This chapter centers on the *technical* dimension of quality, which refers to the correctness of diagnosis, the appropriateness of prescribed interventions based on best evidence, and the competency of the clinical team in delivering those interventions, resulting in an increased likelihood of an improved health outcome at an affordable cost.

The *personal* dimension of quality, including patient satisfaction, is discussed in chapter 4. Briefly, it refers to the responsiveness of care to patients' preferences: the ability to see a preferred clinician, continuity of care, good communication, demonstration of empathy, and respect for privacy contribute to perceived higher QoC. Ensuring the highest standard of quality means that all patients receive the right care, at the right time, in the right setting, every time.

Assessing the Quality of Care

The most salient definition of quality care, by Donabedian (2005), provides a useful framework of structure, process, and outcomes for critically examining problems related to the QoC in China—all three of which provide valuable information for measuring quality:

- *Structural quality* evaluates the relatively stable characteristics of the environment in which care takes place, including infrastructure, equipment, and human resources.
- *Process quality* assesses interactions between clinicians and patients, and whether the clinician follows recommended care or clinical guidelines to reach a correct diagnosis and an appropriate treatment plan, and skillfully delivers treatments.
- *Outcomes* offer evidence about changes in patients' health status as a result of health care.

Failure to adhere to best evidence or professional standards leads to three types of problems in process quality: overuse, underuse, and misuse (for example, of lab tests, procedures, or prescription of drugs). A health intervention is considered appropriate and worthwhile if its expected health benefits exceed its expected health risks by a wide enough margin (Brook 1995). *Overuse* of services occurs when an intervention is given without medical justification—for example, by using antibiotics to treat patients with viral colds or to treat children with simple infections. *Underuse* of services occurs when recommended or necessary care, including effective preventive care, is not delivered to patients. *Misuse* can consist of incorrect diagnosis or inappropriate interventions delivered to patients that may harm their health. In turn, a poor process of care results in poor patient outcomes.

Inappropriate or harmful care occurs across the globe. For example, a landmark RAND study found that adults in the United States received only about 55 percent of the recommended preventive care, acute care, care for chronic conditions, screenings, or follow-up care; these findings indicated a massive underuse of effective interventions, especially cost-effective preventive care (McGlynn and others 2003). In low- and middle-income countries, though evidence needs to be strengthened, inappropriate overuse of antibiotics has been widely documented (Laxminarayan and Heymann 2012).

Low-quality care processes are often associated with poor patient outcomes. A retrospective review of medical records associated with hospital admissions in eight countries (the Arab Republic of Egypt, Jordan, Kenya, Morocco, South Africa, Sudan, Tunisia, and the Republic of Yemen) documented an average adverse event rate of 8.2 percent (ranging from 2.5 percent to 18.4 percent). Of the adverse events, 83 percent were judged to be preventable and 30 percent were associated with death of the patient. One-third were caused by therapeutic errors in relatively non-complex clinical situations (Wilson and others 2012). A systematic review of published studies on health care–associated infections in low- and middle-income countries also found much higher rates than in high-income countries, particularly of nosocomial infections in adult intensive care units; surgical site infections; and methicillin resistance (Allegranzi and others 2011).

Systematic information collection to measure processes and outcomes in a health service plays an important role in generating insights into quality shortfalls, contributing to the development of actionable improvement plans and monitoring arrangements. The World Health Organization and others have done considerable work to develop quality indicators for use at a national level.[1] Because of the complexity and uncertainty of health care, these measures may not be perfect; nevertheless, once endorsed and adopted by health care stakeholders, they serve the purposes of signaling priority areas for quality improvement and respective quality standards and of holding providers accountable to the agreed-upon performance framework.

Improving the Quality of Care: The Need for System Support

International experience suggests that addressing any quality gap will require strong stewardship by government, usually in partnership with nongovernmental stakeholders, to develop national support for sustained quality improvement. Improving QoC is not merely the responsibility of one doctor or one health facility. The capacity of any country to measure and raise QoC is critical to system-wide improvement of health care delivery and patient outcomes.

Health workers and facilities acting alone are often ill prepared or lack incentives to take on such complex tasks. They require support from within their organizations, as well as from the broader health system, to foster a culture of quality improvement. Appropriate policies, regulations, incentives, and monitoring systems are needed to guide continuous quality improvement. Of equal importance, institutions are needed to measure and monitor quality, provide guidance to health care organizations while strengthening their capacity, and support systematic research and evaluation of clinical practices.

System support and institutional leadership are key to creating a high-level vision for quality improvement and a conducive policy environment. In many countries, the lack of an overall vision of QoC has led to wide variations in quality across health care facilities. Leaving quality improvement to the discretion of individual facilities will not produce higher QoC at scale; instead, it may favor facilities that are well endowed with physical, financial, and knowledge resources and thereby exacerbate inequities.

Strong, unified leadership from a national-level professional institution is critical. Institutional leadership in quality assurance and improvement serves at least three essential functions (WHO 2006):

- It leads analysis of quality in health service delivery, including stakeholder involvement and situational analysis, which ultimately contributes to the creation of a unified vision for QoC and confirmation of QoC goals.
- It provides technical leadership in harmonizing and disseminating quality measures and standards, identifying QoC deficiencies, and developing quality improvement strategies.
- It offers high-level oversight of the implementation of quality improvement efforts and allows monitoring of their progress.

Monitoring and evaluation (M&E) is a critical component of the architecture of a health care system, linking health policy and health care practice and providing the essential information to guide quality improvement and enforce accountability. Diligent M&E of quality improvement is indispensable because investments in quality improvement at the system or facility level can only be justified in terms of the positive changes they achieve in support of predefined goals. If an improvement falls short of expectations, evaluation of the existing strategy can be used to shape modifications early on, thus maximizing the likelihood of success. Recognition of progress and celebration of achievements also help to maintain the motivation and commitment of stakeholders in the change process. Public reporting, based on continuous monitoring of indicators, benchmarking, and comparison, has become an increasingly common mechanism to complement monitoring systems.

QoC Challenges in China

China faces increasing public pressure to raise quality. Large disparities exist between the country's elite tertiary hospitals and the vast majority of lower-level facilities in physical and human resources, quality culture, and clinical practices. The government aims to raise the bar of quality for all providers and has invested in expanding and upgrading the health care infrastructure, particularly at the grassroots level, but it has only recently directed attention to improving the processes and outcomes of care. Following the structure-process-outcome framework outlined in the previous section, this section reviews key aspects of China's health care delivery system, briefly examines recent policy initiatives related to quality, and outlines the challenges to achieving higher-quality care.

Evidence on China's QoC is thin. Most people (and stakeholders) rate health care facilities often using subjective assessments based on prestige, possession of high-technology equipment, or the presence of distinguished senior specialists. As a result, evidence on the QoC in most facilities is lacking, and efforts to measure and assess quality are few.

The scope of QoC research also varies. Most assessments of quality are descriptive studies of a single hospital or a handful of tertiary hospitals (for example, Nie, Wei, and Cui 2014; Wei and others 2010). Studies of the quality of inpatient care at tertiary hospitals are more common than studies of secondary hospitals and primary care facilities. Given the conflicting definitions of quality, there is no agreed-upon framework for undertaking a comprehensive quality assessment. The wide range of quality measures and analytical methods in use makes the results hard to compare. Prominent themes of QoC-related studies are the prevalence of inappropriate care and the relation between quality and efficiency (for example, Li and others 2012; Yin and others 2015; Yin and others 2013).

Structure of the Delivery System

Most QoC studies in China focus on structural aspects of the delivery system. After the massive expansion of facilities over the past two decades, China is well endowed with modern infrastructure and state-of-the-art equipment even at the lower levels of its health care system.

The government has done a remarkable job in regulating building standards (for example, setting minimum requirements for total facility areas and floor plans) and establishing an inventory of essential equipment for grassroots facilities such as village clinics, township health centers (THCs), and community health centers (CHCs). In Guizhou, for example, facility surveys show an average

of five pieces of medical equipment valued at RMB 10,000 or above at THCs, including X-ray machines, ultrasound machines, biochemical analyzers, electrocardiogram machines, ventilators, blood-cell-count machines, and urine analyzers. Many THCs have multifunction life monitors, electric suction devices, electric lavage machines, and anesthesia machines (Wang and Xue 2011).

In addition, the 2009 health sector reform (as discussed in chapter 1) prioritized the establishment of a network of urban CHCs that are geographically accessible to any resident within a 15- to 20-minute walk. These measures are laudable, as they aim to improve timely access to health services.

QoC is also a product of the knowledge, attitudes, and practices of health professionals. Like many countries, China faces shortages of well-trained health professionals, especially in grassroots facilities and rural areas. Among all registered (assistant) physicians, only 45 percent have bachelor's degrees or higher; most work at large hospitals. At the grassroots level, about 75 percent of the doctors at THCs and CHCs have vocational high school or two-year college medical education, and only 10–15 percent have a bachelor's degree. Most village doctors are former barefoot doctors who only have a vocational high-school medical education.[2] Continuing medical education (CME) is limited for doctors in grassroots facilities: THC and CHC doctors register 15 days of CME training each year. In addition, most nurses in China are not college educated.

Process of Care

Restricted by shortcomings in the available data, few studies in China have directly examined the mechanisms and procedures used to deliver health care. But existing evidence suggests shortfalls in care processes. Overuse of prescription drugs and health services—particularly high-technology, high-cost interventions—prevails in most facilities. Li and others (2012) studied 230,900 outpatient prescriptions written between 2007 and 2009 in 28 Chinese cities and found that half of the prescriptions were for antibiotics and that 10 percent were for two or more types of antibiotics.

Overprescription of antibiotics is particularly problematic in lower-level facilities and poorer regions, because these facilities rely more heavily on drug revenue. According to a senior health official, the overuse of CT scanning, cesarean section, coronary artery stent implantation, and coronary artery bypass graft are conspicuous problems in China's clinical practice (Liao 2015) (table 3.1).

Underuse of effective care is another concern in China. Underuse of effective prophylaxis was found to have contributed to the occurrence of preventable surgical-site infections (Fan and others 2014). In addition, cost-effective behavioral counseling such as smoking-cessation counseling may be underused; even among physicians, the smoking-cessation rate was found to be low, and the provision of advice to patients on smoking cessation was not common (Abdullah and others 2013). Other researchers found underuse of early beta-blocker therapy among patients with acute myocardial infarction who could benefit from it as well as potential overuse among patients who might be harmed by it (Zhang and others 2015). Both overuse and underuse represent failures to follow best practice.

Chronic diseases have become the major disease burden in China, and studies have found that knowledge and experience in managing common chronic diseases are insufficient among grassroots-level doctors (Liu, Hou, and Zhou 2013; Wu and others 2009; Xu 2010). Wu and others (2009) tested 651 village doctors' knowledge of hypertension treatment. They found that less than 40 percent of village doctors performed the correct procedure to take a patient's blood pressure and that only 7 percent regularly measured patients' blood pressure in their work. Less than 50 percent knew the recommended treatment for hypertension or that hypertension is the single most important risk factor for cardiovascular diseases.

Evidence on appropriate processes of care is mixed for secondary and tertiary hospitals; for example, Wei and others (2010) found a high uptake of secondary prevention of ischemic stroke by doctors in a nationwide sample of urban hospitals. However, Qian and others (2001) showed that obstetric care did not follow best practice in four hospitals in Shanghai and Jiangsu, with three out of six procedures that should be avoided being routinely performed more than 70 percent of the time. Similar results were found regarding medication for patients with acute coronary syndromes (Bi and others 2009).

Outcomes

As in many countries, limited access to medical records, uneven record keeping, and unreliable clinical service data present challenges to outcomes research. The available evidence in China suggests large variations in patient

TABLE 3.1 Overuse of prescription drugs and other health interventions in China

Type of health intervention	Findings
Overprescription of drugs	Average number of drugs per prescription (three) exceeds WHO rational drug use reference level (Yin and others 2015); 50 percent of prescriptions were for antibiotics, and 10–25 percent were for two or more types of antibiotics (Li and others 2012; Yin and others 2013).
Overuse of intravenous injection drugs	Intravenous injection rate (53 percent) exceeds WHO rational drug use reference level (Yin and others 2015).
Overuse of surgical procedures	Cesarean section rate is 46 percent of all deliveries; 50 percent of cesarean sections were unnecessary (Liao 2015).
Overuse of CT scans	True positive rate of CT scans is only 10 percent, compared with global average of 50 percent (Liao 2015).

Note: WHO = World Health Organization.

outcomes in tertiary public hospitals (Xu and others 2015). Reduction in hospital mortality has lagged over time (Li and Wang 2015), and preventable adverse events remain common. A meta-analysis showed that the surgical-site infection rate averaged 4.5 percent between 2001 and 2012 (Fan and others 2014), compared with 1.9 percent in the United States between 2006 and 2008 (CDC 2018).

China's Health Care Regulatory and Policy Environment

The health care sector requires a strong regulatory regime, in part because of the complexity of health services and the information asymmetry between providers and consumers. Some health services can be considered "credence goods," whose utility and impact the consumer finds difficult or impossible to ascertain even after the services have been completed. The government can play an important role in safeguarding the QoC by developing quality standards and mandating providers' compliance. In addition, government can also provide political and financial incentives to promote continuous quality improvement.

Institutional and Policy Mechanisms for Quality Improvement

The government of China has long considered quality assurance a core responsibility of health administration and has been a leader in this regard. Table 3.2 summarizes the main regulatory strategies and policy initiatives in force. Basic regulatory mechanisms to ensure safety and quality have been in place since the late 1970s, specifying minimum equipment and staffing standards by type of facility; governing the qualification of health professionals; and setting out general management principles. Between 1989 and 1998, China implemented a first round of hospital accreditation that was intended to categorize and rank hospitals based on their relative quality.

In part because the 2009 reforms positioned public hospital reform as a priority, the then-Ministry of Health (predecessor

to the NHFPC) created a new Department of Medical Service Management that year. The department's mandate is to develop and implement strategies for improving public hospital management and performance, including quality assurance and improvement. Under the department's leadership, quality standards have been revisited and specific quality issues have been addressed by updating standards and guidelines, promoting investigations, and strengthening regulation.[3] The "Guidelines on Antimicrobial Drug Use" have been updated several times, with the latest version published in 2015.[4] The department has also drafted a set of condition-specific quality control guidelines, measures, and clinical pathways[5] to be piloted in some public hospitals, with substantial inputs from other countries' experience. These efforts have contributed to a more comprehensive, up-to-date set of quality-related regulations.

In addition, the Ministry of Health established national and local committees for medical quality control (MQCCs) to be responsible for developing standards and enforcing quality control within medical specialties at the facility level. Local MQCCs are situated in tertiary or teaching hospitals that are considered technical leaders—which empowers them to undertake quality evaluation. Zhejiang province, for example, currently has 47 MQCCs, and its provincial Medical Quality Control and Evaluation Office serves as a coordinator of quality improvement work and as an external evaluator of medical quality (ZJOL 2011). The office's Continuous Quality Improvement Work Plan (2009–12) has provided a model for other facilities. Based on the plan, many hospitals have established a quality management committee for clinical care, which is typically chaired by the hospital president or a vice president in charge of quality and consists of medical directors from various specialty departments.

Since 2009, the NHFPC has initiated various activities on hospital management, with safety and quality assurance as integral components. These include the Hospital Management Year initiative (2005–09),

TABLE 3.2   Regulations on health care quality in China

Regulatory strategy	Major policy documents or initiatives	Purpose and implementation
Regulatory institutions	• Medical Service Management and Guidance Center (MSMGC) established in March 2015 • National and local medical quality control committees (MQCCs) established since 2009 • Department of Medical Service Management (DMSM) within Ministry of Health (MoH) established in 2008	• MSMGC carries out health technology assessment and provide technical support to local quality improvement efforts. • MQCCs develop standards and enforce quality control within medical specialties. • DMSM provides high-level political authority and leadership in public hospital management and quality regulation.
General regulations	• Clinical Quality Management Regulations (opinion-seeking draft) issued in 2014 • Work plan for comprehensively improving the capacity of county hospitals developed in 2014 • Accreditation Standards for Tertiary Hospitals established in 2011; Accreditation Standards for Secondary Hospitals established in 2012 • General Hospital Evaluation Standards revised in 2009 • Guiding Principles on Clinical Pathway Management issued in 2009	• Traditionally, the MoH only develops and publishes general hospital management regulations that include a quality component.
Clinical practice guidelines and standards	• Chinese Medical Association has developed clinical diagnosis and treatment guidelines and clinical technology and operations standards by specialty since 2006. • Provincial and local medical associations established various local clinical guidelines, specifications, expert opinions, expert consensus, guiding opinions and other advice on specific clinical issues. • NHFPC publishes guidelines on specific issues: for example, "Nosocomial Infection Management" (2011); "Guidelines on Clinical Use of Antibiotics" (2015); and "Evaluation System of Single-Disease Quality Management" (2008).	• Forty-seven such specialty guidelines have been developed and distributed. • However, there is limited monitoring of clinical practice against these guidelines. Only certain secondary and tertiary hospitals are required to report clinical data. • Guidelines cannot be used as a legal basis in malpractice litigation.
Health facility evaluation and quality improvement initiatives	• Two rounds of hospital accreditation (2011–12 and 1989–98) • Further Improving Medical Services Initiative (2015–17) • The 10,000 Miles Medical Quality Inspection Tour annually since 2009 • The Hospital Management Year initiative (2005–09) • "100 Best Hospitals" recognition	• Although new accreditation standards were developed, the NHFPC withdrew accreditation for more than 240 newly accredited tertiary hospitals between 2011 and 2012. Fraud and corruption were suspected during the accreditation process.[a] • On-site survey is the most commonly used method for hospital evaluation.

Source: National Health and Family Planning Commission (NHFPC) website (accessed June 27, 2018), http://en.nhfpc.gov.cn/.
a. *Dajiang Net* 2012.

the 10,000 Miles Medical Quality Inspection Tour (an annual national tour to perform on-site surveys of hospitals), and recognition of 100 Best Hospitals. The Further Improving Quality of Health Care Services

initiative (2015–17), which aims to improve convenience of access and patients' service experience (for example, by enabling online medical appointments and weekend outpatient consultations, reducing waiting times, and providing access to medical records) has been implemented since 2015 with some success. Two recent policy documents on urban public hospital reforms and county hospital reforms have reiterated the call for quality assurance and improvement.[6]

In March 2015, the NHFPC took another important step in developing national institutional infrastructure and leadership in support of quality improvement. It established a national Medical Service Management and Guidance Center (MSMGC) with a range of mandates, including health technology assessment and technical support to local quality improvement efforts.

Challenges for Quality Improvement Policy

The rapid expansion and upgrading of health care infrastructure in China has laid the foundation for delivering higher-quality care, and the NHFPC has made earnest efforts to create the institutional and policy architecture essential to improve quality. The speed of policy change is impressive, but the depth of policy implementation and its impact remain to be seen. In addition, some shortcomings in the existing approach may limit its potential for quality improvement, as follows.

First, QoC regulation and evaluation emphasize entry qualifications and structural readiness (as indicated, for example, by setting up internal quality control committees). These tasks need to be broadened to encompass audit, control, and clinical processes and outcomes. For example, the current standards and assessment criteria cover more items related to structure (and give more weight to structural factors) than to processes and outcomes—that is, to how services are provided and the resulting benefits for patients. Although many health facilities in less-developed areas may still require investment in basic physical and human resources, China as a whole needs to advance its quality agenda with a stronger focus on monitoring and improving clinical processes and patient outcomes.

Second, institutional leadership for quality improvement remains elusive. The local MQCCs are conceived of as technical working groups rather than as permanent agencies with implementation capacity or administrative authority. The MSMGC's current focus is on health technology assessment, and it appears to give less attention to quality assurance, improvement, and M&E. Important functions that the MQCCs and the MSMGC are not set up to perform include harmonizing and mandating the use of national standardized measures of quality, managing quality M&E at the facility level, and coordinating efforts for quality improvement across various stakeholders. Moreover, as part of the NHFPC system, the focus is more on public hospitals rather than on providing institutional support to all providers. Within the NHFPC, the Department of Medical Service Management has the authority and technical capacity but insufficient resources to monitor and evaluate quality as a foundation for continuous quality improvement.

Third, to better support quality improvement across the health care system requires greater efforts to strengthen information systems, quality evaluation, and facility-level improvement initiatives, as follows:

- *Information systems, e-health, and reporting.* Regular reporting of clinical data has room for improvement in China. Facility-based information systems are not set up to collect such data. An undetermined number of tertiary hospitals (and, to a lesser extent, secondary hospitals) are required to report clinical data, albeit limited in scope. Even the available data are not regularly analyzed to provide insights on quality practices and outcomes. Researchers must sample often difficult-to-access medical records for clinical data, which is a costly process. Data are generally lacking on the QoC provided by secondary hospitals and primary care facilities.
- *Quality evaluation.* The government assesses and enforces regulatory compliance through periodic inspections. On their own, these inspections are unlikely to be sufficient to drive continuous

quality improvement on the front lines. The scope of annual on-site surveys is limited in part by the absence of verifiable data on processes and outcomes. As such, the assessments can be subjective, and the results are only shared between the evaluated hospital and the health administration. They are not disseminated to the public or other stakeholders or used to generate financial rewards and penalties.

- *Support for facility-level improvement initiatives.* Incentives and accountabilities for continuous quality improvement can be improved in China. Frontline providers are not incentivized to improve quality processes and outcomes. Health facilities are oriented toward increasing the quantity of services so they can generate revenue and enlarge market share, and their income is not directly affected by quality. The government does not provide funding support or incentives for quality improvement activities, nor (when evidence is available) does it penalize hospitals for having low quality or poor patient outcomes. The lack of an institutional focus on quality means that few hospitals are willing to invest in quality improvement initiatives.

International Experience in Improving Health System Quality

In the past 15 years, many OECD countries have recognized continuous quality improvement as a central goal of health sector development and have implemented systematic reforms to improve QoC. This new wave of quality improvement is occurring in the context of aging populations, an increasing burden of chronic diseases, and surging expenditures on health care. Governments in these countries are increasingly acting as stewards of public health and payers for health care, and they are driving the changes in health care delivery to improve QoC. They have evaluated the cost-effectiveness of new health interventions and technologies, developed quality measures and proposed new quality standards, and popularized modern management tools and practices to improve QoC. Their lessons are relevant for China's fast-evolving health system.

As discussed earlier, certain features and institutional arrangements in a country's health system form critical parts of the supporting infrastructure that is needed for improving quality and sustaining quality improvement. Box 3.1 summarizes

---

BOX 3.1 **Institutional arrangements for quality improvement in France, Germany, and the Netherlands**

The Haute Autorité de Santé (HAS) is the French independent public authority that certifies health facilities and practitioners; draws up best-practice recommendations; and evaluates health products and services, professional practice, and the organization of care and public health (Chevreul and others 2010). The Ministry of Health and HAS together establish a set of quality indicators, and both public and private health facilities are required to publish their quality performance yearly. In France, pharmaceuticals are evaluated for effectiveness and for their added benefits over other pharmaceuticals for the same indicators. Low-value pharmaceuticals are delisted from social health insurance.

In Germany, the Federal Joint Committee is legally authorized to evaluate all new and existing technologies for their appropriateness and cost effectiveness, and the Institute for Quality and Efficiency in Health Care provides technical capacity to scientifically evaluate health services. Their recommendations can lead to restriction of services under social health insurance.

The Netherlands in 2012 set up a Quality Institute that imposes a mandatory framework for the development of care standards, clinical guidelines, and performance measures, including using evidence-based medicine principles to assess established medical science and medical practices.

institutional arrangements in support of quality improvement in three European countries. The experience of Australia, the United Kingdom, and the United States in putting in place these building blocks is then examined in more detail below. The cases examine the countries' overall approaches to quality assurance and improvement, institutional leadership, accountability and control mechanisms, and management innovations.

United States: Public and Private Collaboration for Quality Improvement

The United States has been a leader in modern quality improvement in health care. In the 1980s, a double-digit increase in health spending drove a sense of urgency to strengthen regulations to prevent abusive use of medicine. In 1989, the U.S. Department of Health and Human Services (HHS) established the Agency for Health Care Policy and Research to enhance the quality, appropriateness, and effectiveness of health care services. The HHS used updated clinical guidelines and stringent peer review, combined with financial incentives, but it achieved little buy-in from health professionals and had little impact on QoC.

The IOM has played a critical role in driving the quality improvement agenda in the United States. Established in 1970, the IOM is an independent organization of eminent professionals from diverse fields including health and medicine; the natural, social, and behavioral sciences; and beyond who advise the government and others on medical and health policy issues. In 1996, the IOM convened a National Roundtable on Health Care Quality to review health service delivery and identify QoC-related issues. In a consensus report, the Roundtable concluded that serious and widespread quality problems existed throughout the American medical care system that harmed many people (Chassin and Galvin 1998). It also determined that the quality of health care can be precisely defined and measured with a degree of scientific accuracy comparable to that of most measures used in clinical medicine.

The IOM subsequently published two seminal reports that called for an overhaul of U.S. health care, proposed a strategic but action-oriented framework for quality improvement, and set a goal of a 50 percent reduction in medical errors in five years (IOM 2001; Kohn, Corrigan, and Donaldson 1999). The findings and the proposed improvement strategy in these reports were well received by policy makers, payers, and the medical professionals. The IOM placed quality improvement on the health care agenda; created a vision for quality improvement; and galvanized nationwide campaigns, further research, and quality improvement activities.

In 1999, the Agency for Healthcare Research and Quality (AHRQ) was established within HHS as the U.S. government's lead agency for research in health care quality. The AHRQ finances and acts as a clearinghouse for evidence to make health care safer; of higher quality; and more accessible, equitable, and affordable. It also works with stakeholders to ensure that such evidence is understood and used. For example, the AHRQ develops and updates clinical guidelines for a large and growing number of conditions. It also has produced quality indicators for inpatient and outpatient services, including for preventive measures, inpatient quality, patient safety, and pediatric care.

The AHRQ plays a significant role in the national effort to improve patient safety through national programs to reduce health care–associated infections, "science of safety" training programs, and the production and dissemination of patient safety toolkits. Free software is provided to any hospital to calculate these quality measures, which in turn are reported to the Centers for Medicare & Medicaid Services (CMS) according to quality regulations. In addition, the AHRQ publishes the annual *National Healthcare Quality and Disparities Report* (AHRQ 2017), which is mandated by Congress to measure progress in the national priority areas for improving QoC and reducing disparities in the care received by different racial and socioeconomic population groups.

Other government and nongovernmental organizations that are involved in developing and disseminating quality measures include the National Quality Forum (NQF), the Joint Commission of the National Committee for Quality Assurance, and the American Medical Association's Physician Consortium for Performance Improvement. The NQF is a private, nonprofit membership organization (and a federal government contractor) that was established to coordinate and endorse quality standards and quality measures that are produced by other organizations and agencies and used for public reporting. The NQF has more than 400 member organizations, representing consumers, health plans, medical professionals, employers, the government, pharmaceutical and medical device companies, and other quality improvement organizations. The NQF uses a multistep consensus development process to ratify measures before they are applied (as shown, for example, in its Ambulatory Care Project, described in box 3.2). Its independence and its ability to convene working groups of high-level technical authority have been instrumental to its success.

The NQF is best known for its reporting, first published in 2002, on serious reportable events (SREs), or "never" events—defined as 28 "preventable, serious, and unambiguously adverse events that should never occur" in a health care setting.[7] The Medicare program does not provide payment for the 28 "never" events because, literally, they should never occur.

Although medical professionals once frowned upon the idea of public reporting—and the evidence is still mixed on how it affects QoC—reporting is now a standard practice in the United States. The QoC provided by individual physicians, physician groups, health plans, and hospitals is measured and publicized through various organizations and programs.[8] The hope is that information about providers' quality will help protect consumers' rights, help them make better choices among providers, and hold providers accountable for the safety and quality of their services. In addition to public reporting, major payers (including the government's payer agency, CMS) have added financial incentives for quality performance to their payment schemes.

BOX 3.2   The Ambulatory Care Project of the National Quality Forum

Ambulatory care embraces a wide range of health conditions, services, and settings and is the primary form of care that patients receive. The demand for performance measures to evaluate all aspects of ambulatory care, including various settings of care, is growing rapidly.

Priorities are to ensure the safety, appropriateness, and effectiveness of outpatient care, the coordination of care, timely communication, pediatric urgent care, and the quality of clinicians' performance. Performance measures address issues including timely treatment, antibiotic use, patient admission and discharge, and appropriate documentation by staff.

The National Quality Forum's (NQF) Ambulatory Care Project is a multistage endeavor that seeks consensus on standardized measures of performance in outpatient care. Proposals for standards were solicited

through an open call for measures and were actively sought by NQF staff through literature reviews, a search of the Agency for Healthcare Research and Quality's National Quality Measures Clearinghouse, NQF member websites, and an environmental scan.

Using standardized evaluation criteria including scientific acceptability, usability, and feasibility, the Ambulatory Care Steering Committee evaluated 27 measures for appropriateness as voluntary consensus standards for accountability and public reporting. The chosen measures focus on the care of the following conditions and situations in the ambulatory care setting: heart disease, diabetes, hypertension, obesity, asthma, prevention, depression, medication management, patient experience with care, and care coordination.

Source: NQF 2008.

Private corporations are also exploring how they can support the achievement of better quality and lower cost. For example, in 1987 an experiment was launched, known as the National Demonstration Project on Quality Improvement in Health Care (NDP), in which 21 health care organizations participated in an eight-month study of the applicability of quality improvement methods typically used in industrial settings. Twenty-one companies agreed to support the 21 health care organizations during their studies by providing free consulting, materials, access to training courses, and reviews. The companies participating in this experiment included many of America's leading organizations, such as AT&T, Corning, Ford, Hewlett-Packard, IBM, and Xerox.

The results were impressive (Berwick and others 1990): Fifteen of the health care organizations made significant progress. Other hospitals reduced lengths of stay by nearly half for some procedures, reduced emergency room waiting times by 70 percent, and eliminated 67 percent of the time it took for physical examinations. One facility reduced infections after surgery by more than half.

The NDP was extended for three more years and evolved into the Institute for Healthcare Improvement (IHI), a nonprofit organization that provides leadership in redesigning health care to reduce errors, waste, delay, and unsustainable costs. The IHI takes an approach it calls the "science of improvement," which emphasizes rapid-cycle testing of innovations in the field, followed by rollout to generate learning about what changes, in which contexts, produce what types of improvements.[9]

In sum, the quality improvement efforts in the United States have been driven by the government, nonprofit organizations, and the private sector. Adherence to scientific models for measuring performance and improvement has been crucial for obtaining support from health professionals and for replicating success. The government is an important partner by financially supporting the organizations as well as by backing demonstration projects for quality improvement and knowledge creation.

United Kingdom: Publicly and Centrally Driven Quality Improvement

The quality improvement agenda in the United Kingdom's health sector has been largely led by the government through the Department of Health, which acts as a centralized provider of health sector information, services, and policy initiatives.

Extensive changes in health service delivery and quality regulation have occurred in the past few years. Before 2008, the National Health Service (NHS) focused on building system capacity and reducing patients' waiting time to ensure free access to needed health care for all. The NHS report, *High Quality Care for All: NHS Next Stage Review* proposed to move beyond the centrally driven performance management regime, with its focus on driving activity and meeting targets, to a new quality improvement agenda (DH 2008). The report set out recommendations to tackle variations in the quality of care, champion best practice, and enable greater competition and choice as a way to incentivize a culture of quality improvement (Keown and Darzi 2015). It presented a vision of a service in which quality improvement is driven by local clinicians armed with better data on the effectiveness of their own work, spurred on by financial incentives and by the choices of well-informed patients rather than by top-down targets. Operationally, the report endorsed more and better information about clinical performance and strengthening of incentives to improve quality (Maybin and Thorlby 2008).

Two years later, the Department of Health set out the most significant reorganization plan in NHS history (DH 2010). This removed responsibility for citizens' health from the secretary of state for health, abolished the primary care trusts and strategic health authorities (which had been responsible for enacting the directives and implementing the fiscal policy dictated by the Department of Health at the local and regional levels), and transferred £60–80 billion of health care funds from the primary care trusts to 211 clinical commissioning groups (CCGs) that are partly run by general practitioners. The new plan had significant implications for the regulation of the quality of care because the CCGs are to champion three key principles: putting patients at the center of the NHS, focusing on health outcomes in the measurement and review of QoC, and empowering health professionals.

The U.K. government has established the Health and Social Care Information Center as the national provider of information, data, and information technology systems for commissioners, analysts, and clinicians in health and social care. Its website provides a comprehensive guide to the NHS Outcomes Framework (box 3.3).[10] Established in 2010, this framework is intended to provide national-level accountability for the outcomes of NHS-provided health care as well as to drive transparency, quality improvement, and outcome measurement throughout the NHS. The NHS Commissioning Board's Outcome Indicator Set uses the same five-part structure as the Outcomes Framework (NHS Commissioning Board 2012). Patient-reported outcome measures have been added to the quality review; they focus on measuring health gains in patients undergoing hip replacement, knee replacement, and varicose-vein and groin-hernia surgery.

Besides collecting and maintaining data on health care (such as episode statistics for hospital-based and general practitioners' care), the Health and Social Care Information Center is also mandated to conduct clinical audits. For example, the National Diabetes Audit—the largest annual clinical audit in the world—measures the effectiveness of diabetes care in primary and secondary facilities against clinical guidelines and quality standards in England and Wales, and it publishes its report online. The audit collects and analyzes data for use by a range of stakeholders to drive changes and improvements in the quality of services and health outcomes for people with diabetes.

The well-known National Institute for Health and Clinical Excellence (NICE) is another arm's-length body of the U.K. Department of Health that develops clinical guidelines and care standards based on best evidence and assesses the efficacy and cost-effectiveness of health technologies and interventions used in the NHS. NICE provides technical leadership in government decisions on the allocation of resources for health care, and it supports evidence-based clinical care.

In the United Kingdom, although efforts to improve the quality of care are largely government-driven and top-down, the underlying goals and strategies are similar to those used in the United States. Several institutions and mechanisms in the United Kingdom have a similar structure to their U.S. counterparts. They include technical bodies that review evidence and develop clinical guidelines, develop comprehensive quality frameworks, hold providers accountable, conduct performance reviews and audits, and align incentives in support of quality improvement. In addition, both countries have supported pilots in organizational innovation designed to facilitate quality improvement at the organization level.

BOX 3.3   U.K. National Health Service outcomes indicator set, 2013/14

1. Preventing people from dying prematurely
2. Enhancing quality of life for people with long-term conditions
3. Helping people to recover from episodes of ill health or following injury
4. Ensuring that people have a positive experience of care
5. Treating and caring for people in a safe environment and protecting them from avoidable harm

Source: NHS Commissioning Board 2012.

A recent successful example of such a pilot in the United Kingdom is the centralization of cardiac and stroke services in London, which has led to reductions in mortality and length of hospital stay (box 3.4). It emphasizes that service reconfiguration can improve the quality of care by helping to create a critical mass of high-quality providers, imposing best-practice standards, and facilitating integrated pathways.

Australia: Central and State Government Collaboration for Quality Improvement

Like the United Kingdom, Australia has established a robust institutional infrastructure to promote, support, and guide quality improvement in health care. This includes the Commonwealth (federal) Department of Health (including the Medical Services Advisory Committee), the Australian Commission on Safety and Quality in Health Care, the National Health and Medical Research Council, and the Clinical Excellence Commission. These institutions develop clinical standards and guidelines, monitor and evaluate the performance of health care providers, assess the value of health interventions and technology, and offer quality-related information to providers and the public.

Australian Commission on Safety and Quality in Health Care

The Australian Commission on Safety and Quality in Health Care was established as a corporate Commonwealth entity after the Parliament of Australia passed the National Health Reform Act of 2011. The commission is jointly funded by all state and territorial governments on a cost-sharing basis, and its annual program of work is developed in consultation with the national, state, and territory health ministers. The commission led the development of the Australian Charter of

---

BOX 3.4   An innovative U.K. model to improve care for stroke patients

Receiving appropriate care is the single most important determinant of outcome for patients who have suffered a stroke. In several countries, acute stroke services are being centralized as a means of improving access to critical acute care, including rapid access to brain imaging and anticoagulant drugs, and to create fewer but higher-volume specialist services. Hospitals of different capabilities work together to create a centralized system of stroke care in which patients are taken to central specialist units rather than to the nearest hospital. Research in Australia, Canada, Denmark, the Netherlands, and the United States has shown the cost-effectiveness of this approach.

In 2010, stroke and major trauma were chosen as cases for piloting a new health care delivery model to improve patient outcomes, for two reasons: (a) good evidence on how to improve the quality of stroke care, and (b) a clinical community that desired change to improve such care. The new service delivery model split stroke care into hyperacute, acute, transient ischemic attack, and community care.

In the London pilot, change was governed by a top-down approach led by the regional health authority. The Manchester pilot, by contrast, used a more bottom-up, network-based approach led by local providers and commissioners. In London, 8 of the original 32 acute stroke service providers were converted to hyperacute stroke units (HASUs), and 24 became local stroke units (SUs) that delivered post hyper-acute care; stroke services were withdrawn from 5 hospitals. In Manchester, 3 HASUs and 10 SUs were created, and acute care was not entirely withdrawn from any hospitals. Both models resulted in reduced lengths of hospital stay, while London's also saw reduced mortality.

Moving forward, the establishment of specialist centers for rare diseases will also be considered to improve the coordination of care for patients. As part of the new care model, specialized providers will be encouraged to develop networks of services over a wider area, integrating different organizations and services around patient needs.

Sources: Morris and others 2014; Rudd 2011; Turner and others 2016.

Health Care Rights, the National Safety and Quality Health Service Standards, and the National Safety and Quality Framework.

Being a high-level coordinating and facilitating body, the commission is uniquely placed to advocate collaboration in patient safety and health care quality. The commission's Australian Safety and Quality Framework for Health Care was endorsed by the Australian health ministers in 2010. The framework provides a basis for preparing strategic and operational safety and quality plans, sets out guidance on priority areas, stipulates actions for research and clinical improvement in safety and quality, and promotes discussion among stakeholders about ways to improve partnership and collaboration.

Under the framework, safe, high-quality care should follow three core principles:

- It should be consumer- or patient-centered (so that people have timely and easy access to care and providers respond to their choices and needs).
- It should be driven by information (so that care decisions are guided by knowledge and evidence).
- It should be organized for safety (making safety and quality central to how health facilities are run).

The framework sets out 21 areas for action that stakeholders can take to improve the safety and quality of care provided in all health care settings.

The commission has also funded the National Indicators Project, which developed a set of 55 national indicators of safety and quality: 13 indicators apply to primary and community health services, 25 to hospitals, 6 to specialized health services, 5 to residential care for the elderly, and 11 to all types of health services.[11] The indicators measure safety, appropriateness, effectiveness, continuity, and responsiveness. Most of them focus on the appropriateness of care, responding to the growing emphasis on evidence-based health care and best-practice guidelines, while 25 relate to safety (AIHW 2009). Most of the indicators (40 out of 55) can be reported immediately using existing information systems. The Australian Institute of Health and Welfare reports these quality indicators publicly to (a) provide transparency and to inform decision making about overall priorities and system-level strategies for safety and quality improvement, and (b) shape the quality improvement activities of service providers.

Medical Services Advisory Committee

The Medical Services Advisory Committee (MSAC) is an independent expert group under the Commonwealth Department of Health and plays a role similar to that of the NICE in the United Kingdom. It advises the health minister on more appropriate, higher-value health care based on up-to-date evidence on the comparative safety, clinical effectiveness, and cost-effectiveness of new or existing medical services and technologies. It is also responsible for informing the health minister on whether medical services covered by Australia's publicly funded, fee-for-service Medicare Benefits Schedule (MBS) are sufficiently safe and cost-effective to warrant public subsidies. In addition, it produces technical guidelines on therapeutic and diagnostic services and provider-patient interaction.

In an intensive assessment of health technology in Australia, the MSAC recommended that the government develop a postmarket surveillance system for the MBS (Australian Government 2009). This system involves identifying priority technologies for review regarding appropriateness, efficacy, and cost-effectiveness. Outcomes could include delisting from the MBS, reducing payment fees, limiting the frequency or interval of services, or amending a service description or technology specifications to better capture the patient groups most likely to benefit from it. The MSAC also leads other reviews on primary health care and Medicare compliance rules.

National Health and Medical Research Council

Australia's National Health and Medical Research Council helps clinicians, researchers, policy makers, and consumers to access clinical guidelines via its online portal launched in March 2010. Within the council, the National Institute of Clinical Studies seeks to help close gaps between knowledge and clinical practice in health care.

The institute's publications include statistical analysis of clinical practices as they are currently performed and how they could be improved. Based on these reviews, the institute works in partnership with clinical groups and health care organizations to help improve the application of evidence to practice. It provides access to resources and evidence for health professionals, managers, researchers, and policy makers.

Clinical Excellence Commission

Because the Australian states and territories have independent decision powers for health policies, several have developed their own institutions to monitor and improve the safety and quality of care. An example is the Clinical Excellence Commission (CEC), which was established in 2004 to lead safety and quality improvement in the New South Wales health system.

The CEC's main activities include coordination of systemwide analyses of issues through audits and reviews, working collaboratively with health sector stakeholders, and implementing programs, projects, and initiatives to address identified issues. The CEC's Clinical Practice Improvement Series provides training for clinicians to improve the quality of care delivered and to improve patient outcomes, using an approach similar to the U.S. Institute for Health Care Improvement's "science of improvement" model.

Conclusion

As shown in these international examples, several OECD countries are trying to address the gaps in the quality of their care to deliver safer, more effective, and higher-value care that meets the public's changing demands. The Australian, United Kingdom, and United States cases also show striking similarities in the strategies applied: health technology assessment, dissemination of up-to-date clinical guidelines, clinical practice audit and review, public reporting and disclosure of information on the performance of specific facilities, financial incentives directed at providers, and health information and education. These three countries have created institutional arrangements within the government or in partnership with private organizations and academia to fulfill these functions.

Recommendations to China for Improving the Quality of Care

The challenges China faces with respect to QoC can be successfully addressed by creating unified leadership, suitable institutional architecture, stakeholder participation, and implementation tools to foster continuous quality improvement at all levels of the service delivery system. China may like to consider building a comprehensive strategic framework consisting of three core action areas:

1. Strengthening institutional leadership and system support
2. Establishing quality measurement and feedback mechanisms
3. Transforming organizational management to cultivate continuous quality improvement

Two additional core action areas—provider skills and patient engagement—are addressed in chapters 4 and 6. Table 3.3 displays the core action areas listed above and corresponding implementation strategies.

Core Action Area 1: Organizational Structure to Create Information Base and Develop Strategies for Quality Improvement

Government leadership and stewardship are vital for building capacity to improve the quality of health care. International experience points to three categories of activity that the government

TABLE 3.3   Three core QoC action areas and implementation strategies

Core action areas	Implementation strategies
1: Organizational structure to lead creation of an information base and development of strategies for quality improvement	• Explore options to cultivate a national coordination architecture to oversee systematic improvements to health sector quality • Conduct an in-depth national study of the quality of care and quality improvement initiatives at all levels of the system • Develop a national strategy for quality improvement
2: Systematic QoC measurement and continuous use of resulting data to support quality improvements	• Shift the measurement of quality from structure to process and outcomes • Create and maintain an atlas of variation in process quality and outcomes • Use measures of quality to improve performance • Establish an engagement model to support peer learning and energize collective quality improvement
3: Transformation of management practice to improve QoC in health facilities	• Promote evidence-based standardized care • Embed the "quality culture" in the management philosophy of health care organizations and promote modern managerial techniques • Use e-health innovations to support quality improvements

can consider: (a) expanding the mandate of current bodies or setting up additional ones to lead, oversee, and implement quality improvement initiatives; (b) conducting national reviews; and (c) developing nationwide approaches for quality enhancement.

Strategy 1: Cultivate a national coordination architecture to oversee systematic improvements

This architecture would be publicly responsible for coordinating all efforts aimed at quality assurance and improvement in health care and would actively engage all stakeholders to facilitate the implementation of quality assurance and improvement strategies for this purpose. It would have nine key functions:

• Ensure that national aims for quality are set
• Establish quality standards and develop quality measures
• Continuously measure and report on progress toward those standards
• Develop a standardized national medical curriculum, incorporating the best available scientific knowledge
• Ensure that the medical professions are certified to deliver care in accordance with these standards
• Oversee efforts to accredit and certify both public and private providers

• Define treatments and interventions that are reimbursable under social health insurance, based on cost-effectiveness analysis and ethical considerations
• Assess and promote clinical guidelines
• Conduct research and build the capacity needed to advance the continual improvement of quality care.

Stakeholder organizations, including the NHFPC, the Ministry of Finance, the Ministry of Human Resources and Social Security, key professional and scientific bodies, private providers, and the public could be represented in this coordination architecture.[12] The entity could also serve as the platform for tapping international expertise and sharing knowledge about care improvement. In the long run, it would serve as an important source of scientific information on all quality-related topics for both clinicians and the public. It would become the institutional leader in promoting QoC and ensuring that evidence-based care is consistently delivered to the highest standard.

As discussed earlier, several OECD countries have established such institutions over the past 15 years:

• *United Kingdom:* The NICE is responsible for developing evidence-based clinical guidelines and pathways and evaluating clinical interventions.[13]

- *France:* The national authority for health, HAS, is responsible for the assessment of drugs, medical devices, and procedures; the publication of guidelines; the accreditation of health care organizations; and the certification of doctors (Chevreul and others 2010).
- *The Netherlands:* The Quality Institute has crafted a mandatory framework for the development of care standards, clinical guidelines, and performance measures (VWS 2018).
- *United States:* The AHRQ supports the development of measures of quality, national reporting on quality, and research on quality.[14]
- *Germany:* The Institute for Quality and Efficiency in Health Care (IQWiG) is responsible for reviewing the evidence on diagnosis and therapy for selected conditions, providing evidence-based reports (for example, on drugs, nondrug interventions, and diagnostic and screening tests), and developing recommendations on disease management programs.[15]

Operationally, one option for China would be to broaden the mandate of the MSMGC to incorporate additional government and nongovernment actors and enhance its capacity to perform the recommended functions. Although the MSMGC already has some of these responsibilities, its limited staff (30), lack of stakeholder representation, and narrow focus on public hospitals may be insufficient to perform the proposed functions.

Another option would be to establish a coordination architecture directly under the State Council to ensure the highest-level authority to mobilize various public, private, and professional stakeholders. Importantly, the chosen institution will need to apply the same quality standards to both public and private facilities.

Strategy 2: Conduct a national study of QoC and quality-improvement initiatives at all levels

In many countries, efforts to improve health system performance have been catalyzed by comprehensive, evidence-based reports on quality and performance. These reports contribute to the collection of reliable information on performance and the analysis of problematic areas. They also help focus the attention of leaders and professionals on avoidable shortcomings in quality and on opportunities to do better for patients and communities. Such studies can bring quality issues to the forefront of the policy debate. Moreover, by showing the government's commitment to addressing real needs, they can also help to improve public confidence in the health care system.

For example, prompted by mounting evidence of quality failures, public demands, and increasing costs, several countries have carried out systematic reviews of national approaches to quality, assessed the status quo, and proposed recommendations. As mentioned earlier, two seminal IOM reports—*To Err is Human: Building a Safer Health System* and *Crossing the Quality Chasm: A New Health System for the 21st Century*—exposed the breadth and depth of health care quality issues in the United States and set out a strategy to address these failures (IOM 2001; Kohn, Corrigan, and Donaldson 1999). Another example is the "Quality in Australian Health Care Study" commissioned by the Australian Ministry of Health, which used retrospective clinical auditing methods to assess adverse events in hospitals (Wilson and others 1995). And in the United Kingdom, "A First-Class Service: Quality in the New NHS" highlighted key mechanisms for enhancing accountability, performance measurement, and inspection in health care (DH 1998).

Such studies are not yet available in China. China has piloted the collection of performance data and the monitoring of quality and patient safety in hospitals but has not yet published rigorous analyses of these data (Jiang and others 2015). Led by the proposed national authority for health care quality, similar research in China could systematically document quality problems related to structures, processes, and outcomes. Doing so would help to galvanize quality improvements throughout the nation.

To make this happen, an independent panel including both Chinese and international experts on health care quality, together with Chinese academic research institutions, could be commissioned to conduct the proposed study. The panel would summarize the findings and issue a comprehensive report on the QoC in China and recommend goals and targets for quality improvement and reforms in policy, training, and practice.

Strategy 3: Develop a national strategy for quality improvement

Drawing on the results of the proposed study, a strategy could be developed that would describe an acceptable level of quality, set forth quality goals, clarify the roles and responsibilities of stakeholders, and mandate activities at different levels.

An example along these lines is the U.S. National Strategy for Quality Improvement in Health Care, an annual report launched in 2011 after enactment of the Patient Protection and Affordable Care Act (HHS 2011). The strategy articulated three national aims—better care, healthy people/healthy communities, and affordable care—and six priorities:

- Making care safer by reducing harm caused in the delivery of care
- Ensuring that each person and their family are engaged as partners in their care
- Promoting effective communication and coordination of care
- Promoting the most effective prevention and treatment practices for leading causes of mortality
- Starting with cardiovascular disease, working with communities to promote wide use of best practices to enable healthy living
- Making quality care more affordable for individuals, families, employers, and government by developing and spreading new health care delivery models.

The aims and priorities of the strategy would form the basis for designing local initiatives and for monitoring progress.

The strategy would build on existing work (the national reviews would provide inputs to the strategy) and serve as an evolving guide for the nation. It could be revised annually with increasing refinements.

Core Action Area 2: Systematic QoC Measurement and Use of Data to Support Quality Improvements

A notable feature of quality improvement efforts in the past decade in OECD countries is their widespread use of quantitative data on health care processes and outcomes. Thanks to both proliferation of data and advancements in statistical methods, reliable indicators of quality are much easier to obtain today than in the past. These measures give policy makers a powerful tool to benchmark providers' quality, identify low and high performers, devise incentives to reward higher quality, and evaluate progress over time.

Strategy 1: Shift quality measurement from structure to process and outcomes

Structural quality is relatively easy to measure. Reliable data on infrastructure, equipment, and human resources are readily available in China. But as discussed earlier, although adequate structural quality is necessary, it is not sufficient to ensure better health care outcomes or experiences. Thus, measures are also needed to capture the processes of care between patients and providers. Development of such measures is more complex and should be conducted on the basis of the best scientific and clinical evidence or clinical guidelines. For example, to make evidence-based care the norm, doctors' clinical actions must be measured against recommended processes.

Changes in the quality of processes of care are in turn reflected in changes in outcomes. Measures of outcome, which center on survival rates and the extent of health and functional restoration as a result of health care, are arguably the measures that matter the most to the beneficiaries of any health system, and as such they are critical to measuring the performance of any patient-centered care model. Although data on patient outcomes like mortality and medical complications are collected in China, these data are broad measures and not useful for comparing quality across providers. For example, mortality analysis in China does not typically consider the differences in health risks among the patients admitted to hospitals, leading to estimates that are not comparable across health facilities.

Many OECD countries are making efforts to engage patients in quality assessment and developing tools to measure health outcomes from the patient perspective. Patient-reported outcome measures (PROMs) and patient-reported experience measures (PREMs) constitute feedback on patients' physical, mental, and social health and on how well they are managing their chronic diseases or health conditions. As noted in chapter 2, these measures may be incorporated into the quality measurement frameworks used for both integrated health systems and single health providers.

Strategy 2: Create and maintain an "atlas of variation" in process quality and outcomes

In most nations, China included, the quality of health care and outcomes varies from one place to another and even among clinicians in the same city. This variation derives from differences in professional opinions, habits, training, and application of scientific standards. The use of certain clinical procedures for specific conditions showing these large variations are considered "supply-sensitive" because they are largely due to provider choices (whether providers deem it necessary to admit a patient or perform a surgery), not science or patient preferences.

Controlling variation begins with understanding it. For example, significant variations in elective surgeries (such as tonsillectomy or prostatectomy) and hospitalization associated with chronic diseases have been documented in the United States and internationally (Wennberg 2010). Xu and others (2015) found that after adjustment for differences in patients' risk, variations in patient outcomes are significant among Beijing's tertiary public hospitals.

China may consider developing a Chinese version of the Dartmouth Atlas of geographic variations in health care to inform the public and professionals about differences in practice on important health topics. The Dartmouth Atlas of Health Care is a U.S. map of regional variations in health care quality, outcomes, costs, and utilization.[16] In the United Kingdom, the NHS Atlas series offers similar insights.[17]

Measuring regional variations allows leaders to identify opportunities to improve care through standardization. Regional data can help to uncover best practices that should be spread more widely and can reveal where inappropriate, excessive, or deficient care is occurring. Under the supervision of the proposed authority responsible for quality, a designated team could create an atlas of variation for China.

Strategy 3: Use measures of quality to improve performance

Three ways in which quality measures can be applied to improve frontline quality are accreditation, public reporting, and pay-for-performance incentives. Together they can provide a comprehensive system for providing performance feedback and incentives for improvement.

Accreditation. In the United States, reporting of quality-related data and measures is mandatory for hospital accreditation, which in turn is a prerequisite for hospitals to participate in the public insurance schemes, Medicare and Medicaid. The Joint Commission, an independent organization responsible for accrediting health facilities in the United States, requires accredited hospitals to report data for at least six core sets of measures for specific conditions or processes (such as acute myocardial infarction, perinatal care, stroke, emergency department visits, surgical improvement projects, and venous thromboembolism), drawing from patients' medical charts or electronic medical records.

For public and private hospitals seeking accreditation, China can consider requiring the reporting of data on quality.

Public reporting. Making quality measures publicly available is an effective way to create peer pressure among providers and to encourage them to pursue quality improvement by making them aware that they are being monitored. Public disclosure of quality measures can also help patients make informed choices among providers based on their safety and quality performance. In the past decade, this has become the norm in OECD countries.

For example, in the United States, state-level maps for benchmarking quality can be found on the AHRQ website, and information on quality at the level of individual facilities and health plans can be found on multiple websites, including Hospital Compare, managed by the CMS, and the sites of the National Committee for Quality Assurance and the Joint Commission.[18] In France, similarly, information on the quality of providers is published online on the Scope Santé website,[19] and in Canada, it is provided by the Canadian Institute of Health Information.[20]

The CMS's Hospital Compare site allows users to compare three hospitals at a time on seven quality dimensions: surveys of patients' experiences, timely and effective care, complications, readmissions and deaths, use of medical imaging, payment, and value of care. Patients using the site may choose the most suitable hospital based on their needs and preferences.

Pay-for-performance incentives. Pay-for-quality (P4Q) schemes provide financial incentives to improve quality. Although their impact has been mixed and depends on the design of the incentives, several countries have adopted such schemes.

In the United States, the CMS began in 2004 to financially penalize hospitals that did not report to CMS the same performance data they collected for the Joint Commission; they also decided they would no longer pay for the 28 "never" events (as defined earlier). In addition, the CMS

initiated two P4Q programs: (a) the Hospital Readmission Reduction program, which links payments to a hospital's performance in reducing readmissions for selected high-cost or high-volume conditions like heart attack, heart failure, and pneumonia; and (b) the Hospital Value-Based Purchasing Program, in which Medicare adjusts a portion of its payment to hospitals based on how well they perform on quality measures and how much progress they make in quality improvement.

The U.K. government in 2004 introduced a pay-for-performance scheme to recognize quality in family practice, covering the management of chronic diseases, practice organization, and patients' experience of care. Payments under the scheme make up as much as 25 percent of a family practitioner's income (Doran and Roland 2010; Kroneman and others 2013). Some evidence shows that the impact on quality improvement is enhanced when public reporting is coupled with P4Q incentives (Lindenauer and others 2007; Werner and others 2009).

The concept of pay-for-performance has gained prominence in China in recent years. Although a payment system could be implemented based on practitioners' workloads, service quality, and patient satisfaction, China's lack of standardized measures and the still-dominant fee-for-service incentives for revenue generation make this challenging. P4Q schemes are ideally designed to avoid unintended cost-shifting. This occurred, for example, when an experiment in Guizhou removed incentives for overprescribing medication. Doctors responded by increasing their nondrug services such as injections and unnecessary referrals to hospital care—which in turn raised total health care costs (Wang and others 2013). But there are promising examples. For example, in Ningxia Province, an intervention that combined capitation with P4Q incentives reduced antibiotic prescriptions and total outpatient spending without significant adverse effects on other aspects of care (Yip and others 2014).[21]

Strategy 4: Establish an engagement model to support peer learning and energize collective quality improvement

Besides benchmarking their own quality to that of peer organizations, hospitals should be encouraged to share valuable lessons and to support each other in transforming organizations toward better quality and collectively achieving clearly defined goals. Examples of such mutual support in the United States are the CMS Partnership for Patients and the hospital engagement networks. Physicians, nurses, hospitals, employers, patients and their advocates, and the federal and state governments have joined to form the Partnership for Patients, adopting common goals to make care safer and improve care transitions.

The hospital engagement networks help to identify successful ways to reduce hospital-acquired conditions and work to spread these approaches to other hospitals and health care providers. A form of provider-to-provider peer network to share information and learning is proposed in chapter 10.

Core Action Area 3: Transformation of Management to Improve QoC

Effective organizational management is indispensable for safety and quality assurance. Even capable health professionals can make mistakes in hectic, often overcrowded clinical environments where they are practicing increasingly complex medical interventions. Managers can use known and tested tools to support quality improvement.

Strategy 1: Promote evidence-based standardized care

Clinical guidelines and pathways are valuable tools to standardize care and reduce variations in practice. With technical assistance from the United Kingdom's NICE, China's Ministry of Health has developed evidence-based clinical pathways and applied them in several pilot reforms in rural public hospitals. The intent is to standardize procedures and limit providers' discretionary prescription of services and drugs.

A preliminary evaluation suggests that implementing the pathways reduced patients' average hospital stay and curbed unnecessary services (Cheng 2013). Patients paid less out of pocket, and a substantial improvement in communication and relations between patients and providers raised the satisfaction of both groups.

However, other studies have noted that managers and physicians resisted implementing the clinical pathways because doing so would cause them to lose income. Managers were driven by revenue generation and did not see clinical pathways as a useful managerial instrument (He, Yang, and Hurst 2015). China may consider analyzing lessons from these experiences to inform the further development and adoption of clinical pathways.

China has no standard evidence-based system for ensuring nationwide standardized care, nor for continuously aligning Chinese guidelines with appropriate worldwide clinical standards adapted to China. It is important to develop a larger set of standardized clinical pathways and to mandate their use in all hospitals. Under the guidance of the proposed national authority, and with the assistance of prestigious Chinese hospitals, professional associations, and clinical leadership groups, evidence-based care guidelines can be created or adopted based largely on international standards and then modified to suit the characteristics of the Chinese health system. The standards could focus on evidence-based care protocols, use of appropriate medication, person-centered care, and skills and methods for continuous quality improvement.

Strategy 2: Embed "quality culture" in management philosophy and promote modern managerial techniques

High-quality health care does not arise from inspection alone. To ensure safety and sustain quality improvement requires a "quality culture" and continuous attention to quality improvement from managers and staff. Important elements of a quality culture are an openness toward errors, a relatively flat management hierarchy, collaborative teamwork in a learning environment, and a focus on continuous system improvement.

In contrast, an accountability mechanism that centers on individuals and punishes them for errors by "naming and shaming" discourages providers from reporting errors and reinforces a deeply embedded belief that high-quality care results simply from being well trained and trying hard. Some evidence suggests that "naming and shaming" may still be a common management practice. A survey of employees of six secondary general public hospitals in Shanghai in 2013 found that although hospital staff are generally positive about the safety climate in their workplace, "fear of blame" and "fear of shame" are two important concerns. In the United States, these are among providers' smallest concerns (Zhou and others 2015).

Sound scientific evidence exists for treating many health conditions—evidence that can drive care improvement and, in some cases, reduce costs. But much of this evidence is not fully applied in daily clinical practice. Identifying and filling the gap between what is *known* and what is *done* requires continuous quality improvement efforts at any health facility. Health facilities can improve quality by using some of the modern managerial approaches shown to change health workers' behaviors and optimize the clinical care system (Deming 2000; Langley and others 2009):

- *Continuous quality improvement (CQI) and total quality management (TQM)* approaches emphasize a continuous effort by all members of the organization to meet the needs and expectations of clients; managers and clinicians work together to identify undesirable variations in the process of care and try to eliminate them.
- *Six Sigma* targets aim to reduce error rates to six standard deviations from the process mean, to ensure standardized service where appropriate.
- *The Plan-Do-Study-Act (PDSA) cycle* is a mechanism in which clinical teams learn how to apply key ideas for change to their organizations in a series of testing cycles,

using specific and measurable aims that are tracked over time.

These and other management approaches can be combined and flexibly applied. The need is to use them to cultivate a sense of continuous attention to improving the quality of management practices. Some are already being applied in some large Chinese hospitals. For example, Anzhen Hospital has applied the PDSA cycle to hospital strategic management (Nie, Wei, and Cui 2014), and Peking University People's Hospital has used TQM with PDSA to improve the efficiency of specialist clinic registration (Chen and others 2014). Lessons from these experiences should be examined, and similar initiatives expanded, throughout China.[22]

Strategy 3: Use e-health innovations to support quality improvements

Many nations are investing substantially in (a) electronic health (e-health) and mobile health (m-health) tools, seeking new efficiencies using electronic health records; (b) computerized decision-support systems; (c) picture archiving and communication systems; and (d) remote patient monitoring and other technologies.

Electronic health records. EHRs form the bedrock of e-health systems because they capture fundamental patient data, often including images, patient histories, and relevant nonclinical data. EHR platforms allow data to be captured, manipulated, and shared, potentially reducing errors and improving efficiencies within and across health facilities and systems. EHRs can also form a central IT hub through which other e-health mechanisms (such as computerized order entry for physicians) can be run. Platforms such as electronic workstations accomplish similar goals while increasing clinicians' mobility. In some cases, in addition to improving efficiency, EHRs help to improve clinicians' practice and ultimately yield gains in both quality and safety.

In the United States, for example, an EHR system was shown to have positive effects on the quality of pediatric care

(Adams, Mann, and Bauchner 2003). At the Boston Medical Center's Pediatric Primary Care Center—a clinic with more than 28,000 annual patient visits—clinicians used the Automated Record for Child Health (ARCH), a point-and-click interface reminiscent of the paper records with which they were already familiar. Placed in each examination room, ARCH allowed clinicians to record routine health maintenance; maintain lists of problems and medications; monitor patients' growth; record obstetrical history, medical history, and family history; view limited laboratory data; link to internet-based resources; and print reports. ARCH prompted clinicians to ask about and record certain risk factors that, when tracked over time, provided a longitudinal view of health not provided by the paper-based method. The researchers found that the clinicians using ARCH were significantly more likely than clinicians using paper-based records to address routine health maintenance topics such as diet, sleep, psychosocial issues, smoking in the home, exposure to violence, and behavioral or social developmental milestones. Clinicians who used ARCH reported that the use of the system had improved overall QoC and the guidance they gave families. Although some users noted that the use of the system reduced eye-to-eye contact with patients, they all recommended its continued use.

In Huangzhong in 2013, the Qinghai Provincial Health Department equipped each of 30 village clinics with a general practitioner (GP) workstation: an electronic system that allows physicians to conduct medical examinations, perform tests, download data from their current location, and upload data to the regional health system (Meng and others 2015). The workstations are portable, so practitioners can travel with them and bring high-quality, reliable health care to patients' homes. THC personnel perform routine checks on the system every three months and respond to issues reported by village-level providers as needed. The workstations have improved information sharing between the village and the county level. GPs can use the platform to secure expert knowledge from higher-level health facilities, whose staff can view the data uploaded by the GPs and provide feedback. The workstations have also greatly improved the performance of providers at the village level, who have benefited both from the connection to providers in THCs and from content sources such as the standardized formulary and care standards that are embedded in the system. Users have responded positively to the workstations, noting improved patient satisfaction due to the trusted results of the technology.

Computerized decision-support systems. CDSSs are electronic platforms that integrate clinical and demographic data to support decision making by clinicians. They can serve a number of purposes, such as improving e-prescribing—sometimes considered its own form of CDSS—or providing treatment recommendations. CDSSs generally include active or passive prompts to guide clinicians' decisions with the goal of standardizing care and reducing errors to improve quality and safety (Black and others 2011). Factors that can influence the usefulness of CDSSs include clinician training and the quality of customization based on the intended goals of the system. In the examples below, CDSSs have been successfully used to improve quality and reduce errors.

In Feixi in 2014, the county Bureau of Health introduced a standardized formulary policy to regulate providers' prescribing behaviors and to ensure that medications are used safely in THCs and village clinics. A recommended list of medications for 50 common outpatient conditions THC and village clinic providers might encounter, such as influenza and bronchitis, was integrated into the district's computerized information system. The system also contains predefined prescription packages. When a village provider inputs a particular diagnosis and related symptoms, the computer system proposes medications to recommend. Providers must choose from among the options presented by the system. Feixi's CDSS has standardized the prescription behaviors of primary health care providers and enhanced safety and reliability for patients.

Similar gains through CDSSs have been documented in the United States. In one example, physicians at a university hospital clinic received a CDSS, accessible on their handheld personal digital assistants, to guide the prescription of nonsteroidal inflammatory drugs (Berner and others 2006). The CDSS, called MedDecide, contained a suite of clinical prediction rules based on evidence-based literature. The study found that the physicians who used the system prescribed more safely than those who did not and that they documented more complete assessments of the risks to patients. Though it is a narrowly defined example, this trial highlights how mobile technology and CDSSs can support physicians in making safer treatment decisions and that m-health programs at the point of care can improve clinicians' performance in the ambulatory setting.

Picture archiving and communication systems. PACS are clinical IT systems that allow facilities to acquire, archive, process, and distribute digital images (such as radiological scans) to improve the quality of patient care (Black and others 2011). They are often integrated with EHRs and are designed to encourage the scaling of expertise within and across facilities. Through PACS, physicians can share images with clinicians within the facility or externally and receive expert advice and treatment recommendations via the platform. Some countries have successfully implemented PACS to extend the reach of their specialists.

Hangzhou provides a strong example of such a system in China. The city began in 2013 to better integrate its municipal tertiary hospitals with CHCs (Yan 2015). PACS were used to establish regional e-consultation centers for medical imaging and electrocardiograms. The reform was designed to increase the access of CHC-based primary care providers to the expertise in municipal hospitals, build higher-quality capacity at those CHCs, and increase patients' access to expert imaging services. Hangzhou structured its e-consultation network in four distinct

cooperation groups that were organized by the municipal hospitals. Each hospital provided a site to house one medical imaging e-consultation center and one electrocardiogram (ECG) e-consultation center; it also provided a director, staff, and supporting facilities, along with training and technical support for the physicians at the CHCs.

Much of this program was supported by implementation plans and technical guidance from the Hangzhou government and the Hangzhou Bureau of Health, which sets requirements for e-consultation services and regulates program implementation. Currently, the PACS services are provided free of charge to CHCs and patients and are funded by the bureau. The bureau also compensates municipal hospitals retroactively based on the number of e-consultations performed during the year at the following rates: RMB 30 for each case of ordinary imaging e-consultation, RMB 50 for each case of CT or magnetic resonance diagnosis e-consultation, and RMB 10 for each case of ECG e-consultation. By the end of 2013 in the Xiacheng district, imaging e-consultation services through PACS were available to 46 CHCs, and more than 300 e-consultation cases had been evaluated. Through 2014 in the Jiang-gan district, more than 20,755 ECG submissions and 16,425 imaging submissions had been reviewed through the e-consultation centers.

Remote patient monitoring. Remote patient monitoring is a broad term encompassing technologies that allow clinicians to observe patients outside of conventional settings, such as from the patient's home or from a care setting where the physician is not physically present. Remote patient monitoring has the potential to extend physicians' reach, increase the time physicians have available to treat patients, and more actively engage patients in their care. A number of examples of remote patient monitoring for both inpatient and outpatient care show the positive impact it can have on both quality and safety for patients.

In an outpatient example, a U.S. study shows the potential benefits of a mobile-phone-based self-management aid for adolescents suffering from asthma (Rhee and others 2014). Recognizing the potential benefits of the self-management of asthma, as well as the portability and accessibility of mobile phones, the investigators evaluated whether mobile-phone technology could facilitate symptom monitoring, treatment adherence, and adolescent-parent partnerships for asthma. The system allowed adolescents to communicate via short message service (SMS) text in natural English and to initiate interactions with an automated support system. Participants received reminder texts from the system, such as for taking medication. They could also interact with the system through scheduled or unscheduled communications to share their concerns about symptoms, medications, or other asthma-related activity. The system would automatically generate responses that were evaluated by certified asthma educators who could step in and respond through the system. Parents of participants received automatically generated emails from the system informing them of their adolescent's asthma-control levels, levels of activity, frequency of use of rescue medication (such as albuterol), and use of control medication.

The study found that the response rates from adolescents to the system's text messages were 81–97 percent and that adolescents initiated a message to the system an average of 19 times over a two-week trial period. Post-trial focus groups illuminated how beneficial the m-health intervention had been for adolescents with asthma, indicating that it had raised patients' awareness of symptoms and triggers, improved self-management and medication adherence, and improved their sense of control over asthma. Overall, the mobile support platform improved the quality of asthma care for these adolescents, and illustrates how, for certain patient populations, m-health is a useful lever for promoting QoC.

Conclusion

This chapter has reviewed the challenges China faces in enhancing the quality and value of care and has proposed a set of recommendations based on experience in China and OECD countries. We recommend that the government continue to engage all stakeholders in the health sector to publicly affirm its quality improvement goals, strengthen technical leadership through M&E of clinical care quality, and foster improvement at the front line by supporting innovations in health care delivery and spreading successful experiences. The reforms in the delivery of health care proposed here are aligned with the "supply-side reforms" that were introduced by the Chinese government in 2015 and early 2016, which will be a key lever for building the PCIC model.

Notes

1. For resources on national-level quality indicators, see the following: "Quality Measures," Centers for Medicare & Medicaid Services (https://www.cms.gov/Medicare/Quality-Initiatives-Patient-Assessment-Instruments/QualityMeasures/index.html?redirect=/QUALITYMEASURES); the World Health Organization's Performance Assessment Tool for Quality Improvement in Hospitals (PATH) project (http://www.pathqualityproject.eu and Veillard and others [2005]); and the OECD's Health Care Quality Indicators (HCQI) project (http://www.oecd.org/els/health-systems/health-care-quality-indicators.htm and Arah and others [2003]).

2. Barefoot doctors are "farmers who received a short medical and paramedical training, to offer primary medical services in their rural villages" (Yang and Wang 2017).

3. See, for example, the "General Hospital Evaluation Standards" (revised version) in 2009; "Tertiary Hospital Accreditation Standards" in 2011 (*Weiyiguan Fa* 2011, No. 33); and "Secondary Hospital Accreditation Standards" in 2012. "Requirements on Medical Errors and Adverse Events Reporting" were announced in 2011 (*Weiyiguan Fa* 2011, No. 4).

4. "Guidelines on Antimicrobial Drug Use," NHFPC (2012, No. 84); NHFPC 2015.

5. "Guiding Opinions on the Implementation of Clinical Pathways During the Twelfth Five-Year Plan Period," Department of Medical Service Management, Ministry of Health (*Weiyizhen Fa* 2012, No. 65).

6. "Guidance of the General Office of the State Council on Overall Pilot Reform of Urban Public Hospitals," State Council General Office (*Guo Ban Fa 2015*, No. 38); and "Opinions of the State Council on Comprehensively Scaling-Up Reform of County-Level Public Hospitals," State Council (*Guo Ban Fa* 2015, No. 33).

7. Regarding SREs, see "Serious Reportable Events," National Quality Forum Topics (accessed June 28, 2018), http://www.qualityforum.org/topics/sres/serious_reportable_events.aspx.

8. See, for example, hospital indicators in the Medicare Hospital Compare datasets (https://data.medicare.gov/data/hospital-compare), which enable people to compare the quality of care at more than 4,000 Medicare-certified hospitals across the United States.

9. For more information, see "How to Improve," IHI website (accessed June 28, 2018), http://www.ihi.org/resources/Pages/HowtoImprove.

10. For the NHS Outcomes Framework website, see https://digital.nhs.uk/data-and-information/publications/ci-hub/nhs-outcomes-framework.

11. The National Indicators Project was undertaken by the Australian Institute of Health and Welfare in close consultation with the commission and a wide range of clinical and other stakeholders.

12. Chapter 4 includes a discussion on engaging patients and the public in the development and reporting of quality measures.

13. For details, see the NICE website: https://www.nice.org.uk/.

14. For details, see the AHRQ website: https://www.ahrq.gov.

15. For details, see the IQWiG website: https://www.iqwig.de/en.

16. For more information on the Dartmouth Atlas, see the website: http://www.dartmouthatlas.org/.

17. For details on the NHS Atlas series, see https://www.england.nhs.uk/rightcare/products/atlas/.

18. For these quality-related data features, see "National Healthcare Quality and Disparities Reports," AHRQ, http://nhqrnet.ahrq.gov/inhqrdr/state/select?utm_source=AHRQ-EN&utm_medium=article&utm_campaign=SS2015; "Hospital Compare," CMS, https://www.medicare.gov/hospitalcompare/search.html; "HEDIS & Performance Measurement," National Committee for Quality Assurance, http://www.ncqa.org/HEDISQualityMeasurement.aspx; and "Pioneers in Quality," Joint Commission, http://www.joint-commission.org/accreditation/top_performers.aspx.

19. For France's Scope Santé website, see http://www.scopesante.fr/.

20. For the Canadian Institute of Health Information's "Health System Performance" resources, see https://www.cihi.ca/en/health-system-performance.

21. Capitation is a payment arrangement for health care providers such as physicians or nurse practitioners. It pays a physician or group of physicians a set amount per period of time for each enrolled person assigned to them, per period of time, whether or not that person seeks care.

22. Chapter 10 presents an approach for scaling up care improvement that applies the PDSA cycle.

References

Abdullah, A. S., F. Qiming, V. Pun, F. A. Stillman, and J. M. Samet. 2013. "A Review of Tobacco Smoking and Smoking Cessation Practices among Physicians in China: 1987–2010." *Tobacco Control* 22 (1): 9–14.

Adams, W. G., A. M. Mann, and H. Bauchner. 2003. "Use of an Electronic Medical Record Improves the Quality of Urban Pediatric Primary Care." *Pediatrics* 111 (3): 626–32.

AHMAC (Australian Health Ministers' Advisory Council). 1996. "The Final Report of the Taskforce on Quality in Australian Health Care." AHMAC report, Council of Australian Governments (COAG) Health Council, Adelaide, South Australia.

AHRQ (Agency for Healthcare Research and Quality). 2017. "2016 Healthcare Quality and Disparities Report." AHRQ Publication No. 17-0001, U.S. Department of Health and Human Services, Rockville, MD.

AIHW (Australian Institute of Health and Welfare). 2009. *Towards National Indicators of Safety and Quality in Health Care*. Canberra: AIHW.

Allegranzi, Benedetta, S. B. Nejad, C. Combescure, W. Graafmans, H. Attar, L. Donaldson, and D. Pittet. 2011. "Burden of Endemic Health-Care-Associated Infection in Developing Countries: Systematic Review and Meta-Analysis." *The Lancet* 377 (9761): 228–41.

Andel, Charles. 2012. "The Economics of Health Care Quality and Medical Errors." *Journal of Health Care Finance* 39 (1): 39.

Arah, O. A., N. Klazinga, N. S. Klazinga, D. M. J. Delnoij, A. H. A. Ten Asbroek, and T. Custers. 2003. "Conceptual Frameworks for Health Systems Performance: A Quest for Effectiveness, Quality, and Improvement." *International Journal for Quality in Health Care* 15 (5): 377–98.

Australian Government. 2009. "Review of Health Technology Assessment in Australia: A Discussion Paper." Department of Health and Ageing, Australian Government, Canberra.

Baicker, Katherine, and Amitabh Chandra. 2004. "Medicare Spending, the Physician Workforce, and Beneficiaries' Quality of Care." *Health Affairs* 23 (3): 184–97.

Berner, E. S., T. K. Houston, M. N. Ray, J. J. Allison, G. R. Heudebert, W. W. Chatham, and R. S. Maisiak. 2006. "Improving Ambulatory Prescribing Safety with a Handheld Decision Support System: A Randomized Controlled Trial." *Journal of the American Medical Informatics Association* 13 (2): 171–79.

Berwick, Donald, M. Godfrey, A. Blanton, and Jane Roessner. 1990. *Curing Health Care: New Strategies for Quality Improvement.* San Francisco: Jossey-Bass.

Berwick, Donald, Thomas W. Nolan, and John Whittington. 2008. "The Triple Aim: Care, Health, and Cost." *Health Affairs* 27 (3): 759–69.

Bhattacharyya, Onil, Yin Delu, Sabrina T. Wong, and Chen Bowen. 2011. "Evolution of Primary Care in China 1997–2009." *Health Policy* 100 (2): 174–80. doi:10.1016/j.healthpol.2010.11.005.

Bi, Yufang, Runlin Gao, Steve Su, Wei Gao, Dayi Hu, Dejia Huang, Lingzhi Kong, and others. 2009. "Evidence-Based Medication Use among Chinese Patients with Acute Coronary Syndromes at the Time of Hospital Discharge and One Year after Hospitalization: Results from the Clinical Pathways for Acute Coronary Syndromes in China Study." *American Heart Journal* 157 (3): 509–16.

Black, A. D., J. Car, C. Pagliari, C. Anandan, K. Cresswell, T. Bokun, and A. Sheikh. 2011. "The Impact of e-Health on the Quality and Safety of Health Care: A Systematic Overview." *PLoS Medicine* 8 (1): e1000387.

Brook, R. H. 1995. "The RAND/UCLA Appropriateness Method." Publication No. RP-395 (reprinted by RAND Corp.), U.S. Department of Health and Human Services, Washington, DC.

Campbell, Dennis. 2014. "NHS Wastes over £2bn a Year on Unnecessary or Expensive Treatments." *The Guardian*, November 5.

CDC (Centers for Disease Control and Prevention). 2018. "National Healthcare Safety Network (NHSN): Patient Safety Component Manual." Division of Healthcare Quality Promotion, CDC, Atlanta. http://www.cdc.gov/nhsn/pdfs/pscmanual/pcsmanual_current.pdf.

Chassin, Mark, and Robert Galvin. 1998. "The Urgent Need to Improve Health Care Quality: Institute of Medicine National Roundtable on Health Care Quality." *JAMA* 280 (11): 1000–05.

Chen, Ming, Hongmei Zhao, Saijun Jia, Lihua Wang, and Yue Zhao. 2014. "Total Quality Management: Improving the Procedure of Additional Registration in Specialist Clinic." *Chinese Hospitals* 18 (1).

Cheng, Tsung-Mei. 2013. "A Pilot Project Using Evidence-Based Clinical Pathways and Payment Reform in China's Rural Hospitals Shows Early Success." *Health Affairs* 32 (5): 963–73.

Chevreul, Karine, Isabelle Durand-Zaleski, Stéphane Bahrami, Cristina Hernández-Quevedo, and Philipa Mladovsky. 2010. "France: Health System Review." *Health Systems in Transition* 12 (6).

Dajiang Net. 2012. "Who Will Bear the Rating Consumption of Invalid Tertiary Hospitals?" [title in English translation]. Opinion letter, jxnews.com, August 28. http://jxcomment.jxnews.com.cn/system/2012/08/28/012087450.shtml.

Dayal, Prarthna, and Krishna Hort. 2015. *Quality of Care: What Are Effective Policy Options for Governments in Low- and Middle-Income Countries to Improve and Regulate the Quality of Ambulatory Care?* Policy Brief 4 (1). Manila: World Health Organization, on behalf of the Asia Pacific Observatory on Health Systems and Policies.

Deming, William Edwards. 2000. *The New Economics: For Industry, Government, Education.* Cambridge, MA: MIT Press.

de Silva, D., and J. Bamber. 2014. "Improving Quality in General Practice." Evidence Scan No. 23, The Health Foundation, London.

DH (Department of Health). 1998. "A First-Class Service: Quality in the New NHS." Consultation document, Her Majesty's Stationery Office (HMSO), London.

———. 2008. "High Quality Care for All: NHS Next Stage Review Final Report." Consultation document, Her Majesty's Stationery Office (HMSO), London.

———. 2010. *Equity and Excellence: Liberating the NHS.* London: Her Majesty's Stationery Office (HMSO).

Dlugacz, Yosef D., Andrea Restifo, and Alice Greenwood. 2004. *The Quality Handbook for Health Care Organizations: A Manager's Guide to Tools and Programs.* New York: John Wiley.

Donabedian, Avedis. 2005. "Evaluating the Quality of Medical Care." *Milbank Quarterly* 83 (4): 691–729.

Doran, Tim, and Martin Roland. 2010. "Lessons from Major Initiatives to Improve Primary Care in the United Kingdom." *Health Affairs* 29 (5): 1023–29. doi:10.1377/hlthaff.2010.0069.

Fan, Yunzhou, Zhaoxia Wei, Weiwei Wang, Li Tan, Hongbo Jiang, Lihong Tian, Yuguang Cao, and Shaofa Nie. 2014. "The Incidence and Distribution of Surgical Site Infection in Mainland China: A Meta-Analysis of 84 Prospective Observational Studies." *Scientific Reports* 4: 6783.

He, Jingwei Alex, Wei Yang, and Keith Hurst. 2015. "Clinical Pathways in China: An Evaluation." *International Journal of Health Care Quality Assurance* 28 (4).

Hesketh, Therese, Dan Wu, Linan Mao, and Nan Ma. 2012. "Violence against Doctors in China." *BMJ* 345: e5730.

HHS (U.S. Department of Health and Human Services). 2011. "Report to Congress: National Strategy for Quality Improvement in Health Care." Planning report pursuant to the Affordable Care Act, Agency for Healthcare Research and Quality (AHRQ), Rockville, MD.

IMS Institute for Healthcare Informatics. 2013. "Avoidable Costs in U.S. Health Care: The $200 Billion Opportunity from Using Medicines More Responsibly." Study report, IMS Institute for Healthcare Informatics, Parsippany, NY.

IOM (Institute of Medicine). 2001. *Crossing the Quality Chasm: A New Health System for the 21st Century.* Washington, DC: National Academies Press for the Committee on Quality of Health Care in America.

Jiang, Lixin, Harlan Krumholz, Xi Li, Jing Li, and Shengshou Hu. 2015. "Achieving Best Outcomes for Patients with Cardiovascular Disease in China by Enhancing the Quality of Medical Care and Establishing a Learning Health-Care System." *The Lancet* 386 (10002): 1493–1505.

Keown, Oliver P., and Ara Darzi. 2015. "The Quality Narrative in Health Care." *The Lancet* 385 (9976): 1367–68.

Kohn, Linda T., Janet M. Corrigan, and Molla S. Donaldson, eds. 1999. *To Err Is Human: Building a Safer Health System.* Washington, DC: National Academies Press.

Kroneman, Madelon, Pascal Meeus, Dionne Sofia Kringos, Wim Groot, and Jouke van der Zee. 2013. "International Developments in Revenues and Incomes of General Practitioners from 2000 to 2010." *BMC Health Services Research* 13: 436.

La Forgia, Gerard Martin, and Bernard Couttolenc. 2008. *Hospital Performance in Brazil: The Search for Excellence.* Washington, DC: World Bank.

Langley, Gerald J., R. Moen, K. M. Nolan, T. W. Nolan, and C. L. Norman. 2009. *The Improvement Guide: A Practical Approach to Enhancing Organizational Performance.* New York: John Wiley & Sons.

Laxminarayan, Ramanan, and David L. Heymann. 2012. "Challenges of Drug Resistance in the Developing World." *BMJ* 344: e1567.

Li, Yongbin, Jing Xu, Fang Wang, Bin Wang, Liqun Liu, Wanli Hou, and Hong Fan. 2012. "Overprescribing in China, Driven by Financial Incentives, Results in Very High Use of Antibiotics, Injections, and Corticosteroids." *Health Affairs* 31 (5): 1075–82.

Li, Weiping and Jianxiu Wang. 2015. "China's Public Hospital Governance Reform: Dongyang Case Study." China National Health Development Research Center, Beijing.

Liao, Xinbo. 2015 "An Ethical Analysis of Over-Treatment." *Clinical Misdiagnosis and Mistherapy* 28 (1): 1–5.

Lindenauer, Peter K., Denise Remus, Sheila Roman, Michael B. Rothberg, Evan M. Benjamin, Allen Ma, and Dale W. Bratzler. 2007. "Public Reporting and Pay for Performance in Hospital Quality Improvement." *New England Journal of Medicine* 356 (5): 486–96.

Liu, Dongying, Qingchun Hou, and Haiyan Zhou. 2013 "Appropriate Technology for General Practice in Township Health Centers." *Chinese Journal of General Medical Practice* 16 (12A): 4027–30.

Maybin, Jo, and Ruth Thorlby. 2008. "High Quality Care for All." Briefing, July 2008, The King's Fund, London.

McGlynn, E. A., S. M. Asch, J. Adams, J. Keesey, J. Hicks, A. DeCristofaro, and E. A. Kerr. 2003. "The Quality of Health Care Delivered to Adults in the United States." *New England Journal of Medicine* 348 (26): 2635–45.

Meng, Qingyue, Zhang Luyu, Zhu Weiming, and Ma Huifen. 2015. "People-Centered Health Care: A Case Study from Huangzhong County, Qinghai Province." China Center for Health Development Studies, Peking University. Case study commissioned by the World Bank, Washington, DC.

Morris, Stephen, Rachael M. Hunter, Angus I. G. Ramsay, Ruth Boaden, Christopher McKevitt, Catherine Perry, Nanik Pursani, and others. 2014. "Impact of Centralising Acute Stroke Services in English Metropolitan Areas on Mortality and Length of Hospital Stay: Difference-in-Differences Analysis." *BMJ* 349: g4757.

NCHS (National Center for Health Statistics). 2010. "The National Survey Study on Patient-Doctor Relationship." National Health and Family Planning Commission of the People's Republic of China, Beijing.

NHFPC (National Health and Family Planning Commission). 2014. "The National Health and Family Planning Commission Publicly Solicited Opinions on the 'Measures for the Management of Medical Quality (Draft for Soliciting Opinions)'." Release, August 5. http://www.nhfpc.gov.cn/yzygj/s3586/201405/4b01f1da84f342cb8357b8ecd77f95c9.shtml.

NHS (National Health Service) Commissioning Board. 2012. "The CCG Outcomes Indicator Set 2013/14." Infographic, NHS Commissioning Board, NHS England, Leeds, U.K.

Nie, Xiaomin, Yongxiang Wei, and Xiaoyan Cui. 2014. "Implementation of Hospital Strategic Management under PDCA Cycle." *Chinese Hospital Management* 34 (3).

Nolte, Ellen, and Martin McKee. 2011. "Variations in Amenable Mortality—Trends in 16 High-Income Nations." *Health Policy* 103 (1): 47–52.

———. 2012. "In Amenable Mortality—Deaths Avoidable through Health Care—Progress in the U.S. Lags That of Three European Countries." *Health Affairs* 10: 1377.

NQF (National Quality Forum). 2008. *National Voluntary Consensus Standards for Ambulatory Care, Part 1: A Consensus Report.* Washington, DC: NQF.

Qian, Xu, Helen Smith, Li Zhou, Ji Liang, and Paul Garner. 2001. "Evidence-Based Obstetrics in Four Hospitals in China: An Observational Study to Explore Clinical Practice, Women's Preferences, and Providers' Views." *BMC Pregnancy and Childbirth* 1 (1): 1.

Rhee, H., J. Allen, J. Mammen, and M. Swift. 2014. "Mobile Phone–Based Asthma Self-Management Aid for Adolescents (mASMAA): A Feasibility Study." *Patient Preference and Adherence* 8: 63–72.

Rudd, Tony. 2011. "The Legacy of NHS London Stroke." Presentation at "Progressing Health Care in London" conference, October 11. https://www.kingsfund.org.uk/audio-video/tony-rudd-legacy-nhs-london-%E2%80%93-stroke-programme.

Stranges, Elizabeth, and Carol Stocks. 2010. "Potentially Preventable Hospitalization for Acute and Chronic Conditions, 2008." Statistical Brief No. 99, Healthcare Cost and Utilization Project (HCUP), AHRQ, U.S. Department of Health and Human Services, Rockville, MD.

Turner, Simon, Angus Ramsay, Catherine Perry, Ruth Boaden, Christopher McKevitt, Stephen Morris, Nanik Pursani, and others. 2016. "Lessons for Major System Change: Centralization of Stroke Services in Two Metropolitan Areas of England." *Journal of Health Services Research & Policy* 21 (3): 156–65.

Veillard, J., F. Champagne, N. Klazinga, V. Kazandjian, O. A. Arah, and A.-L. Guisset. 2005. "A Performance Assessment Framework for Hospitals: the WHO Regional Office for Europe PATH Project." *International Journal for Quality in Health Care* 17 (6): 487–96.

Wang, X., and H. Xue. 2011. "Analysis of the Stock of Equipment and Human Resources at Township Health Centers in Guizhou Province." *Chinese Journal of Public Health Management* 27 (2): 117–20.

Wang, Jin-cai, J. Zhen, W. Fan, Q. Zhang, and Guo-li Zhang. 2013. "Investigation and Analysis of the Effects of National Essential Drug

System on Medical Expenses in Different Levels of Medical Institutions." *China Pharmacy* 23: 2982–84.

Wei, Jade W., Ji-Guang Wang, Yining Huang, Ming Liu, Yangfeng Wu, Lawrence K. S. Wong, and Yan Cheng. 2010. "Secondary Prevention of Ischemic Stroke in Urban China." *Stroke* 41 (5): 967–74.

Wennberg, John E. 2010. *Tracking Medicine: A Researcher's Quest to Understand Health Care.* Oxford: Oxford University Press.

Werner, Rachel M., R. Tamara Konetzka, Elizabeth A. Stuart, Edward C. Norton, Daniel Polsky, and Jeongyoung Park. 2009. "Impact of Public Reporting on Quality of Post-Acute Care." *Health Services Research* 44 (4): 1169–87.

WHO (World Health Organization). 2006. *Quality of Care: A Process for Making Strategic Choices in Health Systems.* Geneva: WHO.

Wilson, R. M., P. Michel, S. Olsen, R. W. Gibberd, C. Vincent, R. El-Assady, O. Rasslan, and others. 2012. "Patient Safety in Developing Countries: Retrospective Estimation of Scale and Nature of Harm to Patients in Hospital." *BMJ* 344: e832.

Wilson, R. M., W. B. Runciman, R. W. Gibberd, B. T. Harrison, L. Newby, and J. D. Hamilton. 1995. "The Quality in Australian Health Care Study." *Medical Journal of Australia* 163 (9): 458–71.

Wu, Xianru, Shuxiu Luo, Bin Chen, Yunkang Lu, Cuirong Gan, Yong Yang, and Kaling Wang. 2009. "A Survey of Village Doctors' Knowledge and Clinical Skill in Prevention and Treatment of Hypertension." *Internal Medicine of China* 4 (6): 910–12.

Xu, J. 2010. "Investigation of CPR Knowledge and Skills Training of Village Doctors." *Medical Innovation of China* 7 (21): 18–20.

Xu, Y., T. Shu, W. Yang, M. Liang, and Y. Liu. 2015. "Variations in Quality of Care at Large Public Hospitals in Beijing, China: A Condition-Based Outcome Approach." *PLOS One* 2 (10).

Yan, Fei. 2015. "Integrated Health Services Reform between Community Health Service Centers and Hospitals in Hangzhou, Zhejiang Province." School of Public Health, Fudan University. Case study commissioned by the World Bank, Washington, DC.

Yang, Le, and Hongman Wang. 2017. "Medical Education: What about the Barefoot Doctors?" *The Lancet* 390 (10104): 1736.

Yin, Wenqiang, Zhongming Chen, Guan Hui, Xuedan Cui, Qianqian Yu, Haiping Fan, Xin Ma, and Yan Wei. 2015. "Using Entropy Weight RSR to Evaluate Village Doctors' Prescription in Shandong Province under the Essential Medicine System." *Modern Preventive Medicine* 42 (3): 465–67.

Yin, Xiaoxv, Fujian Song, Yanhong Gong, Xiaochen Tu, Yunxia Wang, Shiyi Cao, Junan Liu, and Zuxun Lu. 2013. "A Systematic Review of Antibiotic Utilization in China." *Journal of Antimicrobial Chemotherapy* 68 (11): 2445–52.

Yip, Winnie, and William C. Hsiao. 2015. "What Drove the Cycles of Chinese Health System Reforms?" *Health Systems & Reform* 1 (1): 52–61.

Yip, Winnie, T. Powell-Jackson, W. Chen, M. Hu, E. Fe, M. Hu, W. Jian, M. Lu, W. Han, and W. C. Hsiao. 2014. "Capitation Combined with Pay-For-Performance Improves Antibiotic Prescribing Practices in Rural China." *Health Affairs* 33 (3): 502–10.

Zhang, Lihua, Jing Li, Xi Li, and Lixin Jiang. 2015. "National Assessment of Statin Therapy for Patients with Acute Myocardial Infarction 2001–11: Insight from the China PEACE-Retrospective Acute Myocardial Infarction Study." *The Lancet* 386: S42.

Zhang, Peipei, Lianyi Zhao, Jing Liang, Yan Qiao, Quanyan He, Liuyi Zhang, Fang Wang, and Yuan Liang. 2014. "Societal Determination of Usefulness and Utilization Wishes of Community Health Services: A Population-Based Survey in Wuhan City, China." *Health Policy and Planning*: czu128.

ZJOL (Zhejiang Online). 2011. "Zhejiang Establishes the First National 'Medical Quality Control and Evaluation Office.'" *Zhejiang Online—Health Network News Network*, March 2. http://health.zjol.com.cn/system/2011/03/02/017334382.shtml.

Zhou, Ping, M. K. Bundorf, Jianjun Gu, Xiaoyan He, and Di Xue. 2015. "Survey on Patient Safety Climate in Public Hospitals in China." *BMC Health Services Research* 15 (1): 1.

4

Lever 3: Engaging Citizens in Support of the PCIC Model

Introduction

The people-centered integrated care (PCIC) model seeks to organize primary health care around the health needs of citizens and communities of China, not simply around the diseases from which they suffer. The model hinges on patients' responsibility and engagement with their health, on their confidence in the system, and on their trust that the system will meet their needs in a responsive, appropriate, and timely manner. At the same time, beneficiaries of the health system need to be empowered with knowledge and understanding of individual health–promoting behaviors that will be amplified through interaction with the formal service delivery system. Such empowerment and engagement of citizens is a foremost strategic direction advocated in the World Health Organization's (WHO) framework on people-centered and integrated health services (WHO 2015b).

In part because of rising incomes, rapid urbanization, and increased demand for health services, the Chinese population has high expectations that health system reforms will improve service delivery. These expectations have only partially been met by increased access to health care and increased reimbursement of health care costs. In fact, public dissatisfaction with the health system

has sometimes led to violence toward providers (Chen 2012; Yuan 2012). Although the response from health authorities focuses on adding security staff to hospitals, outlawing hongbao (red packets given as gifts), and related stopgap measures, the underlying causes of distrust remain unaddressed.

This chapter focuses on core action areas that directly seek to strengthen people's engagement in their health, the health system, and the patient-provider relationship. Patient empowerment and engagement is central to any health system reform that aims to improve efficiency and make providers accountable for the services they deliver. For optimal use of resources, decisions about investment and disinvestment in services must be shaped by patients' preferences (Coulter, Roberts, and Dixon 2013; Mulley, Richards, and Abbasi 2015). Moreover, different outcomes matter to different patients. When clinicians overlook or misunderstand patients' preferences, the consequences can be as harmful as misdiagnosing disease (Mulley, Trimble, and Elwyn 2012).

Outside the hospital and other acute-care settings, much of health care, including disease prevention and health promotion, is a knowledge-intensive service industry where value is coproduced from two-way communication between multidisciplinary clinical teams and the patients they serve (Mulley 2009). This two-way nature of health care underscores the need for approaches and processes that support greater health literacy and sharing of knowledge. Without this exchange, decisions are made with avoidable ignorance at the front lines of care delivery, services fall short of meeting needs while exceeding wants, and efficiency declines over time.

Strengthening patient engagement is a goal relevant for China, as reflected in several state policies[1] that call on the health system and its stakeholders to

- Strengthen health promotion, education, and dissemination of medical and health knowledge; advocate a healthy and civilized lifestyle; promote rational nutrition among the public; and enhance the health awareness and self-care ability of the people;
- Build sound and harmonious relations between health care workers and patients; and
- Promote the transparency of hospital information through regular disclosure of finances, performance, quality, safety, price and inpatient cost, and so on.

The most recent state directive explicitly mentions use of media "to publicize disease prevention and treatment knowledge . . . as well as reasonable selection of medical institutions" and "more publication" to "increase people's understanding" toward diagnosis and treatment.[2]

The 2015 communiqué of the 18th Session of the Central Committee of the Fifth Plenary Session of the Communist Party of China emphasized the need to create a "Healthy China." Seeking to improve outcomes and well-being through a multipronged approach, the concept of Healthy China involves deepening the reform of the health system, rationalizing drug prices, integrating services, improving coverage of basic health services in both urban and rural areas, modernizing hospital management, and implementing a food-safety strategy.

Significantly, though, the communiqué also invokes each individual's responsibility to strive for better health: the concept emphasizes that everybody is responsible for the construction of a Healthy China and that each person should strengthen "the management of self-health" and avoid sickness as much as possible. Thus, the creation of a Healthy China involves not just health care but also changes in people's awareness about health and healthy lifestyles through education to realize personal "health management"—for example, through behavioral changes such as increased physical activity and improved eating habits.

On the basis of these principles, the National Health and Family Planning Commission (NHFPC) initiated the development of a "Healthy China Construction Plan (2016–20)." These policies in turn reflected several initiatives to improve patient engagement, including the following:

- Changshu (Jiangsu Province) has applied diabetes prevention and control measures as part of the WHO Alliance for Healthy Cities, and the approach has shown promise in addressing the spread of diabetes (Szmedra and Zhenzhong 2013).
- The NHFPC released the National Health Literacy Promotion Action Plan, 2014–20, to raise health literacy in China by providing information on basic health knowledge, healthy lifestyles, and basic medical skills (NHFPC 2014).
- The erstwhile Ministry of Health (now NHFPC) and the China Journalists' Association in 2005 launched the China Health Communication Awards; each year this project develops health communication strategies focused on one selected disease, such as hypertension (2005) or cancer prevention (2006).
- In Shanghai, a self-management program for hypertension (centered on a hypertension manual and delivered in the setting of a community antihypertensive club) showed promising reductions in blood pressure (Xue, Yao, and Lewin 2008).

The Shanghai Chronic Disease Self-Management Program improved participants' health behavior, self-efficacy, and health status and reduced the number of hospitalizations (Fu and others 2003).

- A recent *Health News* article argued for the need for shared decision making between provider and patient in China to manage and prevent illness (Zhong 2015).
- The National Clinical Information System, established in 2013, is an official website that provides a platform for news on quality control.

This chapter draws on experience with strengthening patient engagement in health systems in China and around the world and describes a variety of approaches used to engage patients. The chapter is organized as follows:

- *"Challenges to Engaging Citizens"* presents evidence regarding the patient-provider relationship in China, which needs to be improved urgently.
- *"Two Routes to Engaging People to Improve Health Outcomes and Restore Trust"* describes "individual" and "public" routes to engaging patients and citizens in health and explains why this chapter focuses on the latter.
- *"Recommendations: Strengthening Patient Engagement in the Patient-Provider Relationship"* outlines the concepts and core action areas for the individual route to engagement: (1) building health literacy; (2) strengthening self-management practices; (3) improving shared decision making; and (4) using information and communications technology to strengthen patient engagement.[3]

The core action areas presented in this chapter complement, build on, and ultimately reinforce each other. For example, shared decision making cannot take place without a basic level of health literacy among patients—which in turn is linked to and cultivates a certain confidence in the patient's ability to manage his or her own health. This experience is critical to shaping the patient's ability

to provide useful inputs to discussions with health providers when making decisions about care and hence to the patient's range of influence on the outcome of such decisions.

The final core action area is "public" in nature: creating a supportive environment for citizen engagement. Strategies in this area aim to improve the macro-environment to support interventions for engaging patients and to mobilize societal forces to enable people to live a healthy life. Of interest are models such as the WHO's Healthy Cities and Villages (CSDH 2008) and environmental "nudges" to improve healthy behaviors.

Challenges to Engaging Citizens

Although official policy statements indicating a desire to move toward a patient-centered health system are a step in the right direction, a much-needed comprehensive, systemwide approach to engage citizens in health—with well-defined roles for patients and providers—is still missing. China's health system needs to become more patient-centered. In part because of rising incomes, rapid urbanization, and increased demand for health services, the Chinese population has high expectations that health system reforms will improve service delivery performance.

It is important to meet these expectations: public dissatisfaction with the health system has sometimes led to violence toward providers (Chen 2012; Yuan 2012). Recent years have shown an increasing tendency toward medical disputes in China (*China Medical Tribune* 2012, 2013; CMDA 2013; Hesketh and others 2012; Moore 2012); of these, roughly a third of the medical disputes caused direct injuries to medical personnel (*Guangzhou Daily* 2014). The current patient-physician relationship needs to be improved, in particular to avoid violence targeting doctors.

Outbursts of anger and frustration are thought to stem from poor care, medical errors, and exorbitant costs, but relatively few studies examine the direct causes that underlie patient dissatisfaction and ensuing conflict. A 2010 report by the NHFPC Center for

Health Statistics found that only 59 percent of patients were satisfied with outpatient care and 55.8 percent with inpatient care (Center for Health Statistics 2010). The leading reasons for dissatisfaction with doctors included poor attitudes (51 percent), short consultation times and lack of effort (43 percent), and over-prescription of unnecessary medication or exams (23 percent). Dissatisfaction with nurses was due to poor attitude (78 percent), poor nursing skills (24.7 percent), and unprofessional behavior (23 percent).

Echoing these findings, Sylvia and others (2015) documented average patient-physician interaction time of 7.2 minutes in rural clinics, with half the time spent filling prescriptions. On average, clinicians spent only 1.6 minutes consulting with patients, in spite of long wait times. Liang and Bao (2012) found that, in Shanghai, patients on average wait for 13 and 16 minutes for outpatient and inpatient registration, respectively; after that, they need to wait an additional 30 minutes to be seen by a doctor.

Patients at community health centers (CHCs) were more likely to feel satisfied with the convenience, waiting time, and communication with doctors but less likely to feel satisfied with medical charges, drug costs, and medical equipment (Tang and others 2013). From a positive perspective, the Fifth National Health Services Survey shows that 76.5 percent of the outpatient and 67 percent of the inpatient patients were satisfied with their services and experiences (NHFPC 2015).

Tucker and others (2015) studied incidents of conflict at seven hospitals in Guangdong province and found that patient perceptions of injustice stemmed from costs of care (box 4.1), commercialization of medicine, and conflicts of interest. Physicians' intent to heal and cure was perceived to be compromised by a wide range of nonsalary incentives, including indirect favors and all-expenses-paid trips to tourist sites and conferences; incentives from hospitals and clinical departments to generate revenue; direct cash payments from pharmaceutical companies based on the number of branded drugs prescribed; and favors, cash, and gifts received as part of hongbao from patients.

Further, hospitals were perceived as systematically refusing care to poor patients and financially devastating families whose members are suffering from prolonged illness, while rudimentary health insurance schemes alongside an underdeveloped legal infrastructure provided few options for the sick who could not afford health services (Yip and others 2012).

Patient-physician trust is an implicit, fundamental building block of medicine and of achieving better health outcomes. A physician's trust of his patients and a patient's trust of his physician are inherently related, and both are crucial for health care partnerships. Reciprocal trust establishes a moral dimension to healing that is related to, but also distinct from, the biomedical aspects of eradicating disease.

Because satisfaction is premised on expectations—the greater the discrepancy between the perceived service and prior expectations, the greater the patient dissatisfaction (Linder-Pelz 1982)—policy makers should strive to understand and guide the financial, cognitive, and emotional expectations of both patients and doctors. In this context, the findings of the Fifth National Health Survey—which report that 76.5 percent of outpatients and 67 percent of inpatients were satisfied with their care-seeking experiences (NHFPC 2015)—are encouraging.

Two Routes to Engage People to Improve Health Outcomes and Restore Trust

A vast body of literature points to how strengthened patient and citizen engagement in health can improve the quality of their interactions and suggests that satisfaction and health outcomes can be improved through interventions that delineate and enhance the roles of both provider and patient in joint production of good health. Patients are thus not just consumers of health services but are also empowered to act in ways that influence their own health.

BOX 4.1 Understanding citizen mistrust: Perspectives from patients and providers

One study implemented at seven hospitals in Guangdong province recorded 25,000 medical disputes in 2013 and found that the origins of patient-physician mistrust were rooted in strong perceptions of injustice. Patients felt that drug costs and overall medical costs were inflated and that clinical decisions about diagnostic tests and drug prescriptions were skewed toward maximizing revenue instead of improving outcomes.

Several of the remarks by patients and medical personnel are illustrative:

- "Now everything is guided by economics. For physicians, hospital salaries can't come close to matching money from kickbacks and commissions. Maybe because his wallet grows, he is willing to engage in practices that violate his own professional ethics so that he can increase his own profits."—Patient
- "You will find that when some patients see the doctor, they carry with them an extremely distrustful, hostile, and negative tone of speaking. These patients lay it out: newspapers are talking about the violence, hospitals are not to be trusted, and doctors are the worst. If you see a hundred patients and only see one distrustful patient, it matters. It slowly influences your perception of patients."—Physician
- "The biggest problem is that the information between patients and physicians is asymmetric. Physicians have too much information and patients have too little. And physicians' information is very

systematic, while patients' information is disorganized. This information inequality can cause many conflicts."—Physician
- "[Health professional education] is just taught according to the book line by line; it's very rigid and dogmatic. For example, patient-doctor communication isn't sufficient. Actually at the bedside, we learn a lot of these kinds of communication skills. But the kinds of communication skills we were taught in school are not the kinds of skills we can apply."—Nurse

Physicians also perceived injustices within the medical system, pointing to intense workloads (for example, seeing 50 outpatients within a four-hour outpatient clinic shift) and pressures from within the hospital to generate revenue in the face of low salaries, high patient expectations, and sensationalist reports from mass media. Physicians also noted that the training system produced a limited number of subspecialized experts clustered in urban tertiary care settings (transiently evaluating a large volume of patients) rather than a larger number of primary care doctors (longitudinally caring for a smaller volume of patients). Finally, medical training prioritized technical biomedical competence over caregiving (cognitive, behavioral, emotional, and moral support) and empathy for patients.

Source: Tucker and others 2015.

This empowerment can help dislodge a deeply entrenched culture or mindset of helplessness and perceptions of lack of control that lead to the range of adverse outcomes observed in China, from patient dissatisfaction to violent conflict as a last resort in the most extreme cases. Box 4.2 defines the key concepts of empowerment, engagement, and coproduction.

Acknowledging the worsening of patient-physician relations, national Chinese government leaders have identified citizen mistrust as a major problem and sounded calls to action (Hesketh and others 2012; *Lancet* 2012, 2014; Zhong 2015). Policy responses

to date have focused on adding security staff to hospitals, outlawing hongbao, and related stopgap measures.

These measures seek to address the symptoms but not the fundamental issues that underlie mistrust of health services. As seen earlier, drivers of cost and commercialization of health care, overuse and underuse of services, and suboptimal clinical quality all contribute to dissatisfaction with the system. Chapters 3 (on quality of care) and 6 (on provider incentives) propose solutions for these problems. A case can be made that addressing perverse incentives to overprovide care may be a first step to improving provider-patient

---

BOX 4.2   **Defining empowerment, engagement, and coproduction of health**

The terms "empowerment," "engagement," and "coproduction" are often used interchangeably to describe policies or interventions that seek to achieve such goals, but in reality they represent distinct, if overlapping, strategies:

- *Empowerment* is about supporting people and communities to take control of their own health needs. It results in, for example, the uptake of healthier behaviors, the ability of people to self-manage their illnesses, and changes in people's living environments.
- *Engagement* is about people and communities being involved in the design, planning, and delivery of health services. This enables them to make choices about care and treatment options or to participate in strategic decision making on how, where, and on what their health resources should be spent. Engagement is also related to the community's capacity to self-organize and to generate changes in its environment.
- *Coproduction* is about care that is delivered in an equal and reciprocal relationship between (a) the clinical and nonclinical professionals and (b) the individuals using care services, as well as their families, caregivers, and communities. Coproduction therefore goes beyond models of engagement, because it implies a long-term relationship between people, providers, and health systems where information, decision making, and service delivery become shared.

Source: WHO 2015b, 22.

---

engagement. But much more will still need to be done to fix patient-provider interaction and build trust in the long run.

Broadly, interventions to enhance patient engagement can be organized at two levels (box 4.3): engaging people as (a) individual patients—the "individual" route—or (b) as members of the public—the "public" route. These two approaches can also be described as "patient involvement" (which refers to people "making decisions about their own health") and "public involvement" (which engages "members of the public in strategic decisions about health services and policy at a local or national level") (Florin and Dixon 2004). The remainder of this section outlines the differences between the two approaches and presents the rationale for the core actions recommended later in the chapter.

The Individual Route: Engaging Patients in the Micro Context of the Patient-Provider Relationship

The first route to engaging patients in health addresses the relationship between the patient and the medical provider as individuals.

The WHO strategy on People-Centered and Integrated Health Services states that "at the most fundamental level, it is people themselves who spend the most time living with and responding to their own health needs and will be the ones making choices regarding health behaviors and their ability to self-care or care for their dependents. Since people themselves tend to know better the motivations that drive these behaviors, people-centered care cannot be provided without engaging them at a personal level" (WHO 2015b, 22).

Broadly, at the individual level, patient engagement encompasses two key aspects: empowerment and activation. Patients need to be empowered with knowledge and information to make sound health care choices, ranging from generating changes in behaviors, selecting providers to seek services, and weighing the costs and benefits of surgical versus nonsurgical treatment options to accessing timely and effective complaint resolution mechanisms and addressing potential causes of ill health in their living environments. Once equipped with essential information, patients can be "activated" to participate in various activities for managing their health and health

---

BOX 4.3   **Individual and public routes to patient engagement**

Efforts to engage people in health practice and policy can involve them as individual patients or as members of the public. Individual and public engagement can require quite different things from participants. Jones and others (2004) suggest that patient involvement is essentially "private participation" in which individuals promote and protect their own preferences and values. Public involvement, in the context of treatment services and public health, can request citizens to "put aside their particularistic preferences . . . and participate for the common good" (Tenbensel 2010).

Individual routes to engagement

In the clinic, efforts to engage individuals in their own health are evident in initiatives that promote person- or patient-centered care as a way of "refocusing of medicine's regard for the patient's viewpoint" (Laine and Davidoff 1996).

The Institute of Medicine has described patient-centered care as one of six areas that are central to health improvement efforts (IOM 2001). It defines such care as that which "is respectful of and responsive to individual patient preferences, needs, and values and [ensures] that patient values guide all clinical decisions" (IOM 2001).

Others are more specific regarding the ethical content of person-centered care, stating that it "emphasizes patient autonomy, informed consent, and empowerment" (Edwards and Elwyn 2009).

Public routes to engagement

Public participation initiatives associated with health endeavor to make the field more citizen-centered in much the same way that health care provision aims to be patient-centered. Public engagement exercises take a variety of forms: for example, they provide participants with information, ask for their opinion, and incorporate them as active partners within policy formation (Arnstein 1969; Charles and DeMaio 1993; Feingold 1977).

Several countries have taken the ambitious approach of involving patients and the wider public in different levels of the decision-making process, including health services planning and, at the national level, health care policies. Examples include Germany's Institute for Quality and Efficiency in Health Care (https://www.iqwig.de/en), the United Kingdom's National Institute for Health and Care Excellence (https://www.nice.org.uk), and the United States' Patient-Centered Outcomes Research Institute (http://www.pcori.org).

In Australia, the Consumer Health Forum (https://www.chf.org.au) acts as a national voice and collaborative for health consumers. Its mission includes advocacy, research, issue identification, and consumer representation related to a large array of themes including health literacy, consumer-centered regulations and policy making, quality and patient safety, access to information, new technologies, and equitable access to care.

Source: Williamson 2014.

---

care, addressing risky behaviors, and safeguarding their living environment.

Health providers play a vital role in patient engagement by providing information about treatment options, explaining the potential risks and benefits of each option, encouraging patients to deliberate on and express their preferences, and developing plans for long-term self-management. Patient engagement in health care thus requires change and effort from both providers and patients.

Health systems use a variety of approaches to empower and activate patients at the individual level. These include building health literacy, strengthening self-management, and improving shared decision making with enhanced use of technology. These three approaches represent recommended core action areas for strengthening patient engagement and are described in detail in the "Recommendations" section. A substantial body of evidence highlights the effects of patient engagement approaches, with benefits accruing in the form of improved quality of care, appropriate decisions, and good health outcomes (box 4.4).

BOX 4.4   Effects of patient engagement strategies

A Commonwealth Fund survey of 11 Organisation for Economic Co-operation and Development (OECD) countries found that engaging patients can improve quality and patient experience, reduce medical errors, encourage compliance, and ultimately lead to better health outcomes with lower cost (Osborn and Squires 2012). Useful patient engagement strategies include the following:

- *Self-management interventions* improve not only patient knowledge, coping skills, and confidence to manage chronic illnesses, especially among the elderly, but also intermediate health outcomes; in some cases, they even reduce hospitalization rates (Picker 2010).
- *Shared decision making* has the potential to improve patient satisfaction and health care in

multiple settings (Coulter and Collins 2011; Stacey and others 2011) and may also successfully increase the use of less-invasive treatments that are often also less expensive (Deyo and others 2000; Kennedy and others 2002; Morgan and others 2000; National Voices 2014; Wennberg 2010).
- *Electronic health (e-health) and mobile health (m-health) platforms* can be powerful tools for supporting strategies for strengthening patient engagement (Bennett and others 2010; Bove and others 2013; Chen and others 2008; Nolan and others 2011; Rhee and others 2014; Wong and others 2013). In particular, they promote patient engagement by improving patient knowledge, increasing patients' willingness to participate in their own care process, enhancing accountability, and enabling self-monitoring.

The Public Route: The Macro Environment's Role at the Local and National Levels

Targeting patient-provider relationships at the micro level may not be sufficient by itself to improve patient confidence and trust in the health system. This is because these relationships rest in a macro environment influenced and shaped by nationwide and societywide forces. As well as being seekers and consumers of health services, patients are also citizens of nations and states, and as such can be engaged to exert influence on the broader policy environment that shapes the health and well-being of the societies they live in. This is the "public" route to engagement.

Instead of focusing on how patients could be engaged as citizens to improve participation in civic processes shaping health services in China, we focus on how the macro-environment can be shaped by policies and collective activities to support better individual engagement in health. Two "public route" engagement strategies are recommended that broaden the perspective from

the clinical environment and individual patient-provider relationships to include the ecology of individuals, families, communities, and organizations: The first strategy refers to initiatives such as the WHO's Healthy Cities and Villages; the spirit underlying these initiatives is that all societal forces can be mobilized to create conditions that enable people to live a healthy life. The second strategy is informed by insights from recent research in behavioral economics. It entails "nudges" and messages embedded in the physical and social environment that are used to cue people to adopt healthier behaviors. The next section describes each action area in detail.

Recommendations: Strengthening Patient Engagement in the Patient-Provider Relationship

Four core action areas and corresponding implementation strategies can strengthen citizen engagement in support of PCIC (table 4.1). Core action areas 1–4 build patient confidence and trust through patient empowerment and engagement in the individual sphere of the patient-provider relationship.

- *Health literacy* (core area 1) can empower patients with information needed to improve health behaviors and change expectations about what is acceptable treatment, including harm. It also shapes patient expectations for interactions with medical professionals.
- *Self-management* and *shared decision making* (core areas 2 and 3) cultivate a culture of comanaging health with the provider. Together, these interventions help improve the patient-provider relationship, build trust, and empower patients to break patterns of tension and prevent conflict. E-health and m-health solutions can facilitate implementation of these core action areas.
- A *supportive macro environment* (core action 4) focuses on broader, collective activities to foster an enabling environment of citizen and patient engagement.

The recommendations focus mainly on the individual route to engagement. Certainly, the macro environment affects patients' individual experiences as coproducers of health. And proposing strategies to define and strengthen the roles and responsibilities of patients as citizens—and to create an environment that sustains and nurtures civic participation in Chinese society at large to reduce "participatory deficit" (WHO 2015a)—may well be long-term goals for China, but these are topics beyond the scope of a health sector report such as this. To treat them adequately would require delving into the political economy of Chinese governance institutions as well as governance-society relations.

Core Action Area 1: Health Literacy

Health literacy is the ability to understand and act upon health information so that people have greater motivation and ability to control their health. The concept entails the ability to understand basic health knowledge and to use this to make health-related decisions.

Health literacy is essential to good health and fundamental to public health. If people cannot obtain, understand, and use health information, they will not be able to take care of themselves effectively, to navigate the health system without difficulty, or to make appropriate health choices for their own, their family's, and their community's health.

Adults with limited health literacy report having less knowledge about their medical conditions and treatments, worse health

---

TABLE 4.1 Four core citizen engagement action areas and implementation strategies

Core action areas	Implementation strategies
1: Health literacy	• Improve citizen understanding of evidence-based care, the importance of health-related behaviors, and preventive practices • Launch public media campaigns to encourage health promotion and prevention activities
2: Self-management practices	• Train health providers to support and facilitate self-management by patients • Educate and support patients on how to self-manage
3: Shared decision making	• Cultivate an expectation of patient involvement in decisions about their health care • Develop and promote use of decision-aid tools at health facilities
4: Supportive macro environment for citizen patient engagement in health promotion and improvement	• Improve macro environment for health promotion: develop Healthy Cities (and Healthy Villages)[a] • Create environmental "nudges" to improve health choices

a. WHO 1998. Also see "Healthy Cities," Health Promotion Programmes, World Health Organization Western Pacific Region, http://www.wpro .who.int/health_promotion/about/healthy_cities/en/.

status, less understanding and use of preventive services, and a higher rate of hospitalization and use of emergency rooms (Berkman and others 2011; Kindig, Panzer, and Nielsen-Bohlman 2004). Surprisingly, as many as half of all adults in the United States have difficulty understanding and acting upon health information—a problem that leads to ineffective care (Kindig, Panzer, and Nielsen-Bohlman 2004).

Nutbeam (2008a, 2008b) distinguished two perspectives on health literacy: health literacy as a risk factor and health literacy as an asset. These two perspectives differ subtly in their approach to the same concept.

Health literacy as a risk factor. Understanding health literacy as a risk factor leads to a focus on how to mitigate the negative effects of low health literacy on health-related behaviors and health outcomes. To this end, the Institute of Medicine defines health literacy as "the degree to which individuals have the capacity to obtain, process, and understand basic health information and services needed to make appropriate health decisions" (Kindig, Panzer, and Nielsen-Bohlman 2004). Research following this theory has linked health literacy to a range of health behaviors and outcomes, including effective management of chronic disease, compliance with medication and other health advice, and participation in health and screening programs.

Health illiteracy can also be a demand-side barrier: in particular, low health literacy among the poor and among ethnic or racial minority groups is associated with poorer health status, more hospital admissions, more drug and treatment errors, less use of preventive services, and poorer adherence to treatment recommendations (Berkman and others 2011; Kindig, Panzer, and Nielsen-Bohlman 2004). Lower health literacy among seniors is associated with higher mortality (Berkman and others 2011). Tackling gaps in health literacy is considered an important element in optimizing clinical effectiveness and reducing health inequities.

Health literacy as an asset. By contrast, the health-literacy-as-asset approach promotes the positive role of health education and communication in developing competencies for different forms of health action that benefit the health of individuals and the population. Particularly, the WHO Commission on Social Determinants of Health proposed that "health literacy implies the achievement of a level of knowledge, personal skills, and confidence to take action to improve personal and community health by changing personal lifestyles and living conditions" (CSDH 2007). Gaining health literacy as an asset could fundamentally address some of the social determinants of health outside the narrowly defined health care system.

Clearly the two approaches are distinctive in their clinical versus public health perspectives, but both are valuable and complementary for guiding policies to promote health literacy. They imply different strategies in response to low literacy that may supplement each other. In addition to improving access to effective school education and providing adult education to targeted populations with low basic literacy (CSDH 2007), health systems must also enhance the quality of health communications and education and provide greater support and tailored information to increase functional literacy to understand and use health information for managing health and diseases (Coulter and Ellins 2007).

Strategy 1: Improve citizen understanding of evidence-based care, the importance of health-related behaviors, and preventive practices

While health literacy is the outcome of a complex array of individual, social, and economic processes, the health system is a critical intervention point. Patients look to health providers for information and education on how to manage illnesses and long-term conditions. Beyond the information acquired through one-on-one patient-provider interactions, many countries have implemented formal educational approaches to target disadvantaged population groups. These approaches include training courses for small groups, colleges, and adult education institutions as well as one-on-one counseling.

The United Arab Emirates and the United Kingdom provide successful examples. "Skilled for Health," a national program run in part by the U.K. Department of Health, aimed to help people improve their health while boosting their language, literacy, and numeracy skills. The program was intended both to provide useful information and skills and to improve people's confidence to look after their health. The program targeted participants' health knowledge in the areas of healthy eating, smoking, exercise, drinking, and looking after their mental health. Educational sessions on a range of health topics such as healthy eating, exercise, and first aid were delivered to people in deprived areas (ContinYou 2010).

In the United Arab Emirates, student "ambassadors" at universities were trained in the basics of genetic screening and then encouraged to spread the word to their peers about the importance of being screened (Laurance and others 2014).

Strategy 2: Launch public media campaigns to encourage health promotion and prevention activities

Other strategies tackle health literacy across whole populations and focus on improving the provision of high-quality health information. Some media-based campaigns focus on both providers and individuals: in Canada, for example, the National Literacy and Health Program promotes awareness among health professionals and patients of the links between health literacy and health. Many media-based campaigns use printed materials, videos, websites, and formal and informal courses. Quality health information that is timely, relevant, reliable, and easy to understand is an essential component of any strategy to support self-care, shared decision making, self-management of long-term conditions, and health promotion.[4] The following are typical in public media campaigns for health education:

- *Informational materials*, provided at health facilities or electronically, can be tailored to the individual and reinforced by verbal information from clinicians and by web-based interventions as part of an educational program.

- *Newspapers, magazines, and broadcast media* are important vehicles in health education campaigns across the world. Media publicity can be a key component, for example, to discourage smoking; encourage use of folic acid among pregnant women (the Netherlands); raise awareness of excessive and rising hysterectomy rates (Switzerland); diminish stigma associated with depression (United Kingdom); promote uptake of immunization and cancer screening; educate about human immunodeficiency virus (HIV) risk; and publicize appropriate care for suspected myocardial infarction.

- *Social marketing* is used by government departments and health authorities to achieve specific behavioral goals for a social good (French and Blair-Stevens 2007). It typically involves a systematic approach to health promotion using tried and tested techniques that are informed by commercial insights (for example, on segmentation and from marketing theory) and theories of behavioral change. Such marketing interventions aim to help people make healthy choices, adopt healthier lifestyles, or make better use of health services. They have targeted healthy eating, substance misuse, physical activity, workplace health, and well-being. For example, social marketing played a key role in a Chinese campaign to prevent and control hepatitis B (box 4.5).

In China, messaging should focus not only on changing expectations about medications, intravenous therapy, and other diagnostics and therapeutics, but also on making citizens aware of the harm caused by overuse and misuse of treatments. A series of messages and public education efforts should be launched to change public perceptions regarding medications, procedures, and clinical services. It would require a continuous, multiyear, multichannel communication program, and ideally would use the energies of health care professionals as well as civil society agencies. The goal would be to help people understand the salient features of good, evidence-based care.

However, it would also be best for campaign planners to draw on research on why and how people understand and use information in choosing to seek care in China. In particular, this education effort would need to decrease the nonscientific overdependence on procedures such as intravenous infusions, medications, and hospital visits and admissions that the current volume-based payment system has encouraged.

Further, a national appeal to the public to engage in the collective pursuit of health could be explored. This would start with producing a technical review of three to five major evidence-based changes that individual citizens could make in their personal lives that would lead to a healthier future (for example, for smokers this would be smoking cessation; for alcohol drinkers this would be reducing their intake; for overweight or diabetic patients this would be to walk at least a mile a day). Messages advocating these health-enhancing behaviors would be assembled into national or provincial campaigns to get every citizen to engage in one or more of them. Given that people do not have equal access to information, complementary and more targeted interventions may be needed for low-income, elderly, and ethnic population groups.

One example that could serve as a model for China is the Million Hearts Campaign in the United States (box 4.6), a national initiative that set an ambitious goal to prevent

---

BOX 4.5   Social marketing in China: Prevention and control of hepatitis B

China's anti–hepatitis B campaign has been described as an excellent example of social marketing whose design and implementation maximized effectiveness as a result of the ample attention paid to the social, cultural, and regulatory context.

The first public service advertisement (PSA) was aired by a Chinese television station in 1986, and since then the Chinese government and media have been hosting annual national PSA campaigns and presenting awards to outstanding pieces (Cheng and Chan 2009). The Chinese government played a major role in this nationwide campaign, which was cosponsored by the China Foundation for Hepatitis Prevention and Control and the Information Office of the Ministry of Health, with donations of expertise from McCann Health China and airtime and space from many media outlets.

Source: Cheng, Kotler, and Lee 2011.

BOX 4.6   The Million Hearts Campaign

The Million Hearts Campaign rallies communities, health care professionals, health systems, nonprofit organizations, federal agencies, and private sector organizations around a common goal: preventing 1 million heart attacks and strokes by 2017.[a] A small set of changes have served as targeted interventions to achieve this goal (figure B4.6.1).

So far, the campaign's results include the following: (a) More than 100 partners have formally committed to the campaign goal and to specific activities; (b) promoting optimal care with the ABCS strategy (aspirin when appropriate, blood pressure control, cholesterol management, and smoking cessation) has achieved some early success.

The campaign has also helped to pass laws that create a healthier environment (for example, on smoke-free zones, a sodium reduction program in communities, and elimination of trans fats).

(Box continued next page)

BOX 4.6   **The Million Hearts Campaign** (continued)

FIGURE B4.6.1   **Million Hearts targets**

Million Hearts® Targets

By 2017 . . .

Reduce smoking
The number of
American smokers
has declined from
26% to 24%

**Reduce sodium
intake**
Americans consume less
than 2,900 milligrams of
sodium each day

**Eliminate trans
fat intake**
Americans do not
consume any artifical
trans fat

Optimizing Care in the Clinical Setting

Focus on ABCS
Aspirin use when appropriate . . .
Of the people who have had
a heart attack or stroke,
70% are taking aspirin

Blood pressure control
Of the people who have
hypertension, 70% have adequately
controlled blood pressure

**Use health tools
and technology**
Cholesterol management
Of the people who have high
levels of bad cholesterol, 70% are
managing it effectively

**Innovate in care
delivery**
Cholesterol management
Of current smokers, 70% get
counseling and/or medications
to help them quit

Million Hearts® promotes clinical and population-wide targets for the
ABCS. The 70% values shown here are clinical targets for people
engaged in the health care system. For the U.S. population as a whole,
the target is 65% for the ABCS.

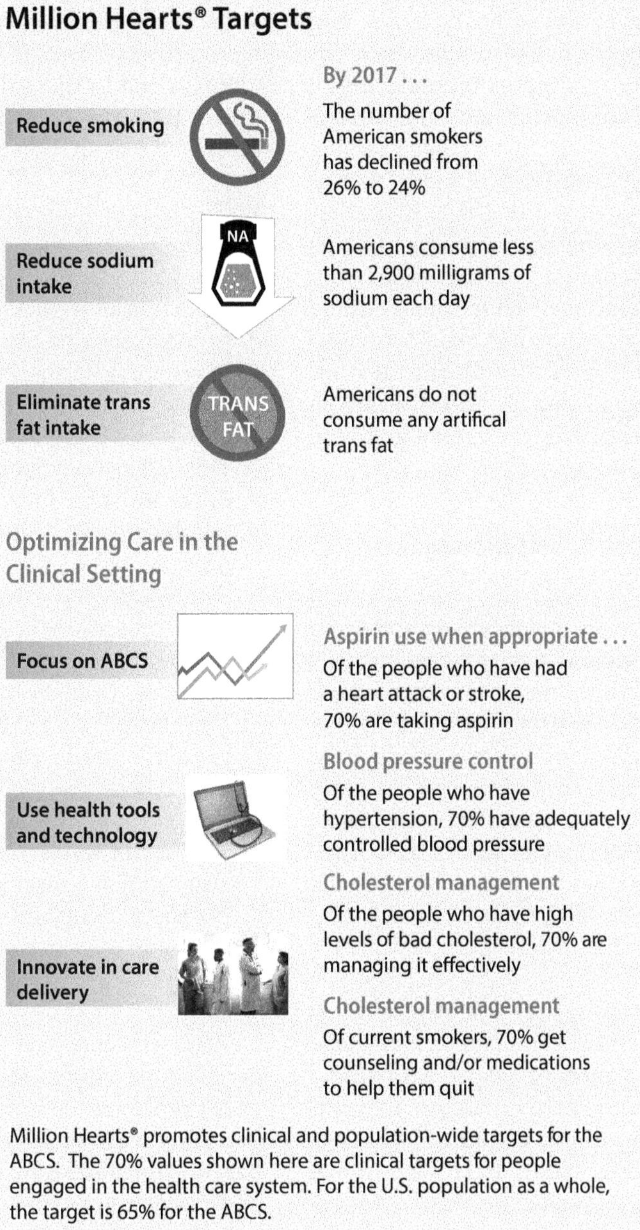

Source: "Infographic: Million Hearts Targets," About Million Hearts, https://millionhearts.hhs.gov/about-million-hearts/targets.html. ©U.S. Department
of Health and Human Services (HHS).
Note: "ABCS" refers to a strategy comprising the following: aspirin when appropriate, blood pressure control, cholesterol management, and smoking
cessation.
a. Million Hearts is an initiative co-led by the Centers for Disease Control and Prevention (CDC) and the Centers for Medicare & Medicaid Services (CMS).
For more information, see the Million Hearts website: https://millionhearts.hhs.gov/about-million-hearts/index.html.

1 million heart attacks and strokes by 2017 by improving access to effective care; raising the quality of care through the ABCS strategy (aspirin, blood pressure, cholesterol, smoking cessation); focusing clinical attention on the prevention of heart attack and stroke; activating the public to follow a heart-healthy lifestyle; and improving prescription and adherence to appropriate medications under ABCS.

Scotland's ongoing Early Years Collaborative, launched in 2012, is another example of this kind of campaign.[5] In this collaborative, Scotland is asking all parents nationwide to read their children a bedtime story each night, which has been shown to improve future literacy and educational attainment. China could use these models as examples while tailoring the campaign to the specific Chinese context.

Core Action Area 2: Self-Management Practices

Barring self-care for instances of short-term minor illness (such as a cold or other common viral infection), much self-care across the world today consists of the day-to-day management of chronic illnesses such as asthma, arthritis, and diabetes. Strictly speaking, people suffering from these conditions "self-manage" most of the time: they manage their daily lives and cope with the effects of their conditions as best they can, mostly without help from their health care providers.

More technically, self-management is defined as "the individual's ability to manage symptoms, treatment, physical and social consequences, and lifestyle changes inherent in living with a chronic condition" (Barlow and others 2002, 178). It is also about enabling people "to make informed choices, to adapt new perspectives and generic skills that can be applied to new problems as they arise, to practice new health behaviors, and to maintain or regain emotional stability" (Lorig 1993, 11). By promoting systems for patient self-management, health systems can empower individuals to reduce their use of

health services; make more informed decisions about office visits, medication, and procedures; and practice behaviors that help control their conditions.

The prevalence of chronic disease and the scope of its consequences have created a dramatically new situation in health care. As Holman and Lorig (2004) describe, patients, health professionals, and the health service must now play new roles:

- *The patient*—who must be responsible for daily management, behavior changes, emotional adjustments, and accurate reporting of disease trends and tempos—becomes the principal caregiver. Expressed in economic terms, health is the product of health care, and the patient, as a principal caregiver, is a producer of health (Hart 1995). As in any production system, a producer must be knowledgeable about the product and skilled in the production process.
- *The health professionals*, in addition to being professional advisers and partners in the design and conduct of medical management, become teachers in developing the patient's management skills. In the present system, physicians, nurses, and public health workers are not trained for this role.
- *The health service* becomes the organizer and financial supporter of the new roles for the patient and health professionals, focusing on assuring continuity and integration of care.

All approaches to self-management include careful elicitation of the patient's view of his or her problems, concerns, values, and preferences; sensitive sharing of relevant evidence-based information by health professionals; and discussion to find common ground. For patients to self-manage their conditions, they and their families need to be systematically educated about their conditions, how to monitor them, and how to incorporate healthy behaviors into their lifestyles.

When people with chronic diseases seek professional advice, they need appropriate help and support to enhance their self-management skills. For example, people with asthma must know when to use their inhalers; people with diabetes must monitor their blood glucose levels; arthritis patients must learn to cope with pain and how to ameliorate it, when possible; and, with self-management, chronic obstructive pulmonary disease (COPD) sufferers can maximize their lung function and improve the quality of their lives (box 4.7).

Strategy 1: Train health providers to support and facilitate self-management

Cultivating appropriate self-management practices among patients often requires a culture shift among health care practitioners. Professionals are urged to stop believing that their goal is to increase the patient's compliance with what they choose to recommend and to instead increase the patient's capacity to make informed decisions. The Five A's Paradigm summarizes this approach (Glasgow, Emont, and Miller 2006):

- *Assess* knowledge, behaviors, and confidence routinely
- *Advise* on the basis of scientific evidence and current information
- *Agree* on goals and treatment plan for improving self-management
- *Assist* in overcoming barriers
- *Arrange* helpful services.

Training for health professionals typically seeks to ensure that, at a minimum, they will

- Inform the patient about the disease, treatment, or management options;
- Educate the patient about effective self-management;
- Train the patient on skills such as how to carry out technical tasks such as testing blood glucose levels for diabetics, monitoring peak flow for asthmatics, and so on;
- Advise on behavioral change—how to modify existing behaviors or adopt new ones;
- Challenge unhelpful beliefs, including beliefs about the causes of illness; and

---

BOX 4.7 Self-management of COPD in the U.S. veterans population

Management of chronic obstructive pulmonary disease (COPD) is complicated because patients with this disease tend to suffer from many other chronic conditions that affect their quality of life. A major challenge is to help patients avoid acute exacerbations that often lead to hospital admissions. In the military veteran population covered by the Veterans Health Administration (VHA) in the United States, for example, COPD is the fourth most common reason for hospitalization. Pulmonary rehabilitation, which includes both exercise and education, helps patients manage their medications and compensate for their disabilities. Two problems are that some patients must travel long distances for rehabilitation and that even among patients who find it more convenient to participate, behaviors learned in the program are not always sustained.

To address these problems, the VHA developed a self-management module "to help COPD patients help themselves" by considering the many elements that improve how patients with COPD perceive their dyspnea and how functional they can be. The self-management module is designed around the principle that many of the goals of pulmonary rehabilitation can be accomplished remotely and that self-management is part of this and helps sustain desired behaviors and the benefits of the program. This, in turn, reduces the likelihood of the need for hospital admissions.

To design the module, the VHA analyzed studies and collected advice from pulmonologists across the United States to create a coherent packet for care teams to facilitate communication of the best and most important strategies. The module focuses on three areas: improving exercise tolerance and patient health status, managing symptoms, and managing or reducing exacerbations. Within these areas, the module addresses strategies such as medication, exercise, and smoking cessation. Overall, the tool is intended to allow patients to work more closely with their physicians to maximize lung function and improve the quality of their lives.

Sources: Ali and Li 2015; Basu 2014.

- Counsel patients on managing emotions—how to cope with the effect of their illness and its effect on their emotions, including how to deal with anxiety and depression.

Training in communication, teamwork, and relationship-building skills should be embedded in medical school curricula, postgraduate clinical training, and continuing medical education. The widely used Calgary-Cambridge framework divides a health care consultation into five stages: initiating the session, gathering information, physical examination, explanation and planning, and closing the session, with a list of tasks that must be accomplished in each (Kurtz and others 2003).

Providers' ability to communicate competently with patients should become a condition for qualification to practice, and due attention should be paid to lessons from research on interpersonal and communication skills. These skills can be learned and improved. For example, trainees can be taught how to express empathy (Bonvicini and others 2009), how to break bad news (Makoul and others 2010), and how to practice shared decision making (Bieber and others 2009).

Providers can be trained to use decision aids[6] (further discussed below) and to be ready to answer questions, especially when communicating with patients about uncertainty, the relative risks of different treatment options, and the specific time frames that define risks and outcomes. An evidence-based educational approach, the Flinders Program, is oriented to chronic-care management. It seeks to assess and improve the relationships between providers and patients that will lead to patients' actively monitoring their conditions while promoting healthy lifestyles (Horsburgh and others 2010).[7] The Flinders Program contains a series of training modules to enhance providers' knowledge of chronic-care management with a focus on communication skills.

Strategy 2: Educate and support patients on how to self-manage

Instituting a culture of self-management among patients requires education. A typical format is short (usually six weekly sessions), peer-led education courses in self-management, in which people with chronic conditions learn from other people with the same chronic conditions (Lorig and others 2001). These courses are often run by voluntary organizations. Educational courses following this format have been used across a wide variety of settings, including Australia, Barbados, Chile, Denmark, Japan, the Republic of Korea, Peru, the United Kingdom, and the United States.

Participants learn how to set goals and make action plans; solve problems; develop their communication skills; manage their emotions; pace their daily activities; manage relationships with family, friends, and work colleagues; communicate with health and social care professionals; find other health care resources in the community; understand the importance of exercise and healthy eating; and manage fatigue, sleep, pain, anger, and depression.

New technologies have been adopted to create interactive approaches delivered electronically. In the United Kingdom, for example, the Expert Patient Program is an internet-based resource with e-mail reminders (Lorig and others 2008). Web-based packages that combine health information with social support, decision support, or behavioral change support have been developed for people with chronic diseases such as asthma, diabetes, eating disorders, and urinary incontinence.

In the United States, health coaching by telephone (providing people with advice and support over the phone as a component of disease-management systems) and telecare technologies (including devices to transmit information over phone lines to sophisticated machines that monitor the patient's vital signs) are also used (Audit Commission 2004; Rollnick, Miller, and Butler 2002). Giving patients access to their medical records—by either enabling them to read and review these or by encouraging them to hold their own copy—can also increase a patient's confidence to self-manage.

Self-management education works best when integrated into the primary and secondary health care systems and when the learning is reinforced by professionals. The most effective self-management programs are those that are longer, more intensive, and well integrated into the health system and where the learning is reinforced by health professionals during regular follow-up. Efforts should focus on providing opportunities for patients to develop practical skills and the confidence to manage their own health. Hands-on participatory learning styles are better than traditional didactic teaching (box 4.8).

Core Action Area 3: Shared Decision Making

Shared decision making is a collaborative process in which providers and patients work together to identify problems, set priorities, establish goals, create treatment plans, and solve issues. As such, it is the essential underpinning for delivering truly people-centered care. Practicing shared decision making is a way to ensure not only that doctors make correct diagnoses based on science, but also that patients receive "the care they need, and no less; the care they want, and no more" (Coulter and Collins 2011, vii). Shared decision making reflects the extent to which citizens feel empowered to engage in their health care.

There are compelling ethical and practical reasons to engage patients in making shared decisions about their health. Patients may have expectations and preferences about treatments and health outcomes that differ from those of their health provider. Recognizing those expectations and preferences is vital to ensuring responsive and respectful care. Studies show that providers consistently overestimate their ability to predict patients' preferences. In one study, doctors reported believing that 71 percent of patients with breast cancer would rate keeping their breast tissue as a top priority, whereas in reality only 7 percent of patients said so (Lee and others 2010). In another, informing patients about the trade-off associated with surgery for benign prostate

---

BOX 4.8   **Encouraging self-management of health: Examples from India and the United Kingdom**

The Year of Care in Diabetes in the United Kingdom was a pilot program launched to actively involve diabetes patients in deciding, agreeing, and working on how their condition is managed. The core idea was to transform the annual review (which often just checks that particular tests have been carried out) into a genuinely collaborative consultation by encouraging patients to share information with their health care team about their concerns, their experience of living with diabetes, and any services or support they might need. Both the patient and the team then jointly agree on the priorities or goals and the actions to take in response to these.

Another self-management resource in the United Kingdom is the Big White Wall, an online mental health community where members can find support managing their care from clinicians, family members, and each other. The initiative provides members with access to immediate support, which may avoid the need for more expensive help later on. The community enables members to measure their mental health through tests and questionnaires, access help on guided support programs, get individual live therapy over a secure Skype-like connection, and track their progress. Although the focus is on self-management, the intervention incorporates elements of health literacy as well.

The Seven-Day Mother and Baby Health Checklist, developed by WHO and implemented in India, helps mothers identify danger signs in the crucial first week after birth. Upon discharge from the health facility, a health care worker explains the list to the mother. Texts and audio messages are sent by mobile phone to remind the mother to check the baby and herself for danger signs. This intervention has elements of health literacy (education on what are the danger signs) and also develops the capacity for self-management (determining when to seek professional help).

Source: Laurance and others 2014.

enlargement led to a 40 percent reduction in the number of patients opting for surgery (Wagner and others 1995). Surgery can ameliorate urinary symptoms associated with the disease, but many informed patients would rather forgo surgery to avoid postsurgical sexual dysfunction.

A Cochrane review found that, compared with usual care, decision aids increased health knowledge, particularly when the decision aid provided detailed rather than simple information (Stacey and others 2011). Exposure to a decision aid that displayed probabilities meant that patients more accurately gauged the risks associated with health interventions. Exposure to a decision aid with explicit value clarification resulted in a higher proportion of patients choosing options that were congruent with their values.

Decision aids were also found to improve patient-provider communication and to increase satisfaction with the decision and the health care process. They reduced patients' decisional conflicts related to feeling uninformed and unclear about their personal values. The Cochrane Review Group on consumers and communication provides continuous updates to effective interventions to enhance patient-provider communication and patient engagement for achieving better health outcomes.[8] The China Cochrane Center in West China Hospital, Sichuan University, may expand its clinical reviews to cover high-quality provider-patient interaction using decision aids.

Just as cultivating the practice of self-management builds a patient's sense of empowerment, shared decision making too leads to a beneficial redistribution of power between patient and provider (Coulter 2011). It can be achieved by changing the ethical and legal requirement of informed consent into a more active standard of informed patient choice (Wennberg 2010). The strategies below outline possible steps toward this goal.

Strategy 1: Cultivate an expectation of patient involvement in health care decisions
Surveys have found that about three-quarters of all patients expect clinicians to consider their preferences and want to have a say in treatment decisions (Coulter and Magee 2003). For example, a U.K. National Health Service survey found that nearly half of hospital patients wanted more involvement in their treatment decisions. Providers should communicate to patients that they are expected to take an active role in their health care, and patients should understand that although they may lack technical knowledge, they bring an equally important form of expertise to the decision-making process.

Internationally, there are several examples of how to improve patient involvement in health care processes at the facility level:

- *In the United States*, under the Program of All-Inclusive Care for the Elderly (PACE) model, patients and health care teams collectively design and agree on the patients' health goals (Ali 2015). Efforts to improve patient-centeredness at the Beth Israel Deaconess Medical Center in the United States provide another example (box 4.9).
- *In Shanghai*, the family doctor system encourages patients and families to jointly set treatment goals with their providers, and monthly patient-satisfaction scores track progress (Ma 2015).
- *In Germany*, a core feature of the Gesundes Kinzigtal system is the joint setting and attainment of goals. Shared decision-making tools augment this process, while case managers support the patients in changing their health conditions and behaviors (Hildebrandt and others 2015; Nolte and others 2015).
- *In Denmark*, the Integrated Effort for People Living with Chronic Diseases (SIKS) project prioritizes patients' involvement in developing their own treatment plans, setting goals through shared care plans, and providing feedback about whether these goals were met in partnership with the care team (Nolte and others 2015; Runz-Jørgensen and Frølich 2015).

BOX 4.9   **Improving patient involvement at Beth Israel Deaconess Medical Center, United States**

At the Beth Israel Deaconess Medical Center in Boston, efforts to improve patient-centeredness incorporated elements of shared decision making, patient literacy, and self-management. A patient-care committee was established, responsible for setting up patient and family advisory councils. The mission was to make sure that the patient's voice is heard, to improve communication, and to foster innovations that enhance the patient's experience of care. Patient and family advisers participated in focus groups and meetings about proposed design changes.

Beth Deaconess also developed a web-based portal that allowed patients to see their test results, communicate with their physician or practice by

e-mail, and request appointments and prescription refills. A "trigger response" system encouraged family members who have a serious concern about the patient to request a review by the care team. Patient education was conducted about patients' right to see test results, read the medical notes made by their physicians, and communicate with their physicians. Strategies employed included dissemination of information packages and provision of support to foreign-language speakers.

Finally, training and education of staff members about building a patient-centered environment began at recruitment, when they were asked to work through patient-oriented scenarios to learn about best practices and Beth Deaconess's standards.

Source: Laurance and others 2014.

Strategy 2: Develop and promote use of decision-aid tools at health facilities

Many health treatment and screening decisions are complicated for a variety of reasons. In some circumstances, there is no single best choice because people vary in the values or in the importance that they place on the benefits versus the harms associated with different treatment or screening options. In other circumstances, there can be uncertainty regarding the scientific evidence about the benefits and harms associated with the different options. Some clinical practice guidelines recommend that people convey their values for outcomes to their practitioners, particularly regarding treatment and screening decisions in which the best course of action depends on the importance the patient places on the benefits versus the harms (ACP 1992; Eddy 1992; Sawka and others 1998).

Decision-support interventions are being developed as an adjunct to practitioners' counseling (Bekker and others 1999; Estabrooks and others 2000; Molenaar and others 2000; O'Connor and others 1997, 1999; RTI 1997). Decision aids vary in their specific aims and in the types of decision they

support (ACP 1992; Entwistle, Sowden, and Watt 1998), but in general they are designed to enable people to

- Understand the probable outcomes of options by providing information relevant to the decision;
- Consider the personal value they place on benefits versus harms by helping clarify preferences;
- Feel supported in decision making;
- Move through the steps in making a decision; and
- Participate in decisions about their health care.

Decision aids in the health sector are being developed in several parts of the world, primarily in North America and Europe. Their development is motivated by factors that include the rise of consumerism, with an emphasis on informed choice rather than informed consent; the evidence-based practice movement's expansion of its audience beyond practitioners to consumers; the use of information strategies targeted at consumers to reduce unwarranted geographic variations in clinical practices; the use of decision-analysis techniques to identify treatment decisions that are highly sensitive to people's values; the interest in cost savings by reserving optional interventions for those people who agree that the treatment benefits outweigh the harms; and the expansion of the criteria used to judge health care quality to include patient satisfaction with the counseling they receive about options. Overall, decision aids provide reliable, balanced, and evidence-based information outlining treatment options, outcomes, and uncertainties and risks associated with treatment options, with the goal of helping patients discuss their preferences with providers.

Patient-decision aids can take a variety of forms, ranging from simple one-page sheets outlining treatment options to more detailed leaflets, computer programs (box 4.10), applications, or interactive websites. An important feature is that the aids are designed not just to inform patients but also to help them think about what the different options might mean for them and to shape their preferences on the basis of scientific information. They can be prescribed to patients before a consultation so that patients can better prepare themselves to discuss their preferences with the doctor and decide how to treat or manage their condition.

Benefits achieved from the use of patient decision aids can be enhanced by patient activation methods such as health coaching and one-on-one interactive interviews with doctors as well as with nurses, pharmacists, psychologists, health educators, or genetic counsellors. These coaching or interview sessions provide opportunities for clarification and decision support, but they also encourage patients to be more confident in managing their own health and to make treatment decisions. Patients can also benefit from question prompts, which are checklists to spark ideas about questions to ask during interactions with health professionals.

Most health coaches are nurses who have received additional training in motivational interviewing—which embodies a shift from "monologue to dialogue" between patients and providers—or specific decision-support techniques. These approaches avoid directive styles of teaching and advice-giving, which can generate resistance or a sense of hopelessness among those on the receiving end. Coaching has also been shown to be highly important in helping patients navigate the health care system so that they can

---

BOX 4.10   Decision aid for stable coronary heart disease by the Informed Medical Decisions Foundation

The decision aid for stable coronary heart disease is an interactive computer-based resource with information tailored to patients' specific clinical circumstances. The aid uses predictive models that help patients to envisage short- and long-term consequences of their choices. Use of the decision aid helps patients to understand that, given its potential complications, surgery can both increase long-term survival rates and reduce short-term survival rates. Based on such information, a patient whose only remaining desire in life is to attend his daughter's wedding six months later might choose to forgo the surgery.

Among other features, the aid also gives patients access to videotaped conversations with other patients who have already lived through various treatments and outcomes. This option is intended to help patients who are struggling to assess how they might feel in the future about health states that they have not yet experienced. The tool also generates printouts that aim to facilitate conversations between patients and caregivers—conversations that make it easier for patients to clearly express their preferences.

Source: Mulley, Trimble, and Elwyn 2012.
Note: For more information, see the Center for Shared Decision Making website: http://med.dartmouth-hitchcock.org/csdm_toolkits.html.

actively choose providers based on their health needs, preferences, and knowledge of providers (box 4.11).

Decision aids differ from health education materials because of their detailed, specific, and personalized focus on options and outcomes for the purpose of preparing people for decision making. In contrast, health education materials are broader in perspective, helping patients to understand their diagnosis, treatment, and management in general terms, but not necessarily helping them to make a specific personal choice among options.

Core Action Area 4: Supportive Environment for Citizen Engagement

The conditions under which people live have a vital influence on their behavior and the state of their health. An informed public is an essential prerequisite for health promotion and improvement, but knowledge cannot be transformed into actions and sustained over time without a supportive environment. This supportive environment pertains not only to clinical settings but also to the ecology of individuals, families, communities and organizations, and society as a whole.

All societal forces can be mobilized to create conditions that enable people to live a healthy life. This important aspect of supporting citizen engagement in health promotion and improvement underlies WHO's

Healthy Settings approach, which is clearly laid out in the 1986 Ottawa Charter for Health Promotion (WHO 1986).

In addition, behavioral economic research (such as Thaler and Sunstein 2008) has shown the importance of the immediate environment in influencing people's behavioral choices. Designing "nudges" that are embedded in the physical and social environment to cue people toward adopting healthier behaviors may be another promising health promotion strategy. These strategies are discussed below.

Strategy 1: Develop healthy cities (and healthy villages)

In the physical and social contexts in which people engage in daily activities, environmental, organizational, and personal factors interact to affect health and well-being. These social determinants of health contribute to the distribution of health in the population and are important targets for health promotion. With China's rapid urbanization, a series of "urban diseases" have emerged, such as environmental pollution, traffic jams, housing shortages, insufficient public services, unsafe drinking water and food, noncommunicable diseases, increased stress, accidents, and injuries. These environmental and societal factors can pose severe threats to people's health. Similarly, environmental degradation and lack of social support in rural

---

BOX 4.11   **Health coaching to coordinate care in Singapore**

To improve the quality and efficiency of care, Singapore implemented a national transitional care program for elderly adults with complex care needs and limited social support called the Aged Care Transition (ACTION) Program. It was designed to improve coordination and continuity of care and reduce rehospitalization and visits to the emergency department.

The program trained and deployed dedicated care coordinators to provide coaching to help individuals

and families understand the individuals' conditions, effectively articulate their preferences, and enable self-management and care planning. These care coordinators are mostly nurses and medical social workers who are hired by the Agency for Integrated Care. The program targeted complex cases: patients older than 65; patients with multiple diagnoses and comorbidities who take more than five different types of medication; or patients with impaired mobility, significant functional decline, or both.

Source: Wee and others 2014.

China are prominent concerns for health. Other countries face similar complex challenges.

WHO promotes the global Healthy Cities movement as a comprehensive strategy to create the supportive environment essential for improving health and addressing social determinants of health problems. The Healthy Cities movement envisages cities with a health-promoting environment that enables people to support each other in performing all the functions of life and developing to their maximum potential (Hancock and Duhl 1986).

The key factors affecting health in cities can be considered within three broad themes: the physical environment, the social environment, and access to health and social services (Galea and Vlahov 2005). Municipal governments will plan, construct, and manage the city in a way that continuously improves the physical and social environment and broadens access to public services that promote health—for example, by modifying the physical environment (increasing urban green spaces or designing wider bicycle lanes) or regulating public health (for example, banning smoking in public areas or requiring safety belts for drivers).

Building a healthy city is by nature an intersectoral endeavor. For example, local government policies on housing, the housing market, citizen action on housing conditions, and local lead-poisoning control programs may all interact to influence the rates of lead poisoning in a particular city (Galea, Freudenberg, and Vlahov 2005); hence, to reduce these rates will involve political commitments by local government along with institutional changes, capacity building, innovations, and partnership. The Healthy Cities movement includes a strong focus on citizen empowerment and participation. The approach promotes participatory governance by empowering individuals and valuing community knowledge in decision making and action on health (CSDH 2008, 18).

Globally, the Healthy Cities movement has attracted many cities to participate (De Leeuw 2009; De Leeuw and others 2008, 2015; Green, Jackisch, and Zamaro 2015).

International Healthy Cities Mayors' Forums in 2008 and 2010 helped to exchange lessons and experiences. The Chinese government has responded positively to the movement. As early as 1994, several cities were selected to participate in the Healthy Cities collaboration project with WHO; more recently, Hangzhou, Dalian, Suzhou, and 10 more cities have joined the Healthy Cities pilot (box 4.12). A policy being drafted to scale up the Healthy Cities movement in China will put health at the heart of the local development agenda and will potentially link local government officials' performance reviews to its progress.

The University College London (UCL)–*Lancet* Commission on Healthy Cities arrived at five key recommendations for achieving Healthy Cities (Rydin and others 2012):

- City governments should work with a wide range of stakeholders to build a political alliance for urban health. In particular, urban planners and those responsible for public health should be in communication with each other.
- Attention to health inequalities within urban areas should be a key focus when planning the urban environment, necessitating community representation in the arenas of policy making and planning.
- Action needs to be taken at the urban scale to create and maintain the urban advantage in health outcomes through changes to the urban environment, providing a new focus for urban planning policies.
- Policy makers at the national and urban scales would benefit from undertaking a complexity analysis to understand the many overlapping relations affecting urban health outcomes. Policy makers should be alert to the unintended consequences of their policies.
- Progress toward effective action on urban health will be best achieved through local experimentation in a range of projects, supported by assessment of their practices and of practitioners' decision-making processes. Such efforts should include practitioners and communities in active dialogue and mutual learning.

BOX 4.12   Changshu: One example of a Chinese Healthy City

Changshu is in the southeastern part of eastern China's Jiangsu province, about 100 kilometers northwest of Shanghai. Situated in the developed Yangtze River Delta, the city has a population approaching 2 million. To implement the Healthy City concept, the Changshu Bureau of Health started with the introduction of lecturer groups made up of medical professionals to provide information and education to both rural and urban residents. Teams made up of medical doctors and nurses as well as clinical researchers provided health education seminars and screenings at regularly held community events and health fairs.

These events demonstrated to citizens that health is something that must be actively pursued and that the individual is key to controlling his or her future health trajectory. Demonstrating that good health and the avoidance of lifestyle illnesses are the responsibility of each individual through conscious actions rather than simply chance, the Healthy Cities program promoted individual empowerment as the first step toward internalizing health responsibility. This is the Healthy Cities message: that all requirements for economic growth can be in place, but the lack of a healthy population cripples growth in its infancy. A healthy population is the essential foundation upon which to build sustainable economic growth.

For its public health cadre, the Changshu Ministry of Health developed standard guidelines entitled "Basic Knowledge and Skill of People's Health Literacy" that contained "The 66 Principles of Health," which provided the content of public health forums. In addition, brochures describing disease management and care, as well as how to avoid disease through lifestyle changes, were distributed during neighborhood visits. To better inform public health policy, the Ministry of Health posed questions that measured the public health knowledge of citizens in the Changshu region. These surveys revealed low levels of information about the 10 most important chronic illnesses facing people in the region.

After establishing baseline levels of chronic disease in the population, the Ministry issued a 2009 white paper, "The Changshu Testing Program for Public Knowledge of Chronic Noncommunicable Diseases Prevention and Control." This document requires all health care institutions in the Changshu region to apply the material contained in a pamphlet (titled "500 Questions to Determine Public Knowledge of Chronic Noncommunicable Disease Prevention and Control") to ensure that the methods that are thought

to increase awareness of chronic disease prevention, management, and control are being applied in clinical settings. The following directives are included in every health care institution's educational mandate:

- Focus on the development of a healthy city through the modernization of rural health and peasant health care services.
- Print and distribute circulars that address health issues, especially those associated with chronic lifestyle illnesses including diabetes, cardiovascular disease, and hypertension.
- Provide the "500 Questions" pamphlet to government organizations, enterprises, institutions, and schools as the principal content reference for lifestyle and chronic diseases.
- Conduct special training in disease management for patients with chronic disease.
- Organize activities promoting chronic-disease awareness in government organizations, enterprises, institutions, and schools.
- Use various methods of publicity to exploit different media types.
- Include the basic learning aspects of the "500 Questions" pamphlet in publicity circulars.

As an example of exploiting various media to promote Healthy Cities through improved levels of public health, the city of Changshu held "a ceremony for promoting public health lifestyles" in December 2011. Through broadcast media, the vice mayor of Changshu promoted public awareness of healthy lifestyles by encouraging the adoption of a rational diet, engaging in moderate exercise, and quitting smoking. He also encouraged rational limits to alcohol consumption and striking a "psychological balance" in life and living. The Ministry of Health awarded prizes to "healthy families": those that demonstrated their commitment to practicing healthy ways of living.

Attendees also received small gifts including health-related books as well as cruets and measuring spoons to accurately measure food portions. Theatrical skits promoting healthy lifestyles were performed. Changshu talk-radio programs invited experts from municipal hospitals to speak about chronic diseases such as hypertension, diabetes, and cancer and to interact with callers. Further, the Ministry organized alternative methods of promoting awareness such as free screening and counseling for diabetes to coincide with World Diabetes Day each November 14.

Source: Case study commissioned by the World Bank.

Strategy 2: Create environmental "nudges" to improve health choices

Most people value their health yet persist in behaving in ways that undermine it. Many psychological reasons underlie this gap between value or cognition and behavior, one being that people's behavior can be subconsciously triggered by environmental or emotional cues that are driven by default, habits, or perception of social norms (Thaler and Sunstein 2008). These inherent human biases offer an opportunity for noncoercive policy interventions to change behavior toward healthier choices. By changing the seemingly subtle cues in the physical, social, and policy environment, so-called "nudging" interventions can signal to people to make better health choices without coercion or material incentive.

Nudges might involve subconscious cues (such as painting targets in urinals to improve accuracy) or correcting misapprehensions about social norms (like telling people that most people do not drink excessively). They can alter the profile of different choices (such as the prominence of healthy food in canteens) or change which options are the default (such as having to *opt out of* rather than *opt into* organ-donor schemes). Nudges can also create incentives for certain choices or impose minor economic or cognitive costs on other options (such as enabling people who quit smoking to bank the money they would have spent on their habit but only allowing them to withdraw it when they test as nicotine-free). Table 4.2 gives examples of nudging strategies as opposed to regulatory strategies (Marteau and others 2011).

Some of these strategies have proven highly effective, as follows:

- Australia, France, Poland, and Portugal have adopted "opt-in" as the default for indicating willingness for organ donation and, as a result, 90–100 percent of their citizens are registered donors, compared with only 5–30 percent in countries that do not use the donor default strategy (Johnson and Goldstein 2003).
- In some states in the United States, the default is that pharmacists can fill written drug prescriptions with generic drugs unless the physician opts out by placing "dispense as written" on the prescription (Blumenthal-Barby and Burroughs 2012).
- An example of making health messages more salient to act on is the requirement for restaurants to put caloric amounts on menus. In New York, this requirement caused people to order meals containing fewer calories and caused restaurants to lower the calorie content of meals (Rabin 2008).

TABLE 4.2 Examples of nudges and regulation to change target behaviors

Behavior	Nudges	Regulations
Smoking	• Make nonsmoking more visible through mass media campaigns communicating that most people do not smoke and most smokers want to stop • Reduce cues for smoking by keeping cigarettes, lighters, and ashtrays out of sight	• Ban smoking in public places • Increase price of cigarettes
Alcohol	• Serve drinks in smaller glasses • Make lower alcohol consumption more visible by highlighting in mass media campaigns that most people do not drink to excess	• Regulate pricing through taxes or minimum pricing per unit • Raise the minimum age for purchase of alcohol
Diet	• Designate sections of supermarket trolleys for fruit and vegetables • Make salad rather than chips the default side order	• Restrict food advertising in media directed at children • Ban industrially produced trans-fatty acids
Physical activity	• Make stairs, not elevators, more prominent and attractive in public buildings • Make cycling more visible as a means of transport, for example through city bicycle-hire schemes	• Increase tax on gasoline year-on-year (fuel price escalator) • Enforce car drop-off exclusion zones around schools

Source: Marteau and others 2011.

- People also respond to a change in perception of a social norm. The State of Montana ran an intensive "Most of Us Wear Seatbelts" media campaign from 2000 to 2003 in which the Department of Transportation let people know that most people (85 percent) wear seatbelts. This resulted in a significant increase in the reported use of seatbelts (Linkenbach and Perkins 2003).
- Finally, a successful technique to increase fruit consumption among school students is to place fruits and vegetables in prominent places in the cafeteria and display them attractively. This demonstrates the behavior-shaping effect of priming cues.

Notes

1. "Opinion on Deepening China's Health Care System Reform," State Council (*Zhong Fa* 2009, No. 6); "The Twelfth-Five Year Plan of Health Care Development," State Council General Office (*Guo Fa* 2012, No. 57); "Guidance of the General Office of the State Council on Overall Pilot Reform of Urban Public Hospitals," National Health and Family Planning Commission (*Guo Ban Fa* 2015, No. 38); "Opinions of the State Council on Comprehensively Scaling-Up Reform of County-Level Public Hospitals," State Council (*Guo Ban Fa* 2015, No. 33); and "Planning of the National Health Service System (2015–2020)." State Council General Office (*Guo Ban Fa* 2015, No. 14).
2. "Guidance of the General Office of the State Council on Promoting Multi-Level Diagnosis and Treatment System," State Council (*Guo Ban Fa* 2015, No. 70).
3. Related e-health themes are discussed in chapter 3.
4. Public education campaigns should be part of a comprehensive strategy for health promotion that includes legislation and regulation—for example, legislative action against smoking through banning cigarette advertisements, banning smoking in public places, taxation of cigarette sales, and so forth. A full treatment of possible options goes beyond the scope of this report.
5. In 2016, the Scottish Government combined the Early Years Collaborative with the Raising Attainment for All program to form the Children and Young People Improvement Collaborative; for more information, see https://beta.gov.scot/policies/improving-public-services/children-and-young-people-improvement-collaborative/.
6. Decision aids are interventions designed to help people make specific and deliberative choices among options by providing information about the options and outcomes that are relevant to a person's health status.
7. For more about the Flinders Program, see https://www.flindersprogram.com.au/.
8. For updates on Cochrane Reviews, see http://cccrg.cochrane.org/our-reviews.

References

ACP (American College of Physicians). 1992. "Guidelines for Counselling Postmenopausal Women about Preventive Hormone Therapy." *Annals of Internal Medicine* 117 (12): 1038–41.

Ali, Rabia. 2015. "Programs of All-Inclusive Care for the Elderly (PACE) in the U.S.: Background and Rationale." Case study commissioned by the World Bank, Washington, DC.

Ali, Rabia, and Rong Li. 2015. "Patient-Centered Medical Home (PCMH) Model of U.S. Veterans Health Administration." Case study commissioned by the World Bank, Washington, DC.

Arnstein, S. 1969. "A Ladder of Citizen Participation." *Journal of American Institute of Planners* 35 (4): 216–24.

Audit Commission. 2004. "Implementing Telecare: Strategic Analysis and Guidelines for Policy Makers, Commissioners and Providers." Public Sector National Report, London.

Barlow, J., C. Wright, J. Sheasby, A. Turner, and J. Hainsworth. 2002. "Self-Management Approaches for People with Chronic Conditions: A Review." *Patient Education and Counseling* 48 (2): 177–87.

Basu, Sandra. 2014. "VHA Emphasizes Self-Management in New COPD Care Tool." *U.S. Medicine*, May 21.

Bekker, H., J. G. Thornton, C. M. Airey, J. B. Connelly, J. Hewison, and M. B. Robinson. 1999. "Informed Decision Making: An Annotated Bibliography and Systematic Review." *Health Technology Assessment* 3 (1): 1–156.

Bennett, G. G., S. J. Herring, E. Puleo, E. K. Stein, K. M. Emmons, and M. W. Gillman. 2010. "Web-Based Weight Loss in Primary Care: A Randomized Controlled Trial." *Obesity* 18 (2): 308–13.

Berkman, Nancy D., Stacey L. Sheridan, Katrina E. Donahue, David J. Halpern, and Karen Crotty. 2011. "Low Health Literacy and Health Outcomes: An Updated Systematic Review." *Annals of Internal Medicine* 155 (2): 97–107.

Bieber, Christiane, J. Nicolai, M. Hartmann, K. Blumenstiel, N. Ringel, A. Schneider, M. Härter, W. Eich, and A. Loh. 2009. "Training Physicians in Shared Decision-Making: Who Can Be Reached and What Is Achieved?" *Patient Education and Counseling* 77 (1): 48–54.

Blumenthal-Barby, Jennifer S., and Hadley Burroughs. 2012. "Seeking Better Health Care Outcomes: The Ethics of Using the 'Nudge.'" *American Journal of Bioethics* 12 (2): 1–10.

Bonvicini, Kathleen A., Michael J. Perlin, Carma L. Bylund, Gregory Carroll, Ruby A. Rouse, and Michael G. Goldstein. 2009. "Impact of Communication Training on Physician Expression of Empathy in Patient Encounters." *Patient Education and Counseling* 75 (1): 3–10.

Bove, A. A., C. J. Homko, W. P. Santamore, M. Kashem, M. Kerper, and D. J. Elliott. 2013. "Managing Hypertension in Urban Underserved Subjects Using Telemedicine: A Clinical Trial." *American Heart Journal* 165 (4): 615–21.

Center for Health Statistics. 2010. "The National Survey Study on Patient-Doctor Relationship." National Health and Family Planning Commission, Beijing.

Charles, C., and S. DeMaio. 1993. "Lay Participation in Health Care Decision Making: A Conceptual Framework." *Journal of Health Politics, Policy and Law* 18 (4): 881–904.

Chen, F. 2012. "At Shenzhen Pencheng Hospital a Nurse Was Attacked by Knife" [title translated from Chinese]. *Shenzhen News*, September 4. http://health.sohu.com/20120904/n352262739.shtml.

Chen, Z.-W., L.-Z. Fang, L.-Y. Chen, and H.-L. Dai. 2008. "Comparison of an SMS Text Messaging and Phone Reminder to Improve Attendance at a Health Promotion Center: A Randomized Controlled Trial." *Journal of Zhejiang University Science B* 9 (1): 34–38.

Cheng, H., and K. Chan. 2009. "Public Service Advertising in China: A Semiotic Analysis." In *Advertising and Chinese Society: Impacts and Issues*, edited by H. Cheng and K. Chan, 203–21. Copenhagen: Copenhagen Business School Press.

Cheng, H., P. Kotler, and N. Lee. 2011. *Social Marketing for Public Health: Global Trends and Success Stories*. Boston: Jones & Bartlett Learning.

China Medical Tribune. 2012. "Medical War in 2012" [title translated from Chinese]. December 16. http://www.cmt.com.cn/detail/111139.html.

———. 2013. "Violent Events against Doctors in the First Half of 2013." (Accessed August 16, 2013.) http://www.cmt.com.cn/detail/270013.html.

CMDA (Chinese Medical Doctor Association). 2013. "Four Doctors Dead within a Week: Who Will Guard the Physicians' Health?" July 14.

ContinYou. 2010. "Skilled for Health Has the 'Heineken' Effect." ContinYou, Coventry, U.K.

Coulter, Angela. 2011. *Engaging Patients in Health Care*. London: McGraw-Hill Education.

Coulter, Angela, and Alf Collins. 2011. *Making Shared Decision-Making a Reality: No Decision about Me, Without Me*. London: The King's Fund.

Coulter, Angela, and Jo Ellins. 2007. "Effectiveness of Strategies for Informing, Educating, and Involving Patients." *British Medical Journal* 335 (7609): 24.

Coulter, Angela, and H. Magee, eds. 2003. *The European Patient of the Future*. Maidenhead, U.K.: Open University Press.

Coulter, A., S. Roberts, and A. Dixon. 2013. "Delivering Better Services for People with Long Term Conditions: Building the House of Care." Report, The King's Fund, London.

CSDH (Commission on Social Determinants of Health). 2007. "Achieving Health Equity: From Root Causes to Fair Outcomes. Commission on Social Determinants of Health, Interim Statement." CDSH, World Health Organization, Geneva.

———. 2008. *Closing the Gap in a Generation: Health Equity through Action on the Social Determinants of Health*. Geneva: WHO.

De Leeuw, Evelyne. 2009. "Evidence for Healthy Cities: Reflections on Practice, Method and Theory." *Health Promotion International* 24: i19–i36. doi:10.1093/heapro/dap052.

De Leeuw, Evelyne, Agis D. Tsouros, Mariana Dyakova, and Geoff Green, eds. 2008. *Healthy Cities: Promoting Health and Equity— Evidence for Local Policy and Practice. Summary Evaluation of Phase V of the WHO European Healthy Cities Network.* Copenhagen: WHO Regional Office for Europe.

De Leeuw, Evelyne, Geoff Green, Mariana Dyakova, Lucy Spanswick, and Nicola Palmer. 2015. "European Healthy Cities Evaluation: Conceptual Framework and Methodology." *Health Promotion International* 30 (Suppl. 1): i8–i17.

Deyo, R. A., D. C. Cherkin, J. Weinstein, J. Howe, M. Ciol, and A. G. Mulley Jr. 2000. "Involving Patients in Clinical Decisions: Impact of an Interactive Video Program on Use of Back Surgery." *Medical Care* 38: 959–69.

Eddy, D. M. 1992. *A Manual for Assessing Health Practices and Designing Practice Policies: The Explicit Approach.* Philadelphia: American College of Physicians.

Edwards A., and G. Elwyn. 2009. *Shared Decision-Making in Health Care: Achieving Evidence-Based Patient Choice.* 2nd ed. Oxford: Oxford University Press.

Entwistle, V. A., A. Sowden, and I. Watt. 1998. "Evaluating Interventions to Promote Patient Involvement in Decision Making: By What Criteria Should Effectiveness Be Judged?" *Journal of Health Services Research and Policy* 3: 100–7.

Estabrooks, C. A., V. Goel, E. Thiel, S. P. Pinfold, C. Sawka, and J. I. Williams. 2000. "Consumer Decision Aids: Where Do We Stand? A Systematic Review of Structured Consumer Decision Aids." Technical report, Institute for Clinical Evaluative Sciences, Toronto.

Feingold, E. 1977. "Citizen Participation: A Review of the Issues." In *The Consumer and the Health Care System: Social and Managerial Perspectives*, edited by H. M. Rosen, J. M. Metsch, and S. Levey, 153–60. New York: Spectrum.

Florin D., and J. Dixon. 2004. "Public Involvement in Health Ethics." *BMJ* 328: 159–61.

French, J., and C. Blair-Stevens. 2007. *Big Pocket Book: Social Marketing.* London: National Social Marketing Center.

Fu, Dongbo, Fu Hua, Patrick McGowan, Shen Yi-e, Zhu Lizhen, Yang Huiqin, Mao Jianguo,

Zhu Shitai, Ding Yongming, and Wei Zhihua. 2003. "Implementation and Quantitative Evaluation of Chronic Disease Self-Management Programme in Shanghai, China: Randomized Controlled Trial." *Bulletin of the World Health Organization* 81 (3): 174–82.

Galea, Sandro, and David Vlahov. 2005. "Urban Health: Evidence, Challenges, and Directions." *Annual Review of Public Health* 26: 341–65.

Galea, Sandro, Nicholas Freudenberg, and David Vlahov. 2005. "Cities and Population Health." *Social Science & Medicine* 60 (5): 1017–33.

Glasgow, R. E., S. Emont, and D. C. Miller. 2006. "Assessing Delivery of the Five 'A's' for Patient-Centered Counselling." *Health Promotion International* 21 (3): 245–55.

Green, G., J. Jackisch, and G. Zamaro. 2015. "Healthy Cities as Catalysts for Caring and Supportive Environments." *Health Promotion International* 30 (Suppl. 1): i99–i107.

Guangzhou Daily. 2014. "Doctor-Patient Disputes Increase 10 Times in 10 Years: Doctors Average 2.4 Minutes to See 1 Patient" [title translated from Chinese]. June 30. http://gd.sina.com.cn/news/m/2014-06-30/0726 109553.html.

Hancock, T., and L. Duhl. 1986. "The Healthy City: Its Function and its Future." *Health Promotion* 1 (1).

Hart, J. T. 1995. "Clinical and Economic Consequences of Patients as Producers." *Journal of Public Health Medicine* 17: 383–86.

Hesketh, T., D. Wu, L. Mao, and N. Ma. 2012. "Violence against Doctors in China." *BMJ* 345: e5730.

Hildebrandt, Helmut, Alexander Pimperl, Oliver Gröne, Monika Roth, Christian Melle, Timo Schulte, Martin Wetzel, and Alf Trojan. 2015. "Gesundes Kinzigtal: A Case Study on People Centered/Integrated Health Care in Germany." Case study commissioned by the World Bank, Washington, DC.

Holman, Halsted, and Kate Lorig. 2004. "Patient Self-Management: A Key to Effectiveness and Efficiency in Care of Chronic Disease." *Public Health Reports* 119 (3): 239.

Horsburgh, M., J. Bycroft, F. Mahony, D. Roy, D. Miller, F. Goodyear-Smith, and E. Donnell. 2010. "The Feasibility of Assessing the Flinders Program of Patient Self-Management in New Zealand Primary Care Settings." *Journal of Primary Health Care* 2 (4): 294–302.

IOM (Institute of Medicine). 2001. *Crossing the Quality Chasm: A New Health System for the*

21st Century. Washington, DC: National Academies Press for the Committee on Quality of Health Care in America.

Johnson, E. J., and D. Goldstein. 2003. "Do Defaults Save Lives?" *Science* 302 (5649): 1338–39.

Jones, I. L., M. Berney, M. Kelly, L. Doyal, C. Griffiths, G. Feder, S. Hillier, G. Rowlands, and S. Curtis. 2004. "Is Patient Involvement Possible When Decisions Involve Scarce Resources? A Qualitative Study of Decision Making in Primary Care." *Social Science and Medicine* 59: 93–102.

Kennedy, A. D., M. J. Sculpher, A. Coulter, N. Dwyer, M. Rees, and K. R. Abrams. 2002. "Effects of Decision Aids for Menorrhagia on Treatment Choices, Health Outcomes, and Costs: A Randomized Controlled Trial." *JAMA* 288: 2701–08.

Kindig, David A., Allison M. Panzer, and Lynn Nielsen-Bohlman, eds. 2004. *Health Literacy: A Prescription to End Confusion*. Washington, DC: National Academies Press.

Kurtz, Suzanne, Jonathan Silverman, John Benson, and Juliet Draper. 2003. "Marrying Content and Process in Clinical Method Teaching: Enhancing the Calgary–Cambridge Guides." *Academic Medicine* 78 (8): 802–09.

Laine, C., and F. Davidoff. 1996. "Patient-Centered Medicine: A Professional Evolution." *JAMA* 275 (2): 152–56.

Lancet. 2012. "Ending Violence against Doctors in China." *The Lancet* 379 (9828): 1764.

———. 2014. "Violence against Doctors: Why China? Why Now? What Next?" *The Lancet* 383 (9922): 1013.

Laurance, Jeremy, Sarah Henderson, Peter J. Howitt, Mariam Matar, Hanan Al Kuwari, Susan Edgman-Levitan, and Ara Darzi. 2014. "Patient Engagement: Four Case Studies that Highlight the Potential for Improved Health Outcomes and Reduced Costs." *Health Affairs* 33(9): 1627–34.

Lee, Clara N., Rosalie Dominik, Carrie A. Levin, Michael J. Barry, Carol Cosenza, Annette M. O'Connor, Albert G. Mulley Jr., and Karen R. Sepucha. 2010. "Development of Instruments to Measure the Quality of Breast Cancer Treatment Decisions." *Health Expectations* 13 (3): 258–72.

Liang, Ying, and Yong Bao. 2012. "Analysis of waiting time in medical visits of Shanghai residents." *Journal of Shanghai Jiaotong University (Medical Science)* 32 (10): 1368–72.

Linder-Pelz, Susie. 1982. "Toward a Theory of Patient Satisfaction." *Social Science & Medicine* 16 (5): 577–82.

Linkenbach, J., and H. W. Perkins. 2003. "Most of Us Wear Seatbelts: The Process and Outcomes of a 3-Year Statewide Adult Seatbelt Campaign in Montana." Presentation, National Conference on the Social Norms Model, Boston, July 17.

Lorig, K. 1993. "Self-Management of Chronic Illness: A Model for the Future." *Generation* 17: 1–14.

Lorig, Kate R., Philip L. Ritter, Ayesha Dost, Kathryn Plant, Diana D. Laurent, and Ian McNeil. 2008. "The Expert Patients Programme Online, a 1-Year Study of an Internet-Based Self-Management Programme for People with Long-Term Conditions." *Chronic Illness* 4 (4): 247–56.

Lorig, Kate R., Philip Ritter, Anita L. Stewart, David S. Sobel, Byron William Brown Jr., Albert Bandura, Virginia M. Gonzalez, Diana D. Laurent, and Halsted R. Holman. 2001. "Chronic Disease Self-Management Program: 2-Year Health Status and Health Care Utilization Outcomes." *Medical Care* 39 (11): 1217–23.

Ma, Jin. 2015. "Primary Care–Centered Care in Two Districts in Shanghai." Shanghai Jiao Tong University. Case study commissioned by the World Bank, Washington, DC.

Makoul, Gregory, Amanda B. Zick, Mark Aakhus, Kathy J. Neely, and Phillip E. Roemer. 2010. "Using an Online Forum to Encourage Reflection about Difficult Conversations in Medicine." *Patient Education and Counseling* 79 (1): 83–86.

Marteau, Theresa M., D. Ogilvie, M. Roland, M. Suhrcke, and M. P. Kelly. 2011. "Judging Nudging: Can Nudging Improve Population Health?" *BMJ* 342: 263–65.

Molenaar, S., M. A. G. Sprangers, F. C. E. Postma-Schuit, E. J. Rutgers, J. Noorlander, and J. Hendriks. 2000. "Feasibility and Effects of Decision Aids." *Medical Decision Making* 20 (1): 112–27.

Moore, M. 2012. "Female Doctor Axed to Death in Chinese Hospital." *The Telegraph*, November 29.

Morgan, M. W., R. B. Deber, H. A. Llewellyn-Thomas, P. Gladstone, R. J. Cusimano, and K. O'Rourke. 2000. "Randomized, Controlled Trial of an Interactive Videodisc Decision Aid for Patients with Ischemic Heart Disease."

Journal of General Internal Medicine 15 (10): 685–93.

Mulley, A. 2009. "Inconvenient Truths about Supplier Induced Demand and Unwarranted Variation in Medical Practice." *BMJ* 339: b4073.

Mulley, Albert, Tessa Richards, and Kamran Abbasi. 2015. "Delivering Health with Integrity of Purpose." *BMJ* 351: h4448. doi: 10.1136/bmj.h4448.

Mulley, A., Chris Trimble, and Glyn Elwyn. 2012. *Patients' Preferences Matter: Stop the Silent Misdiagnosis.* London: The King's Fund.

National Voices. 2014. "Prioritising Person-Centered Care—the Evidence." National Voices, London.

NHFPC (National Health and Family Planning Commission). 2014. "National Health Literacy Promotion Action Plan (2014–2020)." Planning document, NHFPC, Beijing.

———. 2015. "Report on Development of Deepening Health Reform to the 18th meeting of the Standing Committee of the 12th National People's Congress." NHFPC report presented December 22, Beijing.

Nolan, R. P., R. E. Upshur, H. Lynn, T. Crichton, E. Rukholm, D. E. Stewart, and M. H. Chen. 2011. "Therapeutic Benefit of Preventive Telehealth Counseling in the Community Outreach Heart Health and Risk Reduction Trial." *American Journal of Cardiology* 107 (5): 690–96.

Nolte, Ellen, Anne Frølich, Helmut Hildebrandt, Alexander Pimperl, and Hubertus J. Vrijhoef. 2015. "Integrating Care: A Synthesis of Experiences in Three European Countries." European Observatory. Case studies commissioned by the World Bank, Washington, DC.

Nutbeam, D. 2008a. "The Evolving Concept of Health Literacy." *Social Science & Medicine* 67 (12): 2072–78.

———. 2008b. "Health Literacy: Perspectives from Australia." Society for Academic Primary Care—Health Literacy Group, London.

O'Connor, A. M., E. R. Drake, V. J. Fiset, J. Page, D. Curtin, and H. A. Llewellyn-Thomas. 1997. "Annotated Bibliography of Studies Evaluating Decision Support Interventions for Patients." *Canadian Journal of Nursing Research* 29 (3): 113–20.

O'Connor, A. M., V. Fiset, C. De Grasse, I. D. Graham, W. Evans, and D. Stacey. 1999. "Decision Aids for Patients Considering Options Affecting Cancer Outcomes: Evidence of Efficacy and Policy Implications." *Monograph of the National Cancer Institute* 25: 67–80.

Osborn, Robin, and David Squires. 2012. "International Perspectives on Patient Engagement Results from the 2011 Commonwealth Fund Survey." *Journal of Ambulatory Care Management* 35 (2): 118–28.

Picker (Picker Institute Europe). 2010. "Invest in Engagement: Self-Management."

Rabin, R. C. 2008. "New Yorkers Try to Swallow Calorie Sticker Shock." MSNBC, July 16. http://www.nbcnews.com/id/25464987/ns /health-diet_and_nutrition/t/new-yorkers -try-swallow-calorie-sticker-shock/# .WzawCdJKiM8.

Rhee, H., J. Allen, J. Mammen, and M. Swift. 2014. "Mobile Phone-Based Asthma Self-Management Aid for Adolescents (mASMAA): A Feasibility Study." *Patient Preference and Adherence* 8: 63–72.

Rollnick, S., W. R. Miller, and C. C. Butler. 2002. *Motivational Interviewing: Preparing People for Change.* New York: Guilford Press.

RTI (Research Triangle Institute). 1997. "The Effects of Informatics Tools and Decision Aids to Support Shared Patient Decision Making about Medical Screening and Treatment." Report to the Agency for Health Care Policy Research, RTI (formerly Research Triangle Institute) International, Durham, NC.

Runz-Jørgensen, Sidsel Marie, and Anne Frølich. 2015. "SIKS—The Integrated Effort for People Living with Chronic Diseases: A Case Study on People Centered/Integrated Health Care in Denmark." The Research Unit for Chronic Conditions, Bispebjerg Hospital, Denmark. Case study commissioned by the World Bank, Washington, DC.

Rydin, Yvonne, Ana Bleahu, Michael Davies, Julio D. Dávila, Sharon Friel, Giovanni De Grandis, Nora Groce, and others. 2012. "Shaping Cities for Health: Complexity and the Planning of Urban Environments in the 21st Century." *The Lancet* 379 (9831): 2079–2108.

Sawka, C. A., V. Goel, C. A. Mahut, G. A. Taylor, E. C. Thiel, and A. M. O'Connor. 1998. "Development of a Patient Decision Aid for Choice of Surgical Treatment for Breast Cancer." *Health Expectations* 1 (1): 23–36.

Stacey, Dawn, C. L. Bennett, M. J. Barry, N. F. Col, K. B. Eden, M. Holmes-Rovner, H. Llewellyn-Thomas, A. Lyddiatt, F. Légaré, and R. Thomson. 2011. "Decision Aids for People Facing Health Treatment or Screening Decisions." *Cochrane Database Systematic Reviews* 4: CD001431. doi:10.1002/14651858.

Sylvia, Sean, Yaojiang Shi, Hao Xue, Xin Tian, Huan Wang, Qingmei Liu, Alexis Medina, and Scott Rozelle. 2015. "Survey Using Incognito Standardized Patients Shows Poor Quality Care in China's Rural Clinics." *Health Policy and Planning* 30 (3): 322–33. doi:10.1093/heapol/czu014.

Szmedra, Philip, and Li Zhenzhong. 2013. "Implementing a Healthy Cities Plan in China: The Impact of Focused Public Health Education on a Diabetes Epidemic." *Southeast Review of Asian Studies (SERAS)* 35: 230–40.

Tang, C., Z. Luo, P. Fang, and F. Zhang. 2013. "Do Patients Choose Community Health Services (CHS) for First Treatment in China? Results from a Community Health Survey in Urban Areas." *Journal of Community Health* 38 (5): 864–72.

Tenbensel, T. 2010. "Public Participation in Health Policy in High-Income Countries—Why, Who, What, Which, and Where?" *Social Science and Medicine* 71 (9): 1537–40.

Thaler, R., and C. Sunstein. 2008. *Nudge: Improving Decisions about Health, Wealth, and Happiness*. New Haven, CT: Yale University Press; London: Penguin Books.

Tucker, J. D., Yu Cheng, Bonnie Wong, Ni Gong, Jing-Bao Nie, Wei Zhu, Megan M. McLaughlin, and others. 2015. "Patient–Physician Mistrust and Violence against Physicians in Guangdong Province, China: A Qualitative Study." *BMJ Open* 5 (10): e008221. doi:10.1136/bmjopen-2015-00822.

Wagner, Edward H., Paul Barrett, Michael J. Barry, William Barlow, and Floyd J. Fowler. 1995. "The Effect of a Shared Decision-Making Program on Rates of Surgery for Benign Prostatic Hyperplasia: Pilot Results." *Medical Care* 33 (8): 765–70.

Wee, Shiou-Liang, Chok-Koong Loke, Chun Liang, Ganga Ganesau, Loong-Mun Wong, and Jadon Cheah. 2014. "Effectiveness of a National Transitional Care Program in Reducing Acute Care Use." *Journal of the American Geriatrics Society* 62 (4): 747–53.

Wennberg, John E. 2010. *Tracking Medicine: A Researcher's Quest to Understand Health Care*. Oxford: Oxford University Press.

WHO (World Health Organization). 1986. "The Ottawa Charter For Health Promotion." Charter document presented at the First International Conference on Health Promotion, Ottawa, November 21.

———. 1998. "Health Promotion Glossary." WHO/HPR/98.1, WHO, Geneva.

———. 2015a. "People-Centered and Integrated Health Services: An Overview of the Evidence." WHO/HIS/SDS/2015.7, WHO, Geneva.

———. 2015b. "WHO Global Strategy on People-Centered and Integrated Health Services." WHO/HIS/SDS/2015.6, WHO, Geneva.

Williamson, L. 2014. "Patient and Citizen Participation in Health: The Need for Improved Ethical Support." *American Journal of Bioethics* 14 (6): 4–16. doi:10.1080/15265161.2014.900139.

Wong, C. K., C. S. Fung, S. S. Siu, Y. Y. Lo, K. W. Wong, D. Y. Fong, and C. L. Lam. 2013. "A Short Message Service (SMS) Intervention to Prevent Diabetes in Chinese Professional Drivers with Pre-Diabetes: A Pilot Single-Blinded Randomized Controlled Trial." *Diabetes Research and Clinical Practice* 102 (3): 158–66.

Xue, F., W. Yao, and R. J. Lewin. 2008. "A Randomised Trial of a 5 Week, Manual Based, Self-Management Programme for Hypertension Delivered in a Cardiac Patient Club in Shanghai." *BMC Cardiovascular Disorders* 8: 10. doi:10.1186/1471-2261-8-10.

Yip, Winnie, Chi-Man Yip, William C. Hsiao, Wen Chen, Shanlian Hu, Jin Ma, and Alan Maynard. 2012. "Early Appraisal of China's Huge and Complex Health-Care Reforms." *The Lancet* 379 (9818): 833–42. doi:10.1016/S0140-6736(11)61880-1.

Yuan, T. 2012. "Man with a Knife Stabbed Four Doctors in China" [title translated from Chinese]. ChinaNews.com, March 24. http://www.chinanews.com/fz/2012/03-24/3769439.shtml.

Zhong, Nanshan. 2015. "Shared Decision Making Is the Core of Humanistic Spirit." *Health News*, June 19. http://www.jkb.com.cn/medicalHumanities/2015/0619/372485.html.

5

Lever 4: Reforming Public Hospital Governance and Management

Introduction

Reforming hospitals is an integral part of reforming service delivery in favor of people-centered primary care. Hospitals will continue to play an important role, but one that will become less financially dominant and focus more on providing only the specialized services that hospitals alone can offer.

As primary care is strengthened and the patient-centered integrated care (PCIC) model is put in place, a wide range of care processes will need to be shifted from hospitals to ambulatory settings (for example, certain surgeries and diagnostics, chemotherapy) and primary care facilities. Hospitals will become centers of excellence, but with adequate volume to deliver high quality care. They can perform important training and workforce development functions. They can also focus more on biomedical research and on providing clinical support to lower-level providers. As described in chapter 2, many of these changes are under way in China. State Council directives since 2009 have emphasized the importance of governance and management reforms as part of a comprehensive strategy that includes reforms in financing, provider payment methods, pricing, and care integration.[1]

One of the core objectives for reforming public hospitals is the separation of government administration from hospital management. The central government envisages public hospitals as independent entities with legal personality. Hence, policy directives aim to grant hospitals greater managerial autonomy from direct hierarchical control by the government administrative apparatus. However, hospitals are to retain their public institutional identity and maintain their accountability to government priorities, particularly in terms of acting in the public interest.

While relinquishing direct control over hospitals, government agencies would play vital roles in regulating, sector planning, standard setting, and monitoring and evaluation (M&E) of hospital performance. At the same time, policy directives aim to improve managerial practices in hospitals. They promote professionalized management and endorse strengthening of managerial functions such as cost accounting, clinical management, logistics and materials management, patient flows, and nursing management.

Strong hospital governance and management will be needed to alter the roles and responsibilities of hospitals and strengthen their links to the broader health care delivery system. Governance and management are the least understood drivers of hospital performance and the hardest to isolate analytically. Emerging evidence from China and elsewhere suggests that elements of good governance include (a) clearly specified and enforced accountabilities to payers and government, (b) a degree of autonomous decision making, (c) aligned incentives, and (d) effective organizational forms that interface with government (as owners) and hospital management. Management also matters: just as better-managed firms tend to display better performance, the same is true for hospitals. Managers put in place the organizational behaviors and practices that are aligned with the broader governance and incentive environment.

This chapter focuses on two major components of the public hospital reform agenda—governance and managerial practices—and is organized as follows:[2]

- *"Overview and Trends"* presents a brief overview of China's hospital sector.
- *"Public Hospital Governance"* examines hospital governance challenges and lessons learned from reform in China and internationally, drawing on available literature as well as cases and surveys commissioned for this report.

- *"Hospital Managerial Practices"* examines the challenges and lessons learned from managerial practices in China and internationally.
- *"Recommendations for Moving Forward with Public Hospital Reform"* specifies the core action areas for reform and the corresponding strategies for improving governance and managerial practices.

Overview and Trends

Hospitals account for a high proportion of China's total health spending. According to government statistics, hospitals absorbed 70 percent of total health spending in 2013.[3] Using a different methodology, the Organisation for Economic Co-operation and Development (OECD) estimated hospital expenditures to account for 54 percent of total health spending.[4] Both figures exceed the average ratio for OECD countries of 38 percent.

Of more concern is the high growth rate of China's hospital spending, which reflects expanding supply and utilization. While total health spending grew 2.7-fold between 2005 and 2013, hospital spending surged threefold (figure 5.1).

Over that same period, the number of hospitals increased by nearly one-third (from 18,703 to 24,709); the number of beds increased by 83 percent (from 3.37 to 6.18 million); and admissions grew 1.7-fold (from 51.1 to 140.1 million). China currently has more beds per 1,000 population than do several OECD countries, including Canada, the United Kingdom, and the United States (figure 5.2). Although beds-per-population ratios are, on average, decreasing throughout the OECD countries, they continue to rise in China.

With their dominance in the health care landscape, hospitals are the point of entry into the health system for most Chinese seeking care. More than half of patients' first contacts with the delivery system for an illness episode, and 40 percent of all outpatient visits, occur in hospitals. In urban areas, more than half of outpatient visits occur in

FIGURE 5.1 **Growth in total health and hospital spending in China, 2005–13**

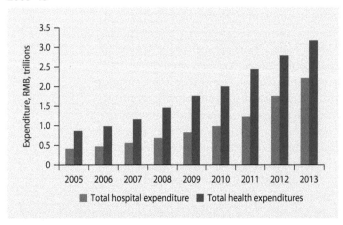

Source: *China Health Statistical Yearbook*, National Health and Family Planning Commission.

hospitals, compared with less than 20 percent in rural areas.

Within the hospital subsector and broader delivery system in China, public hospitals are the major providers of health care. However, official statistics show that in recent years nearly all hospital growth has occurred in the private sector, while the number of public hospitals has declined (figure 5.3). Even so, most of the gains in bed numbers have occurred in public facilities (figure 5.4).

Although public hospitals make up just under half of all hospitals (47.4 percent), they account for the vast majority of beds (80.6 percent, compared with 19.4 percent in private facilities). Similarly, most inpatient admissions (88 percent) occur in public hospitals, which account for more than 85 percent of health professionals. Thus, most public hospitals are relatively large facilities, averaging 310 beds in 2014, while private facilities are much smaller, averaging 67 beds.

Hospital dimensions are trending upward, especially in tertiary hospitals, which are mainly public and located in large urban areas (figure 5.5). These trends are mirrored by statistics on utilization: admissions are growing faster at tertiary hospitals than at secondary hospitals (figure 5.6).

The trend of ever-larger public tertiary hospitals is driven by a number of factors (some of which this report addresses elsewhere), including the following:

- Social insurance systems that favor inpatient over outpatient care
- Demand by a rising middle class for specialty and high-tech care (KPMG 2010), which is heavily concentrated in tertiary hospitals
- Need for improvement in primary care networks that are staffed by less-well-qualified medical professionals
- Need to strengthen functional links (including referral systems) between hospitals and primary care providers
- Investment planning practices that favor hospital construction and expansion (Huang 2009)

FIGURE 5.2   Trends in hospital beds per 1,000 population in China and selected OECD countries, 2000–13

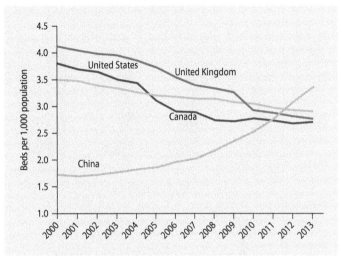

Source: "Statistical Bulletin of Health and Family Planning Development in 2014," National Health and Family Planning Commission.
Note: OECD = Organisation for Economic Co-operation and Development.

FIGURE 5.3   Growth in number of hospitals in China, by ownership type, 2005–13

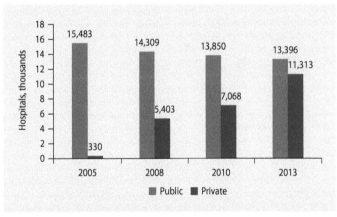

Source: China Health Statistical Yearbook, National Health and Family Planning Commission.

As reviewed in chapter 3, information on the quality of hospital care is sparse. Even less is known about hospital efficiency and productivity. Although the average lengths of stay are declining, they remain longer in China than in most OECD countries (10.4 days and 8.9 days in China's secondary and tertiary facilities, respectively, compared with 8.1 in OECD countries).[5] Moreover, of the 34 countries tracked by the OECD, only 7 registered longer lengths of stay than China. Occupancy rates are generally

FIGURE 5.4   Growth in number of hospital beds in China, by ownership type, 2005–13

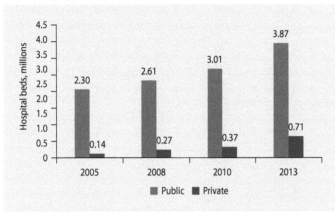

Source: China Health Statistical Yearbook, National Health and Family Planning Commission.

FIGURE 5.5   Trends in average number of beds in Chinese secondary and tertiary hospitals, 2008–14

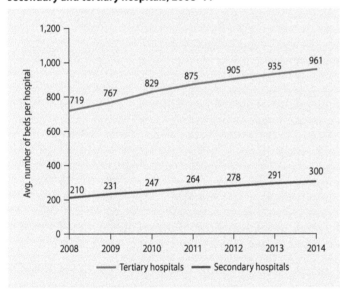

Source: "Statistical Bulletin of Health and Family Planning Development in 2014," National Health and Family Planning Commission.

high—at over 100 percent in tertiary facilities, suggesting overcrowded conditions. Secondary and primary hospitals register lower occupancy rates of 88 percent and 60 percent, respectively.

Micro studies applying robust methods to measure hospital efficiency are inconclusive. For example, using variants of data envelope analysis,[6] researchers examined hospital efficiency in Guangdong province (Ng 2011),

Weifang prefecture (Audibert and others 2013), Shenzhen city (Yang and Zeng 2014), and a panel of regional hospitals across 30 provinces (Hu, Qi, and Yang 2012). In addition, Chu, Zhang, and Chen (2015) applied a directional-distance-function approach to measure technical efficiency.

In general, these studies found huge variations in technical efficiency,[7] with higher-level public hospitals, hospitals in large cities (Beijing, Guangdong, and Shanghai), and private hospitals demonstrating higher efficiency scores. Technical efficiency in public hospitals is yet to be improved, while scale was the source of low efficiency for private hospitals (because of their small size).[8] However, Yang and Zeng (2014) reported that scale inefficiency was also the main source of inefficiency for large public hospitals, suggesting that the aforementioned large expansion of hospital size may reduce productivity. (That is, there is a U-shaped cost curve indicating scale inefficiencies at both ends of the size range.)

The efficiency scores in Chinese hospitals are much lower than those of hospitals in OECD countries measured using similar methods. China's introduction of health insurance is seen to have contributed to efficiency gains, while the use of budgetary subsidies has been associated with lower efficiency. Improvements in efficiency were also found to be related to technological change. More research with larger data sets is needed before conclusive findings can be advanced.

Public Hospital Governance: Challenges and Lessons from Reform in China and Internationally

Governance has many meanings, and the term is used differently across contexts and organizational settings. Hospital governance has been defined as "a set of processes and tools related to decision making in steering the totality of its institutional activity, influencing most major aspects of organizational behavior and recognizing the complex relationships between multiple stakeholders" (Durán, Saltman, and Dubois 2011, 38).

Organizationally, governance consists of an organization's structures and functions that set and enforce policies and exercise the ultimate authority for decisions made on behalf of the organization and its owners. Important functions of hospital governance include defining and reviewing its mission, role, and goals; providing financial stewardship; formulating future strategy; appointing and evaluating the chief executive officer (CEO); ensuring clinical efficiency and quality; and representing the hospital's stakeholder groups (Coile 1994).

Reform of public hospital governance aims to better align the policies and performance objectives of the government (as hospital owner) with the behaviors of hospital managers by providing incentives and accountabilities, which are usually executed through organizational forms such as governing boards and councils. Although public hospital reform is highly complex and context-specific, globally the trend has been to move away from centralized, command-and-control, direct administration of hospitals by government ministries and toward more "arm's-length," indirect oversight, which allows more independent decision making by the hospitals themselves (Huntington and Hort 2015; La Forgia and Couttolenc 2008; Preker and Harding 2003; Saltman, Durán, and Dubois 2011).

Granting greater autonomy to public hospitals requires altering how the government engages with them. It involves putting in place (and enforcing) a new set of accountability mechanisms and crafting incentives to support these accountabilities. Taken together, these accountabilities and incentives foster the alignment of hospital behaviors with government objectives while respecting the increased decision-making autonomy of hospitals.

Following a framework developed to analyze practices in the governance of public

FIGURE 5.6 **Growth in admissions to Chinese tertiary and secondary hospitals, 2006–14**

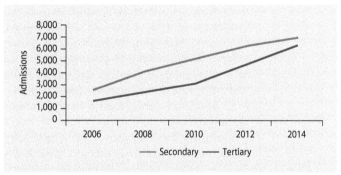

Source: *China Health Statistical Yearbook*, National Health and Family Planning Commission.

hospitals,[9] this section examines four major elements of public hospital reform:

- Accountability mechanisms to ensure that hospitals perform well and to align their performance with public objectives
- Incentives facing the organization to support accountability
- Degree of autonomy or decision-making authority granted to managers
- Organizational makeup and legal status of governance models

A fifth element—the quality of managerial practices to implement decisions and respond to accountabilities and incentives—is taken up in the concluding "Recommendations" section.

Hospital Governance Challenges in China

Public hospital reforms in Shanghai, Zhejiang, and Sanming aim to affect hospital behaviors by linking hospital director income to performance. However, insufficient information is available to judge the impact of this performance assessment system and how it differs from routine systems to evaluate managers' performance.

Anecdotal evidence suggests that Sanming is better at hospital reform implementation because its directors' positions are at risk based on performance assessments. Dongyang's board has established a comprehensive hospital-based performance assessment system that embraces the financial, efficiency, quality, patient satisfaction, and safety domains. Unlike Dongyang, Shanghai and Zhenjiang do not independently assess hospital performance or compliance with rules and standards, and they appear to piggyback on supervisory practices performed by government agencies.

Sanming's leadership group carefully supervises the implementation of human resource, compensation, and pricing reforms. Nevertheless, some observers suggest that influencing managers' behaviors may be difficult because managers appear more accountable to the higher-level leaders who appointed them than to the government agencies responsible for reform implementation or on-the-ground performance.

Public hospitals in China require stronger governance arrangements if they are to drive improvements in quality and efficiency, promote service integration, and act in the public interest rather than respond to vested interests related to revenue generation (Allen, Cao, and Wang 2013; He 2011; Tam 2008; WHO and World Bank 2015).[10] This subsection summarizes the main governance challenges observed in China's public hospitals.

Accountability

Mechanisms to hold hospital managers accountable for efficient and high-quality services or for fulfilling social functions need to be developed. Given many Chinese hospitals' underlying incentives to enhance revenues via treatment choices and drug provision, their managers are oriented toward augmenting service volume and expanding infrastructure, including acquiring high-tech equipment.

Diffuse lines of accountability make it difficult to counterbalance these incentives. Hospital directors are in principle accountable to multiple government agencies at local government levels. For example, the National Health and Family Planning Commission (NHFPC) is responsible for health-related

matters, yet responsibility for setting prices and payment mechanisms, allocating human resources and capital investments, and purchasing services is divided among other ministries.

The main form of oversight of the bureaus is hierarchical; it is usually applied through directives known as "red letters" that instruct hospitals to implement public policies and to follow relevant public administration rules such as for human resource management, use of funds, use of public assets, or product procurement. In practice, these directives often provide ambiguous and sometimes conflicting guidance because (a) the functions, responsibilities, and accountabilities of public hospitals are not clearly defined and (b) the agencies themselves have unaligned policies and diverse interests (Yip and others 2012). Nor are the directives rigorously enforced— partly because supervision itself is divided across different agencies.

Although financial reporting is strong, public hospitals face weak requirements from government and social insurers to improve their safety processes, quality, patient satisfaction, or efficiency. Improvements along these lines are generally not a priority (Tam 2008). Hospital directors are rarely monitored or sanctioned for noncompliance with government directives or for failure to meet agreed-upon targets (He and Qian 2013).

Incentives

Hospitals earn a large share of their revenues by selling services to social insurers and self-paying individuals, usually through fee-for-service payment systems. Surpluses are distributed to staff through nontransparent bonus schemes that are based on service production and revenues, usually at the department level.

Under these conditions, hospitals and their clinicians have strong incentives to maximize revenues by raising service volumes, ordering expensive procedures, selling pharmaceuticals, providing unnecessary care, generating admissions, and extending patients' hospital stays.[11] Given the incentives to capture more patients, hospitals have little interest to integrate with, or shift care to, lower levels of the health care system or to fulfill social functions. Meanwhile, hospitals' revenue-seeking behaviors have led to considerable citizen discontent.

Autonomy

Public hospital autonomy in China has few parallels internationally. Most of the hospitals enjoy considerable autonomy in financial and asset management, retaining their financial surpluses, opening and closing services, expanding or contracting their physical plants and equipment, and entering into and servicing debts. However, the legacy of "command-and-control" remains, both with the appointment of senior managers and in the management (conducted directly by local government leaders or agencies) of "quota" personnel. This legacy means that hospital managers lack full decision-making authority to hire, dismiss, and set compensation for all staff. It may also limit the quality of management practices.

Nevertheless, in light of the weak accountabilities and distorted incentives, some local government officials consider, probably correctly, that merely granting public hospitals more autonomy—or similarly, freeing them from the vestiges of hierarchical government control—will result in chaos (WHO and World Bank 2015).

Organizational arrangements

Most public hospitals in China are governed directly by government bureaus. As mentioned earlier, oversight is exercised through directives issued by different bureaus. It is each bureau's responsibility to assess and enforce implementation and to engage directly with hospital managers. Some bureaus may be reluctant to sanction public hospitals for lack of compliance because they see the hospitals as extensions of the government administrative apparatus. Except in a limited number of pilots, no independent supervisory structures such as

boards or councils have been created or given responsibility to oversee and monitor hospital activities and performance related to quality, efficiency, or fulfillment of social functions.

The central government envisages public hospitals as having full decision-making authority over management and operations so that hospital operation and management are separated from the governments' ownership rights (State Council 2015a, 2015b). Importantly, the central government also envisages putting in place an accountability framework by requiring M&E of several domains of hospital performance (for example, functions, quality, spending, patient satisfaction, access, and efficiency). However, as in the case of previous reform directives, it is not clear how such a framework will be designed or applied, nor who will have the authority to assess (and enforce) performance and compliance. International experience may provide some guidance on reforming governance arrangements for public hospitals.

Hospital Governance Challenges and Lessons from International Experience

In high- and middle-income countries, a range of modalities for hospital governance have emerged that differ in their legal provisions, financing schemes, accountability arrangements, and decision-making rights. All of them operate within and respond to specific incentive environments, which vary considerably across countries (Nolte and Pitchforth 2014). The foundation trusts of the National Health Service (NHS) in the United Kingdom, nonprofit private foundations in the Netherlands, regional health enterprises in Norway, public health care companies and foundations in Spain, and social health organizations in Brazil, to name a few, reflect different aspects and configurations that public hospitals have adopted (Durán and Saltman 2015; La Forgia and Couttolenc 2008; Mossialos and others 2015; Preker and Harding 2003).

The impetus for developing these models arose from concerns over avoidable distortions that resulted from command-and-control political authority, including the following:

- Overlap or conflicts of interest between ownership, regulation, and management (functions that were often consolidated in a single government agency)
- Political interference in hospital operations, especially human resource management
- Restrictive or inflexible administrative rules applied to all inputs
- Undersupply of some services and oversupply of others
- Inefficiencies and budgetary overruns
- Low quality
- Patient dissatisfaction
- Inability to respond to technological change or more generally to change the model of care
- Weak links to the broader delivery system

Another driver of greater hospital independence was a reform movement known as "new public management" (Greenwood, Pyper, and Wilson 2002). Reformers sought to modernize hospitals' organizational culture by introducing a market or quasi-market environment that would enhance competition and motivate entrepreneurship and thereby improve efficiency and responsiveness to patients. In some countries, such as Spain and the United Kingdom, reforms that granted greater autonomy to public hospitals were in part a political compromise to avoid privatization. In several countries, the public hospital reforms were part of broader public administration reforms (as in Brazil) or were a component of health system reforms such as the separation of purchasing from provision and the introduction of alternative provider payment mechanisms.

Reforms that shift decision rights to public hospitals are complex. International experience suggests that to succeed, they require putting in place a legal or regulatory framework; setting up new organizational arrangements (such as boards); establishing a more arm's-length relationship between government and hospital; making use of indirect tools of accountability (such as performance reviews, compliance monitoring, external audits, use of contracts, and contract management) and provisions for their enforcement; and aligning incentives with public objectives (Deber, Topp, and Zakus 2004; La Forgia and Couttolenc 2008; Preker and Harding 2003; Saltman, Durán, and Dubois 2011).

China's experience along these lines is nascent at best (Allen, Cao, and Wang 2013; World Bank 2010). The following discussion summarizes the international experience with organizational arrangements, autonomy, accountability, and incentives. It focuses on three countries: Brazil, the United Kingdom, and Spain.[12]

Organizational arrangements

Nearly all reforms are based on or at least initiated through legislation or regulation. The breadth and depth of legislation or regulatory change varies across countries and over time. In some countries, such as Brazil and the United Kingdom, framework laws were issued that supported a single governance modality that applied to all hospitals participating in the reform. In São Paulo, Brazil, public hospitals with reformed governance were incorporated under civil law as nonprofit social organizations of "public interest," known as social health organizations (OSSs), following statutes that were set out in a 1998 state law.[13] The United Kingdom used a two-step process for legally granting autonomy to public hospitals: self-governing trust status in the mid-1990s superseded by the establishment of foundation trusts in the early 2000s.

In contrast, Spain enacted different laws for different governance modalities. India and Panama limited their reforms to a handful of hospitals that benefited from specific laws enacted to make them independent public entities.

Hospital governance models take a wide range of legal and organizational forms and corresponding nomenclatures (table 5.1) and are specified in regulatory frameworks. The models emerged in the 1990s and early 2000s and vary considerably in terms of the organizational structures (and the degree of independence granted to hospitals) that they established to replace hierarchical government administration.

Most countries legislated some form of board or council that serves as the unit of responsibility between hospital management and government owners. In general, boards are expected to set overall policies and strategies, approve and oversee business plans and financial matters, monitor performance against objectives or targets, appoint managers, and ensure that the hospital acts in the public interest.

Boards can take many roles, forms, and compositions, and they can be responsible for a single hospital, a group of hospitals, and even regional networks of facilities, as several examples show:

- *In the United Kingdom,* the board of governors (BoG) for the NHS foundation trusts (FTs) consists of elected and appointed members. The BoG in turn appoints the hospital governance board consisting of hospital executives and non-executives representing various professional interests.
- *In Brazil,* the Secretariat of Health of the State Government of São Paulo (SES) contracts with nonprofit organizations (NPOs) to manage public hospitals. Each NPO is required to have a board that is legally accountable to the government. Board members can be public officials, representatives of private entities, or private citizens selected by the NPO. Boards have not been formed in specific hospitals.
- *In Spain,* governance boards of various types have been established in hospitals, and members are appointed by the government. Depending on the modality, board members are high-ranking public officials from a specific region, or they can be a mix of public officials and private members. In one model in Spain, a board

TABLE 5.1   Hospital governance models in selected countries

Country	Hospital governance model
Brazil	• Social health organizations (OSSs)
Czech Republic	• Limited liability companies • Joint-stock companies
Estonia	• Joint-stock companies • Foundations
Norway	• State enterprises
Portugal	• Public enterprise entity hospitals
Spain	• Public health care companies • Foundations • Consortiums • Administrative concessions (to a private firm)
Sweden	• Public-stock corporations
United Kingdom	• Self-governing trusts • Foundation trusts

Sources: La Forgia and Couttolenc 2008; Saltman, Durán, and Dubois 2011.

was formed for a regional network consisting of a hospital and ambulatory care facilities run by a private firm under concession.
- *In Norway,* hospitals are organized as independent trusts with boards consisting of appointed elected politicians and regional health authorities.

Autonomy

Although in many countries the new governance modalities for public hospitals have granted their managers considerable decision rights, few public hospitals can be considered fully autonomous and comparable to independent private entities. Across the world, even substantially autonomous public hospitals lack the decision-making flexibility of private hospitals. Experience has shown that decision-making boundaries are a moving target and depend on shifting political and financial conditions. Some well-intended reforms were not fully implemented, the governments proving unwilling or unable to relinquish bureaucratic and political control (Huntington and Hort 2015; Preker and Harding 2003; Saltman, Durán, and Dubois 2011).

The FTs in the United Kingdom and the OSSs in São Paulo, Brazil, enjoy considerable autonomy in hiring, firing, and compensating staff as well as in managing inputs, procurement, and finances as long as their finances are under control and regulators find their health care quality and performance to be acceptable (for the FTs) and compliant with the SES contractual terms (for the OSSs). They can also retain and invest surpluses and borrow commercially.

In both countries, these hospitals are free to hire their CEOs and do so based on merit criteria.[14] CEOs are not appointed by the government. As public facilities, however, the hospitals cannot choose their patient mix, and those in both countries must seek government permission to make major shifts in the services they provide. Similarly, plans for infrastructure expansion and purchases of expensive equipment require government approval.

Some differences between the FT and OSS models are worth noting:

- *Infrastructure planning.* For FTs but not the OSSs, infrastructure expansion usually requires a multiyear planning exercise that is set by the economic regulator and ultimately the national Department of Health.
- *Business ventures and assets.* FTs can set up joint ventures and subsidiary businesses but cannot sell core assets such as land and buildings, because these assets are locked to prevent privatization and cannot be used to guarantee debt or be sold to pay creditors. OSSs are not permitted to sell shares or seek investors.
- *Labor contracts.* FTs have the right to depart from nationally determined labor contracts and pay scales for their medical professionals and unionized staff, though none have done so. OSSs are free to set the labor contracts and compensation for all their staff.
- *Price setting.* For service price setting, FTs supposedly have more freedom, but in practice they are price takers of the centrally determined tariffs and other price

structures that are used to reimburse hospitals for care or ancillary services such as medical education. OSSs do not set prices and are not permitted to charge fees to "public" patients. More recently, however, OSSs have negotiated fees with private insurance plans to provide services to insurance plan members.

In Spain, an administrative concession to a private joint-venture company constitutes a model that probably gives public hospitals more autonomy than in any other model in Europe. The hospital has the right to decide on all its inputs (including capital investments) and on expanding its services, though its profit margins are capped at 7.5 percent. At the time of this reform, staff of the formerly government-run hospital received the right to remain civil servants or to become nonstatutory staff. All new staff are nonstatutory, with compensation and benefits set by the private company awarded the concession.

In the other governance modalities in Spain, hospitals enjoy less autonomy. For example, foundations and consortiums have decision rights over inputs and investments but follow public procurement rules. They have freedom to hire and fire staff but have only limited authority to determine workers' income levels other than bonuses at the margin.[15] Spain's public health care companies have limited autonomy. They employ statutory workers who are subject to civil service rules. Because their boards mainly comprise regional health officials, regional health departments still appear to exercise considerable control.

Accountability

Putting in place sound accountabilities is arguably the essential tenet of governance reforms and is an important driver of results. To be sure, the granting of greater autonomy needs to be accompanied by the implementation of strong and enforceable accountability mechanisms to orient hospital behaviors toward improved performance, compliance with social functions, and alignment with government priorities. International experience suggests that the success—judged by the achievement of public policy goals—of any public hospital reform involving autonomy depends on the effectiveness of accountability mechanisms.

Typically, hospitals are held accountable by a number of agencies (such as government owners, payers, and regulators) in several areas (such as use of resources, performance, compliance with rules, procedures, and standards) through specific checks and balances (such as reporting requirements, inspections, audits, contracts, and citizen involvement). It is worth repeating that the key to checks and balances is their rigorous enforcement, which, as explained below, requires a robust information system. Boards are the usual interface between oversight agencies and the hospitals and are ultimately held accountable for hospital behaviors and performance.

United Kingdom

In the United Kingdom's FTs, oversight focuses on board performance and accountability and is conveyed through three mechanisms: the BoG, Monitor, and annual reports.

Board of governors. The BoG for FTs holds the nonexecutive directors (NEDs) on the hospital governance board (including the chairman) accountable—both individually and collectively—for performance, financial reporting, quality, and other aspects. In turn, the NEDs hold the hospital executive, including the CEO, to account. The roles of board chairman and CEO are separate, which is an essential feature of British governance in both the public and private sectors.

Monitor. The government created two oversight agencies. One is an FT-specific economic regulator, known as Monitor, that is responsible for licensing FTs, monitoring their financial performance, assessing their achievement of nationally set targets (such as for waiting times) and compliance with FT laws, and gauging their quality of governance. Monitor does not oversee (or prescribe) how the targets are met. Monitor also has responsibilities to foster competition, set systemwide prices, and ensure continuity of care. Another oversight agency, the Care Quality Commission, is responsible for ensuring compliance with regulatory standards for quality and patients' safety in all public and private health care facilities.[16] FTs are also answerable to other regulatory bodies in specific areas such as financial management, medical education, and fertility treatment.

Annual reports. Finally, FTs are required to produce publicly available annual reports on financial status, patient engagement activities, and a range of quality measures covering adverse events, infection rates, mortality rates, patient feedback, staff views, and performance against targets. With few exceptions, public hospitals in England have a strong focus on public service and on fulfilling social functions, though this focus is more implicit and embedded in social arrangements than codified.

Spain

In Spain, boards and managers are held accountable by regional health authorities through audits, inspections, and reporting requirements on financial status, quality, and other information. Compulsory minimum data sets established by legislation for all hospitals (autonomous and nonautonomous) are a main feature of information tracking and reporting in Spain that incorporates indicators of activities, accessibility, and performance. The detailed topics covered and the periodicity and comprehensiveness of reporting vary across regions according to rules and procedures set by regional public authorities. Most autonomous models apply a program contract arrangement (contrato programa) between the regional health service executive and facilities as the preferred mechanism for funding and accountability. Contractual terms specify reporting requirements and other documentation that hospitals must send to the regional health service executive.

Accountability arrangements also vary by model; more explicit accountability measures have been put in place for those hospitals granted greater autonomy. For example, in the concession model the contract between the private operator and the government requests specific information from the operator including well-structured reports on monitoring indicators, detailed business and financial records, and clinical reports based on a large set of indicators. Reporting requirements in less autonomous models such as public health care companies and foundations are related to performance assessments for payment purposes. Public health care companies, foundations, and consortiums use some intermediate economic indicators based on statements of income and expenditures, but they give a strong simultaneous role to budget monitoring. Consortiums provide monthly reports on waiting lists and quarterly reports on financial status.

Brazil
Accountability mechanisms for Sáo Paulo's OSSs consist of several interlocking components:

- *Performance measures.* Production targets, quality benchmarks, and rules are specified in a legally binding "management contract" between the SES and each OSS; OSS boards are legally accountable and supervise hospitals' compliance with contractual terms.
- *Purchasing and contract management.* The SES created a dedicated service purchasing and contract management unit that reviews and analyzes OSS performance and rule compliance and negotiates budgets.
- *Contract and performance enforcement.* The contract management unit enforces compliance with the management contract and performance measures through financial sanctions. Poor performance can lead to withholding of funds and cancellation of the government contract (and retendering to another NPO).
- *Audits.* The SES conducts internal audits, and the state's comptroller general conducts external audits to verify the performance data and financial statements submitted by the OSSs.
- *Standardized information system.* The SES developed and installed a standardized information system that links all OSSs with the SES management unit to facilitate performance monitoring; much information is placed in the public domain.
- *Independent review commission.* The SES established an independent review commission consisting mainly of civil society representatives to conduct "social audits" of OSS operations to ensure that hospitals are fulfilling their social obligations (such as not charging patients, not denying care, and not referring patients for unnecessary services) and that their behaviors are aligned with the mission of a public hospital.

Incentives
The behavior of any hospital is driven by incentives, whether monetary or nonmonetary. Some incentives are embedded in the way hospitals and staff are paid, but others are ingrained in the system culture. Examples include the centrality of free care and dedication to public service observed in the United Kingdom's NHS.

United Kingdom
The United Kingdom attaches considerable weight to the use of "codes of behavior." Though these codes appear voluntary and are self-policed, they are laid on top of many rules—for example, on care quality—that have the force of law. Clinical regulations are strong and enforced. FTs are at financial risk for budgetary overruns. If an FT is perceived by Monitor, the economic regulator, to have become financially unviable, it is taken under central control. Importantly, some of the most prestigious hospitals in the United Kingdom have not become FTs, in part because of a poor track record of staying within their financial envelopes.

All FTs are paid using fixed prices under an activity tariff for standard procedures, together with a series of other payment mechanisms for specialized activity, emergency care, medical education, and earnings from research. The standard tariff—calculated from national average retrospective cost information for diagnosis-related groups (DRGs)—is the dominant portion of the revenues of district general hospitals. More-complex tertiary units earn much more of their income from specialized tariffs and from teaching. Such hospitals also inevitably attract the bulk of research funding, whether privately sponsored or public, and benefit from other allowances for such factors as location in major city centers.

To the extent that standardized national DRG-based prices underlie the tariff, there is no incentive—indeed the opposite—to favor expensive treatments, though it remains true that the greater the activity, the greater the revenue. That said, both self-governing trust and FT hospitals have framework contracts with their local purchasing agencies that cap their total revenues (hence the fact that so many U.K. hospitals are now running at a financial loss).

In FTs, hospital professional staff, particularly senior ones, have reasonably high salaries that are little affected by their activity. In general, the FTs (or more broadly, the NHS) have few incentives to order extra diagnostic tests, buy more drugs, or carry out interventions judged unnecessary on clinical grounds. Staff are paid for extra sessions beyond the standard in their contract, and modest bonuses may be paid, but generally clinicians face a broadly flat income throughout the NHS.

Hospital staff also have options to treat private patients within and outside the hospital. A study found that, on average, income from private patients provides about 2 percent of an FT's total income—suggesting that profit-making activities are minimal at best.[17] Equally, staff do not share in profits or surpluses created at the level of the hospital. When a change in internal management or a gain in efficiency reduces costs for a department, most of the resulting surplus will stay on the hospital's central books.

Nor do patient choice and competition appear to be strong incentives for individual clinicians or for organizations. For example, the vast majority of primary care referrals are either to the local facility or, for patients with more serious conditions, to the nearest specialty unit, so it is unlikely that patient choice is a big driver in performance.

Brazil

São Paulo's OSSs face powerful incentives to meet performance (and productivity) targets, improve quality, and align their behavior with public priorities. Importantly, OSSs are at financial risk for budgetary overruns and poor performance.

The global budget is performance-driven in two respects. First, 90 percent of it is paid monthly and is linked to meeting production or volume targets for specific services (such as inpatient, outpatient, diagnostic, and surgical procedures) as specified in the management contract. If hospitals skimp on production, they are financially sanctioned. For example, if a hospital only meets 70 percent of a production target for, say, surgical procedures, its financing is reduced by 30 percent. In contrast, hospitals have few incentives to oversupply services because they do not receive a financial benefit if they exceed production targets (except under extenuating circumstances such as an epidemic). Second, 10 percent of the budget is placed in a retention fund and paid in quarterly allotments against achievement of benchmarks for efficiency and quality (such as for infection control, mortality rates, length of stay, and readmissions).

Importantly, both sets of benchmarks are enforced, and monthly and quarterly budgetary allocations are reduced for an OSS hospital that fails to meet them. The state government pioneered the use of standardized cost accounting systems that were installed in each OSS hospital with a virtual link to the SES's contract management unit. The cost data allow hospital managers to monitor the costs of all inputs in each department and allow the contract management unit to compare costs across all facilities and services, analyze efficiency and productivity, and negotiate global budgets.

The availability of cost data has shifted the nature (and transparency) of annual budget formulation away from the more or less arbitrary setting of ceilings to a calculus based on volume and costs. Having information on volume and costs also allows the SES to monitor potentially opportunistic behaviors such as reducing high-cost services.

OSSs cannot provide bonuses to their managers, who receive fixed salaries; they can provide bonuses to staff, but none have done so. There is no evidence that OSSs pay higher salaries than traditional public hospitals. OSS managers prefer to recruit high-quality staff who "fit" well with the organizational culture, and they quickly dismiss nonperformers (World Bank 2006).

Spain

In Spain, the hospitals managed under the concession model are the only ones that face significant financial risk. The Alzira region in Valencia provides a noteworthy example. This initiative involves a public-private partnership in which the concessionaire, a private company, operates a 300-bed public hospital along with 40 public primary health care centers in a region, serving approximately 250,000 people (NHS European Office 2011).

The concessionaire must offer universal access and is responsible for nearly all care provided to the population; it receives a fixed per capita payment from the regional government. Service obligations and other responsibilities are specified in a contract. The government has the right to audit and inspect facilities to ensure compliance with regulation and contractual terms as well as to impose sanctions. The concessionaire must cover all expenses from the capitation payment, including amortizations, investments, payroll, and other operating expenses for the network of facilities. Medical staff receive salaries that contain a fixed (80 percent) and variable (20 percent) component. The latter is paid depending on achievement of targets for access and quality. If patients seek care outside the region, the concessionaire is responsible for paying the full cost of that care

according to established fees (based on DRGs).

The capitation payment provides a strong incentive to strengthen primary care, avoid unnecessary hospital admissions and services, and integrate hospitals with primary providers to provide cost-effective care at the appropriate location. Given that the concessionaire is at financial risk for covering the cost of patients seeking care outside the region, it faces a strong incentive to strengthen quality and safeguard patients' experiences.

International experience: Ingredients for successful public hospital reforms

International experience suggests that reforms of public hospital governance appear to work best under the following conditions:

- A social consensus on the role of public health care
- A strong legal framework that defines the organizational forms of governance, including roles, functions, and accountabilities
- Full decision rights for hospital managers to hire, fire, promote, and shape workers' incentives (through remuneration, work hours, rewards, and sanctions) and to manage all other inputs
- Sound accountability mechanisms together with effective enforcement measures to ensure performance and compliance with public objectives
- The right incentives to align hospital and staff behaviors with desired performance and outcomes and, most critically, to avoid adverse actions such as private rent-seeking via increasing clinical activity, diagnostic tests, or drug sales

The trend in the United Kingdom has been to promote greater independence of public hospitals but with strengthened accountabilities. The sustainability of Brazil's OSSs and of the two Spanish models (concessions and consortiums) may be related to the strong contractual relationships with private partners, which involve transfers of financial risks. In contrast, public health companies and foundations have been closely linked to politicians and public administrators through board membership; over time, political interference in the management of these hospitals increased, legislation was amended, and managerial autonomy decreased.

In the United Kingdom, where many hospitals are in financial difficulty, the economic regulator, Monitor, is placing less emphasis on converting self-governing trusts to FT status and more emphasis on supporting hospitals in financial distress. Monitor and other government agencies have relied on "NHS providers"—membership-representative organizations of public and private hospitals—that actively support hospitals in the early stages of their transition to FTs to help with the challenges of organizational redesign and to provide training to board members.

In general, though the evidence is not definitive, public hospital reforms that embraced the above components have been shown to increase efficiency, quality, and patient satisfaction (La Forgia and Couttolenc 2008; McKee and Healey 2002; McPake and others 2003; Preker and Harding 2003). A recent study examining hospitals in England and the United States found a strong relationship between the governance practices of hospital boards and quality processes and ratings (Tsai and others 2015). Recent analyses also show that the Alzira concessionaire model in Spain provides more efficient and better-quality care than comparator hospitals, as measured by lower readmission rates, shorter waiting times, higher productivity, and higher patient satisfaction (NHS European Office 2011).

Other studies found that governance reforms involving autonomy had little effect (Allen and others 2012; Govindaraj and Chawla 1996), although it is possible that the reforms featured in these studies involved only limited autonomy and little strengthening of accountability mechanisms to improve performance (Castaño, Bitrán, and Giedion 2004; Preker and Harding 2003). Indeed, several European public hospital reforms have been found to have little effect on

efficiency, in part because they granted hospitals only partial decision-making authority; in these cases, political meddling continued and accountability was lax (Saltman, Durán, and Dubois 2011). But despite their limited effect, the European reforms were deemed "reasonably successful" (Saltman, Durán, and Dubois 2011, 71), and they have been more or less embraced by governments, managers, and citizens. To be sure, in many countries, the movement toward greater hospital independence will be difficult to reverse.

Emerging Models of Hospital Governance Reform in China

Typical of broader Chinese reform measures, local experiments in public hospital reform were to serve as the basis for formulating policies and the subsequent rollout of successful models to address the aforementioned challenges. Seventeen cities were identified to launch public reform pilots in 2010.

This section examines the opportunities and constraints in hospital governance in China, drawing on selected cases commissioned for this report. Following the analytical framework presented earlier, table 5.2 shows the major components and characteristics of governance models being piloted in four mostly urban areas: Shanghai-Shenkang, Zhenjiang-Kangfu, Dongyang, and Sanming.[18] The findings are presented by component.[19]

Organizational arrangements
The Shanghai and Zhenjiang models are typical of governance reforms observed in the hospitals that are piloting reform in China, building upon initiatives that were launched in Wuxi, Wifang, and other cities in the early and mid-2000s (World Bank 2010). These cities legislated the creation of new agencies—usually referred to as hospital management centers or councils (HMCs)—that are led by high-level municipal officials and consist of representatives of public agencies that are involved in health sector operations or in oversight.

TABLE 5.2   **Characteristics of selected reform models for Chinese public hospital governance, 2015**

Component	Shanghai (Shenkang)	Zhenjiang (Kangfu)	Dongyang	Sanming
Organizational arrangement				
Organizational unit or name	Multihospital management center	Multifacility "network" council	Hospital board	Prefecture health reform leadership group
Jurisdiction	Municipal	Municipal	Municipal	Prefecture
Number of hospitals	24	5[a]	1	22
Autonomy				
Hiring and firing hospital director	Partial[b]	No	Yes	Yes
Hiring and firing quota staff	No	No	No	No
Flexibility in setting remuneration for quota staff	No	No	Yes	Yes
Pricing	No	No	No	Yes
Residual claimant	No[c]	No[c]	Yes	Partial
Asset management	Partial[d]	Partial[d]	Yes	Yes
Accountability mechanisms				
Performance assessment of hospital directors[e]	Yes	No	Yes	Yes
Performance assessment of hospital(s)	No	No	Yes	No
Review and enforcement of safety and quality standards	No	No	Yes	No
Compliance supervision	Similar to other public facilities	Similar to other public facilities	Yes	Partial
Incentives				
Realigning staff incentives	Partial	No	Yes	Yes
Governance unit: members' position at risk	No	No	No	No
Hospital directors' position at risk	No	No	Yes	Yes
Sanctions for noncompliance with rules or for low performance	Similar to other public facilities	Similar to other public facilities	Yes	Yes

Sources: Li and Jiang 2015; Li and Wang 2015; Ma 2015; Ying 2014.
a. Network includes nine ambulatory centers.
b. Can recommend to government.
c. Retained at hospital level.
d. In consultation with government agencies.
e. Usually involves signing a "responsibility agreement" between governance unit and hospital director.

Staffed by civil servants, the HMCs were granted legal personality, but their member hospitals also maintained their original legal personalities. The goals of the HMCs in these two cities differ. The one in Shanghai aims to improve the operations and performance of the participating hospitals. The one in Zhenjiang shares this objective but also aims to promote greater vertical integration among a mix of facilities at the tertiary, secondary, and primary levels.

The Dongyang pilot involves a single hospital that formed an independent board with government and nongovernment participation. The board consists of representatives of government agencies, private corporations, and local and foreign medical schools. The hospital has special legal status, and its statutes are similar to those in the corporate governance models observed in private hospitals.[20] The pilot aims to create a corporate governance arrangement that will improve the efficiency, capacity, and quality of services while maintaining the hospital's public nature through "social responsibility" (Li and Wang 2015).

Sanming has not created a new agency but has decreed a fully empowered leadership group (LG) to enact health system reforms with an initial focus on the prefecture's 22 tertiary and secondary hospitals (Ying 2014).[21]

Autonomy

In Shanghai and Zhenjiang, key decisions on human resource management, staff compensation, and service pricing remain with government agencies. Hospitals have largely retained their residual claimant status and their ability to manage their own assets. In Zhenjiang, entities were unwilling to relinquish control to the HMC, which spans independent municipal and district public administrative units (Li and Jiang 2015). As a result, the district administration has retained control of asset management in primary care units and some secondary hospitals, while the municipal administration, together with hospital management, controls asset management in larger hospitals.

In contrast, Dongyang's independent hospital board and Sanming's LG exhibit considerably more decision rights. Dongyang still abides by government pricing policies and rules that govern the hiring and firing of quota staff, but the board determines the full compensation package for all staff (Li and Wang 2015). Sanming's LG has assumed full decision-making authority except over the recruitment and dismissal of quota staff. It has altered compensation

policies for hospital directors and all medical professionals. For example, the government directly pays the salaries of hospital directors, and physicians' income is no longer linked to revenue-based bonuses. The LG also makes all decisions regarding major asset investments, prices, and reimbursement rates for social insurance (Ying 2014).

Accountability

Three of the governance models aim to influence hospital behaviors by linking hospital directors' income to performance. However, it is uncertain how the performance assessment system in force differs from routine systems and whether it is sensitive and specific enough to capture improvements in an objective and reliable way. Another question relates to the observation that hospital directors appear more accountable to the higher-level leaders who appointed them than to the government agencies that are responsible for reform implementation or on-the-ground performance (Qian 2015).

Among the four cases studied here, only Dongyang's board has established a comprehensive hospital-based performance-assessment system that spans the financial, efficiency, quality, patient satisfaction, and safety domains (Li and Wang 2015). In fact, Dongyang's is the only governance arrangement within the group to mandate a continuous quality improvement program—which has entailed establishing a quality management department, a committee to control medical records, and a clinical assessment system for physicians and nurses.

The Shanghai and Zhenjiang HMCs do not independently assess hospital performance or compliance with rules and standards, and they appear to piggyback on the supervisory practices performed by government agencies (Li and Jiang 2015; Ma 2015). Dongyang's board and Sanming's LG are fully empowered to apply sanctions themselves. In practice, however, Sanming's sanctions have centered on noncompliance with LG-initiated reforms. The LG carefully supervises the implementation of the human resource, compensation, and pricing reforms it has crafted, but it relies on government agencies to supervise other domains (Ying 2014).

Incentives

Dongyang and Sanming have placed physicians on salaries and delinked their bonus income from the revenues the hospitals derive from sales of drugs, medical supplies, and diagnostic tests. The salaries contain fixed and variable components, with the latter being unrelated to revenues but linked to a combination of indicators of productivity, cost control, quality, and patient satisfaction (Sanming Prefecture Government 2015). As suggested above, altering physician compensation was a major accomplishment and has addressed a cost-escalating distortion widely observed in public hospitals.

Shanghai has placed a hard budget constraint on total personnel spending, but this measure has not clearly affected the bonus system. Surplus revenues are still distributed to physicians at the discretion of hospital and departmental directors (Ma 2015).

In Shanghai and Zhenjiang, partly because most of the governance units consist of government officials, member facilities' positions are not at risk if they perform poorly or do not comply with government policies (Li and Jiang 2015; Ma 2015). In Dongyang and Sanming, by contrast, hospital directors can be dismissed (by the board or the leadership group, respectively) for poor performance (Li and Wang 2015; Ying 2014).

In terms of residual claimant status, the Sanming LG has set caps on reimbursements for inpatient stays and outpatient visits; if hospitals spend below the caps, the savings are shared with the social insurance schemes (Ying 2014)

The Limits of Hospital Governance Models

These four cases suggest that public hospital governance reforms in China have made important advances but have not conclusively separated hospital management from government administration. An array of organizational arrangements has emerged, but most are pilot initiatives. Each has aimed to consolidate decision making within a single entity by coordinating the actions and policies of diverse government departments responsible for the health sector. The failure to rigorously evaluate these models, and public hospital reform interventions in general, limits the ability to draw lessons from the pilot experiences (box 5.1).

Variants of the HMC model implemented in Shanghai and Zhenjiang are common in other pilots in China (World Bank 2010). In practice, the HMC members are all current or former government officials and appear to behave more as extensions of government than as independent agents. Additional decision rights have not been transferred to the HMCs from government administration. Meanwhile, hospitals under HMC governance maintain their financial autonomy and do not appear to be answerable to the HMCs on financial matters. Arm's-length tools and mechanisms to foster accountability have not been developed, and the HMCs mostly rely on the direct supervisory and oversight mechanisms traditionally operated by the relevant government agencies. Nor do the HMCs have a robust track record in realigning incentives.

In contrast, Dongyang Hospital has many of the features of corporate governance observed internationally. It is operated by an independent board with members from both government and nongovernment bodies and enjoys considerably more decision-making authority than the HMCs. The board has created strong accountability mechanisms and incentives to control costs and improve quality and patient experience. However, the origins of the Dongyang governance model, which involved external partners that provided financing and technical support, may be difficult to reproduce elsewhere in China. After 20 years of existence, the model has yet to be replicated. As in the OSS model in Brazil and the concessions and consortiums models in Spain, having an external partner may help to defend (and advance) the reform model.

BOX 5.1   **Impacts of public hospital reform in China**

Given that none of the following cases has been rigorously evaluated, it is difficult to distinguish the results of public hospital reforms from the results of other health reforms—such as the policy specifying zero markup on drug sales.

Based on available but limited administrative data, salient results of each case are as follows:

- *Shanghai:* Compared with similar hospitals in Shanghai, the HMC's member facilities showed no difference in trends in service volume (inpatient discharges), lengths of stay, or asset expansion from 2003 to 2013.
- *Zhenjiang:* Compared with provincial and national averages between 2009 and 2013, Zhenjiang was able to contain charges and spending, outpatient visits, and inpatient admissions. The reduced growth in spending may relate to the consolidation of sterilization, pathology, and logistics services for all network members by the hospital management council.
- *Dongyang:* Dongyang's income from drug sales was 10–15 percent lower than that of comparator hospitals both before and after the introduction of the zero-markup policy in 2012. Its average outpatient and inpatient costs were significantly lower than those in a sample of comparator hospitals over the same period. Restrictive use of antibiotics has exceeded national standards. The hospital reports a surgical-site infection rate of 1 percent and an overall nosocomial infection rate of 7 percent. These rates are closely monitored.
- *Sanming:* For outpatient visits and inpatient admissions, government reports show significantly lower growth in Sanming's hospital spending between 2009 and 2013 than the average for Fujian province and the national average. The cost of an average inpatient stay fell by 3.9 percent in Sanming, while it rose by 11.6 in Fujian and by 14.7 percent nationally. Drug revenues as a proportion of Sanming's total hospital revenues decreased from 47 percent to 28 percent between 2011 and 2013.

Sources: Li and Jiang 2015; Li and Wang 2015; Ma 2015; Ying 2014.

Facing a financial crisis, high-level leaders in Sanming created the LG with a broad reform mandate, though with an initial focus on addressing cost escalation in the prefecture's hospitals. The LG can best be described as an arrangement for health system governance rather than as a model of hospital governance. The LG was granted full autonomy and authority to alter accountabilities and incentives to foster more efficient use of hospital resources. To its credit, the LG took on the complex and deep-rooted issues that distorted the incentives facing hospitals. The hospitals themselves were not granted greater decision-making authority, nor was a platform of accountability mechanisms formalized. The LG did consolidate decision making across multiple institutional actors. The group lacks institutionalization, and in the future, administrative rotation of key officials may erode its effectiveness and sustainability. Despite intense promotion by the central government, the Sanming model has yet to be replicated in China.

Hospital Managerial Practices: Challenges and Lessons from China and Internationally

How hospital managers respond to the accountabilities and incentives embedded in their governance and organizational environments is a key determinant of hospital performance. Managerial practices can be defined as "the set of formal and informal rules and procedures for selecting, deploying, and supervising resources in the most efficient way possible to achieve institutional objectives" (Over and Watanabe 2003, 122–23). Hospital management entails a wide range of clinical and nonclinical functions related to selecting, using, and supervising resources.

The effectiveness of managerial practices is a key determinant of hospital performance. This section first briefly reviews the international literature on the relationship between hospital management and performance and then examines what is known about managerial practices in Chinese public hospitals. It concludes with a brief review of innovative managerial practices in small subset of private hospitals in China.

Management Matters: International Evidence and Experience

Studies of hospital management in several countries have shown that better management practices are associated with better outcomes, quality of care, and financial performance (Bloom and Van Reenen 2010; Lega, Prenestini, and Spurgeon 2013; McConnell and others 2013; Tsai and others 2015). In a recent systematic review of the literature, Parand and others (2014) found a positive relationship between management and promoting improvement in quality and patient safety, but more research is needed to better understand how this occurs in practice. For example, the impact of managerial practices on outcomes may be mediated by other factors such as the degree of physician engagement with management, leadership styles, commitment, and organizational culture (Curry and others 2011; Kirkpatrick and others 2009; Mannion, Davies, and Marshall 2005; Parand and others 2014).

A recent empirical study of hospitals in England and the United States has shown that good governance is associated with better managerial practices (Tsai and others 2015). Professional management was introduced into English hospitals in the 1980s. High managerial competence contributed to the success of England's FTs and Brazil's OSS-operated hospitals (Edwards 2011; La Forgia and Couttolenc 2008). In contrast, low managerial capacity may be a contributing factor in the poor performance of

public health care companies in Spain and may have led Spanish regional governments to backtrack on governance reforms (Durán 2015).

In sum, although the evidence is inconclusive, there is a broadly held belief that management matters for improving hospital performance and that developing managerial capacities is an important goal for health systems and hospitals. How to develop such capacities and create the enabling organizational environment for their effective application is an important emerging concern of health systems in high-income countries (Lega, Prenestini, and Spurgeon 2013).

In additional to traditional managerial training, managerial measurement and organizational tools borrowed from other industries are increasingly used in hospital settings internationally to improve performance. These tools include total quality management (TQM); the plan-do-check-act (PDCA) cycle; "lean management"; the balanced scorecard (BSC); and the 5S cycle (discard, arrange, clean, standardize, and discipline). While the evidence of their effects is mixed, hospital managers consider these tools effective for fostering organizational and behavioral change (La Forgia and Couttolenc 2008; Mazzocato and others 2012; Naranjo-Gil 2009).

Managerial Practices in Public Hospitals in China

Information on managerial practices in Chinese hospitals is scarce. Available studies are generally qualitative, small in scale (usually based on a single hospital), or focused on a single managerial function such as staff performance, patient-flow management, or application of managerial tools such as balanced scorecards. This section reviews the literature on hospital management practices, drawing on surveys and case studies.[22] We first examine what is known about management in public hospitals and then turn to management practices in successful private hospitals.

A recent pilot study aimed to systematically measure management practices in a small sample of secondary (35) and tertiary (75) public hospitals across 27 provinces (Liu 2015).[23] Researchers applied a methodology known as the World Management Survey (WMS), which was originally developed to measure managerial and organizational practices in manufacturing but has subsequently been applied to and validated in hospitals in several countries (Bloom and Van Reenen 2007, 2010; Bloom and others 2010; McConnell and others 2013). The survey consists of questions on 20 management practices across four major management domains: standardizing care and operations, target setting, performance monitoring, and talent management. The research team interviewed 291 department directors and head nurses. Following the WMS methodology, practices were scored on a scale of 1 to 5 for each of the 20 practices. A higher score indicates better performance.

The weighted average management score in China was found to be 2.68, with a highly dispersed distribution ranging from 1.85 to 3.35. Compared with OECD countries where the WMS has been applied, China is an average performer, scoring lower than the United Kingdom (2.86) and the United States (3.0) but higher than France (2.4) and Italy (2.48).[24]

Figure 5.7 displays the average scores for each management practice across the four domains. Not surprisingly, secondary hospitals scored significantly lower (2.66) than tertiary facilities (2.90), and considerable variation in scores was observed across provinces. Hospitals scored the highest in use of human resources, promotion of high performers, performance review, and attracting talented staff, but they scored the lowest in standardization and protocols, continuous improvement, consequence management, rewarding high performers, and removing poor performers.

The scores, combined with findings from interviews, highlighted several managerial shortcomings:

- Management practices appear reactive in the sense that hospitals lack systems to find and prevent potential problems or to continuously improve their processes and services.
- Because of a lack of autonomy in staffing, managers have little authority to dismiss low performers; talent management is not a high priority, and there are few consequences for poor performance.
- Hospitals do not systematically analyze performance data or use data to provide feedback for improvement.
- Lack of standardization of care may indicate deficient clinical management, which can negatively affect quality and outcomes.
- Performance management is mainly used to allocate staff bonuses, not to improve individual or hospital performance. Interestingly, autonomy (defined as authority to make decisions on human resource, asset, and financial management) was associated with higher management scores.

The research also sought to analyze the determinants of score variation, accounting for the following factors: competition (number of hospitals within a 30-kilometer radius); hospital characteristics (age of facility and average number of beds); location (by region); economics (per capita gross domestic product [GDP]); and autonomy (decision-making authority on human resource, asset, and financial management). The results showed that bed count, competition, and autonomy were associated with higher management scores. How competition may improve managerial practices was not directly examined.

Research on specific management practices supports a subset of the findings from the WMS-based study. For example, surveys show that BSCs are widely applied in China, usually by tertiary public hospitals affiliated with medical schools (Lin, Yu, and Zhang 2014). Typical of BSC application internationally, Chinese hospitals reported that they used BSCs to develop performance measures along four dimensions: financial, patient satisfaction, service quality, and research and

FIGURE 5.7   **Average managerial practice scores of Chinese hospitals, 2015**

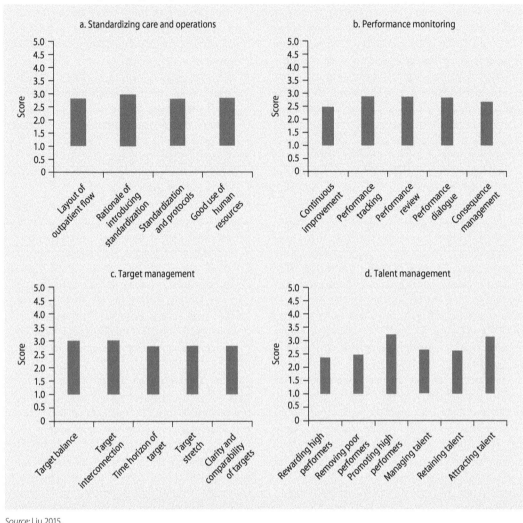

Source: Liu 2015.
Note: Scores obtained using the World Management Survey methodology, which scored practices of 110 hospitals on a scale of 1 to 5 for each of the 20 practices. A higher score indicates better performance.

training. BSCs were found to contribute to improved organizational performance and worker satisfaction. However, another survey, albeit small in scale, found that the use of BSCs in Chinese hospitals focuses on financial performance rather than on quality and patient satisfaction (Gao and Gurd 2014). The tool has mainly been used for assessing physicians' performance to determine their bonuses.

Evidence, mainly from single-site case studies, shows that hospitals in China are using internationally recognized management tools to improve their operations and quality. For example, the provincial hospital in Guangdong has used "lean management" techniques to improve the efficiency and throughput of operating rooms (Guo, Ma, and Zhang 2014). Dongyang Hospital has applied management tools such as TQM, quality-control circles, and the PDCA cycle to improve clinical and nonclinical processes throughout the hospital (Li and Wang 2015). Although TQM and PDCA have been applied in specific Chinese facilities

(Chen and others 2014), the extent to which they are used elsewhere is unknown.

As mentioned earlier, public hospital executives are appointed by higher-level authorities of the party and government, and the appointments are not merit based. Even within hospitals, promotions are usually based on years of tenure and are not determined competitively. Most hospital managers have received little formal training. For example, a 2004 study of managers in 96 hospitals across 21 provinces found that less than one-third had received short-term professional training, while more than half had learned management through their work experience (World Bank 2010). Presidents of public hospitals are typically responsible for all managerial, clinical, and academic activities and tend to manage during their "spare time" or to delegate managerial functions to junior staff. There are no standards or qualification systems for hospital managers, and most see managerial know-how as something that requires investment by government authorities rather than by the hospitals themselves.

Managerial Practices in Private Hospitals

Several elite private hospitals have adopted management practices and service models that set them apart from other private (and public) hospitals in China and make them more similar to hospitals in OECD countries. Three examples are reviewed here: the Aier Eye Hospital Group, Foshan Chancheng Hospital, and Wuhan Asia Heart Hospital. To maintain and expand their market position, these facilities have created enabling organizational and managerial environments of continuous improvement to provide high-quality care efficiently. Though they are not representative of private hospitals in China, these facilities can serve as learning platforms for improving clinical and nonclinical management in public and other private hospitals. Noteworthy management practices are highlighted below.

Though not discussed in the summaries, each case presents evidence that management practices affect quality, patient satisfaction, and finances. However, the evidence has not been independently verified. Similar managerial practices may also be evident in public hospitals, but research is needed to document management innovations. For example, as previously mentioned, the public hospital in Dongyang has pioneered a continuous quality improvement program, and a number of public hospitals use BSCs to monitor performance.

Aier Eye Hospital Group

The Aier Eye Hospital Group (AEHG) is a medical care company operating 70 ophthalmological hospitals across China in 2014 and employing more than 5,000 medical professionals (physicians, nurses, and technicians). The AEHG has adopted corporate-governance arrangements and management structures typical of private hospital systems in OECD countries, in which major decisions and several key functions (such as procurement, human resource management, and asset management) are centralized at the headquarters level (Chen, Gao, and Wang 2015).[25]

A board of directors that oversees all operations of the conglomerate has four specialized committees: strategic, audit, compensation, and managerial supervision. Management is structured in seven main domains: strategic investments, medical devices, marketing, medical management, operations, human resources, and finance. Individual hospital management teams are appointed by the board and are responsible for developing and implementing business plans that are aligned with corporate objectives and policies. The AEHG also applies a "unified management framework" in which individual facilities submit standardized reports, including financial statements, customer analysis, and production and quality, at set intervals. Monthly audits are conducted on five randomly selected hospitals.

AEHG management emphasizes high-quality care and patient satisfaction.

For example, each of the group's hospitals is required to operate six quality-related committees, covering medical quality control, quality of nursing management, ethics, pharmaceutical management, hospital-infection control, and medical-records management. These committees are responsible for monitoring and assessing relevant practices, and they conduct inspections twice a year as well as monthly reviews. Every month each hospital submits a report on medical quality to the leading quality group at headquarters. Each department operates a quality-control team composed of a director, deputy director, and head nurse; the team's responsibilities include reviewing and reporting adverse events. The AEHG also has crafted standard clinical pathways and operating procedures, including checklists for diagnostic services, surgical procedures including for presurgical and postsurgical care, infection control, prescriptions, and medical records.

Several measures are in place to enhance patient satisfaction and communication, including internet-based appointment scheduling; flexible, walk-in appointments for the frail and elderly; WeChat registration; a limit of 40 outpatients per doctor per day; a limit of 20 minutes on patients' waiting time; access to a 24-hour hotline; free shuttle service for people with disabilities; and a patient-service team to inform patients about risks and involve them in their treatment and recovery.

Foshan Chancheng Hospital

In 2004, Foshan Chancheng Hospital (FCH) was converted from a public hospital to a nonprofit facility. Shares are divided among employees and private investors. Although FCH is a general hospital, it is known for specialty care in maternity, pediatrics, orthopedic surgery, and urology. In 2013, the FCH had 700 beds and 1,300 staff.

The FCH has a number of initiatives oriented toward making it more "people-oriented and patient-centered," by developing a hospitalwide culture of fostering positive experiences for patients. For example, it has established a "head nurse home" program in which head nurses engage with patients and their families upon admission, advising about their conditions, treatments, and care processes and responding to any concerns. Head nurses also make arrangements for postdischarge care in outpatient settings.

The hospital also introduced a "one-card solution": a smart card linked to a mobile application (WeChat) that facilitates a number of processes including one-stop payment, appointment making and reminders, access to diagnostic examination results, use of mobile drug-dispensing machines, and inquiries or questions to medical professionals. According to FCH managers, the one-card solution has significantly reduced waiting time for all outpatient services, including diagnostics. A free shuttle bus transports fragile elderly patients to and from their appointments and therapy sessions.

The FCH uses a BSC system to assess staff and departmental performance. This system incorporates a wide range of indicators related to economic efficiency, patient trust, quality of care, patient safety (reduction of medical errors), and staff professional growth. Physicians' and nurses' bonus compensation is tied to their BSC scores. In addition, FCH takes medical complaints from patients and families seriously. It has instituted a root-cause analysis program that investigates complaints, errors, accidents, and factors that contributed to the event and recommends and enforces corrective measures.

Wuhan Asia Heart Hospital

Wuhan Asia Heart Hospital (WAHH) operates a 759-bed facility specializing in the treatment of cardiovascular diseases. In 2014, it had a staff of 2,000, including 450 physicians and 850 nurses. Partly to keep within the reimbursement rates of social insurance schemes, WAHH has established cost-control measures (Chen and Gao 2015):

• Uniform bar coding and tracking of all drugs and consumables, records of which are affixed to a patient's medical record

- Standardized cost accounting, which determines costs per procedure
- A tracking system that identifies deviations of 20 percent or more from standard costs and triggers an audit in such cases (management aims to keep such deviations to fewer than 5 percent of patients)
- Package pricing for ambulatory and short-stay surgical procedures
- Application of clinical pathways
- Strict pharmaceutical procurement and management, which keeps total drug spending to less than 14 percent and 25 percent of treatment costs for inpatients and outpatients, respectively.

Both WAHH and the AEHG use a "differentiated management model" in which clinical and academic responsibilities rest with the facility president and nonclinical matters are handled by a general manager. In public hospitals, the hospital president has both clinical and nonclinical responsibilities. This pattern is replicated at the departmental level: each departmental clinical director has an administrative manager to support nonclinical activities and facilitate coordination with other departments. Each department also has a medical assistant—usually a nurse—who is responsible for communication with patients, post-discharge follow-up, and promotion of patients' self-management. For example, WAHH has established a patient service center that makes appointments, provides medical advice, undertakes triage, and assists patients with navigation among the hospital's service departments.

For long-term postdischarge care, WAHH operates a "life link" follow-up program in which about 60 percent of discharged patients participate. It has also developed standard operating procedures to facilitate patient flows and the division of staff responsibilities in outpatient clinics, diagnostics, wards, and operating rooms.

Recommendations for Moving Forward with Public Hospital Reform

There is broad agreement in China that deeper reforms are needed to improve hospital performance in cost control, quality of care, and patient satisfaction. Alternative models of governance and improvement in managerial practices are only two pieces of a complex hospital reform puzzle that involves reforms in financial arrangements, human resources, planning, and service integration. These latter themes are taken up in other chapters of this volume.

International and Chinese experience suggests that there is no single path to public hospital reform, but emerging models have common elements:

- Establishing (and enforcing) accountability mechanisms
- Crafting strong incentives to align behaviors with performance objectives and public priorities
- Developing sound organizational arrangements for governance
- Increasing the decision rights of hospital managers
- Strengthening managerial capacities

This section recommends specific implementation strategies in each of these core areas, drawing on the Chinese (Shanghai-Shenkang, Zhenjiang-Kangfu, Dongyang, and Sanming) and international (Brazil, Spain, and United Kingdom) case studies as well as the general literature. The core actions and corresponding implementation strategies are summarized in table 5.3.

Like the other types of reforms recommended in this report, public hospital reform requires a unitary vision of comprehensive reforms. The international models described here evolved over time. In the United Kingdom, hospital governance reform benefited from previous health system reforms, including for the professionalization of management, the separation of purchaser from

TABLE 5.3   Five core action areas and implementation strategies for improving public hospital governance and management

Core action areas	Implementation strategies
1: Strong accountability mechanisms for autonomous public hospitals to strengthen performance	• Specify the rules, reporting requirements, and other mechanisms to foster strong hospital accountability to government, including contracts, financial management, audits, patient-safety processes, and performance requirements • Set up institutional arrangement to support monitoring and oversight • Determine the information to be publicly disclosed • Establish effective enforcement mechanisms
2: Incentives aligned with public objectives and accountabilities	• Gradually place hospitals at financial risk for budgetary overruns and low performance (for example, quality, efficiency, and patient satisfaction) • Develop payment systems that promote cost consciousness • Install standardized cost-accounting systems in hospitals and use the results in budget setting
3: Sound organizational arrangements for public hospital governance	• Develop organization form(s) that support the proposed governance model(s) • Codify the model within a legal framework • Set the functions, roles, and composition of governance entities such as boards and councils
4: Gradual delegation of decision rights to hospitals	• Establish a formal application and approval process for hospitals to achieve (more) autonomous status under the to-be-determined governance model • Set a phased timetable for transferring functions that are currently managed by government bureaus but are to be shifted to the (approved) autonomous hospitals • Create formal mechanisms to assist hospitals in developing governance arrangements and subsequently to assess effects and provide feedback for adjustments
5: Managerial capacity building	• Assess the skills of hospital managers, the quality of managerial practices, and their effects on the quality and efficiency of hospital operations and services • Study and adapt managerial practices implemented in leading public and private facilities • Establish an executive management program for upgrading skills along several dimensions • Support demonstration projects that address specific managerial challenges • Develop a career path for professional hospital managers and integrate managerial and leadership competencies into recruitment and promotion practices • Work with academic institutions to strengthen and expand degree programs in hospital management and ultimately to establish centers of excellence in management and leadership development • Create a benchmarking system for hospital management that periodically tracks indicators of various dimensions of management and links them to important indicators of hospital performance—not to evaluate management but to proactively find problems and improve practices as a means to improve hospital performance

provider, and the introduction of managed pricing. It also benefited from high clinician remuneration in hospitals without either fee-for-service or profit making and from strong clinical regulation and enforcement. In São Paulo, Brazil, the OSS model was introduced as part of broader public administrative reforms. Its design took account of lessons learned from failures in earlier hospital governance reforms and involved strengthening the state's mixed delivery system, consisting of public purchasing of private provision. Even with these advantages, São Paulo took more than five years to introduce the accountability arrangements and incentives that support the governance model.[26]

Though it is difficult to disentangle any one of the five core action areas from the others, accountabilities and incentives are clearly crucial. Establishing robust accountabilities and powerful incentives to strengthen performance and align hospital behaviors with public objectives—Core Action Areas 1 and 2, respectively—underpin the remaining core action areas, which relate to putting in place effective organizational governance models (Core Action Area 3), strengthening autonomy (Core Action Area 4), and improving managerial practices (Core Action Area 5).

Without strong (and enforceable) accountabilities and appropriate incentives, it is unlikely that emerging organizational arrangements will represent the interests of government or patients. Instead, greater autonomy may stimulate deviant behaviors and greater distancing from public priorities, and there will be little demand for better managerial practices. Finding a workable balance between decision-making autonomy and accountability is no easy task. Indeed, no hospital, whether public or private, can act outside the interests of its owners. Planners must find a pragmatic formula for combining these elements while accounting for local context and capacities. Implementers must also display a willingness to make the necessary adjustments.

Core Action Area 1: Strong Accountability Mechanisms

A fundamental component of hospital reform is to put in place sound accountability mechanisms to orient hospital behaviors toward improved performance, compliance with social functions, and alignment with government priorities. International experience suggests, for example, that the success of any public hospital reform involving greater autonomy depends on the effectiveness of accountability mechanisms.

In China, many observers consider that granting public hospitals more autonomy, or, similarly, freeing them from direct administrative control, would result in even more unconstrained behaviors. But

experience both in China and internationally suggests that this would not be the case if sound indirect mechanisms for accountability are established and skillfully deployed. It is important that regulations and rules specifying accountability mechanisms are strong and enforceable, and that measures are put in place to support their enforcement.

Recommended strategies to strengthen accountability include the establishment of rules and other mechanisms to foster accountability; the implementation of institutional arrangements to support monitoring and oversight; the determination of publicly disclosed information; and the establishment of enforcement mechanisms.

Strategy 1: Specify rules, reporting requirements, and other mechanisms to foster strong hospital accountability to government
"Arm's-length" accountability mechanisms applied to autonomous public hospitals usually entail rules and compliance monitoring. They include internal and external audits of board appointments and operation, accounting and financial reporting, quality and safety standards, patient outcomes, and fulfillment of social functions.

Reporting requirements, performance targets, and other checks and balances are increasingly embodied in legally enforced contracts between the hospital board (as owner) and government (as the service purchaser). For example, as evident in the British, Brazilian, and Spanish cases examined earlier in this chapter, contracts often are the instrument used to allocate resources, set performance requirements, assess compliance with government regulations, and mandate the integration of care with lower-level providers. The overall content, terms, and management of contracting mechanisms can be specified in regulations. However, as discussed below, good contracts require strong contract management, monitoring, and enforcement.

Strategy 2: Set up institutional arrangements to support monitoring and oversight

Oversight agencies or similar units within current agencies play key roles in fostering accountability and enforcing compliance. Some countries have found it necessary to establish new public units to deploy newly established tools for indirect accountability; some have built contract management units to negotiate, monitor, and enforce accountability requirements deriving from the receipt of public funding; and some have established units to support the establishment and operation of hospital boards.

In the United Kingdom, as noted earlier, Monitor oversees financial performance, legal and regulatory compliance, and the achievement of national targets, while the Care Quality Commission reviews compliance with standards and policies for quality and patient safety. In São Paulo, the SES's purchasing unit manages and monitors compliance with contracts, while an independent review commission comprising citizens, academics, and government representatives conducts social audits of OSS operations that focus on compliance with social functions.

Strategy 3: Determine the information to be publicly disclosed

In the United Kingdom, the FTs are required to produce publicly available annual reports on financial status; patient-engagement activities; and a range of quality, patient safety, and performance measures including adverse events, infection rates, mortality rates, patient feedback, staff views, and performance against targets.

In São Paulo, the OSSs report on unit costs and service production by department, and on metrics related to quality, patient safety, and efficiency. The state government has installed information systems in autonomous public hospitals to enable validated reporting of performance and costs, and it makes all data publicly available on the SES website.

In Spain, hospitals governed under the concession model must provide the government with detailed and updated dashboards of monitoring indicators as well as financial statements.

Strategy 4: Establish effective enforcement mechanisms

The effectiveness of accountability mechanisms depends on their effective enforcement. In São Paulo, every year, the SES refuses payment of all or part of the retention funds (10 percent of a hospital's agreed financing envelope) for OSSs that have not achieved agreed-upon performance benchmarks. Continued poor performance spanning two years results in cancellation of the SES contract with the NPO that operates the OSS hospital and the selection of another NPO through an open tendering process.

In China, many of these tools for indirect accountability are in use, though apparently in only a handful of hospitals. For example, the director of Dongyang Hospital signs a performance agreement with the board, which links the director's salary to performance. Continued underperformance would put the director's position at risk. Financial accounts are audited internally by the hospital board and externally by the Dongyang Audit Bureau. The board assesses the hospital's performance on a series of indicators reflecting cost containment, quality, and efficiency.

Core Action Area 2: Incentives Aligned with Public Objectives and Accountabilities

Hospital behaviors are shaped by incentives, which are usually embedded in how hospitals and staff are paid. As discussed in chapter 6, all payment systems come with a set of underlying incentives. However, hospitals may also respond to nonfinancial incentives that are embedded in the culture and behaviors of medical care organizations and the broader delivery system. For example, the United Kingdom's NHS contains embedded incentives, apparently shared by all or most of its personnel, that support a culture of public service, free care, and to a certain extent, ethical practices. Such a culture may not be so evident in other systems. Professional staff also respond to incentives related to growth and career paths.

The following strategies are recommended to support the alignment of incentives with public objectives: (a) gradually placing hospitals at financial risk for budgetary overruns and low performance in quality, efficiency, and patient satisfaction; (b) developing payment systems that promote cost consciousness; and (c) creating the institutional capacity in government to monitor performance and enforce sanctions.

Strategy 1: Place hospitals at financial risk for budgetary overruns and low performance

The United Kingdom's FTs and São Paulo's OSSs are at financial risk for budgetary overruns and for meeting performance goals. However, each country takes a different approach.

Like many other OECD countries, the United Kingdom pays its hospitals, including FTs, using a DRG-based payment system with a cap or ceiling on total spending. DRGs bundle discrete services provided to a patient with a specific diagnosis into a single payment and thereby promote the efficient use of services. Use of this system gives little incentive to offer more intensive treatment, extend a patient's length of stay, or favor expensive therapies. A ceiling on total spending also provides a disincentive for a hospital to increase the number of patients (and thus the volume of DRG payments).[27]

Several countries have also integrated criteria on quality and outcomes into DRG systems to allow payments to vary according to performance. In the United Kingdom, for example, a percentage of a hospital's annual income (from DRG payments) is adjusted according to the hospital's performance in meeting the quality goals specified in its contract with regional authorities (Mason, Ward, and Street 2011). As reviewed in chapter 6, DRG-like initiatives are already under way in China.

São Paulo's OSSs have taken a different approach to aligning financial incentives. The state government establishes a global budget that is performance-driven and sets targets for volume, quality, and efficiency. Hospitals have no incentive to either oversupply or undersupply services. For example, if hospitals skimp on production, they are financially sanctioned; if they exceed production targets, they are not financially compensated except under extenuating circumstances such as an epidemic. As mentioned earlier, 10 percent of a hospital's budget is placed in a retention fund and paid in quarterly allotments against meeting efficiency and quality benchmarks (such as for infection control, mortality rates, length of stay, and readmissions). These benchmarks are strictly enforced.

To facilitate oversight, each OSS has a standardized cost-accounting system with a virtual link to the SES's purchasing and contract management unit. This unit helps hospital managers to monitor the costs of all inputs in each department and uses the data to compare costs across all facilities and services, analyze efficiency and productivity, and negotiate global budgets. The availability of cost data has shifted the nature (and transparency) of annual budget formulation away from more or less arbitrary setting of ceilings to a calculus based on volume and costs. Countries using DRG-based systems have also strengthened and standardized their cost-accounting systems, and France and Germany provide financial incentives to hospitals to comply with cost-accounting standards (Busse and Quentin 2011).

Core Action Area 3: Sound Organizational Arrangements for Public Hospital Governance

Organizational arrangements or forms such as boards or councils serve as the organizational interface between government (as owners) and hospital management and staff (as service providers). Though they may vary considerably in their composition, size, roles, functions, and degree of independence from government, they constitute the key organizational element of the broader accountability framework for public hospital governance. The nature of any organizational form is woven into the fabric of the governance model itself and codified in a legal or regulatory framework. Boards or councils legally exercise the ultimate authority for decisions made by or on behalf of the owners. In China, developing such arrangements is necessary to achieve reform objectives related to the "separation of government administration from hospital management" (Burns and Liu 2017).

Recommended strategies in this core action area are the following:

1. Develop organizational form(s) that support the proposed governance model(s)
2. Codify the model within a legal framework
3. Set the functions, roles, and composition of governance entities such as boards and councils.

Strategy 1: Develop organization forms that support the proposed governance models

Legislation usually specifies the major elements of a new public hospital model including the components outlined in this chapter: organizational forms, accountabilities, incentives, and autonomy. It characterizes the legal structure of the model as a legal entity separate from government.

Depending on national law, different legal forms have emerged in different countries, including nonprofit corporations, public benefit corporations, nongovernmental organizations, joint ventures, public foundations, and trusts. In nearly all cases, hospitals under these legal models are considered government entities but are governed separately and independently from the government. The degree of government participation varies significantly.

Strategy 2: Codify the governance model within a legal framework

Legislation in the United Kingdom created a new single national model of hospital governance, the FT, which is established as a public benefit corporation. In Brazil, in the context of a national legal framework for public administrative reform, the State of São Paulo legislated the OSS as a new governance model, constituting it as a nonprofit organization of "social interest" (utilidad publica)—a form of public benefit organization. In Spain, whose government is heavily decentralized, multiple models for the governance of public hospitals have emerged, supported by regional legal frameworks. In many countries, individual public hospitals have been granted independence through special and facility-specific legislation.

Internationally, governance reform models specify an organizational form that is formally and legally responsible for hospital behaviors and performance. Nearly all countries have legislated a hospital-level body—and, in some cases, a multihospital body—to replace the direct government administration of public hospitals. Composition, tenure, and selection criteria (and process) are also specified in law or in corresponding regulations.

The degree of separation from the government administrative apparatus varies, as evidenced by board membership. In Spain, government officials dominate board membership in the public health companies and foundations, suggesting strong government participation in decision making. The governance bodies of the OSSs in Brazil and the concession models in Spain mainly draw their members from private companies and nongovernmental organizations. Other countries have a mix of public, private, and citizen representation, as in the FTs in the United Kingdom and Dongyang Hospital in China. The FTs represent a special case in which local people, staff, and patients can become FT members and elect board members, while the other board members are appointed by government.[28]

In China, most hospital boards established thus far (such as those for hospital management councils) consist exclusively of public officials. However, a recent State Council policy directive requires that governance boards or councils should consist of a broader range of participants, including representatives of government agencies, delegates of the People's Congress, members of the

Communist Party of China, and representatives of relevant stakeholders.[29]

Strategy 3: Set the functions, roles, and composition of governance entities

Finally, the functions and responsibilities of hospital boards or councils must be clearly delineated. The vast literature in hospital trade and practitioner journals includes manuals and codes that provide guidance on board functions, responsibilities, and operational procedures (Bjork 2006; Bley and Shimko 1987; Cuervo-Cazurra and Aguilera 2004; Gage, Camper, and Falk 2006; Gill, Flynn, and Reissing 2005; Holland, Ritvo, and Kovner 1997; Rice 2003).

The major board functions include (a) providing financial stewardship, including approval of business plans, budgets, and capital spending; (b) formulating strategies; (c) evaluating management; (d) monitoring hospital performance (for example, to ensure efficient service production and clinical quality and compliance with social functions); and (e) responding to stakeholders such as government, payers, and patients (Coile 1994; Edwards 2011).

It is important that the regulatory framework as well as hospital governance statutes specify responsibilities such as determining the organization's mission and objective; selecting the CEO and assessing the CEO's performance; ensuring effective planning and adequate resources; monitoring programs and services; ensuring ethical integrity; maintaining accountability to government and other stakeholders; and recruiting, training, and assessing new board members (Ingram 1996). It is recommended that governance bodies (boards or councils) recruit and select hospital managers based on merit criteria and according to processes that are specified in regulations and hospital statutes.

Core Action Area 4: Gradual Delegation of Decision Rights to Hospitals

International experience suggests that granting public hospitals greater autonomy is not an all-or-nothing endeavor and that

implementation is highly complex. Decision-making boundaries vary considerably, can shift over time, and depend on political and financial conditions. Relative to autonomous public hospitals elsewhere, public hospitals in China already enjoy a high degree of financial autonomy, but they have less freedom of action in human resource management.

Some observers consider autonomy to be the "acid test" of public hospital governance because it involves drawing a line between, on the one hand, higher-level policy decisions and, on the other hand, frontline operational decisions involving quality, efficiency, and responsiveness that should be exempt from higher-level scrutiny, oversight, and political interference (Saltman, Durán, and Dubois 2011). As seen in the Brazilian and British cases, implementation of autonomy requires years of negotiation and adaptation while putting the accountability and incentive framework in place.

Recommended strategies to implement greater decision-making autonomy include the following:

1. Establish a formal application and approval process for hospitals to achieve (more) autonomous status.
2. Set a phased timetable for transferring functions currently managed by government bureaus to the (approved) autonomous hospitals.
3. Create formal mechanisms to assist hospitals in developing governance arrangements and subsequently to assess effects and provide feedback to shape the inevitable adjustments.

Strategy 1: Establish an application and approval process for (more) autonomous status

Once the governance model and corresponding legal form(s) are in place (see Core Action Area 3), China may consider developing a formalized process for hospitals to apply for more autonomous status according to the governance model adopted. This process will specify which functions are to be transferred from the public administrative apparatus to the (approved) hospitals; the timetable for their transfer; and approval procedures by government agencies and regulators. Functions can include hiring, firing, and compensating staff; managing inputs; opening and closing services; procurement and financial management; investments; borrowing; and so forth.

Strategy 2: Set a timetable for transferring functions from the government to autonomous hospitals

Of equal importance, it is the government's role to set the prerequisites that a hospital must satisfy to gain fully autonomous status. China may want to examine processes used for this purpose in other countries. For example, the United Kingdom has established an application and approval process for hospitals to achieve FT status, which qualifies them for greater decision-making autonomy. The process specifies a three-phased approach involving approval procedures and responsibilities of government agencies and regulators (Monitor).

The process is based on the FT model codified in law. Applicants are appraised against criteria in domains that include the quality of care, financial viability, business strategy, governance structure, service performance, and stakeholder relations. Once a hospital has met the criteria, a formal agreement is signed setting out the accountabilities, roles, and responsibilities of the FT, government, and regulators.

China will need to set a selection and approval process and to define stages or degrees of autonomy, with corresponding criteria for each. Transparency in selection and approval is critical.

Strategy 3: Create mechanisms to help hospitals develop governance arrangements, assess effects, and provide feedback

Finally, the government may consider providing active technical support to hospitals to assist with their introduction of new governance arrangements, helping them to prepare the way for more autonomous decision making and to comply with more rigorous

accountability mechanisms than they are accustomed to—particularly at the early stages. Support will be needed to establish the design and composition of the governance organization (board or council), member selection and tenure and preparation of internal statutes (aligned with the legal and regulatory framework).

The government may also want to consider developing programs for induction of, and continuing support for, board members. Such programs would focus on major governance themes including strategic and business planning, performance monitoring, financial management, conducting legal and regulatory responsibilities, and interacting with managers.

China could consider examples of how OECD countries provide technical support and training for governance arrangements in public and nonprofit organizations. In the United Kingdom, NHS Providers (a membership organization and trade association of NHS health care organizations) provides technical and training support for the FTs, including training programs for NHS FT governors, preparation programs for hospitals seeking FT status, and activities and courses to help FT boards fulfill their functions and responsibilities.[30]

In the United States, a company called the Governance Institute provides training, workshops, and "how-to" materials to help board members successfully perform their roles at U.S. nonprofit hospitals.[31] And in New Zealand, a specialized group within the Treasury Department supports the effectiveness of newly appointed board members. It advises and manages the selection and induction process for board members of state-run enterprises through its "Appointment, Induction, and Professional Development Program" (COMU 2011).

Core Action Area 5: Managerial Capacity Building

Hospitals in China face challenges to improve their efficiency and quality. China is moving forward with reforming hospital governance and separating hospital operations from the government's administrative apparatus. Reforms that seek gains in efficiency and quality are unlikely to succeed without high-quality hospital management (and leadership).

Hospital managers require strong skills in planning; setting organizational goals and annual and multiyear plans; allocating resources efficiently; monitoring performance; setting a functional command chain with corresponding accountabilities; and ensuring effective systems for managerial functions related to financing, human resources, information and data flows, logistics and material management, and quality assurance. Management can be professionalized through a variety of short- and long-term measures, many of which can be implemented in parallel fashion.[32] The following are specific actions to professionalize management and improve managerial practices.

Strategy 1 (short-term): Assess the skills of hospital managers, the quality of managerial practices, and their effects on the quality and efficiency of hospital operations and services

The aforementioned World Management Survey, as well as other available instruments, can be applied for this purpose. These surveys would provide valuable information to shape government commitment to managerial improvement and set the stage for corresponding strategies and actions.

Strategy 2 (short-term): Study and adapt managerial practices implemented in leading public and private facilities

For example, case work commissioned for this study examined managerial practices in high-end private hospitals that introduced a variety of such practices to deliver high-quality and efficient care. Much can be learned from the innovations in these hospitals. Many of the same skills and practices used in private hospitals are appropriate for their public counterparts.

Table 5.4 provides examples of best managerial practices for hospitals.

Strategy 3 (short-term): Establish an executive management program for upgrading skills

Skills should be upgraded along several dimensions: (a) standardizing care (for example by using checklists, handoff protocols, and discharge protocols); (b) refining target setting (for example, scope of targets, links among targets, and difficulty of achievement); (c) measuring performance (for example, by monitoring errors and adverse events and using continuous performance-improvement processes); and (d) improving talent management (by assessing senior managers and policies for internal recruitment, retention, dismissal, and promotion). The development of capabilities applies to both clinical and nonclinical executive managers, both of whom need first-rate managerial and leadership skills.

Strategy 4 (short-term): Support demonstration projects that address specific managerial challenges

Managerial challenges to be addressed include care standardization, infection control, and materials management. Pilot projects can apply tools such as the PDSA cycle, TQM, and "lean management" to improve efficiency, raise quality, and improve patients' satisfaction.

Strategy 5 (long-term): Develop a career path for professional hospital managers

Recruitment and promotion practices should also integrate managerial and leadership competencies.

Strategy 6 (long-term): Create a benchmarking system for hospital management

A benchmarking system periodically tracks indicators of various dimensions of management and links them to important indicators of hospital performance. It should be used not to evaluate management but to proactively find problems and improve

TABLE 5.4   **Best practices in hospital management**

Management area	Sample of specific themes	For more information
Training and development programs	• Accounting for staff demands for training • Clinical training for different learning styles • Computer-based modules • Interactive programs • Developing physician leaders	• *Becker's Hospital Review* (2012)
Building leadership	• Identifying capability gaps • Expanding the management team • Experimenting with different organizational approaches • Promoting clinician engagement in quality and efficient improvement	• HRET (2014)
Talent management and succession planning	• Link between talent management, candidate assessment, and succession planning • Use of leadership competency model • "Stretch" job assignments • Professional development plans • Rigorous and repeated assessment of leadership against key metrics	• NCHL (2010)
Health care scheduling, appointments, and patient flows	• Reducing waiting time • Designing patient flow pathways • Maximizing appointment utilization • Promoting effective dialogue with patients	• Brandenburg and others (2015) • Willyard (2006) • *Becker's Hospital Review* (2010) • Drazen and Rhoads (2011)
Clinical management	• Integrated approach to improving clinical quality, efficiency, and service excellence • Establishing goals and setting priorities • Using data and strategies • Improving patient safety	• Potash (2011) • AHRQ (2017) • Jefferson University Hospitals (n.d.)
Patient-centered hospital care	• Improving responsiveness to patients' needs • Improving discharge experience • Improving pain management	• Aboumatar and others (2015)
Medical teams in hospitals	• Providing evidence-based feedback of team performance • Creating a supportive learning environment • Enhancing physician-nurse teamwork and relationships	• Salas and others (2008) • Cocchi (2012) • Rice (2014)

management practices as a means to improve hospital performance.

Strategy 7 (long-term): Work with academic institutions to strengthen and expand degree programs in hospital management
Ultimately, the goal is to establish centers of excellence in management and leadership development. This may entail revising and updating curricula, introducing internships and in-service training for recent graduates, and developing competencies across recognized management and leadership domains.

Notes

1. The directives include State Council (2012); "Guidance on Comprehensive Pilot Reform of Urban Public Hospitals," National Health and Family Planning Commission (*Guo ban fa* 2015, No. 38); and "Guidance on Comprehensively Scaling-Up Reform of County-Level Public Hospitals," State Council (*Guo ban fa* 2015, No. 33).
2. Other components of the public hospital reform agenda, related to payment methods, financing, and human resources, are the themes of chapters 6 and 7.

3. Except where noted, the sources of the data in this section are *China Health Statistical Yearbook* (National Health and Family Planning Commission, various years) and the "Statistical Bulletin of Health and Family Planning Development in 2014" (NHFPC 2015).

4. Estimate of health expenditures as a share of total health spending is from OECD Health Statistics (database), OECD, Paris, http://www.oecd.org/els/health-systems /health-data.htm.

5. Data on average lengths of hospital stays by country are from OECD Health Statistics (database), OECD, Paris, http:// www.oecd.org/els/health-systems/health -data.htm.

6. Data envelope analysis is a commonly used method for estimating efficiency that involves the use of linear programming to rank firms according to a score of relative efficiency. It is based on the idea that production units—or decision-making units—seek to maximize their output for a given quantity of inputs or, alternatively, to minimize the quantity of inputs for a given output.

7. Technical efficiency is associated with internal factors such as management and control of the production process. It is generated with a given quantity and combination of inputs— or, the fewer inputs that are used to turn out a given quantity of product, the more efficient is the process in the technical sense.

8. Scale efficiency is determined by operational size or scale. Small hospitals are usually inefficient because small scale results in higher unit costs.

9. The framework to analyze governance practices is adapted from La Forgia and others (2013).

10. In addition, see "Guidance of the General Office of the State Council on Promoting Multi-level Diagnosis and Treatment System," State Council (*Guoban fa*, No. 70). The issue of misaligned incentives is discussed in chapter 6. Although public hospitals are owned and operated by the government and financed through a combination of direct subsidies, social insurance payments, and user fees, there has been a wholesale transfer of decision making on income generation to hospital management and clinicians, who tend to act as private agents to maximize their own income.

11. The incentive structure facing providers is the subject of chapter 6.

12. The discussion draws on cases prepared by Durán (2015); La Forgia and Couttolenc (2008); Saltman, Durán, and Dubois (2011); and Wright (2015).

13. The state law was based on a national framework law that aimed to reform the Brazilian administrative apparatus. The goal was to transfer to private managerial functions for social activities that had been wholly and partially funded by the state government, though managed directly by the state administration.

14. English hospitals have hired (and fired) CEOs since the 1980s, and FTs continue this practice.

15. Management teams were allowed to make decisions regarding performance-related incentives amounting to a substantial part of the salary (for clinical staff, amounting on average to 8 percent in consortiums and 15 percent in public health care companies, and, for administrative staff, up to 40 percent of their salary).

16. The Department of Health (and its secretary of state) has overall and political responsibility for strategic direction.

17. The Department of Health's own numbers suggest that, on average, hospitals derive 0.9 percent of their income from private patients, though some derive much more (four units in cancer care, eye care, and children's care derive more than 10 percent). (*Source:* "Private Services in Foundation Trusts," *NHS Privatisation* (blog) [accessed April 7, 2015], https://nhsprivate.wordpress.com /executive-summary/).

18. As already suggested, a number of local governments have launched pilots involving alternative governance arrangements for public hospitals. Some are official pilots sanctioned by the central government; others are not. Shanghai and Zhenjiang are official pilots. Dongyang and Sanming are local initiatives.

19. Unfortunately, verifiable data on the effects of the pilots are unavailable. None of these cases (or any of the official pilots) has been rigorously or independently evaluated.

20. This arrangement was part of a special agreement between city leaders and a Taiwanese businessman who made a substantial donation to rebuild the hospital in 1993.

21. A prefecture is an administrative unit common to all China's provinces and usually consisting of both urban and rural areas. Located

in Fujian Province, the Sanming Prefecture has a population of about 2.7 million and consists of 2 districts and 10 counties. The prefecture had 166 health care facilities in 2013, of which 22 were secondary and tertiary hospitals, with a total of about 8,000 beds.

22. Single-site studies do not provide sufficient information or analysis of the overall quality of management practices, and therefore caution is advised in making inferences about the hospital system.

23. The survey was commissioned by the World Bank, and the preliminary findings are reported here.

24. Country comparisons should be interpreted with caution; 79 percent of the hospitals that the researchers originally contacted in China refused to participate. This may have contributed to a sampling bias in which the surveyed hospitals were those with the best management practices. The researchers did not examine the association between management scores and hospital performance indicators because the latter were impossible to validate.

25. Eighty percent of the procurement of goods and services is managed centrally and the remainder by the hospitals.

26. For example, the establishment of a purchasing and contract management unit within the SES that effectively separated purchasing from provision was a major facilitating step for the OSS reforms. The hospital "administrative" unit that directly managed non-OSS hospitals was incapable of making the transition to arm's-length oversight and monitoring.

27. Countries using DRGs have also introduced measures to counteract two perverse incentives that are embedded in DRGs. They are strengthening auditing systems to detect hospitals' gaming or upcoding to increase revenues. And to deter hospitals from skimping on care to reduce costs or refusing care to high-cost patients, most countries, including the Spain and the United Kingdom, provide additional payments to cover high-cost patients and other services and activities such as intensive care, special therapies, and medical education (Cots and others 2011).

28. For example, FT board members consist of a chairman, hospital CEO, deputy CEO, chief nurse, medical director, finance director, workforce directors, and five nonexecutive elected members.

29. "Guidance on Comprehensive Pilot Reform of Urban Public Hospitals," National Health and Family Planning Commission (*Guo ban fa* 2015, No. 38).

30. For more information, see the NHS Providers website (accessed January 30, 2016), https://www.nhsproviders.org.

31. For more information, see the Governance Institute website (accessed January 30, 2016), http://www.governanceinstitute.com.

32. The measures to strengthen and professionalize management and improve managerial practices are based on Frenk and others (2010); Lega, Prenestini, and Spurgeon (2013); MSH (2005); Shaw (1998); and case studies commissioned for this report.

References

Aboumatar, Hanan J., Bickey H. Chang, Jad Al Danaf, Mohammad Shaear, Ruth Namuyinga, Sathyanarayanan Elumalai, Jill A. Marsteller, and Peter J. Pronovost. 2015. "Promising Practices for Achieving Patient-Centered Hospital Care: A National Study of High-Performing U.S. Hospitals." *Medical Care* 53 (9): 758–67.

AHRQ (Agency for Healthcare Research and Quality). 2017. "Improving Patient Safety in Hospitals: A Resource List for Users of the AHRQ Hospital Survey on Patient Safety Culture." Reference document, AHRQ, U.S. Department of Health and Human Services, Washington, DC.

Allen, Pauline, Qi Cao, and Hufeng Wang. 2013. "Public Hospital Autonomy in China in an International Context." *International Journal of Health Planning and Management* 29 (2): 141–59. doi:10.1002/hpm.2200.

Allen, P., J. Keen, J. Wright, P. Dempster, J. Townsend, A. Hutchings, and R. Verzulli. 2012. "Investigating the Governance of Autonomous Public Hospitals in England: Multi-Site Case Study of NHS Foundation Trusts." *Journal of Health Services Research & Policy* 17 (2): 94–100.

Audibert, Martine, Jacky Mathonnat, Aurore Pelissier, Xiao Xian Huang, and Anning Ma. 2013. "Health Insurance Reform and Efficiency of Township Hospitals in Rural China: An Analysis from Survey Data." *China Economic Review* 27: 326–38.

Becker's Hospital Review. 2010. "Quint Studer: Four Best Practices for Improving Emergency

Department Results." January 25. https://www.beckershospitalreview.com/news-analysis/quint-studer-four-best-practices-for-improving-emergency-department-results.html.

———. 2012. "7 Best Practices for Hospitals' Training and Development Programs." December 12. https://www.beckershospitalreview.com/hospital-management-administration/7-best-practices-for-hospitals-training-and-development-programs.html.

Bjork, David A. 2006. "Collaborative Leadership: A New Model for Developing Truly Effective Relationships between CEOs and Trustees." Collaborative Leadership Tools for CEOs brief, Center for Healthcare Governance, Chicago.

Bley, Charles M., and Cynthia T. Shimko. 1987. "A Guide to the Board's Role in Hospital Finance." Chicago: American Hospital Publishing.

Bloom, Nicholas, and John Van Reenen. 2007. "Measuring and Explaining Management Practices across Firms and Countries." *Quarterly Journal of Economics* 122 (4): 1351–1408.

———. 2010. "Why Do Management Practices Differ across Firms and Countries?" *Journal of Economic Perspectives* 24 (1): 203–24.

Bloom, Nicholas, Rebecca Homkes, Raffaella Sadun, John Van Reenen, Stephen Dorgan, and Dennis Layton. 2010. "Management in Healthcare: Why Good Practice Really Matters." Research report, McKinsey & Company and the Centre for Economic Performance, London School of Economics and Political Science.

Brandenburg, Lisa, Patricia Gabow, Glenn Steele, John Toussaint, and Bernard J. Tyson. 2015. "Innovation and Best Practices in Health Care Scheduling." Discussion paper, Institute of Medicine, National Academy of Sciences, Washington, DC.

Burns, Lawton Robert, and Gordon G. Liu, eds. 2017. *China's Healthcare System and Reform.* Cambridge: Cambridge University Press.

Busse, Reinhard, and Wilm Quentin. 2011. "Moving towards Transparency, Efficiency, and Quality in Hospitals: Conclusions and Recommendations." In *Diagnostic-Related Groups in Europe,* edited by Reinhard Busse, Alexander Geissler, Wilm Quentin, and Miriam Wiley, 149–74. Berkshire, U.K.: Open University Press, World Health Organization,

and European Observatory on Health Systems and Policies.

Castaño, Ramón, Ricardo Bitrán, and Ursula Giedion. 2004. "Monitoring and Evaluating Hospital Autonomization and its Effects on Priority Health Services." Paper for the Partners for Health Reform*plus* project of the U.S. Agency for International Development, prepared by Abt Associates, Bethesda, MD.

Chen, Ming, Hongmei Zhao, Saijun Jia, Lihua Wang, and Yue Zhao. 2014. "Total Quality Management: Improving the Procedure of Additional Registration in Specialist Clinic." *Chinese Hospitals* 18 (1).

Chen, Vivian, and Yue Xia Gao. 2015. "Wuhan Asia Heart Hospital Case Study." Unpublished report commissioned by the International Finance Corporation, World Bank, Beijing.

Chen, Vivan, Yue Xia Gao, and Yuan Wang. 2015. "Aier Eye Hospital Case Study." Unpublished report commissioned by the International Finance Corporation, World Bank, Beijing.

Chu, Kejia, Ning Zhang, and Zhonfei Chen. 2015. "The Efficiency and its Determinants for China's Medical Care System: Some Policy Implications for Northeast Asia." *Sustainability* 7: 14092–14111.

Cocchi, Renee. 2012. "Best Practices for Enhancing Doctor/Nurse Relationships." *Healthcare Business & Technology* (e-newsletter), May 7. http://www.healthcarebusinesstech.com/best-practices-for-enhancing-doctornurse-relationships/.

Coile, R. 1994. *The New Governance: Strategies for an Era of Health Reform.* Ann Arbor, MI: Health Administration Press.

COMU (Crown Ownership Monitoring Unit). 2011. "Board Appointments, Induction, and Professional Development." COMU, New Zealand Treasury, Wellington.

Cots, Francis, Pietro Chiarello, Xavier Salvador, Xavier Castrells, and Wilm Quentin. 2011. "DRG-Based Hospital Payment: Intended and Unintended Consequences." In *Diagnostic-Related Groups in Europe,* edited by Reinhard Busse, Alexander Geissler, Wilm Quentin, and Miriam Wiley, 75–92. Berkshire, U.K.: Open University Press, World Health Organization, and European Observatory on Health Systems and Policies.

Cuervo-Cazurra, Alvaro, and Ruth V. Aguilera. 2004. "Codes of Good Governance Worldwide: What Is the Trigger?" *Organization Studies* 25 (3).

Curry, Leslie A., Erica Spatz, Emily Cherlin, Jennifer W. Thompson, David Berg, Henry H. Ting, Carole Decker, Harlan M. Krumholz, and Elizabeth H. Bradley. 2011. "What Distinguishes Top-Performing Hospitals in AMI Mortality Rates? A Qualitative Study." *Annals of Internal Medicine* 154: 384–90.

Deber, R., A. Topp, and D. Zakus. 2004. "Private Delivery and Public Goals: Mechanisms for Ensuring that Hospitals Meet Public Objectives." Background paper commissioned by the World Bank, Washington, DC.

Drazen, Erica, and Jared Rhoads. 2011. "Using Tracking Tools to Improve Patient Flow in Hospitals." Issue brief, California Health Care Foundation (CHCF), Oakland and Sacramento, CA.

Durán, Antonio. 2015. "New Roles for Hospitals in China; Lessons from Public Hospital Governance Reforms in OECD: Spain." Case study commissioned by the World Bank, Washington, DC.

Durán, A., and R. B. Saltman. 2015. "Governing Public Hospitals." In *The Palgrave International Handbook of Healthcare Policy and Governance*, edited by E. Kuhlmann, R. Blank, I. L. Bourgeault, and C. Wendt, 443–61. London and New York: Palgrave McMillan.

Durán, Antonio, Richard B. Saltman, and Hans F. W. Dubois. 2011. "A Framework for Assessing Hospital Governance." In *Governing Public Hospitals: Reform Strategies and the Movement towards Institutional Autonomy*, edited by Richard B. Saltman, Antonio Durán, and Hans. F. W. Dubois, 35–53. Copenhagen: World Health Organization on behalf of the European Observatory on Health Systems and Policies.

Edwards, Nigel. 2011. "England." In *Governing Public Hospitals: Reform Strategies and the Movement towards Institutional Autonomy,* edited by Richard B. Saltman, Antonio Durán, and Hans F. W. Dubois, 113–40. Copenhagen: World Health Organization on behalf of the European Observatory on Health Systems and Policies.

Frenk, Julio, Lincoln Chen, Zulfiqar A. Bhutta, Jordan Cohen, Nigel Crisp, Timothy Evans, and Harvey Fineberg. 2010. "Health Professionals for a New Century: Transforming Education to Strengthen Health Systems in an Interdependent World." *The Lancet* 376 (9756): 1923–58.

Gage, Larry S., Anne B. Camper, and Robert Falk. 2006. "Legal Structure and Governance of Public Hospitals and Health Systems." National Association of Public Hospitals and Health Systems, Washington, DC.

Gao, Tian, and Bruce Gurd. 2014. "Meeting the Challenge in Performance Management: The Diffusion and Implementation of the Balanced Scorecard in Chinese Hospitals." *Health Policy and Planning* 30 (2): 234–41. doi:10.1093/heapol/czu008.

Gill, Mel, Robert J. Flynn, and Elke Reissing. 2005. "The Governance Self-Assessment Checklist: An Instrument for Assessing Board Effectiveness." *Nonprofit Management and Leadership* 15 (32).

Govindaraj, Ramesh, and Mukesh Chawla. 1996. "Recent Experiences with Hospital Autonomy in Developing Countries: What Can We Learn?" Comparative case study report, Data for Decision Making (DDM) Project, Department of Population and International Health, Harvard School of Public Health, Boston.

Greenwood, J., R. Pyper, and D. Wilson. 2002. *New Public Administration in Britain.* London: Routledge.

Guo, Jinshuai, Shijun Ma, and Xun Zhang. 2014. "Lean Management to Transform a Chinese Hospital." *Planet Lean: The Lean Global Network Journal*, September 17.

He, Jingwei Alex. 2011. "Combating Healthcare Cost Inflation with Concerted Administrative Actions in a Chinese Province." *Public Administration and Development* 31: 214–28. doi:10.1002/pad.602.

He, Alex Jingwei and Jiwei Qian. 2013. "Hospitals' Responses to Administrative Cost-Containment Policy in Urban China: The Case of Fujian Province." *China Quarterly* 216: 946–69. doi:10.1017/S0305741013001112.

Holland, Thomas P., Robert A. Ritvo, and Anthony R. Kovner. 1997. *Improving Board Effectiveness: Practical Lessons for Nonprofit Health Care Organizations.* Chicago: American Hospital Publishing.

HRET (Health Research & Educational Trust). 2014. "Building a Leadership Team for the Health Care Organization of the Future." Signature Leadership Series report, HRET, Chicago.

Hu, Hsin-Hui, Quinghui Qi, and Chih-Hai Yang. 2012. "Analysis of Hospital Technical Efficiency in China: Effect of Health Insurance

Reform." *China Economic Review* 23: 865–77.

Huang, Yanzhong. 2009 "An Institutional Analysis of China's Failed Healthcare Reform." In *Socialist China, Capitalist China: Social Tension and Political Adaptation under Economic Globalization*, edited by Guoguang Wu and Helen Landsowne, 75–86. New York: Routledge.

Huntington, Dale, and Krishna Hort, eds. 2015. *Public Hospital Governance in Asia and the Pacific*. Comparative Country Studies Vol. 1, No. 1. Geneva: World Health Organization, Asia Pacific Observatory on Health Systems and Policies.

Ingram, T. T. 1996. *Ten Basic Responsibilities of Nonprofit Boards*. Washington, DC: National Center for Nonprofit Boards.

Jefferson University Hospitals. n.d. "Keeping Our Patients Safe." Thomas Jefferson University Hospitals, Philadelphia. https://hospitals .jefferson.edu/quality-and-safety/keeping -our-patients-safe/.

Kirkpatrick, I., P. K. Jespersen, M. Dent, and I. Neogy. 2009. "Medicine and Management in a Comparative Perspective: The Case of Denmark and England." *Sociology of Health and Illness* 31 (5): 642–58.

KPMG. 2010. "The Changing Face of Health Care in China: Changing Public Policies and Resulting Opportunities." Infrastructure, Government & Healthcare report, Publication No. HK-Pl10-0005, KMPG, Hong Kong.

La Forgia, Gerard Martin, and Bernard Couttolenc. 2008. *Hospital Performance in Brazil: The Search for Excellence*. Washington, DC: World Bank.

La Forgia, Gerard, April Harding, Loraine Hawkins, and Eric Roodenbeke. 2013. "A Framework for Developing and Analyzing Public Hospital Reforms in Developing Countries that Involve Autonomy." Working draft, World Bank, Washington, DC

Lega, Federico, Anna Prenestini, and Peter Spurgeon. 2013. "Is Management Essential to Improving the Performance and Sustainability of Health Care Systems and Organizations? A Systematic Review and a Roadmap for Future Studies." *Value in Health* 16 (1 Suppl): S46–S51.

Li, Weiping, and Mengxi Jiang. 2015. "China's Public Hospital Governance Reform: Case Study of Zhenjiang." Unpublished case study commissioned by the World Bank, Washington, DC.

Li, Weiping, and Jianxiu Wang. 2015. "China's Public Hospital Governance Reform: Dongyang Case Study." China National Health Development Research Center, Beijing.

Lin, Zhijun, Zengbiao Yu, and Liqun Zhang. 2014. "Performance Outcomes of Balanced Scorecard Application in Hospital Administration in China." *China Economic Review* 30 (C): 1–15.

Liu, Gordon. 2015. "Quality of Hospital Management Practices in China—China Hospital Management Survey (CHMS)." Unpublished manuscript, World Bank, Washington, DC.

Ma, Jin. 2015. "China's Public Hospital Governance Reform: Case Study of Shanghai." Case study commissioned by the World Bank, Washington, DC.

Mannion, R., H. T. O. Davies, and M. N. Marshall. 2005. "Cultural Characteristics of 'High' and 'Low' Performing Hospitals." *Journal of Health Organization and Management* 19 (6): 431–39.

Mason, Anne, Padraic Ward, and Andres Street. 2011. "England: The Health care Resource Group." In *Diagnostic-Related Groups in Europe*, edited by Reinhard Busse, Alexander Geissler, Wilm Quentin, and Miriam Wiley, 197–200. Berkshire, U.K.: Open University Press, World Health Organization, and European Observatory on Health Systems and Policies.

Mazzocato, P., R. J. Holden, M. Brommels, H. Aronsson, U. Bäckman, M. Elg, and J. Thor. 2012. "How Does Lean Work in Emergency Care? A Case Study of a Lean-Inspired Intervention at the Astrid Lindgren Children's Hospital, Stockholm, Sweden." *BMC Health Services Research* 12: 28. doi:10.1186 /1472-6963-12-28.

McConnell, K. J., R. C. Lindrooth, D. R. Wholey, T. M. Maddox, and N. Bloom. 2013. "Management Practices and the Quality of Care in Cardiac Units." *JAMA Internal Medicine* 173 (8): 684–92.

McKee, Martin, and Judith Healy, eds. 2002. *Hospitals in a Changing Europe*. European Observatory on Health Care Systems Series. Buckingham, U.K.: World Health Organization and Open University Press.

McPake, Barbara, Francisco Jose Yepes, Sally Lake, and Luz Helena Sanchez. 2003. "Is the

Colombian Health System Reform Improving the Performance of Public Hospitals in Bogota?" *Health Policy and Planning* 18 (2): 182–94.

Mossialos, Elias, Martin Wenzl, Robin Osborn, and Chloe Anderson, eds. 2015. "International Profiles of Health Care Systems, 2014: Australia, Canada, Denmark, England, France, Germany, Italy, Japan, The Netherlands, New Zealand, Norway, Singapore, Sweden, Switzerland, and the United States." Annual publication, The Commonwealth Fund, New York.

MSH (Management Sciences for Health). 2005. *Managers Who Lead: A Handbook for Improving Health Services*. Cambridge, MA: Management Sciences for Health.

Naranjo-Gil, D. 2009. "Strategic Performance in Hospitals: The Use of the Balanced Scorecard by Nurse Managers." *Health Care Management Review* 34 (2): 161–70.

NCHL (National Center for Healthcare Leadership). 2010. "Best Practices in Health Leadership Talent Management and Succession Planning: Case Studies." Case study report, NCHL, Chicago.

NHS (National Health Service) European Office. 2011. "The Search for Low-Cost Integrated Healthcare: The Alzira Model—from the Region of Valencia." Research paper, NHS Confederation, Brussels.

Ng, Y. C. 2011. "The Productive Efficiency of Chinese Hospitals." *China Economic Review* 22: 428–39.

Nolte, Ellen, and Emma Pitchforth. 2014. "What Is the Evidence on the Economic Impacts of Integrated Care?" Policy Summary 11, World Health Organization Regional Office for Europe, Copenhagen (acting as the host organization for, and secretariat of, the European Observatory on Health Systems and Policies).

Over, M., and N. Watanabe. 2003. "Evaluating the Impact of Organizational Reforms in Hospitals." In *Innovations in Health Service Delivery: The Corporatization of Public Hospitals*, edited by Alex Preker and A. Harding, 105–51. Washington, DC: World Bank.

Parand, Anam, Sue Dopson, Anna Renz and Charles Vincent. 2014. "The Role of Hospital Managers in Quality and Patient Safety: A Systematic Review." *BMJ Open* 4 (9): e005055. doi:10.1136/bmjopen-2014-005055.

Potash, David L. 2011. "Accountable Clinical Management: An Integrated Approach."

Healthcare Financial Management 65 (10): 94–98, 100, 102.

Preker, Alex, and A. Harding, eds. 2003. *Innovations in Health Service Delivery: The Corporatization of Public Hospitals*. Washington, DC: World Bank.

Qian, Jiwei. 2015. "Reallocating Authority in the Chinese Health System: An Institutional Perspective." *Journal of Asian Public Policy* 8 (1): 19–35. doi:10.1080/17516234.2014 .1003454.

Rice, J., ed. 2003. "Hospital Boards: An International Journey for World-Class Governance Effectiveness: Global Trends Survey 2003." International Health Summit, Minneapolis.

Rice, Sabriya. 2014. "Top-Performing Hospitals Know How to Use Teamwork." *Modern Healthcare*, November 8. http://www.modern healthcare.com/article/20141108/MAGA ZINE/311089980.

Salas, Eduardo, Cameron Klein, Heidi King, Mary Salisbury, Jeffrey S. Augenstein, David J. Birnbach, Donald W. Robinson, and Christin Upshaw. 2008. "Debriefing Medical Teams: 12 Evidence-Based Best Practices and Tips." *Joint Commission Journal on Quality and Patient Safety* 34 (9): 518–27.

Saltman, Richard B., Antonio Durán, and Hans F. W. Dubois, eds. 2011. *Governing Public Hospitals: Reform Strategies and the Movement towards Institutional Autonomy*. Copenhagen: World Health Organization on behalf of the European Observatory on Health Systems and Policies.

Sanming Prefecture Government. 2015. "Summary of Public Hospital Comprehensive Reform in Sanming Municipality." Case study commissioned by the World Bank, Washington, DC.

Shaw, Jane. 1998. *Hospital Management: Training and Professional Development*. Geneva: World Health Organization.

State Council. 2012. "The Twelfth Five-Year Plan for Health Care Development." *Guo ban fa* 2012, No. 57. http://www.wpro.who.int /health_services/china_nationalhealthplan.pdf.

Tam, Wai-keung. 2008. "Failing to Treat: Why Public Hospitals in China Do Not Work." *China Review* 8 (2): 103–30.

Tsai, T. C., A. K. Jha, A. A. Gawande, R. S. Huckman, N. Bloom, and R. Sadun. 2015. "Hospital Board and Management Practices are Strongly Related to Hospital Performance on Clinical Quality Metrics." *Health Affairs* 34 (8).

WHO (World Health Organization) and World Bank. 2015. Technical Roundtable Discussions. Joint Health Study.

Willyard, David. 2006. "Hospital Revenue Cycle Best Practices." *The Health Care Biller* (Oct. 2006): 1+.

World Bank. 2006. "Brazil. Enhancing Performance in Brazil's Health Sector: Lessons from Innovations in the State of São Paulo and the City of Curitiba." Brief, Report No. 35691 -BR, World Bank, Washington, DC.

———. 2010. "Fixing the Public Hospital System in China." China Health Policy Notes Series, No. 2, World Bank, Washington, DC.

Wright, Stephen. 2015. "New Roles for Hospitals in China: Lessons from Public Hospital Governance Reforms in OECD, MICs, and China: Analysis of Governance Arrangements in England: the Foundation Trust Model." Case study commissioned by the World Bank, Washington, DC.

Yang, Jinqiu, and Wu Zeng. 2014. "The Trade-Offs between Efficiency and Quality in the Hospital Production: Some Evidence from Shenzhen, China." *China Economic Review* 31: 166–84.

Ying, Yachen. 2014. "Achieve Win-Win-Win Situation by Jointly Reforming the Drug Sector, Health Service Sector, and Health Insurance Sector: Field Study Report on Public Hospital Reform in Sanming." Case study, Health Development Research Center (NHFOC), Beijing.

Yip, Winnie Chi-Man, William C. Hsiao, Wen Chen, Shanlian Hu, Jin Ma, and Alan Maynard. 2012. "Early Appraisal of China's Huge and Complex Health-Care Reforms." *The Lancet* 379 (9818): 833–42. doi:10.1016 /S0140-6736(11)61880-1.

Lever 5: Realigning Incentives in Purchasing and Provider Payment

Introduction

People centered integrated care (PCIC), which lies at the core of China's efforts to build a high-quality and value-based health system, has three key elements (as discussed in chapter 2):

- It is organized around the population's needs.
- It promotes primary care as patients' first point of contact for most of their health care needs and is thus based on a strong primary health care foundation.
- It prioritizes integration and coordination of services across all levels of care, from promotion and prevention to curative and palliative needs, to reduce fragmentation and wasteful use of resources across a health system.

Realigning the purchasing and provider payment incentives to reinforce and strengthen PCIC development and adoption therefore entails modifying how providers are paid in ways that correspond with, conform to, and result in these three fundamental PCIC outcomes. This is the focus of this chapter.

Incentives in the health sector refer to "all the rewards and punishments that providers face as a consequence of the organizations in which they work, the institutions under which they operate and the specific interventions they provide" (WHO 2000, 61). Defined thus, incentives are conditions within the work environment of health professionals that enable and motivate them to stay in their jobs, come to work every day, and devote the necessary time and effort as dictated by the demands of their profession and the needs of their clients.

Provider payment methods create powerful incentives affecting provider behavior and the efficiency, equity, and quality outcomes of health finance reforms. The amount and type of payment to health care practitioners and organizations affect the amount and type of health goods and services received by consumers and, ultimately, the aggregate costs to all payers, including the government, insurers, employers, and individuals. The amount and type of payment also have an impact on the behavior of health care organizations and individuals with respect to the quality of care they deliver to consumers. At the same time, the amount and type of payments made by consumers for health care affects their health and preventive-care-seeking behavior, choice of health professional, and quantity of care they seek.

The most critical determinant of incentives is whether the provider payment method is retrospective or prospective, because it affects who bears the risk of the cost of provision, which in turn has implications for treatment choices. Other determinants include (a) the breadth of provider payments (that is, whether the providers are paid narrowly for their own services or broadly for bundles of related services such as laboratory tests and other provider services) and (b) the generosity of the payments (that is, whether the payments are low or high).

Collectively and individually, these dimensions affect providers' incentives and thus their behavior regarding a host of variables, such as volume and intensity of care rendered (including preventive care), efforts to keep costs down, treatment of low- and high-risk patients, number of referrals, provision of quality care, and so on.

Incentives are also affected by the decisions of payers—defined as entities that pay not only premiums (such as individuals, businesses, and the government) but also those who control the premiums before they are paid to the providers (that is, insurance companies and governments). Although patients and businesses function as ultimate purchasers, insurance companies and the government serve a processing or payer function.

Purchasers also worry about financial management, including withholding a certain percentage of premiums to provide a fund for committed but undelivered health care, setting aside resources for uncertainties such as longer hospital utilization levels than expected, overutilization of referrals, accidental catastrophes, and other financial liabilities. Likewise, payers are concerned with benefits (that is, specific areas of insurance coverage such as outpatient visits, hospitalization, and so forth) that make up the range of medical services that a payer markets to its subscribers.

All these functions—carried out in the execution of normal business functioning of payers (related to determination of benefits and resource management) and purchasers (related to financial management, benefit design, contracting, and monitoring)—affect provider incentives and behavior.

The rest of this chapter is organized as follows:

- *"Evolution of Health System Incentives"* briefly discusses the evolution of health system incentives over the years.
- *"Challenges and Lessons Learned from Select Studies"* presents lessons learned from select case studies in China that were carried out in order to assess opportunities and challenges in purchasing practices and identify roadmaps for strengthening capacities of social insurance agencies.
- *"Provider Payment Reforms in China"* discusses challenges and lessons from recent provider payment reform pilots.
- *"Core Action Areas and Implementation Strategies to Realign Incentives"* concludes with a discussion of four core action areas and associated strategies to deepen reform through realignment of incentives.

Evolution of Health System Incentives

From Socialism to a Market Economy: 1949–2009

In the first decades after the People's Republic of China was established in 1949, the health care system was built within the socialist planned economy and characterized by public production, with public financing in urban areas and community financing in rural areas. The rural collectives and urban work units (danwei) purchased and provided health care for their members.

In an environment marked by a shortage of doctors and medicines, the health care system made innovative use of part-time doctors to provide extensive preventive and primary health care (Manuel 2010). Fees in public hospitals were set at low levels, and because the hospitals were protected against deficits through a flexible government budget system, they had no incentives to provide unnecessary care that would increase the economic burden on patients (Jing 2004). This period saw extraordinary improvements in population health achieved at very low levels of spending (Liu 2004).

Two other policies, undoubtedly introduced with good intentions, met with unfortunate consequences. First, to motivate high performance, bonus schemes were introduced that linked physician incomes with generated revenues. Second, to improve access, basic medical services and pharmaceuticals were priced artificially low while expensive procedures and drugs were marked up for high profit margins.

The consequences of these inappropriate incentives are by now well-known: to maximize incomes, physicians resorted to demand inducement to generate higher revenue; and to maximize profits, hospitals began encouraging overprescription of drugs and expensive diagnostic tests. These reinforcing actions led to massive inefficiencies and further increased the financial burden on patients (Chen 2009; Feng, Lou, and Yu 2015; Ma, Lu, and Quan 2008). These and related misaligned incentives became embedded in the health system, contributing to escalating costs, medical impoverishment, and large-scale public discontent.

At the same time, wanting health facilities to survive financially, the government priced some new, high-tech procedures above cost and allowed hospitals a 15 percent markup on drugs. The consequences were unsurprising: to generate higher revenues, hospitals began encouraging overprescription of drugs and expensive diagnostic tests, and physicians in turn prescribed more drugs and provided more high-profit services. As public facilities turned into profit-seeking entities, a perverse dynamic ensued in which a "provider [had] to dispense seven dollars' worth of drugs to earn one dollar of profit" (Yip and Hsiao 2008, 462). These reinforcing incentives and actions led to massive inefficiencies and further increased the financial burden on patients. These and related misaligned incentives became embedded in the

health system, contributing to escalating costs, medical impoverishment, and large-scale public discontent (Blumenthal and Hsiao 2005; Liu and Mills 1999; Yip and Hsiao 2008).

These policies created a bias in China's financing and service delivery system toward more costly services delivered in hospitals. The pricing systems of provincial pricing bureaus favored hospitals and reinforced the overuse of more expensive care settings and higher-priced technology. They also exacerbated the general trend among providers to invest, upgrade facilities, and provide higher levels of care in ways that were more responsive to potential profits than to health care needs and potential improvements in health. The fee-for-service provider payment mechanisms stimulated service delivery and fueled rapid growth of health spending. Massive public investments enabled national insurance schemes to rapidly enroll people (Meng and others 2012), and at the same time, reimbursement of individual services by fees encouraged health institutions to provide patients with more health care than required. Further, reimbursement rates were increased to lower out-of-pocket payments (copays), which led to greater consumer demand (Babiarz and others 2012; Lei and Lin 2009; Liu and Zhao 2014; Meng and others 2012; Yip and others 2012; Yu and others 2010; Zhang, Yi, and Rozelle 2010). The result was double-digit spending growth.

Health Care Reform: 2009–Present

Responding to the rapidly rising costs and demand for high-quality, affordable health care, the government of China launched one of the biggest health policy interventions in recent times in 2009. Targeted to reach 1.3 billion people, the reform invested more than RMB 3 trillion into the health system between 2009 and 2014 to support five pillars of change: expanding coverage of social insurance schemes, establishing a national essential medicines system, advancing public hospital reforms, improving the primary care system, and increasing the equality and availability of public health services (Chen 2009). This investment doubled government spending on health and signaled the government's increased role in financing health care.

As noted, the 2009 health care reform made public hospital reforms one of five pillars of change. Specific areas targeted for reform included hospital governance, hospital financing, provider payment methods, and, more recently, encouraging the growth of the private hospital sector. Subsequently, the Twelfth Five-Year Plan (TFY) (covering 2011–15) stated clearly that the objective of a public hospital was to pursue the public interest and introduced a package of policies aimed at realigning incentives in public hospitals with serving the public interest and increasing efficiency (State Council 2011).

These policies included delinking hospital income and staff remuneration from drug revenues, changing provider payment methods, promoting rational drug use, testing alternative governance structures, improving human resource management, and adopting more efficient internal management. A zero-markup drug policy was introduced, which delinked income of public hospitals from drug sales. However, the policy only applied to drugs on the Essential Drug List (EDL), and hospitals continued to charge a markup on drugs not on the EDL. To compensate hospitals for the loss in drug revenue, local governments were encouraged to increase their direct subsidies to public hospitals. In addition, the schedule of hospital prices was revised, and prices for high-tech diagnostic tests were lowered while the prices of more labor-intensive services, which were previously underpriced, were raised.

The Ministry of Human Resources and Social Security (MoHRSS) issued the "Opinions on Further Improving the Reform of Health Insurance Payments" and the "Opinion on Implementing the Control of Total Medical Insurance Payment" in 2011 and 2012, respectively, which state the objectives and implementation pathways for the global budget payment method.[1] In line with the MoHRSS guidelines, a global budget payment method has been implemented nationwide. Moreover, a mixed payment system has been established to introduce case-based capitation and per diem payment methods. The payment system incentivizes the health providers to control costs and provide quality health care services to allocate resources efficiently.

Persistent Weaknesses in Incentives

Despite impressive gains in achieving near-universal insurance coverage in a short time, China still needs to further correct the underlying incentive system that governs provider behavior and influences the nature and scope of purchased health goods and services. The large-scale reforms initiated in 2009 have not aggressively attempted to correct the misaligned supply-side incentives that have carried over from the past three decades. Therefore, hospitals seek help from physicians by offering them bonus schemes linking their performance with hospital revenues. The net result is a situation almost diametrically opposite to PCIC, in that health sector resources get reallocated to profit centers for hospitals and away from patient-centered provision and physicians get drawn into revenue generation, which influences their treatment choices.

The fee-pricing schedule widely used by purchasing agencies prices some services below cost (such as health promotion, prevention, and consultations) and other services above cost (such as expensive diagnostics). This motivates oversupply of services with higher price margins and steers public providers away from prioritizing the public interest. Because this fee schedule yields the lowest profit for providers of health promotion and prevention services, such services get neglected and physicians favor overprescription of antibiotics and intravenous injections, even for simple health problems, to generate revenues. Unsurprisingly, 75 percent of patients suffering from a common cold and 79 percent of all hospital patients in China are prescribed antibiotics—numbers that are more than twice the international average and that have contributed to growth in health spending (Zhou n.d.).

At the same time, the fee schedule incentivizes even public hospitals to profit from expensive procedures, and thus hospitals invest heavily in new technologies and medical devices and get a high initial stock of patients to defray the fixed costs. Reinforced by the profit motivation, higher-level hospitals, which are at an advantage for capital investment, keep expanding and drawing in more and more physical, financial, and human resources at the expense of lower-level hospitals, which cannot compete at the same level of technology.

The net result is a resource-rich tertiary hospital base that stands together with poorly resourced lower-level facilities, a situation that adversely affects the ability of lower-level hospitals to provide quality medical services and motivates doctors to seek employment in tertiary facilities where their income prospects are brighter. Patients get directed to higher-level facilities, resulting in an inefficient situation in which congested higher-level facilities coexist with idle resources in lower-level hospitals. Unsurprisingly, while hospitals' share of total health spending in China rose from 56 percent in 1990 to 63 percent in 2012,

the share of township hospitals fell from 11 percent to 6 percent, and the share of ambulatory health facilities fell from 21 percent to 9 percent during this period (figure 6.1).

In the absence of a strong primary care system and an effective referral system, patients could themselves choose at which level and where in the hospital chain they could seek care. Copayments are differentiated across levels, with higher reimbursement at lower levels (that is, reimbursement is higher at secondary facilities than at tertiary facilities for the same procedure), but the difference is not sufficient to deter patients from bypassing the secondary facilities for tertiary levels because of the perceived quality difference.

And finally, because higher-level facilities typically attract more specialists and are better equipped with high-technology devices, patients show a strong preference for seeking even basic care at these high-level facilities. The net result of this choice process is congestion, long waiting times, higher marginal cost of production, shorter physician time, more high-tech diagnostics, and related inefficiency- and cost-enhancing outcomes.

FIGURE 6.1   Composition of total health expenditure in China, by facility or provider type, 1990–2012

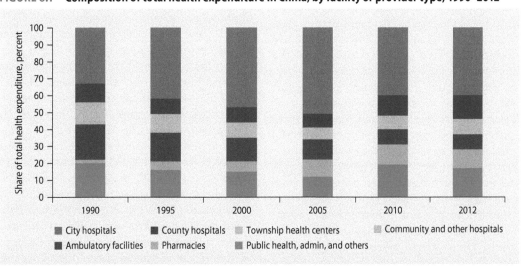

Source: *China Health Statistical Yearbook 2013*, Ministry of Health.

Challenges and Lessons Learned From Selected Case Studies

Overview of Health Insurance and Assistance Schemes

As described in chapter 1, the medical security system in China consists of three basic health insurance schemes: Urban Employee Basic Medical Insurance (UEBMI), Urban Resident Basic Medical Insurance (URBMI), and the New Cooperative Medical Scheme (NCMS). A medical financial assistance (MFA) program for the poor includes urban and rural MFA schemes. By the end of 2015, UEBMI, URBMI, and NCMS covered 289 million, 377 million, and 670 million residents, respectively.[2]

In addition, the Insurance Program for Catastrophic Diseases (IPCD) provides financial protection for the high medical expenses of patients with catastrophic diseases, covering 50 percent or more of eligible expenses over and above the ceiling of basic insurance.[3] Finally, the Emergency Rescue and Financial Assistance System for Disease, established in 2013, provides emergency health expenses for patients who lack identity documents as well as for patients who have identity documents but who cannot pay.[4]

The three health insurance schemes differ in how they are financed and operate. UEBMI is a compulsory scheme to which employers and employees contribute 6 percent and 2 percent of the employees' wages, respectively, to enroll. Contributions are divided into two parts: two-thirds of the employer's contribution is allocated to a risk-pooled fund (the "social pooled fund"), while the remaining one-third is combined with the 2 percent from employees and deposited in an individual savings account owned by the employee. In some cases, the savings account is used to pay for outpatient services while the risk-pooled fund is used to pay for inpatient care. In other cases, funds in the savings account can pay both inpatient and outpatient deductibles before using risk-pooled funds. On average, patients can get 65–70 percent of total inpatient expenses reimbursed.

URBMI is designed to cover children, students, the elderly, people with disabilities, and other nonworking urban residents. The scheme is financed mainly by the insured along with a government subsidy, which increased from RMB 40 in 2007 to RMB 420 in 2016. Local governments have the authority to decide premium and benefit levels for different populations according to affordability and public financing.[5] Initially, URBMI covered inpatient care only, but local governments have now established pooled funds for outpatient services. On average, patients can get 45–50 percent of total inpatient expenses reimbursed.

The NCMS provides insurance coverage to rural residents. Premiums are heavily subsidized (RMB 420 in 2016), while individual contributions are much lower (RMB 120). Most NCMS models initially covered only inpatient services, although some covered inpatient plus several selected outpatient services for major acute illnesses, and a small proportion covered both inpatient and outpatient services. In the western and central regions, the most commonly found model combines a medical savings account (MSA) for outpatient services and high-deductible catastrophic insurance for inpatient services. Since 2010, a growing number of regions have ended MSAs and begun to reimburse both outpatient and inpatient services from the pooled fund, based on predefined drug and service formulas. On average, the NCMS reimburses 55 percent of inpatient costs and 50 percent of outpatient costs.

All three schemes have their own formulas for reimbursing drugs and services. UEBMI and URBMI are the most generous, covering more than 2,000 drugs. The NCMS is much less generous than the other two. The reimbursed lists are similar for UEBMI and URBMI, though UEBMI reimburses larger amounts. The EDL (520 drugs in 2012) is included in the drug list of the three insurance schemes and has a higher reimbursement rate than other drugs. Primary health care institutions can only provide and sell essential drugs, which limits the actual benefit packages at these institutions.

The rest of this section presents results of a specially commissioned study conducted in selected provinces and counties, representing each insurance scheme and each geographic region of the country, to assess opportunities and challenges in purchasing practices and identify road maps for strengthening the capacities of social insurance agencies. Strategic purchasing functions include strategic planning and policy development, financial management, benefits design, contracting with providers, and performance monitoring.

The sample included the following cities or counties, by region:

- *East:* Beijing, Hangzhou in Zhejiang province, Changshu and Jiangyin counties in Jiangsu province, Shanghai, Tianjin, and Zhuhai in Guangdong province
- *West:* Jiulongpo county in Chongqing, Puding county in Guizhou province, Yanchi county in Ningxia province, and Xining county in Qinghai province
- *Central:* Xi county in Henan province.

Most reforms have been accompanied by investments in the capacity of purchasing agencies, especially for the main functions of maintaining fund balance and increasing coverage and reimbursement rates. However, purchasing agencies still have limited capacity to leverage contracting, develop and manage effective provider payment systems, and monitor provider performance. Many purchasing and provider payment innovations build on historical claims and rely on the technical contribution of external experts rather than on routine in-house capacity, and purchasing agencies continue to have limited ability to monitor the case mix and quality of services.

Weak Purchasing Capacity in Basic Medical Insurance Agencies

The mandate of the purchasing agencies of China's three insurance schemes is to balance revenue with expenditure while maintaining and expanding financial protection for the insured. Although the 2009 and 2012 reform guidelines acknowledged the need to better leverage strategic health purchasing and stimulate changes in provider behavior, the performance of the purchasing agencies continues to be assessed mainly on balancing revenues with claims and on ensuring fund safety while increasing reimbursement rates.

The obligations and functions of an NCMS management office are to develop local NCMS policies; organize and mobilize implementation under the framework of provincial NCMS policies, project revenues, and expenditures; enroll the target population; and train subordinate entities in the towns to collect revenues, examine provider qualifications, monitor health services, audit expenses, and publish financial reports. NCMS offices in most counties are thinly staffed and lack the capacity to perform all of these functions. As a result, about one-fourth of all NCMS management offices in the country have hired commercial insurance companies to do some routine tasks. Local NCMS offices have more authority for strategic planning and policy making under the national and provincial requirements released by the National Health and Family Planning Commission (NHFPC). The study of selected provinces shows that in Puding, Xi, Jiangyin, and Changshu counties, for instance, local NCMS offices make decisions on issues related to the benefits package, provider payment, and monitoring and contracting rules.

Revenues Not Always Easy to Forecast

In general, all three schemes have similar financial management processes: projecting the budget, collecting revenue, allocating and using funds, dealing with surplus and debts, auditing, and monitoring. At the end of a fiscal year, each purchasing agency is required to project revenues and expenses for the next year, and the projections need to be approved by the Financial Department.

NCMS and URBMI revenues are difficult to predict because enrollment is voluntary and government subsidies are not announced until the beginning of the new fiscal year. Revenues are not all received until the middle of the year because contributions come from different sources and the appropriation of government subsidies takes time.

In contrast, because UEBMI premiums are mandatory and automatically collected from employers' income and employees' wages, they are usually received in a stable, predictable, and timely way. Revenue forecasts for UEBMI are based on predicted economic growth, insurance coverage, employees' average wages, and contribution rates. Estimated payouts are based on the age structure of the insured, the spectrum of disease, inflation, benefit packages, and fund balances.

All agencies analyze expenditures during the year—usually monthly, but sometimes in real time in places with modern information systems, such as Shanghai, Tianjin, and Changshu county. Surpluses and debts are managed according to guidelines issued by the central government, which suggest a balance of at least 15 percent of annual requirements in NCMS and of six to nine months of payments in UEBMI and URBMI. Payments to providers are usually regular but may be suspended if reserves are inadequate (as occurred in Puding county and Beijing in 2013) or if the payer needs more time for performance assessment (as was the case in Yanchi county).

Benefit Packages Fragmented Across Insurance Schemes

Each NCMS office can decide on benefits, cost sharing, and other arrangements, and so many different models exist. The provincial health bureau generally takes responsibility for designing the disease scope, health care package, drug list, and reimbursement rates for each level of providers. The local county office can adjust the packages and set the cost-sharing arrangements under the leadership of the county government and the county health bureau to reflect the population's needs and preferences. When deciding coverage of services, NCMS should take into account the burden of disease, cost-effectiveness, and provider capacities.

The services and medicines in the benefit packages reflect national policy priorities and resource constraints. In recent years, the NHFPC has called upon pooled NCMS

offices to cover the 22 catastrophic diseases (including leukemia, multidrug-resistant tuberculosis [MDR-TB], and breast cancer) and has set the minimum reimbursement rate at 70 percent. The central government also sets the number of reimbursable drugs (500–800 for township health centers, 800–1,200 for county hospitals) and has set reimbursement rates 5–10 percent higher for essential drugs.

MoHRSS determines the national basic insurance drug list. Provincial and local MoHRSS bureaus define the formularies for health services and medical technology and equipment. The provincial bureaus can also adjust the national drug list (only for Category B drugs, though) according to the local context. Both the national and provincial basic insurance drug lists are reviewed by an expert panel, members of which have a pharmaceutical, clinical, pharmacoeconomic, or health care management background. The drugs are listed by their generic names, and province-based competitive bidding and bulk purchasing systems run by the provincial NHFPC are used to determine the actual drug types, volumes, and providers. The provincial and the lower-level basic medical insurance schemes (BMIs) have the right to decide on disease scopes and cost-sharing arrangements, which usually exempt the elderly and patients with chronic or catastrophic diseases with higher reimbursement rates and higher ceilings.

Since 2012, the central government has mobilized each province to initiate a new insurance scheme in addition to URBMI. Operated by commercial insurance institutions, this scheme targets the urban unemployed who have high out-of-pocket expenditures and offers them an extra minimum 50 percent reimbursement. This scheme is also suggested to be adopted in addition to the basic NCMS.

Selective Contracting Not Used Effectively

In theory, both the NCMS and the urban BMIs can selectively contract with public and private providers annually to deliver the defined list of services and drugs to the insured population. In practice, however, all public providers in the city are contracted, and their contracts are renewed almost every year, raising the question of whether URBMI uses selective contracting effectively as an incentive mechanism.

Besides, the contents of agreements are usually the same for each provider and are in the form of broad principles, which are more like general policies without specific terms and payment figures. In this way, providers are "forced" to undertake the agreement rather than accept it after mutual negotiation. Finally, the legal positions of the purchaser and the providers and the regulatory foundations are not clear, compromising enforcement of the contracts.

Until a few years ago, provider payment under UEBMI and URBMI was largely fee-for-service. In 2012, MoHRSS launched provider payment reforms—shifting postpayment to prepayment and introducing blended payment methods—to control program expenditure, improve efficiency, and enhance quality. Payment rates were set on the basis of growth-adjusted historical prices and negotiations with providers. Providers were allowed to keep residuals, while purchasers and providers shared reasonable levels of overspending.

Within two years, more than 80 percent of the regions had initiated pilots and adopted capitation or global budgets for outpatient services and case-based or per diem payment for selected inpatient care. However, without analysis of volume and quality, it is difficult to determine whether these reforms have yielded the desired benefits, either in controlling expenditures or in enhancing quality of care.

Provider Performance Inconsistently Monitored

Most NCMS purchasers play a passive third-party payer role, and although there have been some efforts to introduce performance evaluation, the indicators are largely tied to the number of visits and volume of services provided and less to the quality of these services. In general, NCMS offices emphasize

auditing of claims and paying of bills; they do not routinely collect data on performance. There are exceptions, however. Ningxia province's Yanchi and Haiyuan counties routinely measure outcome and system indicators, such as the antibiotics usage rate, and withhold 40 percent of the capitation fee contingent on suitable performance.

Most BMIs have the authority to set standards, verify that standards are followed, and determine the consequences for poor quality. Jiangyin and Changshu counties not only monitor providers' performance but also help them to improve. The performance assessment system in Yanchi county focuses on quality, clinical outcomes, and a competitive pay-for-performance scheme that is professionally managed by an external expert team.

Most BMIs strictly monitor the indicators that readily flow from the information system, such as budget execution, actual patient reimbursement, expenditure per visit or admission, length of stay, total volume, ratio of total hospital visits to total patients, readmission rate, and so on. They also monitor expenditures on drugs and consumables because providers can make high profits on these items. In addition, they monitor certain efficiency indicators—for example, the extent of "upcoding" (assigning an inaccurate billing code to a medical procedure or treatment to increase reimbursement) in Xi County and the expenditure consumption index (expenditure for treating the same disease category) and case-mix index in Beijing—to ensure that the diagnosis-related groups (DRGs) provide appropriate payment (that is, there is some, but not excessive, cost variation within groups).

Insurance agencies also pay attention to prescribing practices—an important cost driver. The most common indicator they track is drug expenditure as a proportion of total expenditure. Some counties track other indicators as well, such as the standard prescription rate (Xi county); the antibiotic use rate and rate of "split prescriptions" to track single prescriptions that are intentionally split into two or more separately billed orders (Yanchi and Changshu); prescription doses, to track illegal acquisition of prescription drugs for personal use or profit (Beijing and Jiulongpo); the intensity of antibiotic use, the hormone use rate to determine whether the lowest necessary dose of hormones is being used for the shortest needed time, and the fluid infusion rate (Changshu); and whether community health centers use only NCMS-listed medicines (Jiangyin).

Several counties and provinces monitor quality and clinical outcome indicators, such as coherence of clinical practice with guidelines (Xi); positive rates of medical tests (Xi, Hangzhou, Jiangyin, Changshu); diagnostic accuracy and prescription accuracy (Changshu); treatment according to indication (Hangzhou); hospitalization in accordance with indication (Jiangyin); cesarean section rate (45 percent or less in tertiary hospitals and 20 percent or less in community centers [Jiangyin]); mortality (Yanchi); readmission rate (Hangzhou, Xining, Shanghai, Changshu); and referral rate (Xining and Changshu).

Different performance indicators are used in different ways. When the proportion of surplus or overspending is set as a performance indicator in a prospective payment system (as in Xi, Hangzhou, Xining, and Zhuhai), it is usually used to decide how much the providers can be paid when there is a surplus or deficit. Some agencies (Jiulongpo, Beijing, Tianjin, and Zhuhai) use indicators of efficiency and cost containment to adjust the budget at the beginning of the next year. Others (Xi, Yanchi, Jiangyin, and Changshu) set aside a fixed proportion of the final budget to link with performance—usually quality, efficiency, clinical outcomes, or patient satisfaction indicators. In Beijing and Changshu, the copay rate over the budget cap also depends on the assessment results, and the agency only shares the surplus with providers who perform well in the performance assessment.

Provider Payment Reforms in China: Lessons From Recent Pilots

Globally, payers are moving away from fee-for-service, volume-driven health care services and toward value-based payment models that incentivize providers (hospitals, physicians, and other professional health care providers) on the basis of quality, outcomes, and cost containment. In promoting patient value and efficiency, these payment methods shift some risk to the provider. (Box 6.1 contains a typology of payment methods.)

Several local experiments are also going on in China that use payment incentives in support of some aspect of PCIC. Some of these experiments are aimed at integrating care between town and village providers, while others focus on creating incentives for county hospitals to become effective gatekeepers. Lessons from these pilots are relevant to the discussion of PCIC.

Provider payment reforms in China started over 15 years ago when, in a policy issued in 1999, the former Ministry of Labor and Social Security (MoLSS) promoted global budgets, fee-for-service, and per diem payment methods for UEBMI.[6] Five years later, in 2004, the Ministry of Health (predecessor to the NHFPC) introduced case-based payment in seven pilot provinces.[7]

Innovations in payment mechanisms started after 2009, when the State Council issued an opinion on deepening health reforms and encouraged pilots on case-based payment, capitation, and global budgets.[8] In 2011, MoHRSS issued specific policy guidelines on provider payment reform, offering a road map for achieving a series of national requirements:[9]

- Expenditure control, based on insurance fund revenue and expenditure projections
- Global budget prepayment for specific providers, considering institutional characteristics and service volumes
- Capitation for outpatient services
- Case-based payment for inpatient and catastrophic outpatient services, or per diem payments for inpatient bed-days in areas where case-based payment or capitation for outpatient care could not be implemented
- A negotiation mechanism between insurance funds and providers to decide payment rates.

BOX 6.1 **A typology of health care provider payment methods**

Payment methods can be summarized as follows:

- *Per time period*, that is, a fixed payment per year, such as in a salary
- *Per beneficiary*, or capitation, in which the provider receives a fixed amount per beneficiary
- *Per recipient*, which is like capitation except that it covers specific services a patient might receive
- *Per episode*, that is, bundled payments or prospective, diagnosis-related group–based payments
- *Per day*, in which a provider receives a fixed amount per day irrespective of services provided
- *Per service*, that is, payment according to number of services
- *Per cost*, or cost-based reimbursement
- *Per charge*, that is, cost plus a set profit markup

Risk-based payment models

Risk-based arrangements are based on estimates of expected costs to treat a particular condition or patient population; they include capitation, bundled payments, and shared savings arrangements. These models put the onus on providers to manage utilization and treatment expenses.

Two types of risks are inherent in a risk-based contract: insurance risk and performance and utilization risk. Insurance risk entails the financial costs of diseases, accidents, or injuries spread out over a covered population. Carriers of insurance risk typically hold sufficient financial reserves to cover the insurance risk. Performance or utilization risk

involves managing the rates of utilization of medical services by a defined population. Providers typically have considerable control over utilization of services, particularly unnecessary services, as well as over the quality and services they provide.

Under risk-based contracting, the performance risk is shifted wholly or partially to the provider. Risk-based models include "upside risk" if the provider only shares in the savings and not the risk of loss. A "downside risk" arrangement is one in which providers share in the savings and are responsible for a portion of any losses.

Bundled payments

Bundled payments are a type of prospective payment. Under bundled payments, providers share one payment for a specified range of services as opposed to each provider being paid individually. The intent of bundled payment is to foster collaboration among multiple providers to coordinate services and control costs, reducing unnecessary utilization and improving patient care.

Bundled payments share risk between the payer and providers and are the middle ground between fee-for-service (in which the payer assumes the risk) and capitation (in which the provider assumes the risk). Providers tend to be a little apprehensive about bundled payments because heterogeneity might not be fully reflected in reimbursements and because the lack of accurate cost data at the condition level could create financial exposure.

Sources: Frakt 2016 and "Alternative Payment Models: Frequently Asked Questions," American Academy of Pediatrics (accessed January 19, 2016), https://www.aap.org/en-us/professional-resources/practice-transformation/getting-paid/Pages/Payment-Models.aspx.

The regulations encouraged establishment of new payment mechanisms with reference payment rates based on historical fees, fund affordability, and current payment policies. They also suggested rate adjustments based on social economic development, provider service capacity, suitable technology application, the consumer price index, and medical input price changes. Further, the regulations suggested a global cap on all payment arrangements for different providers. In 2012, MoHRSS, the Ministry of Health, and the Ministry of Finance issued a policy on a

global cap for payment to providers by the BMIs, determined on the basis of a number of factors, including premium collection, fund risk considerations, price level, and historical utilization of health care.[10] In the same year, State Council policy directives mandated that facilities implement payment reforms involving global budgets, case-based payments, or per diem payments.[11]

Issued over the years, these directives have spawned local experiments involving a switch from fee-for-service payment to global budgeting, capitation, case-based payment, per diem payment, or pay for performance, as a result of which financial risks have begun to shift to providers.

Global Budgets

Global budgets that support integration of care and cap expenditures are being implemented in a few provinces and counties, and they have been effective in slowing the growth of insurance expenditures. In Shanghai, for instance, UEBMI switched from fee-for-service to global caps in 2003 and introduced mixed methods, including fee-for-service, per diem payment for mental diseases and case-based payment for diseases or treatment procedures, to make settlements. Global budget prepayment was adopted for all providers in Shanghai in 2009.

Likewise, Hangzhou determines the global budget of each hospital based on its historical fee claim data, institutional level, and service characteristics, with adjustments for inflation and policy changes. The profits and losses of the prepaid budget are shared between UEBMI and providers.

Capitation

There have been several promising pilots with capitation as well. In Zhenjiang (Jiangsu province), capitation is set for primary care providers under the budget cap, based on yearly treatment costs, including medicines and tests. An incentive rule is set up for primary care providers, and full payment is made only when the fee for chronic treatment reaches 70 percent of the chronic capitation.

Likewise, Changde in Hunan province uses capitation for inpatient services even in tertiary hospitals. URBMI allocates 87 percent of the fund for capitation payments to providers, and the balance is kept as a reserve and risk adjustment fund. A 2008–10 evaluation found that this reduced inpatient out-of-pocket costs by 19.7 percent, the out-of-pocket share by 9.5 percent, and the length of stay by 17.7 percent. However, the total inpatient cost, the drug cost ratio, treatment outcomes, and

patient satisfaction differed little between the fee-for-service and capitation models.

Case-Based Payments

Despite a decade of experimentation, the use of case-based payments (that is, negotiated rates per treated case) remains limited. Further, rate setting commonly reflects past trends in caseloads, service volumes, and prices under the fee-for-service system, which also remains the basis for setting patient copays.

There are notable exceptions, however. In Beijing, UEBMI pioneered the first DRG system in China in six hospitals in 2011, covering 108 groups. An evaluation using hospital discharge data from the six pilot hospitals and eight other hospitals that continued to use fee-for-service (and served as controls) found that DRG payment led to reductions of 6.2 percent in health expenditures and 10.5 percent in out-of-pocket payments per hospital admission. However, hospitals continue to use fee-for-service payments for older patients and patients with more complications.

In Shanghai, the insurance agency pays the provider a fixed case rate regardless of actual expenses. An evaluation of the Shanghai experiment showed that to safeguard profits, hospitals engaged in several opportunistic behaviors, including reducing patients' length of stay. Hospitals also used cost-shifting tactics, resulting in uninsured patients incurring higher expenditures to compensate for reduced revenues from insured patients.

In some instances, global budgets included a pay-for-performance (or activities) element, as in Changshu and Hangzhou and in the Jiulongpo district of Chongqing, but without addressing the possible negative impact on quality of care.

Per Diem Payments

Some counties are experimenting with per diem payments. One example is Shenzhen in Guangdong province, which pays per diems for inpatient services. The total payment is determined as a rate per inpatient day, adjusted for inpatient volume calculated as real inpatient volume multiplied by the inpatient-outpatient ratio. The gap between the payment rate and the fee calculated using the fee schedule is shared.

Another example is Changshu in Jiangsu province, where URBMI has set up specific per diem rates based on disease severity, treatment period, and institutional level. The rates for surgeries vary with presurgical hospitalization, surgical procedure, and post-surgical care, and the rates decrease when inpatient days increase.

Mixed Methods

Some counties are experimenting with mixed provider payment methods. Guizhou province introduced a salary-plus-bonus payment for village doctors instead of fee-for-service and removed the incentives for overprescribing medications. An evaluation showed that both outpatient costs and spending on drugs fell, but doctors increased nondrug services such as injections and had more incentive to refer patients to hospital care, which in turn increased total health care costs.

In Ningxia province, an intervention targeted at primary care providers combined capitation with pay-for-performance incentives. An evaluation showed that both antibiotic prescriptions and total outpatient spending declined without major adverse effects on other aspects of care.

In Xi county (Henan province), the NCMS categorizes all diseases treated by public county hospitals into three groups (A, B, C) according to the clinical characteristic of the diagnosis and case mix. For frequent and less-severe cases (groups A and B), case-based payment rates are set to include services prescribed in clinical guidelines. The case payment rate is based on actual average fee-for-service rates over the past three years and is negotiated with providers. More complicated cases (group C) remain under the fee-for-service payment. The NCMS prepays 40 percent of total payments to providers, with the remaining 60 percent based on performance.

The main indicators used to assess performance in Xi include antibiotic and steroid use compliance with regulations (more than 95 percent), positive rate of tests done on large equipment (more than 70 percent), compliance with hospitalization diagnostic criteria (more than 90 percent), and patients' satisfaction level (more than 95 percent). Experts are invited to assess provider performance, and institutions with assessment scores of 85 or higher are paid 100 percent of their claimed payments. Institutions scoring 80–85 points receive 95 percent payment, scores between 75–80 points receive 90 percent payment, and so on. Institutions scoring 60–65 points receive only 75 percent of their claims and a warning. Those that score below 60 three years in a row are not contracted by the Xi NCMS again.

Performance Indicators and Monitoring Systems

In Xining county (Qinghai province), URBMI collects information on efficiency indicators (such as rehospitalization rates, referral and transfer rates, average inpatient bed days, and large equipment cost ratios); patient economic burden indicators (such as the share of medicines in total expenditures and share of out-of-pocket expenditures); and patient satisfaction rates. If hospitalization rates or referral and transfer rates exceed 1 percent of the standard, annual payment is reduced by 0.2 percent; if the medicine cost share and out-of-pocket proportion exceed 1 percent of the standard, the fund payment is reduced by 1 percent. There are similar penalties for other indicators.

Jiangyin county and Changshu (Jiangsu province) have also defined performance indicators for outpatient and inpatient services. Besides indicators of diagnostic and examination accuracy, as in Jiangyin, the Changshu NCMS uses outside treatment referral rates as an indicator of provider service capacity and quality. It also focuses on prescription behavior, looking at antibiotics and combined use, hormone use, intravenous fluid use, and divided prescriptions.

Use of technology and information management in performance monitoring has improved in Jiulongpo, Zhuhai, Xi, and Xining counties and in the Beijing, Hangzhou, and Shanghai municipalities. In particular, Xi county has developed a well-functioning provider performance monitoring system that combines routine performance indicators generated by the information technology (IT) system with random clinical audits. Progress in most agencies has been constrained, however, by fragmented IT systems, limited staff capacity, and poor connectivity. Some of the more innovative purchasing agencies reported that they have built capacity through a combination of well-trained staff and more demanding recruitment requirements, strategic investment in IT and data analytics capacity, and exposure to Chinese and international learning and exchange programs.

Incentive Reforms in Sanming: A Case Study

Sanming, a city in northwest Fujian province, has a population of 2.74 million. It is an old industrial municipality and has a high percentage of retirees in its population. The health expenditures of Sanming's 22 public hospitals increased steadily from RMB 856 million in 2008 to RMB 1.69 billion, as a result of which UEBMI in Sanming has been running a deficit since 2009 (which had accumulated to RMB 17.5 million by 2011).

Against this backdrop, Sanming launched widespread reforms in February 2012, notably the following (Ying 2014):

- *Established the Sanming Public Health Insurance Fund Management Centre* (PHIFMC) to manage important decisions including drug procurement, utilization review, and cost monitoring
- *Centralized provincial drug procurement* under the PHIFMC, with drug suppliers chosen through an online bidding process managed by the PHIFMC, not the hospital
- *Implemented a zero-markup policy* for prescription drugs and consumables,

which separated hospital revenue from prescriptions
- *Increased hospital fees*, as a result of which the 22 public hospitals recouped 87 percent of their losses due to the zero markup on prescription drugs
- *Raised the incomes of hospital directors and health professionals* by increasing salaries as well as performance bonuses

As a result of these interventions, health expenditures fell across the board, UEBMI made a surplus (after years of deficits), and incomes of health professionals increased. Some notable results are as follows:

- *Expenditures on prescription drugs* fell 18 percent, from RMB 680 in 2011 to RMB 560 in 2013, in the 22 public hospitals. The average cost of drugs per outpatient visit fell below provincial and national averages.
- *Expenditures on inpatient services* fell by 6.6 percent in 2013 compared with 2011, after having grown at an average annual rate of 6.2 percent in the preceding five years.
- *Expenditures on outpatient services* saw no significant change between 2011 and 2013, but their rate of growth was the slowest in the whole province.
- *UEBMI gained surpluses* (after several years of deficits) of RMB 26.3 million in 2012 and RMB 116.8 million in 2013.
- *Revenue from drugs and consumables* dropped from 60.1 percent of all revenues in 2011 to 38.3 percent in 2013 across the 22 public hospitals.
- *Revenue from health care services* rose from 39.9 percent of all revenues in 2011 to 61.7 percent across the 22 public hospitals.
- *Salaries of health care professionals* increased significantly. The total salary bill of the hospitals increased by 42 percent, from RMB 498.4 million in 2012 to RMB 709.2 million in 2013. Physicians' average annual income increased by 48 percent, to RMB 99,800.

Core Action Areas and Implementation Strategies to Realign Incentives

Implementing health financing reforms can be challenging, even in the most advanced and organized of economies. One common feature of most health systems is that of flow of finances from the population and the government, via a variety of agencies, to a large, disparate group of providers of health goods and services. Each transfer involves a trade of sorts, an exchange of trust, in which the payer entrusts money to an agent in exchange for some desired aspect of health care delivery. Sometimes the trade is instantaneous, as when an individual goes to the pharmacy and buys an over-the-counter drug. Many times, the exchange takes the form of a promise, as when households entrust their money to an agency that they trust will buy and deliver the best health care for them whenever in the future they may need it.

Each transfer in the health system gives rise to a principal-agent situation in which one party is being paid by another to do something, a situation that can rapidly turn into a problem if the agent is motivated to act in its own best interest instead of that of the principal. This is relevant to several key health financing elements: raising finance, transferring funds to providers at different levels, and purchasing of health services by different agents, to name just a few. Each poses a real danger that the interests of the actors in the health system—especially consumers—are compromised.

The abnormal economic features of the health sector further complicate the situation (Hsiao 1995). The problems related to uncertainty, externality, and information asymmetry are well known. Indeed, the peculiarities of health care provision are so unusual that the usual tenets of neoclassical economics—assumptions of rational, utility maximizing behavior and stable preference functions—are not very useful. And finally, the high degree of variety and idiosyncrasy in the acts of seeking health care and of producing and delivering health goods and services generates huge transaction cost problems for a market system and challenging incentive specification problems for a centrally planned system (Hodgson 2008).

In China, it is widely accepted that effectively leveraging the power of strategic purchasing, contracting, and paying providers could improve the value of the government's large investment in the health sector. Significant steps have been taken in recent years to build the role of health purchasing agencies, develop their institutional capacities, and test innovative contracting and provider payment approaches. Now deeper reforms are required to overcome the legacies of earlier policies, support the PCIC approach, and yield better value for money. China can build on the experiences of the many successful pilots and experiments both within and outside the country to leverage the power of strategic purchasing and put in place a set of incentives that motivates providers at all levels to provide the best-quality health services at lowest cost for all citizens of the country.

The proposed health financing reforms fall into four broad thematic categories, each with its own distinct objective and associated action points (table 6.1):

1. Implement provider payment reforms in support of PCIC.
2. Bring about coherence and consistency in incentive mechanisms and strengthen integration of care.
3. Rationalize distribution of services by level of facility.
4. Strengthen capacity of purchasing agencies.

Translating these strategic intents into individual operating unit plans requires identification of critical drivers and decomposition of the complex health financing system into discrete, manageable elements across functions and across time. The resulting road map, presenting the interaction of multiple forces over time, will help bring together the many diverse issues that need to be managed through various processes.

TABLE 6.1   Four core action areas and implementation strategies to realign health system incentives

Core action areas	Implementation strategies
1. Provider payment reforms in support of PCIC	• Evaluate ongoing reform experiments with prospective payments, and systematically replicate successful efforts in all provinces and cities • Switch from fee-for-service to prospective payments for the portion of expenditure that is borne directly by patients • Put in place mechanisms for concurrent evaluation of ongoing and new provider payment reforms
2. Coherent, consistent incentives and stronger integration of care	• Analyze incentive mechanisms across different insurance schemes within each province to understand areas of consonance and dissonance • Develop a strategy for vertical and horizontal consolidation as necessary • Establish a designated unit at central and provincial levels to oversee implementation and concurrent evaluation
3. Rational distribution of services by facility level	• Determine, standardize, and list procedures at their commensurate level of care (community, township, county, and level 2 and 3 city hospitals) • Reassess copayments across different levels and set significantly higher deductibles and out-of-pocket payments for basic procedures that are being demanded at the tertiary level
4. Capacity building of insurance agencies	• Develop staff expertise and data analytics capability • Empower purchasing agencies and hold them accountable for results • Strengthen cost accounting systems

Note: DRG = diagnosis-related group; PCIC = patient-centered integrated care.

This process is laborious but useful and necessary for implementers and decision makers in the health system and the government in China to determine which aspects of the internal and external environments need to be brought together to initiate coherence in ideas and actions. Health financing reforms are complex by nature, and organizing frameworks help to align activities and steer actions necessary for achieving the desired objectives.

Core Action Area 1: Provider Payment Reforms in Support of PCIC

Provider payment reforms are a central part of health financing reforms, principally because payment methods create powerful incentives that influence provider behavior and have a direct bearing on the efficiency, equity, and quality outcomes of health finance reforms.

There is no one optimal method of paying providers: depending on the market and institutional context, provider payment methods generate incentives that increase or lower health spending, improve or compromise efficiency, enhance or worsen equity, and positively or adversely affect consumer satisfaction. Which approach to use in which context requires a deep understanding of the market in which providers work, sound judgment, and strong administrative and supervisory capacity of regulators.

Strategy 1: Evaluate reform experiments with prospective payments and systematically replicate successful efforts in all provinces and cities

China's contracting and provider payment innovations provide an experience base that needs to be harmonized and deepened to create an effective incentive environment across levels of care (box 6.2).

The experience of ongoing pilots suggests that a combination of case-mix-adjusted, volume-based global budgets for inpatient admissions; capitation payment for primary care with performance incentives; and capped, episode-based payment for outpatient

BOX 6.2   **Examples of provider payment reforms in China**

Global caps

- *In Shanghai,* Urban Employee Basic Medical Insurance (UEBMI) switched from fee-for-service to global caps in 2003 and introduced mixed methods, including fee-for-service, per diem payment for mental diseases, and case-based payment for diseases or treatment procedures, to make settlements. Global budget prepayment was adopted for all providers in 2009.
- *Hangzhou* determines the global budget of a single hospital based on historical fee claim data, institutional level, and service characteristics, adjusted for inflation and policy considerations. The profit and loss of the prepaid budget are shared between UEBMI and providers.

Capitation

- *In Zhenjiang (Jiangsu province),* capitation is set under the budget cap and is based on yearly treatment costs, including medicines and tests. An incentive rule is set up for primary care providers, and full payment is made only when the fee for chronic treatment reaches 70 percent of the chronic capitation.
- *Changde (in Hunan province)* uses capitation for inpatient services even in tertiary hospitals. Urban Resident Basic Medical Insurance (URBMI) uses 87 percent of the fund as the capitation to providers, and the balance is kept as a reserve and risk adjustment fund. A 2008–10 evaluation found that this payment reform reduced inpatient out-of-pocket cost by 19.7 percent, the out-of-pocket ratio by 9.5 percent, and the length of stay by 17.7 percent. However, the total inpatient cost, drug cost ratio, treatment effect, and patient satisfaction showed little difference between fee-for-service and capitation models.

Case-based payment

- *In Shanghai,* the insurance agency pays the provider a fixed case rate regardless of actual expenses. An evaluation of the Shanghai experiment shows that to safeguard profits, hospitals engaged in several opportunistic behaviors, including reducing patients' length of stay. Hospitals also engaged in cost-shifting tactics by raising outlays on uninsured patients to compensate for reduced revenues from insured patients.

- *In Beijing,* UEBMI pioneered China's first diagnosis-related group (DRG) system in China in six hospitals in 2011, covering 108 groups. An evaluation using hospital discharge data from the six pilot hospitals and eight other hospitals, which continued to use fee-for-service and served as controls, found that DRG payment led to reductions of 6.2 percent and 10.5 percent, respectively, in health expenditures and out-of-pocket payments by patients per hospital admission. However, hospitals continued to use fee-for-service payments for patients who were older and had more complications.

Per diem payment

- *Shenzhen (Guangdong province)* pays for inpatient services by per diem payment. The total payment is determined by a rate per inpatient day and adjusted inpatient volume (calculated as real inpatient volume multiplied by inpatient-outpatient ratio). The gap between the payment rate and the real fee (based on fee schedule) is shared.
- *In Changshu (Jiangsu province),* URBMI has set up a specific per diem rate based on disease severity, treatment period, and institutional level. In the case of surgeries, the rate varies among presurgical hospitalization, surgical procedure, and postsurgical care, and decreases as inpatient days increase.

Pay for performance

- *Guizhou province* introduced a salary-plus-bonus payment method for village doctors in lieu of fee-for-service payment and removed the incentives for overprescribing medications. An evaluation showed that both outpatient costs and drug spending fell, but doctors increased nondrug services such as injections and gained more incentives to refer patients to hospital care, which in turn increased total health care costs.
- *In Ningxia province,* an intervention targeted at primary care providers combined capitation with pay-for-performance incentives. An evaluation showed that both antibiotic prescriptions and total outpatient spending declined without major adverse effects on other aspects of care.

Sources: Feng and Hairong 2014; Gao, Xu, and Liu 2014; Hong 2011; Hu 2013; Jian and others 2015; Jiang and others 2011; Liang, Wang, and Jing 2013; Liu and others 2012; Wang 2011; Wang and others 2013; Yip and others 2014; Zhang 2010; Zhang and Wu 2013; Zhang and Xu 2014; Zhen 2009.

specialty services may be the most appropriate approach to manage cost escalation, limit unnecessary referrals, and shift basic services delivery to primary care in the short and medium term.

Replicating the successful efforts systematically across China's provinces and cities would not only incentivize improved physician-patient contact at the primary care level but would also strengthen primary care overall.

Provider payment systems are undergoing a paradigm shift globally as well, and health care payers are moving away from passively reimbursing providers to pursuing a variety of policies to improve the quality and efficiency of care. In Organisation for Economic Co-operation and Development (OECD) countries, for example, payments for primary care have become more blended, with countries using capitation and budgets and adding elements to drive quality or increase productivity.

OECD countries use a variety of ways of setting fees for primary care providers (table 6.2). In countries like Chile, Ireland, and the Netherlands, fees are set unilaterally by the central government. In Greece, Sweden, and Switzerland, fees are set by key purchasers. In other countries, such as the Czech Republic, Germany, the Republic of Korea, and the United Kingdom, fees are negotiated at the central level between the purchaser and provider groups. Chile uses a third-party negotiator, while Australia, Austria, and Canada negotiate at the regional level.

Inpatient care in many OECD countries is paid on the basis of DRG payments alongside other policies to constrain overall budgets and stimulate competition, with a focus on productive efficiency. In many countries, payment systems have evolved beyond fee-for-service and budgets and shifted to finance services on the basis of activity using DRGs. Furthermore, payment methods vary by hospital type (public or private) and whether the payment is being made by social health insurance (table 6.3) or tax-based systems (table 6.4).

Strategy 2: Switch from fee-for-service to prospective payments for the portion of expenditure borne directly by patients

In implementing global budgets, one pressing priority is the development of the case-mix-adjusted, volume-controlled approach to effectively control the growth of hospital expenditures. This will enable insurance agencies to shift savings into primary care.

One possibility is to develop a simple set of DRGs for case-mix adjustments to minimize provider cherry picking, complemented by rigorous monitoring and pay-for-performance elements that ensure access and quality of care. The approach could build on the experience of Beijing, where the DRG system is used to adjust the global budgets of all 263 health care institutions for their case mix. In addition, local pilots across the country offer a wide range of experiences and lessons in monitoring and creating incentives for appropriate provider behavior.

It is important that contracting and payment methods share financial risks between insurers and providers while improving the quality of care and safeguarding the financial protection of patients. As a first step, rate setting for provider payments needs to shift from historical claims to cost information. The way that provider payment rates are set influences how services are produced, so linking payment rates to costs can drive more efficient cost structures. Setting payment rates above costs for high-priority services and below costs for low-priority services, for example, can improve the efficiency of the service mix.

There has been increasing experimentation with new ways of paying providers, especially payment systems that span across levels of care. One option that China may like to consider is that of bundled payments (box 6.3), especially since no single method directly rewards improving the value of care. Capitation, especially global capitation—that is, a single payment to cover all of a patient's needs—decouples payment from what providers can directly control and rewards providers for spending less but not specifically for improving outcomes or value.

TABLE 6.2 Primary care remuneration systems in OECD countries, 2014

Predominant primary care	Countries	Remuneration of provider setting					Remuneration of physicians			
		Cap	FFS	P4P	GB	Other	Salary	FFS	Cap	Other
Private group staffed by physicians and other health professionals	Australia	○	●	●	○	○	○	●	○	●
	Denmark	●	●	○	○	○	○	●	●	○
	Ireland	●	●	○	○	○	○	●	●	○
	Japan	○	●	○	○	○	○	○	○	○
	Netherlands	●	●	●	●	○	○	●	●	●
	New Zealand	●	●	●	○	○	●	●	○	●
	Norway	●	●	○	○	○	○	●	●	○
	Poland	●	○	○	○	○	○	○	●	○
	United Kingdom	●	●	●	○	●	●	●	●	●
	United States	●	●	●	○	●	●	●	●	●
Private group staffed by physicians	Canada	●	●	○	○	○	●	●	●	●
	Italy	●	○	○	○	○	○	○	●	○
Private solo practice	Austria	○	●	○	○	○	○	●	○	○
	Belgium	●	●	○	○	○	○	●	●	○
	Czech Republic	●	●	●	○	○	○	●	●	○
	Estonia	●	●	●	●	○	○	●	●	●
	France	○	●	●	○	●	○	●	○	●
	Germany	○	●	○	○	○	○	●	○	○
	Greece	○	●	○	○	○	○	●	○	○
	Korea, Rep.	○	●	●	○	○	○	●	○	○
	Luxembourg	○	●	○	○	○	○	●	○	○
	Slovak Republic	●	●	○	○	○	○	●	●	○
	Switzerland	●	●	○	○	○	○	●	●	○
Public primary group staffed by physicians and others	Chile	●	●	○	○	○	●	○	○	○
	Finland	○	○	○	●	○	●	●	○	○
	Hungary	●	○	●	●	○	○	○	●	○
	Iceland	○	○	○	●	○	●	○	○	○
	Israel	●	○	○	●	○	●	○	○	○
	Mexico	●	○	○	●	○	●	○	○	○
	Portugal	●	○	●	●	○	●	○	○	○
	Slovenia	●	●	○	○	○	●	○	○	○
	Spain	●	○	●	○	○	●	○	●	○
	Sweden	●	●	●	○	○	●	○	○	○
	Turkey	●	○	●	○	○	●	○	○	○

Source: Questions 27 and 33, OECD Health System Characteristics Survey 2012 and Secretariat's estimates. (For database and questionnaire, see http://www.oecd.org /els/health-systems/characteristics-2012-results.htm.)
Note: Cap = capitation; FFS = fee-for-service; GB = global budget; OECD = Organisation for Economic Co-operation and Development; P4P = pay for performance.

TABLE 6.3   Hospital remuneration systems in OECD countries with social health insurance

Country	Public hospitals	Private not-for-profit hospitals	Private for-profit hospitals
Austria	DRG	DRG	DRG
Belgium	Prospective global budget	Prospective global budget	n.a.
Chile	DRG	DRG	Line-item remuneration
Czech Republic	DRG	DRG	DRG
Estonia	DRG	n.a.	n.a.
France	DRG	DRG	DRG
Germany	DRG	DRG	DRG
Greece	DRG	DRG	Procedure service payment
Hungary	DRG	DRG	Procedure service payment
Israel	Procedure service payment	Procedure service payment	Procedure service payment
Japan	DRG	DRG	n.a.
Korea, Rep.	Procedure service payment	Procedure service payment	n.a.
Luxembourg	Prospective global budget	Prospective global budget	n.a.
Mexico	Prospective global budget	Procedure service payment	Procedure service payment
Netherlands	DRG	DRG	n.a.
Poland	DRG	DRG	DRG
Slovak Republic	Procedure service payment	Procedure service payment	Procedure service payment
Slovenia	DRG	DRG	DRG
Switzerland	DRG	DRG	DRG
Turkey	Prospective global budget	Prospective global budget	Prospective global budget
United States (Medicare)	DRG	DRG	Procedure service payment

Source: Question 31, OECD Health System Characteristics Survey 2012 and Secretariat's estimates. (For database and questionnaire, see http://www.oecd.org/els/health-systems/characteristics-2012-results.htm.)
Note: DRG = diagnosis-related group; OECD = Organisation for Economic Co-operation and Development; n.a. = not applicable.

TABLE 6.4   Hospital remuneration systems in OECD countries using a tax-based system

Country	Public hospitals	Private not-for-profit hospitals	Private for-profit hospitals
Australia	DRG	Procedure service payment	Procedure service payment
Canada	Prospective global budget	Prospective global budget	Prospective global budget
Denmark	Prospective global budget	n.a.	DRG
Finland	DRG	n.a.	n.a.
Iceland	Prospective global budget	n.a.	n.a.
Ireland	Prospective global budget	Prospective global budget	n.a.
Italy	Prospective global budget	DRG	DRG
New Zealand	Prospective global budget	n.a.	n.a.
Norway	Prospective global budget	Prospective global budget	DRG
Portugal	Prospective global budget	Procedure service payment	Procedure service payment
Spain	Line-item remuneration	Prospective global budget	n.a.
Sweden	Prospective global budget	Prospective global budget	Prospective global budget
United Kingdom	DRG	Procedure service payment	Procedure service payment

Source: Question 31, OECD Health System Characteristics Survey 2012 and Secretariat's estimates. (For database and questionnaire, see http://www.oecd.org/els/health-systems/characteristics-2012-results.htm.)
Note: DRG = diagnosis-related group; OECD = Organisation for Economic Co-operation and Development; n.a. = not applicable.

<table>
<tr><td>BOX 6.3</td><td>**Bundled payment models**</td></tr>
</table>

The proliferation of bundled payment models is transforming the way in which care is delivered. Governments, insurers, and health systems in many countries are trying bundled payment approaches, as in these examples:

- *In Sweden,* the Stockholm County Council adopted bundled payments in 2009 for all total hip and knee replacements. The result was lower costs, higher patient satisfaction, and improvement in some outcomes.
- *Germany* uses bundled payments for hospital inpatient care, which has helped control the rise in spending on inpatient care. (No additional payment is made for rehospitalization related to the original care.)

- *In the United States,* bundled payments are used extensively for organ transplant care, as in the University of California, Los Angeles kidney transplant program.

   Some U.S. employers have also embraced bundled payments, including Walmart, which introduced a program that encourages employees who need cardiac, spine, and selected other surgery to obtain care at one of just six providers nationally, all of which have high volumes and track records of excellent outcomes. The hospitals are reimbursed in a single bundled payment that includes all physician and hospital costs associated with all inpatient and outpatient preoperative and postoperative care.

Source: Porter and Lee 2013.

Fee-for-service rewards providers for increasing volume, but that does not necessarily increase value. Bundled payments that cover the full care cycle for acute medical conditions, overall care for chronic conditions for a defined period, or primary and preventive care for a defined patient population, are perhaps best aligned with value.

Strategy 3: Put in place mechanisms for concurrent evaluation of ongoing and new provider payment reforms

Rigorous scientific assessment of provider payment reform pilots is essential to judging the effectiveness and replicability of the reform in other parts of the country. China may like to commission a systematic evaluation of the various reform initiatives in different parts of the country.

   Such an evaluation will require an independent, dedicated, and fully funded autonomous mechanism established at an arm's length from the government to finalize the list of indicators, gather the relevant data, evolve sustainable systems for tracking and data collection, maintain baseline assessment of the indicators at the provincial and central

levels, conduct periodic review at the provincial and national levels to monitor progress, and establish credible external review mechanisms. This review and evaluation will require a complex set of coordinated actions at multiple state levels within the provincial and central governments. This process is necessary to arrive at an impartial and scientific assessment in support of the scaling-up of a reform.

   Insurance agencies also need to integrate learning from successful provider payment experiments as they are scaled up. For example, global budgets have been introduced to control the growth of expenditures in hospitals but have not shifted significant resources into primary care. Capitation payments have been introduced in many instances for outpatient care but not always with pay-for-performance components to mitigate adverse impacts on service volumes and quality. Further, rate setting in new mechanisms has commonly reflected past trends in caseloads and service volumes. This historical approach is one reason why pilots of global budgets have had limited effect on cost containment.

At the same time, flaws persist that distort payment methods, old and new. Most importantly, in the absence of proper cost information, rates continue to reflect pricing systems that reinforce the overuse of more expensive care settings and higher-priced technology and exacerbate the general trend among providers to invest in and upgrade facilities. For example, global budgets are typically calculated based on historical rate systems that pay higher rates for the same service to more specialized service providers (such as secondary and tertiary care hospitals). Together with reforming financial incentives for providers, efforts need to focus on changing the financial incentives facing patients so as to steer them away from higher levels of care.

Core Action Area 2: Coherent, Consistent Incentives and Stronger Integration of Care

How health financing is arranged across different levels of the system may also be a source of inefficiency, especially if it is marked by fragmentation, contradictory incentives at different points of interaction between the providers and patients, and high administrative costs. Establishing a coherent incentive environment that is internally consistent is a necessary step for steering payers and providers of health care toward greater efficiency and quality.

Strategy 1: Analyze incentive mechanisms across insurance schemes to understand areas of consonance and dissonance
Health providers in China receive payments from multiple sources: out-of-pocket payments by patients who pay on a fee-for-service basis; health insurance payments, also largely on a fee-for-service basis, although payment mechanisms are changing rapidly; and direct government funding linked to public health goods and input-based subsidies. If a common provider payment mechanism were used for the first two of these revenue streams, it would make the positive incentivizing effect of prospective payment methods much more powerful. If one payer changes the way it pays providers, the presence of multiple payers allows providers to transfer costs to other payers not included in the payment reform (Yip and Hsiao 2008).

For many health conditions, treatment involves providers at different levels at different stages of the treatment cycle. If the system's incentive structure motivates each level of provider to hold on to patients rather than refer them to the appropriate level of care based on clinical need, patients could potentially receive suboptimal care. A situation of internally inconsistent incentives could also emerge if different methods being used to pay providers at different levels of care result in conflicting or mutually reinforcing but perverse incentives. For example, primary care providers who are paid by capitation may be motivated to refer high-cost patients to specialists who, if paid under a fee-for-service system, may readily welcome them.

It is important, therefore, to ensure coherence and internal consistency in the way that the incentive structures are set up across the health system. As Shortell (2013) notes, "the largest limiting factor is not lack of money or technology or information or people, but rather the lack of an *organizing principle* that can link money, people, technology and ideas into a *system* that delivers more cost-effective care (i.e., more value) than current arrangements."

Strategy 2: Develop a strategy for vertical and horizontal consolidation
Horizontal and vertical consistency and coherence—within and across a facility alliance or network—increase the likelihood that payment mechanisms will achieve the desired changes in provider behavior. Provider payment mechanisms work best when they are defined and applied consistently across the full continuum of health care production and delivery, from primary care to tertiary interventions, and are compatible in the sense that all providers—including hospitals; physicians; and town, community, and village health centers—face similar types of incentives.

Within the proposed organized networks or alliances for PCIC implementation at the county and district levels, for example, networks could receive a prospective global budget based on capitation plus other revenues. The global budget will necessarily entail a hard budget constraint along with measures to avoid cost shifting by providers to patients. The global budget may be based on current spending levels initially but have a focus on controlling future spending growth across the entire network. The global budget could include a "withhold" of a predefined percentage of funding, which could be paid upon compliance with PCIC-related indicators such as quality improvement, integrated care, reducing unnecessary care, and shifting inappropriate care out of the hospital.

Such consolidation would require that the network redefine hospital and primary provider roles and establish formal links. Network management would need to channel incentives to hospitals and primary care providers through, for example, risk-adjusted, facility-specific global budgets. This would be especially important to align incentives of hospitals and primary care providers to work together to implement PCIC.

Another option could be to consider incentive payments outside of the global budget (such as additional funding) that would need to be earned (box 6.4). Hospital performance indicators could focus on patient safety, quality, and efficiency improvements. Measures of this sort would promote the integration of services across the health system and would also incentivize the network to direct the flow of patients to the appropriate levels of care. Any savings generated by the network could be shared by hospitals and primary care providers within that network.

The insurance agencies may also benefit from taking a closer look at their budgets, benefits, and fees to better balance hospital-based care for catastrophic diseases with primary care for common diseases. Specific measures are needed to limit the overuse of hospitals and to shift resources into primary care as its delivery capacity is developed. A combination of regulatory measures and payment incentives is needed to shift service delivery to the appropriate level of care.

BOX 6.4   Quality-compatible modified global payment systems in the United States

In the United States, two health care insurance providers have successfully implemented payment schemes among networks of providers to improve quality and reduce waste and unnecessary utilization. Both programs offer useful lessons for China.

Alternative quality contract

In January 2009, Blue Cross Blue Shield of Massachusetts launched a new payment arrangement called the alternative quality contract. The contract stipulates a modified global payment arrangement: fixed payments for the care of a patient during a specified time period. The model differs from past models of fixed payments or capitation because it explicitly connects payments to achieving quality goals and defines the rate of increase for each contract group's budget over a five-year period, unlike typical annual contracts. All groups participating in the alternative quality contract earned significant quality bonuses in the first year.

Patient-centered medical home

CareFirst's patient-centered medical home (PCMH) program began in 2011, and within three years, over 80 percent of all primary care providers in the CareFirst service area—including parts of Northern Virginia, the District of Columbia, and Maryland—had begun to participate in the program. Since the program began, CareFirst's overall rate of increase in medical care spending for its members has slowed from an average of 7.5 percent per year in the five years before the program's launch to 3.5 percent in 2013. In addition, CareFirst members under the care of participating PCMH physicians fare well when measured on key quality indicators.

Sources: Chernew and others 2011; Murray 2015.

International experience indicates that as long as hospitals are permitted to deliver basic outpatient services—and to financially benefit from such service delivery—shifting the delivery system to a PCIC delivery model is nearly impossible. Options include a mix of regulatory, administrative, and contracting instruments. *Regulations* could specify which services can (and cannot) be delivered at each level of the delivery system and could install primary care providers as gatekeepers. *Budgetary allocations* could be earmarked for primary, secondary, and tertiary care to direct volume and resources toward lower levels of care. And *contracting arrangements* could specify which services will be reimbursed at each provider level.

Strategy 3: Establish a designated unit at central and provincial levels to oversee implementation and concurrent evaluation

Fuenzalida and others (2010) note that effective coordination across various subfunctions of health financing is necessary for successful reform design and implementation. The three subfunctions that are key for successful implementation of financing reforms in China's health sector are alignment between revenue collection and pooling, alignment between revenue collection and purchasing, and alignment between pooling and purchasing. Several important observations made earlier regarding these important subfunctions and internal alignment are summarized here for ready reference:

- Empowering insurance agencies to act as strategic purchasers of health services can significantly improve the returns on the government's large investment in the health sector. China has already taken many important steps to strengthen the institutional capacities of health insurance agencies, but deeper reforms are necessary to yield better value for money.
- The legal mandate and legislative framework governing the insurance agencies must explicitly state that the agencies are responsible for selectively contracting

providers and creating incentives to enhance provider performance. Moreover, as local government institutions, insurance agencies and public health care providers are part of the same legal entity, which compromises the legal enforceability of contractual relationships. Under these arrangements, local insurance agencies tend to concern themselves with balancing their revenue with competing demands from public providers for increases in funding.

- Efforts need to be made to streamline the incentives from different flows of public funds so as to shape provider behavior. Local governments, for instance, provide direct subsidies to public providers, often in the form of block grants paying for the salaries of regular employees, among other items.
- Insurance agencies need urgently and aggressively to build capacities to monitor service access, quality, and provider responsiveness. Currently, insurance agencies are primarily invested in building capacity to process claims and detect fraud.
- It is important that all insurance agencies build strong monitoring capacity and establish a core set of indicators across key performance dimensions.

Integrating, or at least harmonizing, the varied benefits, scheme management, and purchasing practices—as well as channeling supply-side subsidies through the insurance system—is essential to improving pooling of funds, enhancing equity, and creating streamlined incentives for providers. The integration of the NCMS and URBMI schemes has started with some pilots, and Hangzhou's HRSS, like several others, is managing all three schemes and harmonizing purchasing practices. Such experiences could be studied further, and the emerging trends in integrating and harmonizing health insurance schemes and reducing supply-side subsidies could be accelerated.

In China, the fragmentation of insurance agencies across and within schemes limits their leverage over the behaviors of provider organizations. Within each scheme, the purchasing function is typically decentralized to the municipal or county level, as a result of which literally thousands of insurance agencies contract and pay health care providers across the country. For example, in Changshu (Jiangsu province), URBMI pays providers a capitation fee for general outpatient care, with 5 percent of the payment subject to meeting quality of care standards, while UEBMI beneficiaries pay providers on a fee-for-service basis out of personal MSAs. Greater coordination across the three insurance agencies would help remove many of these kinds of incongruities in purchasing. Merging the three insurance schemes is not necessarily a solution because it would create a large single unit, which would be difficult to manage and administer. In fact, the benefits of merging could equally be obtained from enhancing coordination of purchasing across the three agencies—without creating a large insurance monopoly.

The government is committed to integrating the three health insurance schemes, although the huge variations in financing, benefit packages, reimbursement rates, and management structures among different schemes in different areas make this difficult. URBMI and the NCMS have similar financing sources (insured and public finance), benefit packages (inpatient and catastrophic outpatient services), and reimbursement rates, but the differences from UEBMI make integration with the latter problematic. Nevertheless, integration of URBMI and the NCMS into UEBMI has begun, and pilots are under way in Chongqing, Guangdong province, Ningxia province, and Tianjin.

URBMI has two forms of integration: (a) *overall integration* of premium collection, benefit packages, reimbursement rates, fund pooling, payment methods, and management authority and (b) *partial integration*, in which the two schemes are managed by the same authority but with different fund pooling and benefit policies. In some URBMI schemes, different premium levels have been set up for the insured to choose among.[12]

In January 2016, the State Council released the "Opinions" on the merger of URBMI and NCMS to ensure equal access to medical services and reimbursement among urban and rural residents as well as to improve overall service efficiency in the insurance system. Governments at the provincial and municipal level were required to make specific plans for the integration before the end of June 2016.

China may also like to look at some other experiences with these kinds of reforms. One example is Korea, which merged all statutory health insurance funds into a single insurer in July 2000 (Kwon 2015). Before this, there was no competition among the insurance funds to enroll the insured, and each insurance fund covered a well-defined population group. Except for reviewing and assessing claims submitted by providers, health insurance funds did not actively exercise their purchasing power and did no selective contracting with providers. The 2000 merger not only introduced a new single insurer agency—the National Health Insurance Company, which later changed its name to the National Health Insurance Service (NHIS)—but also created a new insurance review agency, the Health Insurance Review and Assessment Service (HIRA).

The NHIS handles premium collection, fund pooling, and reimbursement to providers. HIRA makes decisions related to purchasing (such as claim reviews) and to the design of the benefits package and provider payment system. After the merger, the NHIS expanded health insurance benefits and coverage, started covering cancer screening, reduced coinsurance rates for catastrophic conditions, introduced ceilings for cumulative out-of-pocket payments for covered services for every six months, and so on. The savings in administrative expenses due to economies of scale in management after the merger helped enable the benefits expansion (although it is difficult to confirm the causal relation).

Taiwan, China, also consolidated its fragmented labor insurance market into a single-payer system and set up the National Health Insurance Administration (NHIA) covering health care for all (Leung 2015). With the formation of the NHIA, significant investments were made to develop the resources and technology to enable efficient administration and effective policy making that propelled progress in building purchasing functions and capacities. The reform benefited from strong commitment and advocacy on the part of top political leaders, a growing economy, and a team of knowledgeable and informed health policy advisers. The strong organization and infrastructure become the bedrock for building the NHIA's strategic capacities for influencing the use and delivery of health services in Taiwan, China, which include the ability to design the benefit package, develop provider payment systems, and monitor provider performance.

The monopsony power to set fees, draw up and enforce contracts, and monitor providers, as granted by law, has enabled the NHIA to manage health care resource allocation while controlling costs and improving the quality of health care. The single-payer approach not only has the administrative advantage of uniform systems and procedures but also offers equitable access to quality health care for patients across all demographics and geographies. A large amount of resources was devoted to developing the NHIA's claims system. Once set up, the system enhanced the NHIA's ability to monitor health care utilization and spending, reduced resource requirements for claims processing, and paved the way for other program and technology developments. Up-front investments in technology systems and infrastructure increased the efficiency and effectiveness of the administrative processes and enhanced the purchaser's capacities for managing the insurance program.

Core Action Area 3: Rational distribution of Services by Facility Level

The production and delivery of health care in China is characterized by an "outsized" service distribution system, which creates high costs and compromises its value base. The fee-for-service payment system, dominant in the last few decades of the 20th century, incentivized organizations to offer a full line of services in their communities. In the absence of rationalization of the overall network, this system duplicated expensive services across its operations, overinvested in hospital capacity, and underinvested in delivery of primary care. In switching to a value-based system, it will be important for China to reduce inappropriate utilization and provide patients with the right care at the right place and at the right time to meet quality, cost, and access targets.

Strategy 1: Determine, standardize, and list procedures at their commensurate level of care by facility level

The starting point of this rationalization is to define the scope of services that could be provided at different levels of care across provinces, counties, and cities. For lower levels of care, this would imply exiting from complex service lines where available expertise and infrastructure may compromise ability to deliver high-quality care. For tertiary levels of care, this would imply minimizing routine services, delivered at much higher cost than community providers. This would result in providers at all levels concentrating on delivering care at the best combination of cost and quality.

Strategy 2: Reassess copayments and set significantly higher deductibles and out-of-pocket payments for basic procedures being demanded at the tertiary level

For services covered by the BMI system, China may like to consider setting up reimbursement rates for specific services according to the cost of producing and delivering those services at the agreed-upon and designated level of care. In other words, if a certain service is deemed best delivered at the district hospital level, and the district hospitals have the capacity to deliver, the case-mix-adjusted per case rates estimated for that level could be applied universally across the hospital system. However, if only the highest tertiary-level hospital has the capacity to deliver that service, a prospectively determined case-mix-adjusted rate is set and paid to that hospital but under an agreed-upon ceiling determined by the global budget.

For services not covered by health insurance, payment methods need to be revised to have a much closer relationship with costs. This is consistent with the May 2015 government policy directive that requires health insurance to cover most medical expenditures and sets the target for out-of-pocket payments paid by each patient at below 30 percent by 2017.

A big advantage of this arrangement is that health services would be delivered at the locations where the value is highest. The lower-cost facilities at the primary and secondary levels would take care of relatively less complex conditions and routine services, with charges set accordingly. High-intensity services, such as cardiac and oncological care, would be delivered at well-resourced, well-staffed facilities by subject-matter experts, and charges would be set accordingly.

In several examples globally, matching complexity and needed skills with institutions' resource intensity has resulted in huge value improvements. In the United States, for instance, Children's Hospital of Philadelphia shifted routine tympanostomies (insertion of tubes into children's eardrums to reduce fluid collection and risk of infection) and simple hypospadias repairs (a urological procedure) from its main facility to suburban ambulatory surgery facilities. This move cut costs and freed up operating rooms and staff at the teaching hospital for more complex procedures, resulting in estimated savings of 30–40 percent (Porter and Lee 2013).

There are several examples as well of consolidation of services in fewer locations. In 2009, 32 London hospitals had hyperacute stroke units staffed by dedicated state-of-the-art teams that include neurologists to take care of stroke patients. Having so many facilities offering the same service did not allow any one or two to amass a high volume and enjoy scale benefits. UCL Partners, a delivery system comprising six well-known teaching hospitals that serve North Central London, decided to consolidate the stroke units and

moved them all to the University College facility. Later, they consolidated and moved all emergency vascular surgery and complex aortic surgery to the Royal Free hospital, a different facility. The results were immediate: The number of stroke cases treated at University College climbed from about 200 in 2008 to more than 1,400 in 2011. Mortality associated with strokes at University College fell by about 25 percent, and costs per patient dropped by 6 percent (Porter and Lee 2013).

Capital investments also need to be better aligned with incentives to deliver fewer high-frequency services at tertiary levels and to push a larger share of services to lower levels. International experience indicates that the shift of service delivery to primary care is often accompanied by large investments in infrastructure and human resources at the primary care level to create a "push-pull" effect, so that as incentives push services to the primary care level, better capacity pulls patient demand at the same time. Developing and strengthening the quality of human resources is key: China has already invested a lot in infrastructure in recent years, and adding more infrastructure without concomitant increases in the quality of human resources will not be very productive.

Core Action Area 4: Capacity Building of Insurance Agencies

Strengthening the institutional and human resources capacity of purchasing agencies is critical to transform them from passive payers of health care to active and strategic purchasers of health goods and services on behalf of the covered population.

Strategy 1: Develop staff expertise and data analytics capability

The experience of purchasing agencies in China and globally demonstrates four of the most effective steps to build capacity:

- *Develop staff expertise.* Ensuring that the staff recruited to the purchasing agencies are well versed and trained in the specific duties of their positions and also in the theoretical and practical underpinnings of health financing and purchasing policy is key. A standardized set of training modules could be developed and adapted for ongoing training at the local level.

- *Establish data analytics capability.* Strategic investments in IT and data analytics capacity to manage information and data in-house would help inform decision making. Indeed, investment in IT infrastructure, software development, and programming, as well as staff training in data analytics and research, is one of the most critical aspects of purchasing capacity development.

- *Learn from domestic and international experiences.* Some of the most effective purchasing agencies globally, such as those in Korea and Thailand, have developed or are closely affiliated with highly sophisticated research institutes dedicated to studying the operation, impact, and improvement of their health insurance systems. Exposure to Chinese and international learning and exchange programs is necessary to stay abreast of best practices. Many of China's own ad hoc learning and exchange programs could be built upon and made available to a wider range of purchasing agencies more systematically. In addition, partnerships with local research institutions and think tanks are a common source of capacity building and should continue to be promoted and possibly funded through grants or other financial resources.

- *Develop capability to assess the quality of care.* Finally, the ability and expertise to assess quality is fundamental to the design of any performance-oriented payment mechanism. Providers need to be held accountable for delivering high-quality services efficiently and without shifting costs to patients. Monitoring efforts by purchasing agencies have focused on fragmented aspects of provider performance, including claims expenditures against caps, drug expenditures, and some limited clinical process indicators. The highly automated claims system could be exploited better to develop comprehensive automated provider monitoring systems that generate routine reports on volume, service intensity, referrals, adherence to clinical guidelines, and financial protection, and the information could be used to inform adjustments in purchasing and provider payment strategies.

Strategy 2: Empower purchasing agencies and hold them accountable for results

To improve the value of the Chinese government's enormous investments in the health sector, the power of health purchasing needs to be more effectively leveraged. The purchasing agencies need to have to have the mandate, capacity, and market power to exert real influence over provider behavior and the volume and quality of services delivered. The overarching mandate and accountability of China's BMI schemes need to shift toward strategic purchasing and getting value for money. Although previous reform guidelines have acknowledged the need to better leverage strategic health purchasing and stimulate changes in provider behavior, purchasing agencies should be held accountable for results that go beyond their fiduciary responsibilities to ensure the safety of insurance funds and maintain or increase enrollment and reimbursement rates, to improving the quality of care and patient health outcomes.

In this context it is important that the purchasers of health services differentiate between performance and quality. There are many examples of pay-for-performance in China, but because in most cases "performance" still equates to "activities" and is not related to enhancing quality of care or to improving patient health outcomes, the current pay-for-performance mechanisms have put in place strong incentives to increase volume.

Strategy 3: Strengthen cost accounting systems

Significant long-term returns can be expected from investing in cost accounting systems. Accurate cost information is vital to set realistic payment rates, which is critical to minimize provider cherry picking. Indeed, it would allow the purchasers of health services to set prices below or above average costs, thus creating incentives to improve the efficiency of the service mix and encourage delivery of services in the most appropriate care setting. Cost information also helps providers plan budgets, benchmark within and across health care institutions, and monitor the delivery of services.

Almost all OECD countries have cost accounting systems that generate cost information used for setting payment rates. Typically, cost data are collected and pooled from a selected number of providers that use comparable cost accounting systems that meet predefined quality standards. In addition, these countries make cost accounting mandatory or use cost accounting guidelines to encourage providers to account for their costs and use them for management.

Notes

1. "Opinions on Further Improving the Reform of Health Insurance Payments" (*Renshenbu fa* 2011, No. 63) implements payment reforms in the UEBMI scheme. "Opinion on Implementing the Control of Total Medical Insurance Payment" (*Renshebu fa* 2012, No. 70) suggests implementation of payment reforms across all insurance schemes to control the increase of medical expenditures.
2. Coverage statistics from *China Health and Family Planning Statistical Yearbook 2016* (Beijing: Peking Union Medical College Press).
3. "Notification of the Opinion to Comprehensively Scale Up Urban and Rural Residents' Catastrophic Medical Insurance," General Office of the State Council (*Guo ban fa* 2015, No. 57).
4. "Opinion on Establishing an Emergency Medical Assistance System," General Office of the State Council (*Guo ban fa* 2013, No. 15).
5. "Opinion on Inclusion of College Students in URBMI," State Council Office (2008, No. 119); "Guidelines on Cost Allocation Methods in Health Services Pricing," Pricing Department of China Planning Committee (2001, No. 1560).
6. "Opinion on Enforcement of Payment Management for UEBMI," MoLSS (1999, No. 23).
7. "Notice on Pilots of Cased-Based Service Pricing Management," Ministry of Health (Peking Union Medical College University Press, 2004).
8. "Opinion on Deepening China's Health Care System Reform," State Council (*Zhong fa* 2009, No. 6).
9. "Opinion on Promoting Payment Reform of Medical Insurances, MoHRSS (2011, No. 63); "Opinion on Setting Up Pooling Fund for Outpatient Services for URBMI," MoHRSS (2011, No. 59).
10. "Opinion on Carrying Out Global Control on Basic Medical Insurance Payment," MoHRSS (2012, No. 70).
11. "Guidance on Promoting Reform of the NCMS Payment System," State Council (*Wei nong wei fa* 2012, No. 28).
12. "Opinion on Promoting Payment Reform of Medical Insurances," MoHRSS (2011, No. 63).

References

Babiarz, Kimberly S., Grant Miller, Hongmei Yi, Linxiu Zhang, and Scott Rozelle. 2012. "China's New Cooperative Medical Scheme Improved Finances of Township Health Centers but Not the Number of Patients Served." *Health Affairs* 31 (5): 1065–74. doi:10.1377/hlthaff.2010.1311.

Blumenthal, David, and William Hsiao. 2005. "Privatization and Its Discontents—The Evolving Chinese Health Care System." *New England Journal of Medicine* 353 (11): 1165–70.

Chen, Zhu. 2009. "Launch of the Health-Care Reform Plan in China." *The Lancet* 373 (9672): 1322–24.

Chernew, Michael E., Robert E. Mechanic, Bruce E. Landon, and Dana Gelb Safran. 2011. "Private-Payer Innovation in Massachusetts: The 'Alternative Quality Contract.'" *Health Affairs* 30 (1): 51–61.

Feng, Jin, Pingyi Lou, and Yangyang Yu. 2015. "Health Care Expenditure over Life Cycle in the People's Republic of China." *Asian Development Review* 32 (1): 167–95.

Feng, Lin, and Hairong Wang. 2014. "Exploration of Chronic Disease Management and Payment Reform of Medical Insurances in Zhenjiang." *Chinese Health Resources* 3: 211–12.

Frakt, Austin B. 2016. "A Typology of Payment Methods, Part 1." *AcademyHealth* (blog), January 19. http://academyhealth.org /node/1836.

Fuenzalida, H., S. O'Dougherty, T. Evetovits, C. Cashin, G. Kacevicius, and M. McEuen. 2010. "Purchasing of Health Care Services." In *Implementing Health Financing Reform: Lessons from Countries in Transition*, edited by J. Kutzin, C. Cashin, and M. Jakab, 155–86. Copenhagen: World Health Organization.

Gao, Chen, Fei Xu, and Gordon G. Liu. 2014. "Payment Reform and Changes in Health Care in China." *Social Science & Medicine* 111: 10–16.

Hodgson, Geoffrey M. 2008. "An Institutional and Evolutionary Perspective on Health Economics." *Cambridge Journal of Economics* 32 (2): 235–56. doi:10.1093/cje/bem033.

Hong, Yao. 2011. "Discussion on Case-Based Payment Practice in Shanghai." *Health Economic Research* 4: 30–31.

Hsaio, W. C. 1995. "Abnormal Economics in the Health Sector." *Health Policy* 32 (1–3): 125–39.

Hu, Shanlian. 2013. "Piloting the Global Control." *China Social Security* 2: 73.

Jian, Weiyan, Ming Lu, Kit Yee Chan, Adrienne N. Poon, Wei Han, Mu Hu, and Winnie Yip. 2015. "Payment Reform Pilot in Beijing Hospitals Reduced Expenditures and Out-Of-Pocket Payments per Admission." *Health Affairs* 34 (10): 1745–52.

Jing, F. 2004. "Health Sector Reform and Reproductive Health Services in Poor Rural China." *Health Policy and Planning* 19 (Suppl 1): i40–i49.

Ji-yuan, Jiang, Sun De-yao, Qi Qi, and Sun Yi. 2011. "Research on Payment System Based on Diagnosis Related Groups in Beijing." *Chinese Journal of Hospital Administration* 27 (11): 587–89.

Kwon, Soonman. 2015. "Institutional Capabilities for Health Service Purchasing—Case Study of Korea's National Health Insurance Service (NHIS) and Health Insurance Review and Assessment Service (HIRA)." Case study commissioned by the World Bank, Washington, DC.

Lei, Xiaoyan, and Wanchuan Lin. 2009. "The New Cooperative Medical Scheme in Rural China: Does More Coverage Mean More Service and Better Health?" *Health Economics* 18 (S2): S25–S46. doi:10.1002/hec.1501.

Leung, Alexander T. 2015. "Health Services Purchasing: A Review of Taiwan's Development and Experience." Case study commissioned by the World Bank, Washington, DC.

Liang, Hong, Luan Wang, and Li-mei Jing. 2013. "The Process and Enlightenment from Payment Reform of the Basic Medical Insurance for Urban Workers in Shanghai City." *Chinese Health Resources* 4: 265–67.

Liu, Hong, and Zhong Zhao. 2014. "Does Health Insurance Matter? Evidence from China's Urban Resident Basic Medical Insurance." *Journal of Comparative Economics* 42 (4): 1007–20. doi:10.1016/j.jce.2014.02.003.

Liu, X., and Anne Mills. 1999. "Evaluating Payment Mechanisms: How Can We Measure Unnecessary Care?" *Health Policy and Planning* 14 (4): 409–13.

Liu, X., Zhan Chang-chun, Zhou Lv-ling, and others. 2012. "Empirical Research on the Effect of Payment System on Medical Insurance Expense Control Sampled with Zhenjiang City." *Chinese Health Service Management* (12): 909–12.

Liu, Y. 2004. "Development of the Rural Health Insurance System in China." *Health Policy and Planning* 19 (3): 159–65.

Ma, Jin, Mingshan Lu, and Hude Quan. 2008. "From a National, Centrally Planned Health System to a System Based on the Market: Lessons from China." *Health Affairs* 27 (4): 937–48.

Manuel, Ryan. 2010. "China's Health System and the Next 20 Years of Reform." In *China: The Next Twenty Years of Reform and Development*, edited by Ross Garnaut, Jane Golley, and Ligang Song, 363–91. Canberra: ANU E Press.

Meng, Qun, Ling Xu, Yaoguang Zhang, Juncheng Qian, Min Cai, Ying Xin, Jun Gao, Ke Xu, J. Ties Boerma, and Sarah L. Barber. 2012. "Trends in Access to Health Services and Financial Protection in China between 2003 and 2011: A Cross-Sectional Study." *The Lancet* 379 (9818): 805–14. doi: http://dx.doi .org/10.1016/S0140-6736(12)60278-5.

Murray, Robert. 2015. "The CareFirst Blue Cross–Blue Shield Patient-Centered Medical Home Model, Maryland, U.S.A." Case study commissioned by the World Bank, Washington, DC.

Porter, Michael, and Thomas Lee. 2013. "The Strategy that Will Fix Health Care." *Harvard Business Review*, October 13.

Shortell, Sam M. 2013. "Bridging the Divide between Health and Health Care." *JAMA* 309 (11): 1121–22.

State Council. 2011. "The 12th Five-Year Plan for Economic and Social Development of the People's Republic of China (2011–2015)." Translated by the Compilation and Translation Bureau, Central Committee of the Communist Party of China. Beijing: Central Compilation & Translation Press.

Wang, Kun, Wu Hua-zhang, Du Yu-kai, and others. 2013. "Analysis on the Modes of Medical Insurance Payment of Mental Health Institutions." *Chinese Journal of Social Medicine* (1): 57–59.

Wang, Xiang. 2011. "The Strategy Choices of Payment Reform: Based on 17 Years Reform in Zhenjiang." *China Health Insurance* 7: 35–36.

WHO (World Health Organization). 2000. *The World Health Report 2000: Health Systems—Improving Performance.* Geneva: WHO.

Ying, Yachen. 2014. "Achieve Win-Win-Win Situation by Jointly Reforming the Drug Sector, Health Service Sector, and Health Insurance Sector: Field Study Report on Public Hospital Reform in Sanming." Case study, Health Development Research Center (NHFOC), Beijing.

Yip, W., and W. C. Hsiao. 2008. "The Chinese Health System at a Crossroads." *Health Affairs* 27 (2): 460–68.

Yip, Winnie, Timothy Powell-Jackson, Wen Chen, Min Hu, Eduardo Fe, Mu Hu, Weiyan Jian, Ming Lu, Wei Han, and William C. Hsiao. 2014. "Capitation Combined with Pay-For-Performance Improves Antibiotic Prescribing Practices in Rural China." *Health Affairs* 33 (3): 502–10. doi:10.1377/hlthaff.2013.0704.

Yip, Winnie, Chi-Man Yip, William C. Hsiao, Wen Chen, Shanlian Hu, Jin Ma, and Alan Maynard. 2012. "Early Appraisal of China's Huge and Complex Health-Care Reforms." *The Lancet* 379: 10. doi:10.1016/S0140-6736 (11)61880-1.

Yu, Baorong, Qingyue Meng, Charles Collins, Rachel Tolhurst, Shenglan Tang, Fei Yan, Lennart Bogg, and Xiaoyun Liu. 2010. "How Does the New Cooperative Medical Scheme Influence Health Service Utilization? A Study in Two Provinces in Rural China." *BMC Health Services Research* 10: 9.

Zhang, J. 2010. "The Impact of a Diagnosis-Related Group-Based Prospective Payment Experiment: The Experience of Shanghai." *Applied Economics Letters* 17 (18): 1797–1803. doi:10.1080/13504850903317347.

Zhang, Linxiu, Hongmei Yi, and Scott Rozelle. 2010. "Good and Bad News from China's New Cooperative Medical Scheme." *IDS Bulletin* 41 (4): 10.

Zhang, Ying, and Wu Yong-ling. 2013. "Changshu URBMI (NCMS) Payment Reform Practice and Exploration." *Business* 22: 238–39.

Zhang, Zai-sheng, and Ai-hao Xu. 2014. "Evaluation of Capitation Reform of Payment System on Diabetes Mellitus." *Chinese Rural Health Service Administration* 9: 1058–60.

Zhen, Jie. 2009. "Multiple Payment Practice of Medical Insurance in Beijing." *China Health Insurance* 5: 34–35.

Zhou, R. n.d. "Responsible Utilization of Antibiotics Should Be a Societal Responsibility." Sanmenxia Central Hospital Paper No. 223 (in Chinese), Sanmenxia, China.

7

Lever 6: Strengthening the Health Workforce

Introduction

Transforming China's health service delivery system to provide people-centered integrated care (PCIC) has several implications for China's health workforce.

First, in the PCIC model, primary health care (PHC) plays a central role in providing a continuum of services for patients who have noncommunicable diseases. The current PHC workforce in China would need to be strengthened and expanded to enable PHC facilities to act as gatekeepers and to coordinate health care within the entire health system.

Second, the PCIC model changes the way health care is organized and managed. It relies on general practitioner (GP)-based multidisciplinary teams; strong links to community-based and social care; effective coordination across providers at different levels of the health care system; and a strong focus on prevention, risk stratification, and health maintenance. China's significant imbalance in its workforce composition and considerable shortage of these health professionals pose enormous challenges that will require medium- and long-term strategies to overcome.

Third, the PCIC model emphasizes patient engagement and self-management. In this more collaborative approach, providers and patients work together to identify problems, set priorities, establish goals, create treatment plans, and solve issues. This implies a new way for providers and patients to interact that requires clinicians to have better communication and interpersonal skills when dealing with patients.

Adopting a PCIC approach will also have profound implications for the training, deployment, composition, and management of the Chinese health workforce. International experience suggests that transforming the health workforce to meet the challenges of PCIC would include redefining the scope of practice and functions of different categories of health workers; composing new teams representing a variety of specializations; developing new sets of skills and competencies; achieving a well-balanced distribution of the workforce across different levels of care; improving performance management systems; instituting appropriate incentive structures; and transforming preservice and in-service training. Applying these core principles to guide health workforce reform in China implies changing the institutional, financial, and management systems governing the health workforce.

This chapter examines the main challenges related to the health workforce in China in the context of PCIC and recommends policies to successfully address these challenges.

The rest of the chapter is organized as follows:

- *"The Chinese Health Labor Market"* assesses the current health labor market challenges in the context of China's institutional and policy environment and identifies sources and causes of disequilibrium.
- *"Recommendations for Human Resources Reform"* presents four core action areas and associated strategies for implementation of the recommended reforms.
- *"An Implementation Road Map"* concludes by setting forth short- and medium-term steps for implementing the recommended reforms as well as complementary measures that may be needed to support these actions and their desired outcomes.

The Chinese Health Labor Market: Trends and Challenges

The Health Professional Education System

The health labor market in China has experienced huge changes in recent years. In 1998, China started an ambitious reform of the world's largest educational system for health care professionals. Universities of western medicine that were previously governed by the Ministry of Health were merged into universities supervised by the Ministry of Education. China has also gradually established a comprehensive medical education system of undergraduate and postgraduate education and continuing professional development: students enroll directly from high school into clinical medicine courses of either three years (for a diploma), five or six years (for a bachelor's degree), seven years (for a master's degree), or eight years (for a medical doctorate).

This system produced more than twice as many graduates overall in 2013 than in 2003 and more than four times as many graduates of higher medical education (Liu 2015). About half a million nurses graduated in 2013, the large majority of them with vocational degrees (table 7.1).

The rapid expansion of health professional education has raised important concerns. These include lack of coordination between medical education and labor market demands; rapid expansion in the numbers of students without corresponding efforts to strengthen the quality of training; and curricula that focus narrowly on biomedicine, medical technology, and hospital care with little exposure to community and primary care or rural practice. There is a need for better cooperation between the Ministry of

TABLE 7.1   **Enrollment of medical students and medical graduates in China, 2013**

Student category	Students enrolled			Graduates		
	Higher education	Vocational education	Total	Higher education	Vocational education	Total
Clinical medicine (including TCM)	124,279	108,947	233,226	107,904	108,382	216,286
Public health	9,593	—	9,593	6,793	—	6,793
Nurses and midwifery	42,646	521,159	563,805	34,145	534,502	568,647
Pharmacists (including TCM)	38,904	27,216	66,120	31,404	24,249	55,653
Medical technicians	21,167	52,353	73,520	11,091	40,568	51,659

Source: Liu 2015.
Note: TCM = traditional Chinese medicine; — = not available.

Education, which is now in charge of health professional education, and the National Health and Family Planning Commission (NHFPC). A study found that medical universities decide on their enrollee numbers not on the basis of need or demand for health professionals but mostly based on the number of teachers or even dormitory rooms (Liu 2015). Faculty numbers have not kept pace with the expanding numbers of medical students (figure 7.1)

The massive increase in admissions has considerably increased student-teacher ratios and shortages of clinical internship positions (Daermmich 2013), which has likely affected the quality of medical education. Medical training focuses on clinical biomedicine and hospital practice, with little exposure to community and primary care or rural practice (Hou and others 2014).

Until recently, China did not have a standardized resident training system at the national level; medical graduates usually went directly to work in a hospital or PHC facility after graduation. Internationally, the norm is that medical graduates undergo training in clinical practice (usually for three years) as a resident doctor in a hospital before they can practice medicine independently. This is considered important to ensure the quality of clinical care. In December 2013, the NHFPC and six other ministries issued a joint policy directive, "Guidance . . . on the Establishment of a Standardized Resident Training System," which requires medical graduates to complete a three-year standardized residency in an accredited institution (after five years of medical university study).[1] Funding for training institutes and subsidies for resident trainees are provided by the central and local governments.

Imbalances in Workforce Composition

The government's efforts to increase the training of health professionals have produced a steady expansion of the health workforce and significantly changed its composition. The compensation structure has also changed, notably as a result of the new zero-markup policies on drug prescription. At the same time, the regulatory framework has been modified to enhance the mobility of health workers across regions and providers. These changes reflect institutional transformations in the Chinese labor and health care markets that combine features of a dynamic and fast-growing market economy with rigid state control and intervention.

FIGURE 7.1   Numbers of medical students and faculty and faculty-student ratios in China, 1998–2012

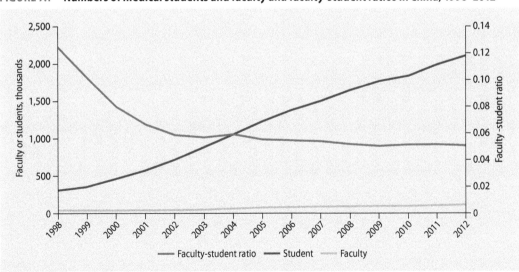

Source: Hou and others 2014, 823.

However, health workforce challenges continue to pose a major challenge in China's bid to strengthen its public and primary health care services (Yip and others 2010). Specialists outnumber GPs, and there are few doctors at the PHC level. Compensation levels are unattractive, and the underlying incentives in physician contracts with hospitals are perverse. The governance structure of the health workforce is characterized by the headcount quota system, and physician licensing is linked with facilities, introducing rigidities and limiting mobility. Managerial autonomy in hiring health workers at the facility level is low, resulting in a mismatch between staffing needs and available skills. This chapter will discuss these issues in detail.

Despite the remarkable increase in the total supply of health workers, many challenges remain in the composition of the health workforce.

First, even though the total number of health workers in China increased from 6.2 million in 2011 to 7.21 million in 2013, the number of health care professionals per 1,000 population in China at the end of 2013 was only 5.3, including 2 licensed physicians

(and assistant physicians) and 2 registered nurses (NHFPC 2014), which is below the Organisation for Economic Co-operation and Development (OECD) country average of 3.2 doctors and 9.6 nurses per 1,000 population (figure 7.2).

Second, among all health workers, there is a huge shortage of nursing staff across the country. Despite the doubling in total numbers and a huge increase in the recruitment of nursing students, the ratio of nurses to doctors in China is only 1 to 1, significantly lower than the average of 2.8 nurses per doctor in OECD countries (Qin, Li, and Hsieh 2013).

What is encouraging, however, is the increase in recruitment of nursing students: in 2013 alone, nursing schools recruited 0.56 million students, 62 percent of them in three-year vocational nursing schools. As a result, the number of nurses per 1,000 population increased from 0.98 in 2003 to 2.04 in 2013 (figure 7.3).

Third, China has a critical shortage of several key specialties: pediatricians, psychiatrists, and GPs constitute only 3.9 percent, 0.9 percent, and 5.2 percent, respectively, of all licensed physicians. The relatively lower

FIGURE 7.2   Ratio of nurses to physicians in OECD countries, 2012 (or nearest year)

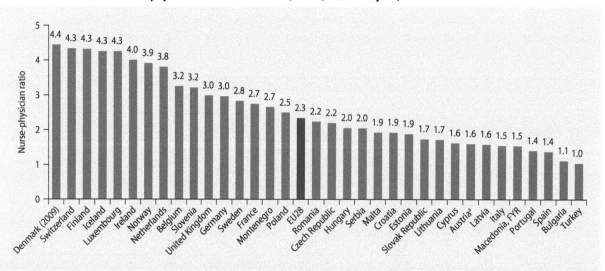

Sources: Eurostat, OECD Health Statistics 2014, and WHO European Region "Health for All" databases.
Note: OECD = Organisation for Economic Co-operation and Development; EU28 = 28 member states of the European Union; WHO = World Health Organization.
a. Austria reports only nurses employed in hospitals.

FIGURE 7.3   Number of health professionals per 1,000 population in China, 2003–13

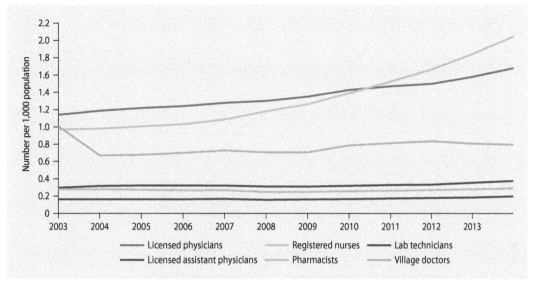

Source: Liu 2015.

income and higher occupational risk of these posts make them less attractive than other specialties. The 5.2 percent share of GPs is well below international norms of 30–60 percent.

A 2011 State Council policy proposes to establish a GP-based primary health care delivery system with two to three GPs per 10,000 population (international practice is one GP per 2,000 population).[2] To meet this target, China needs at least 300,000 to 400,000 GPs, or more than double the current GP workforce (172,597 in 2014) (NHFPC 2015). In China, as in many other countries, being a GP is less attractive than being a specialist. GPs' lower social status and income and limited career development path affects the recruitment of new medical graduates. By 2016, the government had already enrolled 70,000 medical graduates into the standardized three-year residency training programs, with 8,637 slots for GP training.

Fourth, despite an increase in recent years in the number of health workers practicing in rural areas, health professionals are still heavily located in cities. The urban-rural ratio of health workers per 1,000 population increased from about 2.0 in 2005 to about

2.5 in 2013 (figure 7.4; also see annex 7A, table 7A.2). In 2013, urban areas had 2.3 times as many physicians per 1,000 population than rural areas and 1.8 times as many nurses. Likewise, the shortage of nurses is especially severe in rural areas and at the PHC level, where the nurse-physician ratios are 0.82 to 1 and 0.55 to 1, respectively.

The distribution of health workers across the public and private sectors has also changed in recent years (Liu 2015). The share of health professionals practicing in the private sector increased from 14 percent in 2010 to 15.8 percent in 2013 (figure 7.5). The category with the largest proportion in the private sector is assistant licensed physicians (20.1 percent); technicians have the smallest (12.3 percent).

These imbalances in the distribution of the Chinese health workforce result in critical shortages at the PHC level and in rural areas. The number of health professionals working in PHC settings has been increasing, but overall the PHC workforce is still limited. In 2013, only 30 percent of all health professionals and 21 percent of registered nurses worked in PHC settings (including township health centers [THCs] in rural areas and community health centers [CHCs] or stations

FIGURE 7.4   Health professionals per 1,000 population in China, by rural or urban location, 2003–13

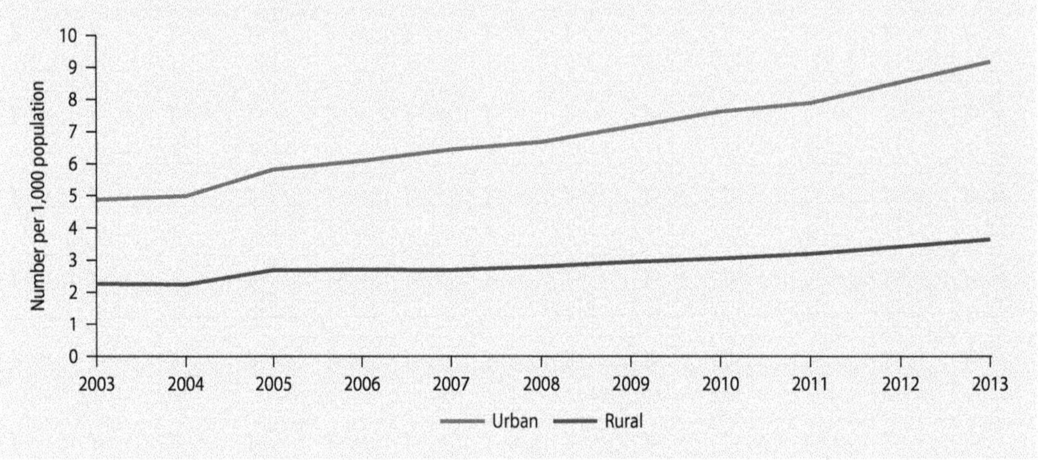

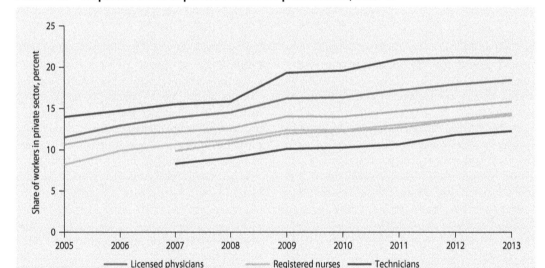

Source: Liu 2015.

FIGURE 7.5   Proportion of health professionals in the private sector, 2005–13

Source: Liu 2015.

in urban areas). Although the overall health workforce expanded, the share of PHC workers declined, from more than 40 percent in 2009 to less than 30 percent in 2013. A recent survey revealed that nearly 50 percent of the assistant physicians and registered nurses who left THCs went to work in hospitals at the county level or above.

In addition, health professionals at the PHC level and in rural areas have less education than those in higher-level facilities and in towns and cities. In 2012, 20 percent of the health professionals in urban areas and only 6 percent in rural areas had a bachelor's degree or above.[3] Most PHC workers in CHCs and THCs have received only post-high-school training and secondary school training, respectively. PHC facilities and poor rural areas continue to have difficulty recruiting and retaining qualified health professionals. The lack of qualified health professionals at the PHC level, especially in the rural areas, is the major reason why patients bypass PHC and seek care directly at hospitals.

Unattractive Compensation Levels and Perverse Financial Incentives

One possible explanation for the persistent shortcomings in China's primary health workforce is unattractive compensation. Earnings in the health sector—which typically include a basic salary, a performance bonus, and a hardship allowance—show

significant variation, with PHC workers earning the least. Average earnings in China's regulated health sector rank ninth among all sectors, only 13 percent above the economy-wide average (figure 7.6), and annual rates of increase have been low relative to those in other sectors.

The compensation structure is also an issue: on average in 2012, the basic salary in the health sector accounted for 23 percent of total compensation, allowances for 20 percent, and performance bonuses for 57 percent.[4] Health care workers—especially doctors—are encouraged to seek additional income from bonuses based on the overall

FIGURE 7.6 Annual average wages of urban employees in China, by sector, 2005 and 2012

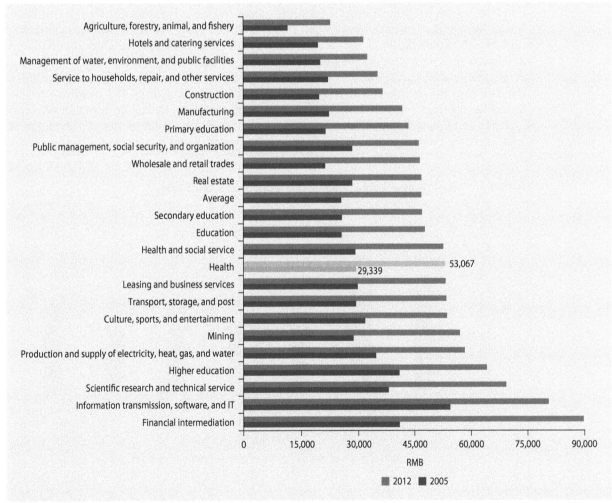

Source: NHDRC 2014a.

revenue that hospitals receive from the services they provide (such as admissions and medical procedures); commissions for prescribing drugs and ordering tests; informal payments from patients (hongbao, or "red envelopes"); and private practice ("moonlighting") (Woodhead 2014; Yip and others 2010). In responding to these perverse incentives, physicians generate demand for their services and overprescribe diagnostic tests and expensive branded drugs.

Compensation levels also differ widely across levels of care. Earnings in public hospitals—especially urban public hospitals—are higher than in PHC facilities and in rural areas (figure 7.7). The average compensation in urban public hospitals is 1.6 times the sector average. Staff working in PHC institutions and THCs earn 76 percent and 72 percent, respectively, of the health sector average. The differentials across cadres of health workers are smaller than what their different education requirements would suggest. For example, doctors earn on average 1.1 to 1.96 times more than nurses.

Large earnings differences between hospitals and PHC settings are incompatible with the government's reform strategy of strengthening PHC. Low compensation, combined with other factors, makes it difficult to recruit and retain good, well-qualified health workers to work in PHC settings.

Additionally, medical schools reportedly face difficulties in attracting students who achieve high scores on the national university entrance exam (gao kao). Instead, they often attract those whose first career choice was not medicine (Hou and others 2014; Waldmeir 2013). A 2013 survey of students with the highest national exam scores from 1977 through 2012 revealed that less than 2 percent chose to major in health or medicine; in contrast, 38 percent chose economics or business management.[5]

Moreover, university recruitment of medical students dropped significantly in 2014. For example, Southern Medical University planned to enroll 200 students but had only 50 applicants. Guangdong Traditional Chinese Medical University planned to enroll 1,807 but had only 485 applicants. The Chinese Medical Doctor Association's regular survey of physicians includes the question, "Would you like your children to go to

FIGURE 7.7   Health worker compensation across levels of care, China 2013

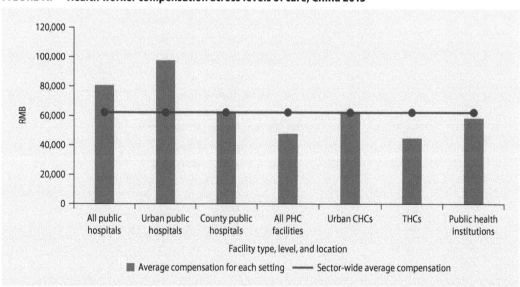

Source: NHDRC 2014a.
Note: CHC = community health center; PHC = primary health care; THC = township health center. "PHC facilities" refers to urban CHCs and rural THCs. "Public health institutions" refers to centers for disease control and hygiene inspection stations.

TABLE 7.2 Share of Chinese doctors who hope their children will attend medical school, 2002–11
Percentage of respondents

Survey year	Yes	No
2002	10.9	54.0
2004	10.4	63.0
2009	11.9	62.5
2011	6.8	78.0

Source: National surveys of the Chinese Medical Doctor Association, http://www.cmdae.org.
Note: Survey question: "Would you like your children to go to medical school"?

medical school?" The percentage of negative responses has been above 50 percent and increasing (table 7.2).

The public perception of medical practice has been deteriorating, and the recent surge of violence against health professionals (experienced by a third of doctors, as further discussed in chapter 5) is also making medical professions progressively less attractive.[6]

Restrictive Headcount Quota System

The policy framework for managing the health workforce follows the governance structure in place for all public service units (PSUs), which is centered on the headcount quota system.[7] The headcount quota system defines the total number of personnel assigned to a PSU; it is a special human resources management arrangement for civil servants and public institutions. The quota framework is formulated by the government's Post Establishment Office (PEO). PSUs must have a quota approved by the PEO, which is also the basis on which the Bureau of Human Resources and Social Security (and not the health facility manager) establishes posts. Quota-based employees have permanent jobs with pensions and other social security benefits, and it is difficult for health facility managers to fire them.

Staffing quotas for public hospitals are based on the number of beds. The national guideline sets the bed-staff quota at 1 to 1.3–1.4 for hospitals with fewer than 300 beds; 1 to 1.4–1.5 for hospitals with 300–500 beds; and 1 to 1.6–1.7 for hospitals with

more than 500 beds (see annex 7A, table 7A.5).[8] For THCs, staff quotas are, in principle, 1 percent of the total population in the THC catchment area; the actual number is calculated considering the ease of transport to the THC and the fiscal capacity of the local government. The current quota in a survey of 12 counties in six provinces covering the east, central, and west regions is 1.2 per 1,000 population. The quota standard for CHCs is two to three GPs and one public health specialist per 10,000 residents, as well as a GP-nurse ratio requirement of 1 to 1.

Many issues related to quotas have been reported from across the country. The quota system has not kept pace with the needs to improve health service provision and to constantly adapt to growing demand and changing technology. For example, headcount standards for various hospitals, including maternity and child care hospitals, were formulated in the 1980s and never updated. Headcount standards no longer meet the changing needs of health facilities.

The result is significant quota shortages in almost all health facilities regardless of level or location. Facilities have to hire additional health workers who are not on quota. A recent survey of health facilities in 10 provinces by the Health Human Resources Development Center (under the Ministry of Health) and Shandong University found that 15 percent of the employees in CHCs, 11 percent in maternity and child care institutions, and 8 percent in THCs are not quota-based. For example, PHC facilities in Yunnan province had to hire so many temporary (nonquota) health workers that, in 2013, 31 percent of all their health workers (13,502 of 43,595) were not on quota.

Hospitals must pay their salaries and benefits out of their own revenues. This adds pressure on hospitals to generate extra revenue and creates a "second class" of employees with different contracts and compensation systems but often undertaking the same roles and tasks. It is broadly reported that nonquota staff are paid less and get fewer benefits; for example, they do not receive a pension.

Limited Mobility and Market Entry

Two processes—qualification certification and practice licensing—govern entry into health service provision by physicians and by assistant physicians, nurses, pharmacists, and rural village doctors in China.[9] Health professionals who meet the eligibility requirements can take the annual national qualification examination, and those who pass the examination obtain a qualification certificate as a physician, nurse, or pharmacist. (There is no national exam for village doctors.) Those who obtain the certificate can then apply for a practice license from the local health authority, which grants permission to practice.

The recertification process has some limitations. Current regulations specify that nurses need to update their licenses every two years and that licensed doctors need to attend inservice training every two years, though doctors face no specific requirement regarding recertification. Several quality assurance initiatives are in place. For example, the Chinese Medical Doctor Association has created a program of reevaluation examinations for physician qualification and requires physicians to take it every two years. The NHFPC's Science and Education Department, in charge of inservice training, has issued a policy requiring physicians to take training that earns them a certain number of points. However, these quality assurance measures are not linked with the relicensing process, and therefore health professionals do not always comply, limiting the impact of the measures.

Current labor regulations compound the limiting effects of the quota system on the mobility of health workers. Under Chinese law, a medical practitioner's license to practice must specify the medical facility where the professional will work; the category (such as clinical medicine, traditional Chinese medicine, dentistry, or public health); and the specialty. The licensing regulation allows health professionals to practice only in the facility specified in the license. This strongly restricts the mobility of doctors, most of whom are employees of public hospitals, and adds to the difficulties that PHCs and private hospitals face in recruiting qualified health workers.

To address this constraint, the government launched the pilot Physician Dual Practice Policy in 2009 (further discussed in box 7.1). This new policy allows a physician to register to practice in up to three hospitals or clinics in the same city if the physician (a) obtains the agreement of the first facility; (b) obtains approval from the local health administration authority; and (c) signs a legal agreement with all health facilities where he or she works regarding malpractice disputes and litigation.[10]

Although the government expanded the pilot in 2011, the policy has not achieved its intended results. By June 2011, only 166 doctors had registered for multiple practices. In Guangdong province (the initial pilot site), about 100 physicians had registered. Three reasons explain the low participation rate:

- Public hospitals are overloaded, so their physicians do not have time to work elsewhere as well.
- The policy requires physicians themselves to bear the risk in case of a medical accident or dispute.
- The current quota-based human resource management system links physicians' pensions, employment benefits, professional title, and access to research and training opportunities directly to the hospital where they work, and physicians fear that dual practice might affect their performance evaluation and opportunities for promotion and clinical research and training at their primary hospital of affiliation.

Lack of Managerial and Decision-Making Autonomy in Hiring Health Workers

Since 2006, all technical professionals, managerial staff, and logistics support staff in health facilities have been hired through an open recruitment system. A March 2000 policy directive directed PSUs to reform their personnel systems, abolish tenure status for management and professional technical staff, and hire health workers to fill posts through open recruitment.[11] Health institutions established an employment relationship with employees

BOX 7.1   History of the Physician Dual Practice Policy in China

"Moonlighting" by physicians emerged significantly in the 1990s in China, without any regulations or policies to assure service quality and safety. In 1999, the Law for Licensed Doctors of the People's Republic of China went into effect, stipulating that a physician may work at only the one site specified by his or her license to practice medicine. This law controlled moonlighting by physicians but also greatly restricted their mobility and significantly affected the ability of private sector and PHC facilities to recruit qualified doctors, most of whom were employed at public hospitals.

Fully aware of this negative effect, the government took steps to counter it. The first Physician Dual Practice Policy was promulgated in September 2009 to start a pilot in selected areas that allowed physicians to register to practice in more than one hospital or clinic on the condition that the physician (a) obtain the agreement of the first facility; (b) obtain approval from the local health administration authority; (c) sign a legal agreement regarding malpractice disputes and litigation with each health facility where the physician works; and (d) have the title of associate chief physician or higher.

In July 2011, the Ministry of Health issued a new policy that (a) expanded the pilot to more prefectures, and (b) changed the minimum professional title from associate chief physician (senior level) to attending doctor (middle level).[a]

In November 2014, six ministries and agencies jointly issued a new policy directive to further promote dual practice. This has opened dual practice to clinical, dental, and traditional Chinese medicine doctors with a middle-level professional title (or above) who have worked in their specialty for more than five years. In addition, physicians no longer need written approval from the first facility or approval from the local authority. The policy also emphasizes that hospitals should not discriminate against dual-practice physicians in professional title, promotion, or access to clinical research opportunities.

Provinces have formulated local policies based on national guidelines. For example, Guangdong province's dual-practice policy does not limit the number of facilities where a physician can practice, though it specifies a certain area such as a county or city. Physicians do not need approval from their primary hospital but need only file an application at the local health bureau when they apply for a license. Since the issuance of this new, more favorable policy, some public hospital physicians reportedly have opened independent clinics.

Nationwide, the number of physicians applying for dual practice has increased only slightly. The most important reason is that employment benefits are determined by the headcount quota and are attached to the health facility to which the physician belongs. The quota system is the root cause of restrictions on physicians' mobility.

a. "Notification on Expanding Pilot of Physicians' Dual Practice," Ministry of Health (2011, No. 95).

through contracts that specify the responsibilities, rights, and benefits of both parties.

The major problem associated with recruiting health workers is health facilities' lack of autonomy. Within the public service, the government defines the number, structure, and responsibility of all posts in all three major categories: technical, managerial, and logistics. The Ministry of Human Resources and Social Security (MoHRSS) and local Bureau of Human Resources and Social Security (BoHRSS) set and manage the posts in PSUs and are responsible for policy development and guidance, macro control, supervision, and final clearance. Once the

local quota establishment office and the finance bureau have defined the staffing quota of each public facility (including the number for each major category such as GPs and nurses), the facility's human resources department, guided by the BoHRSS, formulates the post-setting plan and submits it to the BoHRSS for approval.

Under current practice, the local government defines quotas and, in some cases, limits the issuance of new quotas. Thus, health facilities may not be able to hire the new staff they need. Additionally, "open recruitment" is managed by the local BoHRSS rather than by the health facility. The standardized qualification examinations, recruitment procedures, and evaluation standards formulated by the BoHRSS are also often unsuited to the health sector's special characteristics. For example, the examination questions and evaluation standards do not reflect the functions and skills of PHC workers and GPs, putting them at a disadvantage and sometimes making it impossible to hire them. Moreover, a minimum education of three years of college is required, whereas most THC staff only have training equivalent to secondary school. And the requirement of at least three applicants for each position is difficult to meet for THC positions.

This post management system creates rigidity in the management of the health workforce. First, the widely reported quota shortages imply shortages of official posts in health facilities. The shortages affect PHC facilities more than hospitals because PHC facilities rely more on government funding. Second, it restricts the highest-level post and the number of posts at PHC facilities—which constrains the career prospects of PHC health professionals. Third, health facilities lack autonomy to define what and how many posts they would need to meet the service needs of their local communities. Any changes to the approved post-setting plan need approval from the BoHRSS.

There have been some recent movements to reform human resource management policies in China. In February 2014, the State Council issued a new policy directive, "Personnel Management Regulations for Public Service Units," and formally launched the Post Management System in Public Institutions.[12] The new regulations state that public institutions should set posts according to duties, tasks, and needs, following relevant national regulations. Each post should have a specific title, clearly defined responsibilities, evaluation standards, and qualification criteria. One goal of this reform is to shift from identity-based (headcount quota) to post-based human resources management. Under the new policy, the government defines the category and grade of posts, and then the health facility is responsible for recruitment, evaluation, salary setting, and training for the posts.

Professional Title Evaluation

Professional titles are designed to represent the technical capacity of professional health workers. There are three levels of professional title for physicians in China: at the junior level are resident doctors, at the middle level are attending doctors, and at the senior level are associate chief physicians and chief physicians. Advancement of professional title is an important component of career development; it is linked to salary and often to pension and other benefits.

China's evaluation system for professional titles was established in 1955. For junior-level and middle-level health professionals, there is a national syllabus, and a national technical qualification examination is held at a fixed time once a year across the country with national evaluation criteria. Evaluation for senior-level titles consists of an exam and individual assessment at the provincial level. The provincial evaluation committee is set up by the provincial health and human resources bureaus.

The professional title evaluation system has three major issues: it overemphasizes publication; it does not reflect differences across positions, specialties, and levels of health care providers; and professional associations have only limited involvement.

In 2015, the MoHRSS and NHFPC jointly issued an executive order providing guidelines for improving the professional title evaluation for the PHC workforce.[13] This policy order aims to build a professional title evaluation system that corresponds to the features of medical professionals. Following the policies of differentiated functions and the tiered care system, the requirements for dissertation writing and foreign languages were softened as reference rather than compulsory conditions. The policy order places more emphasis on clinical skills and requires each province to make context-specific implementation plans to improve the professional title evaluation system.

Recommendations for Human Resources Reform

An adequate, well-functioning health workforce is critical to implement and maintain the PCIC model. Human resources for health are a key component of health systems and play a central role in delivering quality care at affordable prices to the population. Issues related to availability, distribution, and performance of health workers pose big challenges, and the extant literature is rich in country experiences with different ways of addressing these concerns.

This section outlines a set of recommendations to address the current health workforce challenges in China and the changes needed to implement PCIC. The recommendations are based on a review of international experience in strengthening the health workforce to implement or expand PHC as well as of China's ongoing initiatives to reform its health workforce. The review sought to understand how selected countries and regions have adapted their health workforces

in the course of implementing a PHC model of service delivery and to identify lessons that could be applied in the Chinese context.

The international review covered Australia; Brazil; Canada; Norway; Taiwan, China; Turkey; and the United Kingdom. Each has made significant efforts to expand PHC coverage and to change how their health workforces are educated, deployed, managed, and regulated in support of the expansion.

The four core action areas and corresponding implementation strategies include the following (table 7.3):

1. Build a strong enabling environment for PHC workforce development to implement PCIC.
2. Improve workforce composition and competency for PHC service delivery.

TABLE 7.3   Four core action areas and implementation strategies to strengthen the health workforce

Core action areas	Implementation strategies
1. Strong enabling environment for development of PHC workforce to implement PCIC	Establish general practice as a specialty, with equivalent status to other medical specialties. Introduce a gatekeeping mechanism to direct patients to primary care providers as first point of contact, and mandate this arrangement once the PCIC system is well established. Introduce career development prospects to develop and incentivize PHC workforce, including separate career pathways for GPs, nurses, mid-level workers, and community health workers. Raise compensation of PHC workers commensurate with other prestige specialties to increase recruitment, retention, and motivation.
2. Balanced workforce composition and competency for PHC service delivery	Scale up the standardized training for resident doctors and GPs. Accelerate ongoing successful efforts to increase supply of GPs and nurses. Reform the curriculum to upgrade medical training and build new skills and competencies required for PCIC. Improve on-the-job training to strengthen competency of current workforce and build new PHC competencies. Set up alternative cadres of health workers (such as clinical assistants, assistant doctors, clinical officers, and community health workers) to strengthen PHC delivery.
3. Compensation system with strong incentives for good performance	Increase basic wages of health workers, linking the exact level of increase to general labor market trends in China to keep the health profession attractive. Increase the percentage of basic salary vis-à-vis performance bonuses in physicians' total income package. Increase the subsidy, and introduce or increase nonfinancial incentives, for health workers in rural and remote areas. Revise the system of incentives by linking income with performance assessment built on comprehensive performance indicators rather than revenue generation.
4. Headcount quota system reform to enable a more flexible health labor market and efficient health workforce management	Give managers autonomy in human resources issues, including post-based recruitment, salaries, deployment, evaluation, and training. Delink physicians' licenses to practice from the facilities of employment. Delink health workers' employment benefits from the quota as well as from health facilities. Work toward abolishing the headcount quota system.

Note: GP = general practitioner; PCIC = people-centered integrated care; PHC = primary health care.

3. Reform the compensation system to provide strong incentives for good performance.
4. Reform the headcount quota system to enable a more flexible health labor market and efficient health workforce management.

International experience shows that large-scale, rapid maintenance or expansion of PHC coverage is possible if there is political commitment and adequate investment. Increasing the availability and accessibility of PHC personnel is a priority, but it is equally important to ensure that health workers produce high-quality and responsive services. This requires that health workers acquire a professional culture in which evaluation and self-assessment are regarded as powerful tools to improve quality. This acculturation process starts during basic professional education and is maintained throughout a career, ensuring continuing professional development. Table 7.4 summarizes the main characteristics of the health systems of some of the countries covered by the review.

Core Action Area 1: Strong Enabling Environment for the Development of PHC Workforce

Strategy 1: Establish general practice as a specialty with status equivalent to other medical specialties

It is imperative to improve the status of PHC to address the challenges in the PHC workforce. It is important to build consensus among government, health providers, and the general public that PHC is as important as hospitals and that the facilities at different levels of the system simply have different roles and functions in providing a continuum of care to citizens.

Strategy 2: Direct patients to PHC providers as the first point of contact

A consensus about the importance of PHC implies a change in the service delivery model to ensure that PHC is the patient's first point of contact with the health system. Such a change would play a key role in the coordination and integration of services to implement PCIC. A gatekeeping mechanism could be introduced to ensure that patients are first directed to PHC providers, and this arrangement could be mandated once the PCIC system is well established.

Strategy 3: Introduce career development prospects to develop and incentivize the PHC workforce

PHC-specific career paths need to be introduced for GPs, nurses, mid-level workers, and community health workers to better develop and incentivize the PHC workforce. General practice must be established as a specialty with equivalent status to other medical specialties and with the same strong attributes of well-regulated standards of practice. China's current pilots of separate accreditation for rural assistant physicians and of a separate professional title-promotion system for PHC are good examples; these should be evaluated and scaled up across the country.

Strategy 4: Raise compensation of PHC workers to be commensurate with that of other prestige specialties

China has significantly increased its government funding of PHC through its subsidy for a package of essential public health services, but raising the compensation of PHC workers to the level of other specialties would require significant additional funding. The government could consider directing its annual incremental health financing toward PHC. Most countries include high coverage of preventive and PHC services in their health insurance benefit package, usually with a fixed copayment or 80 percent reimbursement rate.

China is revising its health insurance policies to expand coverage of outpatient and PHC services, financing the expansion with part of the annual increase in the insurance premium and government subsidy. (In 2015, the per capita subsidy rose from RMB 320 to RMB 380 and the individual contribution rose from RMB 90 to RMB 120.) This would incentivize the use of outpatient services at

TABLE 7.4 Health system characteristics in selected countries

Country	Health system	Dominant mode of PHC provision	Dominant mode of specialist services provision	Gatekeeping by GPs or PHC	GPs' compensation compared with specialists'
Australia	Tax-financed universal health insurance supplemented by a small, compulsory, tax-based health insurance levy	Private group practices	Private group practices, public hospitals, or private hospitals	Yes: GP referral required for the specialist to get reimbursed	Lower
Brazil	Tax-based health system with supplementary private health insurance; decentralized, with states, and municipalities having autonomy for service delivery	Public health centers	Private hospitals	Yes	Higher
Canada	Universal health system providing tax-financed hospital and physician services for all residents; highly decentralized with provinces and territories responsible for planning and delivering health services as well as providing three-fourths of total health financing	Private group practices or private solo practices	Public hospitals or private group practices	Yes	20 percent lower on average
Turkey	Social health insurance schemes	Private group practices or solo units	Public hospitals or private hospitals	Yes	Close
United Kingdom	Highly centralized, tax-financed national health service	Private group practices	Public hospitals	Yes	Close

Note: GP = general practitioner; PHC = primary health care.

the PHC level, reduce reliance on hospitals, and increase financing for PHC facilities.

Core Action Area 2: Balanced Workforce Composition and Competency for PHC Service Delivery

Implementing people-centered health care in China requires rebalancing the workforce and induction of PHC workers with the needed skills and competencies. The skill mix and scope of practice will need to be reviewed, and education programs will be needed to strengthen health workers' cultural and psychosocial competencies, communication skills, and capacity to work in multidisciplinary teams and to support patients in managing their health better. Quality assurance mechanisms such as accreditation of programs and educational institutions and certification of health professionals will need to be implemented or strengthened.

Strategy 1: Set up alternative cadres of health workers to strengthen PHC delivery

One trend across many countries is that of introducing cadres of nonclinician physicians, clinical assistants, assistant doctors, and clinical officers to help expand access to basic PHC services. International experience shows that these cadres can be as efficient and cost-effective as traditional cadres in delivering health services within the limits of their training when they work in supportive, supervised, multidisciplinary teams.

Community health workers (CHWs), sometimes hired from local communities, have been widely used to provide outreach and preventive services. Brazil, for instance, made CHWs a key part of its PHC service delivery model (Johnson and others 2013). Its health sector reform focused on PHC expansion, rapidly deploying its Family Health Strategy (FHS) and Community Health Agents Program (Programa de Agentes Comunitários de Saude [PACS]). The FHS uses multiprofessional health teams composed of a physician, nurse, nurse assistant, and four to six CHWs. PACS became important after the reorganization of health service delivery around the FHS.

The community health agents are recruited from the neighborhoods where they are deployed, trained for three months, and employed by municipal health authorities. They are responsible for a wide range of PHC services: chronic disease management, triage, child development, and public health (screening, immunizations, and so forth). Wherever the FHS is not fully implemented, PACS is a transition model. Brazil has 234,767 community health agents in rural and urban peripheral areas around the country (Johnson and others 2013).

In 15 years (1998–2013), Brazil raised the number of its family health teams 6.9-fold and the population covered 7.8-fold to reach more than 60 percent of the total population (figure 7.8). Registration with a FHS care team is determined by whether a person lives within the FHS team catchment area, not by individual choice. In heavily populated areas, there may be more than one FHS team per health facility; each team is assigned a specific territory and list of families to serve. FHS expansion proceeded unevenly across Brazil; coverage is higher in small municipalities than in large ones, but it now reaches more than 90 percent of Brazil's 5,565 municipalities (Gragnolati, Lindelow, and Couttolenc 2013).

China may like to explore the possibility of producing and integrating alternative cadres of health workers, especially CHWs. The village doctors, for instance, could play a similar role if they could be better integrated into the system and provided with improved training, compensation, and supervision.

Strategy 2: Accelerate successful efforts to increase supply of GPs and nurses

Another trend across several high-income countries (Australia, Canada, Germany, the Netherlands, and the United Kingdom) is that of delivering team-based PHC through the inclusion of more nurse practitioners, registered nurses, and other health staff to work alongside physicians (Freund and others 2015). Australia, Canada, and the United Kingdom have added incentives

FIGURE 7.8   **Community health agents' coverage in Brazil's Family Health Strategy, 1998–2014**

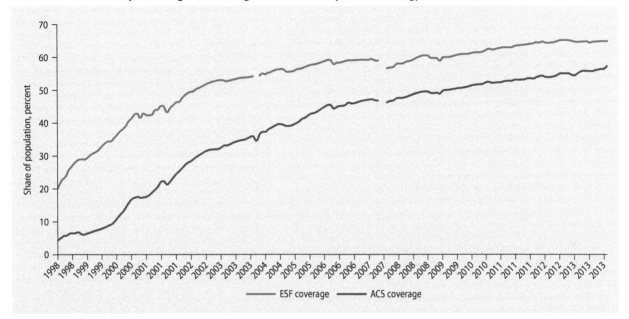

Source: DATASUS database, Brazil Ministry of Health, http://datasus.saude.gov.br/.
Note: Gaps indicate missing or unavailable data. ACS = community health agent (agente comunitário de saúde); ESF = Family Health Strategy (Estratégia de Saúde da Família).

in their GP reimbursement schemes to employ nurses to deliver PHC services. Most high-income countries give greater recognition to family medicine and nursing, and most have many family physicians.

In the United Kingdom, strategies to improve the accessibility and quality of PHC services have included expanding nurses' scope of practice. Its National Health Service Plan of 2000 introduced "new working practices" as a major step toward advanced-level nursing practices. Debate on expanding the functions of nurses went on for more than a decade, and in April 2012 a new law came into effect allowing the more than 20,000 nurses who have undertaken a specialist degree-level course and hold a separate registered qualification to prescribe from the same list of medicines as doctors within their specialty and competence. The Health and Social Care Act of 2012 promotes integrated, personalized, and proactive care by better coordinating the National Health Service's (NHS) hospital- and community-based health services, including PHC and social care.

Furthermore, GPs in the United Kingdom increasingly work in multipartner practices. A typical practice team consists of 5–6 GPs, 1 nurse practitioner, 2–3 nurses, and 6–10 administrative staff (Roland, Guthrie, and Thomé 2012). Teams may also include district nurses, health visitors, midwives, community psychiatric nurses, and allied health professionals and social workers. The patient's first point of contact is usually a practice of self-employed GPs because the NHS requires people to register with a GP or a GP practice. GP practices are responsible for referring patients to specialist services in hospitals or to community-based professionals. Financial incentives are offered to GPs based on 75 quality-of-care indicators, many of which relate to the care of patients with chronic conditions (Roland, Guthrie, and Thomé 2012). There is no restriction on public-private multiple practice, though consultants (as specialists are known) must inform employers of their private practice commitments and obtain NHS authorization to use NHS facilities or staff for private purposes.

Canada has increased its federal and provincial public investments in PHC since 2003. To increase the number of multi-disciplinary teams providing primary care, provinces committed to providing at least 50 percent of their population with 24/7 access to multidisciplinary PHC teams by 2011. Each province designed its own model. Progress has been slow and unequal across provinces, although nurse practitioners have become better integrated into the primary care sector (Freund and others 2015). An estimated three-quarters of Canada's family physicians now work within multiprofessional practices (Marchildon 2013).

Worldwide, numerous policies have been adopted to improve the geographical distribution of physicians and nurses. Recruitment and retention of qualified health workers to work in rural and deprived areas is a challenge even for high-income countries such as Canada and the United States. Financial incentives—increased salaries and benefits—have been used with some success, but they are recognized as only part of the solution to attract and retain health workers in rural and remote areas. Examples of efforts to address geographical disparities in health care include the following:

- *In Brazil,* the challenge of scaling up access to medical services in rural and remote regions remains daunting. Practice in Brazil's urban areas remains more attractive, partly because multiple jobs (highly prevalent in Brazil) are only possible in urban areas, where private insurance and care delivery schemes coexist with Brazil's publicly funded health system (Sistema Único de Saúde) and offer attractive complementary income opportunities.
- *In Taiwan, China,* a recently developed, detailed strategy includes mobile clinics and communication technologies to provide access to quality services in remote regions.
- *In Turkey,* a compulsory service law was reintroduced in 2005 to address persistent shortages of hospital specialists and GPs in certain regions. It requires recent graduates from public medical schools to practice in the public health sector for one to two years, and recent graduates from medical specialty training to serve two to four years

depending on regional socioeconomic characteristics. Failure to complete mandatory service can result in prohibition on practicing medicine in Turkey (Aran and Rokx 2014). The effect on retention of professionals after completion of the compulsory service is not known.

Strategy 3: Scale up standardized training for resident doctors and GPs

Because health workers from rural backgrounds are more likely to practice in rural areas after completing their studies, one strategy is to decentralize professional schools, especially in remote and rural areas, and to recruit local students, as has been done in the far north of Norway. In another approach, Taiwan, China, has developed programs in offshore islands. And many Chinese provinces have implemented special targeted training programs to recruit and train medical students to work in PHC and rural areas. In 2015, for example, Jiangxi province started recruiting 200 high school graduates each year for three years to receive three-year college degrees in clinical medicine with no tuition fees. The provincial government provides a financial subsidy (RMB 5,000 per year) to the trainees. After graduation, these students will work as public health specialists in rural THCs.

From a practical perspective, policy solutions may need to differentiate according to local context and provide special modalities for rural deprived areas. For example, China's current "5+3"-year standard training (five years of medical university training followed by three years of resident training) for GPs and other physicians would not be viable for rural THCs in deprived areas because doctors who are qualified at this level will quickly move to cities and work in urban hospitals. A "3+2"-year training model might be more realistic for recruiting and retaining health workers for THCs (three years of college-degree medical school training followed by two years of resident training).

An approach called "integrated human resource management" has been used in some provinces of China, such as Shaanxi, to recruit and retain qualified health professionals for rural THCs that cannot recruit certified (assistant) physicians. This approach allows the county hospitals to recruit doctors as county hospital employees and rotate them to work in THCs or village clinics.

Strategy 4: Improve on-the-job training to strengthen and build PHC competencies of current workforce

Health professional education and training should be reformed to improve the competencies of the current workforce and build new PHC competencies. Measures for this purpose would include the following:

- Introducing new education concentrations for new types of cadres such as clinician assistants and CHWs
- Reforming medical and nursing curricula toward PCH competencies such as communication skills and patient-centered services (Hou and others 2014)
- Revising clinical training to include more exposure to community-level and primary care and to encourage multidisciplinary team work
- Developing cohorts of trainers who can support the development of new competencies and scaling-up of standardized resident training for GPs and other physicians
- Linking in-service training with recertification of health professionals

Strategy 5: Reform the curriculum to upgrade medical training and build new skills required for PCIC

All countries have used curriculum reforms and continuing education to equip professionals with PHC competencies. In Brazil, new recruits must do induction training in PHC; in Turkey, all must undergo special training when family medicine centers and community centers are established.

Core Action Area 3: Compensation System Reform to Provide Strong Incentives for Good Performance

Strategy 1: Increase the share of basic salary relative to performance bonuses in health workers' total income packages

In general, the official pay of health workers in China is not attractive, in particular at the grassroots level and in the rural areas. The health workers' income relies heavily on the revenues they can generate for the hospital as reflected in their salary structure. On average, the basic salary accounted for an average of 23 percent of total compensation, allowances for 20 percent, and performance for 57 percent.[14]

The structure is even more skewed in urban hospitals. An NHFPC national salary survey (implemented by the National Health Development Research Center) in secondary and tertiary urban hospitals found that for health workers in public hospitals, basic salary accounts for only 13–14 percent of the total salary; allowances and subsidies for 14 percent; and performance-based pay and bonuses, which are linked to hospital service income, for 74 percent.

Although a combination of fixed payment with variable performance-based payments is desirable, China may like to revise its compensation system to reduce reliance on service revenue-based bonuses and to increase base salary and hardship allowances. On average, this percentage is below 30 percent—far below the international norm of more than 50 percent.

Strategy 2: Increase basic wages in line with labor market trends to keep health profession attractive

Raising PHC workers' compensation to levels similar to those in other prestigious specialties would make a PHC career more attractive and competitive. Almost all countries where PHC is a priority have significantly improved PHC workers' compensation.

In countries with strong PHC, as in Canada and the United Kingdom, GPs tend to earn more than specialists (reflecting their more comprehensive role). Increasing GPs' relative earnings also affects the medium- and long-term supply of GPs. Countries such as Brazil, Turkey, and the United Kingdom have removed or reversed the differential between compensation of hospital specialists and PHC doctors (figure 7.9). In China, the differential remains large.

FIGURE 7.9   Ratio of hospital specialist pay to primary GP pay, selected countries and years

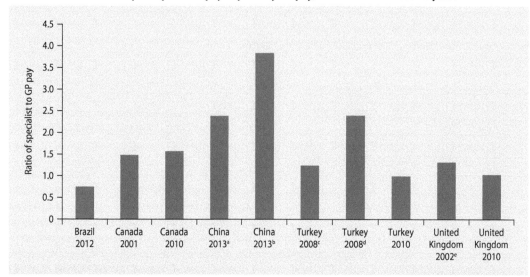

Sources: McPake and others 2015.
Note: GP = general practitioner.
a. "China 2013ᵃ" compares public hospital in an average and primary health institution.
b. "China 2013ᵇ" compares national-level hospital "professional and technical posts" with primary health institution "health institutional in-service staff."
c. "Turkey 2008ᶜ" shows the relative pay of hospital specialist to primary GP (within the country's Family Medicine Program).
d. "Turkey 2008ᵈ" shows the relative pay of hospital specialist to primary GP (outside the family medicine program), better reflecting the historical divergence (that is, before the 2005 launch of the country's Family Medicine Program, which assigns each Turkish citizen to a state-employed family physician).
e. "United Kingdom 2002ᵉ" data are from DH (2010): consultant (specialist) net earnings are as estimated from graph, p. 23.

The size of the increase needs to be linked to general labor market trends in China. Figure 7.10 shows how different categories of health workers are paid relative to their country's income distribution. These data are not directly comparable because they are not disaggregated by type of health professional. However, they show health workers' place within the income distribution of several countries, as follows:

- *In the United Kingdom,* the 10 percent of population at the top of the income distribution has an average per capita annual income of US$111,252. A hospital consultant (specialist) earns US$164,345, approximately 1.5 times the average income of the highest income decile.
- *In Brazil,* family physicians are paid 4.5 times the average income of the highest income decile.
- *In Turkey and the United Kingdom,* doctors in general earn around the average income level of the top decile.

- *In Canada,* family physicians earn twice as much.
- *In Canada and the United Kingdom,* nurses earn about 50 percent of those levels, placing them between the fourth and fifth quintiles of their populations' average per capita income.

As for China, pay is significantly worse for workers in the country's PHC institutions, who earn less than 30 percent of the top decile's average income—putting them a little above the population's average income (between the third and fourth quartiles of the per capita income distribution). However, hospital workers overall earn 1 to 1.5 times the top decile's average income.

Strategy 3: Revise the incentive system by linking income to comprehensive performance assessment rather than revenue generation
Countries like Australia, Canada, and the United Kingdom include incentives within

FIGURE 7.10   Ratio of health professionals' pay to average income per capita of 10th richest decile, China and selected countries

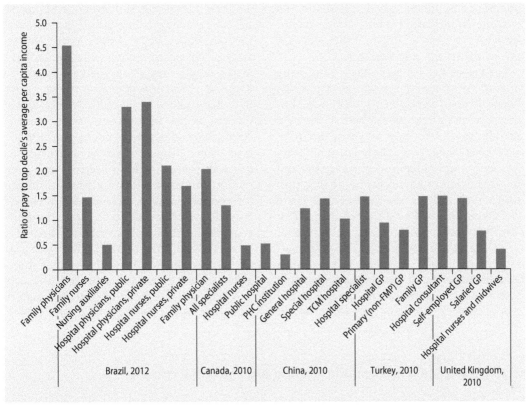

Source: World Bank data.
Note: FMP = Family Medical Program (Turkey); GP = general practitioner; PHC = primary health care; TCM = traditional Chinese medicine.

reimbursement schemes for GPs to encourage them to employ nurses to deliver primary care. Another trend seen in many European countries is that of contracting GPs as entrepreneurs, with remuneration topped up through various pay-for-performance incentives (Kringos and others 2013). This has resulted in a surge of practices run as partnerships of several physicians or by private companies.

Similar experiments are being carried out in Australia where, because of inherent weaknesses in the fee-for-service payment scheme for GPs, the government introduced a Practice Incentive Payment program in 1998. This pay-for-performance scheme provides incentives around three areas: quality of care, capacity strengthening, and support in rural areas. The quality-of-care component provides incentive payments for diabetes care,

cervical screening, asthma care, and indigenous health (Cashin and others 2014).

In China, the comprehensive compensation reforms in Sanming prefecture of Fujian province offer a successful example (box 7.2).

In recent years, remuneration systems have become quite complex globally, especially as countries experiment with innovative payment methods to find new ways of incentivizing health workers. As a result of this continuous trial process, countries typically adopt a combination of payment methods, including salary, fee-for-service, capitation, performance bonuses, and so on.

For example, in countries where the compensation method was primarily fee-for-service, elements such as salaries (Canada), capitation fees (Belgium and France), performance (France), and integrated fees (Belgium and Denmark) are being introduced as additional payments. In countries where GPs were traditionally salaried, capitation and fee-for-service are being added (Finland and Sweden). To increase efficiency and quality of services, the United Kingdom introduced a pay-for-performance scheme (box 7.3).

Fee-for-service payment has traditionally been the predominant mode of remuneration for most physicians in Canada, but alternate remuneration methods have been introduced over the past 10 years. In 2013, the largest category of physician remuneration was a mixed method of payment, and the proportion of physicians being paid predominantly by fee-for-service fell from 51 percent in 2004 to 38 percent in 2013. Family physicians have a higher rate of blended payments (46 percent) than specialists (37 percent).[15] Blended payments in Canada have been associated with some positive effects on preventive care, collaboration, and recruitment and retention in

provinces with low population density (Wranik and Durier-Copp 2010).

At the same time, the new payment methods are raising costs and putting pressures on the financial capacity of the country's health system. Physician incomes in Canada have increased substantially in the past decade (to four and a half times that of an average salary in Canada), aided by the collective bargaining model that has put pressure on provinces to continually increase compensation. Public support has guided the relative strength of the different parties in the collective bargaining process in Canada over the years (Ontario, for example, has been able to freeze remuneration for doctors due to the shift in public support), but doctors have generally been able to successfully negotiate higher wages at times when the public felt that doctor shortages created long waiting times.

There is also a trend of general practices being run as partnerships of several GPs or

---

BOX 7.2   Sanming's comprehensive public hospital compensation reform

In 2013, Sanming prefecture (Fujian province) introduced comprehensive public hospital compensation reform with three major components:

- *New governance structure:* Hospital directors are directly appointed and paid by the government. They are given management autonomy over daily operations. The government assesses hospital directors' performance according to the extent to which the hospital has achieved annual performance targets and tasks set by the government.
- *New criteria for hospital salary budgets:* The government ended reliance on revenue generated from lab tests, physical exams, and drug sales (fully implementing a zero-markup policy on drug sales). It now defines the total amount of funds that can be used for salary for each of the 22 hospitals in the prefecture, using three determining criteria:
  - The hospital's labor-based medical service revenue, excluding income from lab tests, physical exams, and medical supplies

- Salary weights that reflect the capacity of different types of hospitals to generate labor-based service income
- The director's performance assessment results.
- *Salaries comprising a basic allowance plus performance incentives:* The salary of each hospital staff member consists of the following:
  - Basic allowance defined by technical grade, seniority, and managerial position
  - Payment for services provided, such as number of outpatient services performed and number of inpatients discharged—the workload being adjusted considering the service complexity as defined by diagnosis-related groups
  - Awards or sanctions based on patient satisfaction rates, malpractice, additional working hours, and emergency medical aid.

Source: Ying 2014.

BOX 7.3   GP pay-for-performance incentives in the United Kingdom

The United Kingdom comprehensively reformed the remuneration of general practitioners (GPs) in 2004. Contracts and payments went from being independent GP-based to practice-based and from largely capitation-based to a significant proportion of pay-for-performance (Doran and Roland 2010; Kroneman and others 2013). The main objectives of the reform were to improve the quality of care; help recruit and retain GPs; improve GPs' job satisfaction, pay, and working conditions; improve the unequal distribution of personnel; and increase primary health care (PHC) productivity (Doran and Roland 2010).

Before the reform, GP contracts included a basic allowance (with a gradient by seniority) supplemented by allowances based on the number and characteristics of patients on the GP's list. The reform introduced a pay-for-performance component for quality requirements that are outlined in the Quality and Outcomes Framework (QOF). The QOF has four domains:

- *Clinical standards,* emphasizing noncommunicable diseases such as cancer and hypertension
- *Organizational standards,* including information, communication, patient education, and so forth
- *Additional services standards,* such as cervical screening, child health, maternity and contraceptive services)
- *Patient experience standards.*

QOF revenues were expected to increase practice revenue by 15–20 percent. The key components of the new contract were payments for essential services (global sum), enhanced services, out-of-hours care, and the QOF (Boyle 2011).

GP incomes rose 58 percent between 2002–03 (before the reform) and 2005–06 (after the reform), and they are now closer to the incomes of hospital specialists, especially for nonsalaried partners in general practice. In addition, the number of GPs (particularly salaried GPs) increased in line with population growth, and vacancy rates fell (Doran and Roland 2010). The number of nurses employed in primary care also increased as a result of the pay-for-performance incentive linked with chronic disease management. (The use of nurses has been associated with increased quality of care in chronic disease management [Freund and others 2015].) Performance against the QOF's quality indicators improved in the first three years (Doran and Roland 2010).

One potential perverse incentive was that care for nonincentivized diseases and activities might be neglected, and the evidence on this has been mixed. There remain concerns that quantifiable aspects of care may be prioritized over nonquantifiable aspects, that external incentives may replace internal motivation, and that the incentives might undermine professionalism (Doran and Roland 2010). The United Kingdom started a scheme in 2008 in which an element of GP pay was based on patient satisfaction surveys, but this proved problematic and was withdrawn in 2011 (Roland, Guthrie, and Thomé 2012).

---

by private providers. Table 7.5 provides an overview of how primary care and specialist care are organized in selected countries, and how physicians are paid.

Strategy 3: Increase the subsidy, and introduce or increase nonfinancial incentives, for health workers in rural and remote areas
China will also need nonfinancial incentives to attract and retain PHC workers, especially in rural and remote areas. International experiences suggest that financial incentives alone often cannot provide sufficient motivation, and nonfinancial incentives can help meet the needs and expectations of health professionals.

Commonly used options include housing, job opportunities for spouses, education allowances for children, and opportunities for further training (such as in-service training and scholarships for postgraduate studies).

Changes in health workforce compensation also require changes in the approach to setting compensation in China, which can vary from a rigid bureaucratic process to a more flexible and negotiated process between employers and employees. The former approach often requires executive and legislative action to change compensation practices. The latter approach depends on the extent to which employers are required to bargain with

TABLE 7.5   **Physician payment and predominant service provision mode, selected countries**

Country	Primary care physician payment	Outpatient specialist payment	Inpatient specialist payment	Predominant mode of primary care provision	Predominant mode of specialist services provision
Australia	FFS	FFS	Salary	Private group practices	Private group practices or public hospitals
Brazil	Salary	Salary	Salary	Public health centers	Private hospitals
Canada	FFS	FFS	FFS	Private group practices or private solo practices	Public hospitals or private group practices
Turkey	Capitation	PFP and salary	PFP and salary	Private group or solo units	Public hospitals
United Kingdom	Salary, capitation, FFS	Salary	Salary	Private group practices	Public hospitals

Sources: McPake and others 2015; Paris, Devaux, and Wei 2010.
Note: FFS = fee-for-service; PFP = pay for performance.

unions, the availability of arbitration procedures to solve disputes, and whether workers have the right to strike as part of the compensation-setting process (Gregory and Borland 1999).

The structure of unions and employers' organizations influences the degree of collectivization in the compensation-setting process; these organizations can be defined by geographical scope or by the type of workers (nurses, doctors, and so forth) or activities that they cover. Trade unions and professional associations are recognized actors for representing health workers, and agreements usually cover the entire health workforce in specific occupations or sectors, regardless of membership status (Buchan, Kumar, and Schoenstein 2014).

Buchan, Kumar, and Schoenstein (2014) reviewed wage-setting mechanisms for hospital staff in eight OECD countries (Canada, France, Germany, New Zealand, the Netherlands, Norway, Portugal, and the United Kingdom). Their study looked at three features of wage setting (table 7.6):

- *Collective bargaining:* the extent to which wages are determined collectively, normally in agreement with professional associations and trade unions
- *Centralization:* the level or levels at which wages are set, as an indicator of the extent to which the wage-setting process is centralized or localized

- *Coordination:* the extent to which wage setting is coordinated across sectors or companies, the level of national government involvement, and the frequency of wage setting.

The impetus to change the approach to wage setting can come from a range of factors. In OECD countries, labor market concerns (such as shortages or a geographic maldistribution of health workers) have spurred overall pay increases or called into question the responsiveness of a national standardized approach to varied and localized shortages in occupations, geographic regions, or specialties. High-cost central urban areas as well as remote rural areas are often identified as meriting "more" than the national average pay rates to offset recruitment and retention challenges; and certain specialties that are relatively difficult to recruit to may also be identified as "deserving" above-standard rates of pay.

Other pressures have included pay equity issues, particularly given the high numbers of women workers in nonmedical professions; structural changes in pay systems (for example, to increase flexibility or to delink pay in the health sector from pay in the broader public sector or service); attempts to improve organizational productivity and the quality of care; and improving the international competitiveness of pay.

TABLE 7.6   Characteristics of compensation setting for hospital staff, selected OECD countries

Type of characteristic	Findings

Collective bargaining (collectivization)	• All countries recognize trade unions and professional associations as representing the hospital workforce.
	  – The level of union membership (coverage) varies significantly across countries, but collective agreements normally cover all the workforce in designated occupations or sectors, irrespective of their membership status.
	• In all countries, employers are involved directly in negotiating and achieving collective agreements.
	  – In Canada, New Zealand, the Netherlands, Norway, and the United Kingdom, employers are represented in national wage setting by some type of employers' association that has a specialist wage-setting capacity.

Centralization of wage setting	• Most countries have a core national or sectorwide model.
	  – In France, New Zealand, the Netherlands, Norway, Portugal, and the United Kingdom, the primary focus is at the national level, either across the whole health sector or in subsectors or specialties within health.
	• Although national agreements are at the heart of policy, France, Norway, and the United Kingdom (to an extent) provide scope for "top-up" wage setting at the local level.
	  – New Zealand also has some separate regional or local collective agreements, which are in part a legacy of a previous decentralized wage-setting model.
	• Of the eight countries, Canada has the greatest focus at the province level.
	• Germany has a mixed pattern between national and regional approaches as well as a trend toward fragmented wage setting.

Coordination and government involvement	• All countries reported some degree of coordination of wage setting across the health or hospital sector.
	  – Coordination is based on national health sector (or subsector) collective frameworks (France, the Netherlands, Norway, Portugal, and the United Kingdom), or occurs at the province level (Canada) or across central and local governments (Germany).
	• Cross-sectoral coordination within the broader public sector was reported in some countries (for example, New Zealand).
	• Norway uses a broader cross-sectoral coordinated approach based on "front runner" industries setting the benchmark for wage setting.
	• Reflecting the high level of public provision, most countries reported direct or indirect government involvement in wage setting.
	  – In Portugal and the United Kingdom, the government is the main funder or employer of the hospital workforce.
	• France, Portugal, and the United Kingdom have an annual wage-setting cycle; Norway has a biannual process; in the other countries, the wage-setting cycle varies between 18 months and 3 years.

Source: Buchan, Kumar, and Schoenstein 2014.
Note: OECD = Organisation for Economic Co-operation and Development. Eight OECD countries were studied: Canada, France, Germany, New Zealand, the Netherlands, Norway, Portugal, and the United Kingdom.

Core Action Area 4: Headcount Quota System Reform for a More Flexible Health Labor Market and Efficient Health Workforce Management

The headcount quota system leads to inefficiencies in the management of the Chinese health workforce and needs to be improved to be consistent with broad health sector reform trends including increasing hospital autonomy, increasing health labor market mobility, and performance- or results-based

financing policy. As noted earlier in this chapter, the Chinese government is aware of this issue and is taking action to reform the system. The reform would require at least four sets of related actions.

Strategy 1: Give managers autonomy on human resources issues

First, health facility managers would need to be given the necessary autonomy on human resources issues and be left to manage their staffs on the basis of the post rather than quota. This approach would end differences between workers with and without a quota post.

Each health worker would have a standardized labor contract with the health facility that would describe the responsibilities, scope, and accountability of the post. The government would continue to define the categories and grades of common posts but would grant health facility managers the autonomy to decide their workforce composition in term of posts, grades, technical qualifications, and professional titles.

Health facility managers would be responsible for post-based recruitment, post-based deployment, post-based evaluation, post-based salary setting, and post-based training. They would be able to fire a worker who fails to perform according to the contract. In turn, managers would be evaluated by the government and held accountable for the performance of their staff and that of the health facility.

Many OECD countries practice *centralized wage setting* simultaneously with *decentralized recruitment*. Fourteen OECD countries set medical staff remuneration in public hospitals at a national or subnational level while giving responsibility to hospital managers for recruitment (Buchan, Kumar, and Schoenstein 2014). In five countries (Greece,

Ireland, Israel, Italy, and Spain), central or subnational governments are responsible for recruitment of staff for public hospitals. In Australia and Portugal, recruitment is done by public hospitals but requires approval from the central or subnational government (Buchan 2015).

As for wage setting, in more than half (19) of the OECD member countries, salaried medical staff negotiate work contracts directly with the public hospital. This pattern probably reflects specific administrative arrangements unique to these countries and need not imply that salaries are set by public hospitals themselves. However, it is worth noting that the three countries with hospital autonomy over pay levels (Poland, Sweden, and the United States) also have contracts at the hospital level (Buchan 2015).

Table 7.7 provides an overview of responsibility for hospital recruitment and remuneration in the same five countries reviewed for comparison throughout this chapter.

Strategy 2: Delink physicians' licenses to practice from the facility of employment

To increase the mobility of health workers, China may wish to consider delinking a physician's license to practice from the facility of employment. The country's 2009 Physician

TABLE 7.7   Hospital staff recruitment and remuneration in five countries

Country	Recruitment of medical staff	Remuneration level of medical staff	Recruitment of other health professionals	Remuneration level of other health professionals
Australia	Hospital managers have complete autonomy	Hospital managers have autonomy within state-level negotiated pay scales	Hospital managers have complete autonomy	Hospital managers have autonomy within state-level negotiated pay scales
Brazil	Decentralized, with state and municipal governments having autonomy	Decentralized, with state and municipal governments having autonomy	Decentralized, with state and municipal governments having autonomy	Decentralized, with state and municipal governments having autonomy
Canada	Hospitals must negotiate with local authorities	Pay scale set or negotiated at national level	Central or subnational government decides	Pay scale set or negotiated at national level
Turkey	Central or subnational government decides	Pay scale set or negotiated at national level	Central or subnational government decides	Pay scale set or negotiated at national level
United Kingdom	Hospital managers have complete autonomy	Pay scale set or negotiated at national level	Hospital managers have complete autonomy	Pay scale set or negotiated at national level

Sources: McPake and others 2015; Paris, Devaux, and Wei 2010.

Dual Practice Policy has already paved the way for this transition. For example, Guangdong province no longer limits the number of facilities where physicians can work as long as they can reach agreement with each facility. Physicians are only required to file a record with the local health bureau to indicate the health facilities where they work. However, this is not the practice for the whole country, and in Guangdong it only applies to physicians at the middle level and above.

Although multiple practice can increase mobility and retention, it can negatively affect the quantity and quality of care provided in the public sector. Especially among physicians, the higher earnings and better working conditions associated with private practice (as in Brazil) can make it difficult to retain workers in the public sector. Many countries that allow multiple practice also have a problem with doctors channeling patients from the public facility to their private practice instead. Turkey passed a law in 2010 prohibiting multiple practice for all doctors (except university-based doctors, who can engage in multiple practice provided they fully meet their daily commitments in the public sector) and raising public sector salaries.

Some countries prohibit dual practice (whereby doctors combine part-time private practice with a public sector job), while others regulate or restrict it with different intensities and regulatory instruments. Ultimately, the success of each approach depends on the institutional context, resources, and the government's ability to enforce regulations.

Strategy 3: Delink health workers' benefits from the quota and from health facilities

China might also consider delinking the employment benefits of health workers from the quota as well as from health facilities, a process that has already started with the delinking of pensions as part of recent reforms. This would relieve an important constraint on mobility in China's health sector. Currently, as noted earlier, the employment benefits associated with a post are determined by the headcount quota and attached to the health facility.

As also noted earlier, if a health worker leaves the facility, he or she loses all associated employment benefits, including his or her pension. Ending the quota system and delinking benefits from the health facility where individuals are employed, thus making the benefits portable, would remove a large penalty for mobility. The government has already started pension reforms to link pensions with PSUs so that the workers outside of the headcount quota could qualify for the employment pension pooling scheme.

Strategy 4: Work toward abolishing the headcount quota system

Reforming and eventually abolishing the headcount quota system is a critical step to enable efficient health workforce management and for doctors to evolve from being "hospital property" to becoming independent practitioners. Abolishing the headcount quota system would require complementary reforms as preconditions or building blocks—reforms in the pension system, the post-management system, the professional-title-promotion system, the government's fiscal inputs, and the management of opportunities for clinical research and in-service training. Such reforms take time to implement well, though many local pilots have begun. A platform would need to be established to replace the PSU in performing some of the human resource management roles.

Professional associations could take on many of these roles. In many countries, they play important roles in governance. Their most common function is to set standards and assure quality through accreditation and certification. They also are well positioned to manage professional title promotion and continuing education. In many countries, professional associations represent their members in developing legislation and compensation-setting processes as well as in advocacy for patients' rights.

However, these roles may conflict with broader health system or social objectives— as happened, for example, in Canada when professional associations pressed the government to increase compensation by more than the consumer price index, or in Brazil, when the medical association blocked reforms to expand nurses' scope of practice. As China considers a more engaged role for professional associations in the governance of its health workforce, it should also be aware of potential negative impacts.

An Implementation Road Map

The core action areas and associated strategies address the main elements of the health workforce: production, recruitment, deployment, management and regulation, performance evaluation, and compensation. Implementing these strategies would entail both short- and long-term steps. Some need immediate action because they set the stage for others. Others, like improving quality, will take longer to implement.

Several principles are useful to keep in mind in implementing human resource policy reforms:

- The scale of the human resources challenges and the vital importance of overcoming this bottleneck require high-level attention and commitment. Human resources for health should be on the agenda of groups leading the health system reform and be an integral part of the overall health reform action plan.
- Human resources issues are at the root of the challenges faced by health care reform in China. They are interwoven with reforms in other areas and cannot be dealt with as if they are separate. For example, reforms in financing and payment systems are preconditions for changing the compensation system of health professionals. Salary increases will need increased funding for personnel costs. The coherence and full alignment of reform policies in a comprehensive package of reforms is critically important for success.
- There is no "one size fits all" solution. Policy designs as well as reform implementation will need to adjust and adapt to local contexts. Rural and urban regions may need different reform models at different times because their needs in relation to the health workforce differ; policy solutions will need to be matched to the needs in different situations in the country.
- The transformation of a health workforce takes time. Good sequencing and coordination of actions will contribute to successful reform outcomes. Implementation will require a long-term vision plus an implementation pathway defining short-, medium-, and longer-term action plans.

Table 7.8 summarizes the specific actions, designates the responsible agencies to lead implementation, and notes the complementary measures that may be necessary to support implementation and maintenance of the human resource reform actions and desired outcomes.

TABLE 7.8 Road map for implementation of health workforce reforms

Recommendation (core action area)	Short-term actions	Medium-term actions	Responsible agencies	Complementary reforms needed
1: Build a strong enabling environment for the development of the PHC workforce to implement PCIC	• Establish independent system of professional titles and career development prospects for PHC workforce (particularly for GPs) • Introduce PHC-specific career development paths to develop and incentivize PHC workforce • Include separate career pathways for GPs, nurses, mid-level workers, and CHWs.	• Establish general practice as a specialty (family medicine) with equivalent status to other medical specialties • Enhance compensation system (monetary and nonmonetary) for PHC workforce relative to other specialties to make PHC careers more attractive and competitive	• State Council • MoF • MoHRSS • NHFPC	• Ensure full functioning of PHC by putting in place a gatekeeping mechanism to ensure PHC is the patient's first point of contact • Shift health care financing toward PHC • Revise health insurance policy to expand coverage for PHC • Target government incremental health sector funding to PHC
2a: Improve workforce composition (skill mix) for PHC service delivery	• Continue to expand training for GPs and nurses • (Re)train village doctors (to upgrade their scope of practice) • Develop specific policy package of qualification and promotion for rural PHC workforce to improve recruitment and retention of PHC workers • Adopt regulatory measures to mandate rural or PHC service (for example, in return for training, requiring a period of service after training is completed) • Target recruitment of students from rural areas to increase recruitment to rural and remote settings • Integrate recruitment: county hospitals recruit doctors as county hospital employees and rotate them to work in THCs or village clinics	• Produce and integrate new and alternative cadres of health workers, such as clinical assistants, assistant doctors, clinical officers, and CHWs • Increase salary for specialties in shortage, such as pediatricians and psychiatrists, to attract medical students	• NHFPC • MoHRSS	• Raise status of the PHC workforce (see Recommendation 1) • Introduce payment mechanisms that incentivize the use of multidisciplinary teams • Establish medical alliances among hospitals and PHC facilities that enable rotation of health workers within an alliance

(Table continued next page)

TABLE 7.8 Road map for implementation of health workforce reforms *Continued*

Recommendation (core action area)	Short-term actions	Medium-term actions	Responsible agencies	Complementary reforms needed
2b: Improve workforce competencies for PHC service delivery	• Scale up standardized training for resident doctors and GPs • Reform curriculum to upgrade medical training to add PCIC skills and competencies (such as communication skills) and education and training for multidisciplinary team practice • Improve current in-service training to improve competency in current workforce and to build new PHC competencies • Link in-service training requirements with relicensing and re-certification	• In vocational training schools and medical universities, introduce new medical education programs and courses for new workforce types such as clinical assistants, assistant doctors, clinical officers, and CHWs	• MoE • NHFPC • MoHRSS	• Introduce quality assurance mechanism for health professionals' education through accreditation of training schools
3: Reform compensation system to provide strong incentives for good performance	• Increase basic compensation of health workers to change current incentive structure (based on quantity of services) • Increase subsidy for rural and remote area health workers • Introduce or increase nonfinancial incentives (such as housing) to attract and retain health workers in rural and remote areas	• Rationalize compensation structure (increase percentage of basic salary relative to performance bonuses)	• State Council (including MoHRSS, MoF, NHFPC, NDRC)	• Adjust pricing schemes to increase charges for labor-based services, such as doctor consultations, surgeries, and nursing services • Increase percentage of hospital expenses allocated for personnel costs to bring China's average (below 30 percent) closer to international practice (50 percent) • Integrate fragmented financing, especially financing for PHC, to increase leverage for payment and purchasing • Reform payment system to link payment with improved quality of services rather than with revenue generation • Reform payment system to incentivize new PCIC service delivery approach

(Table continued next page)

TABLE 7.8 Road map for implementation of health workforce reforms *Continued*

Recommendation (core action area)	Short-term actions	Medium-term actions	Responsible agencies	Complementary reforms needed
4: Reform headcount quota system to enable a more flexible health labor market and efficient health workforce management	• Grant autonomy to health facility managers on HR management (including post setting, recruitment, deployment, performance evaluation) by moving from quota-based to post-based management • Apply realistic recruitment policies for recruiting health workers for rural PHC centers • Delink the practice license from a specific health facility, to increase mobility of health workers • Establish performance evaluation system to increase accountability of health facility managers • Define an appropriate regulatory policy for health worker multiple practice	• Delink health workers' employment benefits from the quota and from health facilities through pension reform • At urban and rural county level, gradually reform quota system to transform the physician from "hospital property" to "individual practitioner" • Enhance the function and roles of professional associations	• State Council (including MoHRSS, MoF, NHFPC)	• Change the way the government provides its subsidy to health facilities—moving away from paying for a fixed headcount of health workers to paying for tasks and performance, or link the subsidy to per capita demand-side financing • Reform government pension system to delink the pension from PSUs and merge it with social pension pooling schemes • Institute other complementary reforms to delink practitioners from the quota system, including professional title promotion, opportunity for clinical research, and continuous training—establishing a platform to replace the PSU in performing some HR management roles • Define the private sector's role in provision and financing of health services (to define best policy related to health worker multiple practice)

Note: CHW = community health worker; GP = general practitioner; HR = human resources; MoE = Ministry of Education; MoF = Ministry of Finance; MoHRSS = Ministry of Human Resources and Social Security; NDRC = National Development and Reform Commission; NHFPC = National Health and Family Planning Commission; PCIC = people-centered integrated care; PHC = primary health care; PSU = public service unit.

Annex 7A   Supplementary Tables

TABLE 7A.1   China's health workforce: Classifications, numbers, and percentages of total, 2012

Primary classification	Secondary classification	Tertiary classification	Description
Health professional 6,675,549 73.2%	n.a.	n.a.	Includes licensed physician; registered nurse; pharmacist and assistant pharmacist; medical laboratory technician and inspector; medical imaging technician; health supervisor; intern doctor (including pharmaceutical intern, student nurse, and intern technician); and other health professionals. Health professionals working in management (hospital director and associate director, party secretary, and so on) are not included. This group of health personnel usually receives higher medical education.
n.a.	Physician 2,616,064 28.7%	n.a.	Includes licensed physicians and assistant licensed physicians.
n.a.	n.a.	Licensed physician 2,138,836 23.5%	Includes staff whose title is "licensed physician" on their certificates as medical practitioners and who work in medicine, prevention, and health care; excludes those working in management. This group has a bachelor's degree or higher, majoring in medicine, from a college or university. There are four categories of licensed physicians: clinical, traditional Chinese medicine, stomatology, and public health.
n.a.	n.a.	Assistant licensed physician 477,228 5.2%	Includes staff whose title is "assistant licensed physician" on their certificates as medical practitioners and who work in medicine, prevention, and health care; excludes those working in management. They graduate from colleges, universities, or junior colleges with a medical vocational degree. Assistant licensed physicians can be divided into four categories: clinical, traditional Chinese medicine, stomatology, and public health.
n.a.	Registered nurse 2,496,599 27.4%	n.a.	Includes health professionals registered as practicing nurses and with a Practicing Nurse Certificate, engaging in nursing according to the statutory nursing regulation: "to protect life, relieve patients' pain and improve health."
n.a.	Pharmacist, including assistant pharmacist 377,398 4.1%	n.a.	Includes professionals responsible for providing knowledge of drugs and pharmaceutical services: chief pharmacist, associate chief pharmacist, pharmacist-in-charge, pharmacist, and assistant pharmacist. Apothecary is not included.
n.a.	Lab technician 249,255 2.7%	n.a.	Includes medical laboratory technicians and medical imaging technicians: chief technician, associate chief technician, technician-in-charge, and technician.
Village doctor 1,094,419 12%	n.a.	n.a.	Originally called "barefoot doctor"; includes people working in village clinics who have a Village Doctor certificate. Those who work in village clinics without the certificate are called "health workers."
Other technician 319,117 3.5%	n.a.	n.a.	Includes nonhealth personnel who engage in repairing medical equipment, health education, scientific research, teaching, and other technical work.

(Table continued next page)

TABLE 7A.1   China's health workforce: Classifications, numbers, and percentages of total, 2012 *Continued*

Primary classification	Secondary classification	Tertiary classification	Description
Manager *372,997* *4.1%*	n.a.	n.a.	Includes staff in charge of health care management, disease control, health supervision, medical research and teaching, and so on, especially those engaged in administration.
Supportive worker *653,623* *7.2%*	n.a.	n.a.	Includes skilled or unskilled staff engaged in operation, maintenance, logistic support, and so on. Skilled workers include inspector, toll collector, registrar, and so on. Excludes two kinds of staff: (a) those classified as "other technicians" (laboratory technician, technician, and research assistant), and (b) those classified as "managers" (finance person, accountant, and statistician.

Note: n.a. = not applicable.

TABLE 7A.2   Urban and rural distribution of China's health workforce, 2003 and 2013

Classification	2003			2013		
	Urban	Rural	Ratio	Urban	Rural	Ratio
Total health workers	3,515,780	1,759,006	2.00	4,488,500	5,291,983	0.85
All health professionals	2,828,419	1,478,052	1.91	3,680,276	3,520,302	1.05
Certified physicians and assistant physicians	1,216,003	651,954	1.87	1,360,118	1,434,636	0.95
Certified physicians	1,026,607	459,422	2.23	1,261,432	1,024,362	1.23
Certified nurses	928,367	337,592	2.75	1,603,913	1,179,208	1.36
Per 1,000 population						
Health workers	4.88	2.26	2.16	9.18	3.64	2.52
Certified physicians and assistant physicians	2.13	1.04	2.05	3.39	1.48	2.29
Certified nurses	1.59	0.50	3.18	4.00	1.22	3.28

Sources: NHFPC 2004, 2014.

TABLE 7A.3   Average salaries in China, by occupational category, 2005–12
Nominal RMB

Occupation	2005	2006	2007	2008	2009	2010	2011	2012	2012 rank
Agriculture, forestry, animal husbandry, fishery	8,207	9,269	10,847	12,560	14,356	16,717	19,469	22,687	19
Mining	20,449	24,125	28,185	34,233	38,038	44,196	52,230	56,946	5
Manufacturing	15,934	18,225	21,144	24,404	26,810	30,916	36,665	41,650	14
Utilities	24,750	28,424	33,470	38,515	41,869	47,309	52,723	58,202	4
Construction	14,112	16,164	18,482	21,223	24,161	27,529	32,103	36,483	15
Transport, warehouse, postal services	20,911	24,111	27,903	32,041	35,315	40,466	47,078	53,391	7
Information technology	38,799	43,435	47,700	54,906	58,154	64,436	70,918	80,510	2
Wholesale and retail	15,256	17,960	21,074	25,818	29,139	33,635	40,654	46,340	12

(Table continued next page)

TABLE 7A.3   Average salaries in China, by occupational category, 2005–12   *Continued*
Nominal RMB

Occupation	2005	2006	2007	2008	2009	2010	2011	2012	2012 rank
Lodging and restaurants	13,876	15,236	17,046	19,321	20,860	23,382	27,486	31,267	18
Finance	29,229	35,495	44,011	53,897	60,398	70,146	81,109	89,743	1
Real estate	20,253	22,238	26,085	30,118	32,242	35,870	42,837	46,764	11
Rental and leasing	21,233	24,510	27,807	32,915	35,494	39,566	46,976	53,162	8
Science and technology service	27,155	31,644	38,432	45,512	50,143	56,376	64,252	69,254	3
Irrigation, environment, and public facilities management	14,322	15,630	18,383	21,103	23,159	25,544	28,868	32,343	17
Community services	15,747	18,030	20,370	22,858	25,172	28,206	33,169	35,135	16
Education	18,259	20,918	25,908	29,831	34,543	38,968	43,194	47,734	10
Health and social protection	20,808	23,590	27,892	32,185	35,662	40,232	46,206	52,564	9
Culture, sports, and entertainment	22,670	25,847	30,430	34,158	37,755	41,428	47,878	53,558	6
Public administration and social organization	20,234	22,546	27,731	32,296	35,326	38,242	42,062	46,074	13
Total	18,200	20,856	24,721	28,898	32,244	36,539	41,799	46,769	n.a.

Source: China Labor Statistics Yearbook, 2006–13.
Note: n.a. = not applicable.

TABLE 7A.4 Governance framework for health human resources management in China

| Subject | Task or area | Law or regulation | Governing bodies | | | | | Major issues or challenges |
			Central govt.	Local govt.	Public service unit	Professional association	Health institute (hospital or clinic)	
Medical education and training	College or university medical education	n.a.	MoE, in consultation with NHFPC	n.a.	n.a.	n.a.	n.a.	Mismatch between educational investments and labor market demand
	Postgraduate training; resident doctor or GP standardized training	Guidelines for Standardized GP Training, NHFPC, 1999	NHFPC	n.a.	n.a.	n.a.	n.a.	None
	In-service training	Guideline and Planning for GP In-Service Training, NHFPC, 1999 In-Service Training Requirement for THC Health Professionals, NHFPC, 2004 In-Service Training Requirements for Village Doctors, NHFPC, 2004	NHFPC	n.a.	n.a.	Develop training courses and curricula	n.a.	None

(Table continued next page)

TABLE 7A.4 Governance framework for health human resources management in China *Continued*

Subject	Task or area	Law or regulation	Governing bodies					Major issues or challenges
			Central govt.	Local govt.	Public service unit	Professional association	Health institute (hospital or clinic)	
Entry	Establishing qualification standards, qualification examinations, and certification practice licensing	Physicians: Chinese Law of Licensing Medical Practice, 1999	NHFPC formulates exam procedures	Licensing: health authority at county and higher levels	National Medical Exam Center implements the national exam	n.a.	n.a.	Standardized qualification exam does not differentiate across positions, specialties, and levels of health care providers
		Nurse Management, MoH, 1993 Nurse Regulations, State Council, 2008	Market entry, NHFPC	Licensing: health authority at county and higher levels	n.a.	n.a.	n.a.	Pharmacist market entry qualifications not standardized because of different management agency
		Guideline on Qualification of Pharmacist and National Qualification Exam, MoHRSS and SFDA, 1999	MoHRSS and SFDA	Licensing: FDA at city and higher levels	n.a.	n.a.	n.a.	
		Village Doctor Management Regulation, State Council	NHFPC formulates management rules	Licensing is with county health bureau	n.a.	n.a.	n.a.	
Quota	n.a.	Guideline on Quota-Setting Standards for General Hospitals, 1978 Guideline on Quota-Setting Standards for Traditional Chinese Medicine Hospitals, 1986 Guideline on Quota-Setting Standards for MHC Institutions, 1986 Guideline on Quota-Setting Standards for Urban Community Health Centers, 2006 Guideline on Quota-Setting Standards for Township Health Centers, 2011 Guideline on Quota-Setting Standards for CDCs, 2014	Central post establishment office, MoF, and NHFPC jointly set standard for headcount quota	Each province, prefecture, and county sets local standards in compliance with national standards	n.a.	n.a.	n.a.	Quota standards cannot keep pace with changing health service needs or progress in positions and functions of health professionals Huge differences in pay and benefits for health professionals with and without quota

(Table continued next page)

TABLE 7A.4 Governance framework for health human resources management in China *Continued*

Subject	Task or area	Law or regulation	Central govt.	Local govt.	Public service unit	Professional association	Health institute (hospital or clinic)	Major issues or challenges
					Governing bodies			
Post management	n.a.	Guideline on Post-Setting Management in Health Service Institutes and Facilities, Ministry of Personnel and MoH, 2007	MoHRSS and MoH formulate guidelines on post-setting management in health service institutes and facilities	Local HR and health bureaus set number and structure of posts for every public health institution	n.a.	n.a.	Health institutes and facilities have no autonomy on post setting	Health facilities have no autonomy on post setting Limited promotion space for PHC health workers
Recruitment	Open competitive recruitment	Guideline on Deepening HR Management Reform in Health-Service Units, Central Party HR Ministry, Ministry of Personnel, MoF, and MoH, 2000	The national level formulates the guideline and recruitment procedures	Local HR bureau implements required recruitment	n.a.	n.a.	Some institutes participate in the process, some do not	Health facilities have no autonomy in recruitment Rigid recruitment procedures
Professional title evaluation	Professional title setting and professional title evaluation	Guideline on Strengthening Health Professional Titles Evaluation, Ministry of Personnel and MoH, 2000	MoHRSS and NHFPC formulate management procedures HR central of NHFPC organizes the national exam for middle– and junior-level professional titles	Provincial bureau of HR responsible for setting evaluation procedure for high-level professional titles; health bureaus implement	n.a.	n.a.	In provinces that separate professional title evaluation and recruitment, health facilities have autonomy over recruiting In provinces that integrate professional title evaluation and recruitment, health facilities have no autonomy to recruit	Professional title evaluation allows limited space for career development for PHC workers

(Table continued next page)

TABLE 7A.4 Governance framework for health human resources management in China *Continued*

Subject	Task or area	Law or regulation	Central govt.	Local govt.	Public service unit	Professional association	Health institute (hospital or clinic)	Major issues or challenges
				Governing bodies				
Performance evaluation	Includes government evaluation of health facilities and health facility evaluation of staff	Guideline on Implementing Performance-Based Evaluation in Health Service Institutions, 2010 Implementation Plan of Performance-Based Evaluation in Community Health Centers, 2011 Guideline on Implementing Performance-Based Evaluation in Township Health Centers and Village Clinics, 2011 Guideline on Implementing Performance-Based Evaluation in County Maternal and Child-Health Institutions, 2010 Guideline on Implementing Performance-Based Evaluation in Emergency Rooms, 2010 Guideline on Implementing Performance Based Evaluation in Health Promotion Institutions, 2011	NHFPC formulates the implementation plan for performance evaluation management	Local health bureau formulates local plan accordingly	n.a.	n.a.	Health facilities formulate own implementation plans	Assessment indicator system needs improvement Third-party evaluation system yet to be established HMIS system yet to be incorporated to support monitoring and evaluation Feedback and use of evaluation results need enhancement to incentivize performance

(Table continued next page)

TABLE 7A.4 Governance framework for health human resources management in China *Continued*

Subject	Task or area	Law or regulation	Governing bodies					Major issues or challenges
			Central govt.	Local govt.	Public service unit	Professional association	Health institute (hospital or clinic)	
Compensation	n.a.	Guideline on Internal Income Distribution, Reform of Health Service Institutes and Facilities, MoH, 2002 Guideline on Implementing Internal Income Distribution, Reform Action Plan of Health Service Institutes and Facilities, Ministry of Personnel, MoF, and MoH, 2006 Guideline on Implementing Performance-Based Salary in Public Health Institutes and Primary Health Care Facilities, Ministry of Personnel, MoF, and MoH, 2009	MoHRSS formulates wage standards for public institutions, including public hospitals	Local bureau of HR formulates local implementation plan based on central guideline and sets the total wage ceiling for each public institution	n.a.	n.a.	n.a.	Fixed wage level cannot provide incentives for good performance Salary structure needs adjustment; a large portion is from revenue-based bonus Wage gaps too narrow between different positions; disparity significant between rural and urban income

Note: CDCs = centers for disease control and prevention; FDA = State Food and Drug Administration; GP = general practitioner; HMIS = health management information system; HR = human resources; MCH = maternal and child care institution; MoE = Ministry of Education; MoF = Ministry of Finance; MoH = Ministry of Health; NHFPC = National Health and Family Planning Commission; PHC = primary health care; SFDA = State Food and Drug Administration; THC = township health center.

TABLE 7A.5 Headcount quota formulation standards for Chinese health institutions

Scope of application	Issue date	Policy directives	Standards
Urban general hospitals, university teaching hospitals, county hospitals, county specialty hospitals, and outpatient clinics	1978	Draft Principles on Organization and Quota System of General Hospitals (trial)	The state estimates staff quotas for public hospitals according to the number of beds. In accordance with national requirements, hospitals with fewer than 300 beds are calculated to have a staff-bed ratio of 1 to 1.3–1.4; those with 300–500 beds, 1 to 1.4–1.5; and those with more than 500 beds, 1 to 1.6–1.7. Of the total staff, administrative management are 8–10 percent; support workers are 20 percent; and health care technical personnel are 70–72 percent. Among the latter, doctors and TCM doctors account for 25 percent; nursing staff, 50 percent; pharmacy staff, 8 percent; inspection staff, 4.6 percent; radiation inspection personnel, 4.4 percent; and other staff, 8 percent.
Traditional Chinese medicine hospitals	1986	Formulation Standards on Organizational Structure and Manning Quota of National Traditional Chinese Medicine Hospitals (trial)	The bed-staff ratio is 1 to 1.3–1.7. Management personnel, other technical staff, and workers account for 28–30 percent, of whom management personnel are 6–8 percent and other technical staff are, 2 percent. Medical technical staff should account for 70–72 percent of the total. TCM personnel should be more than 70 percent of all medical staff.
Township health centers	2011	Guidance on Quota Formulation Standards for Township Health Centers	In principle, the number of staff is equivalent to 1 percent of the total target population; the actual number is set according to population, traffic conditions, and financial capacity. Professional and technical personnel account for not less than 90 percent of the total quota, and public health personnel for not less than 25 percent of professional and technical staff. The priority is to ensure the number of GPs. Management work, if possible, should be done by medical staff, and managerial positions should be set according to the actual situation.
Community health centers	2006	Guidance on Quota Formulation Standards for Community Health Centers	Community health service centers are staffed with two to three GPs and one public health physician per 10,000 residents; TCM practitioners are provided in each community health service center within the total staff quota. The GP–nurse quota should be 1 to 1, and other personnel should be no more than 5 percent of the total. The actual quota can be set according to the tasks, responsibilities, population served, service radius, and other factors. Centers serving a population of 50,000 residents or more can reduce the standards appropriately in setting the quota.
Centers for disease control and prevention	2014	Guidance on Quota Formulation Standards for Centers for Disease Control and Prevention	The staff quota for CDCs, based on the unit of provinces (autonomous regions and municipalities), is allocated in accordance with their control, classification of approval, and coordination roles. In principle, the proportion is 1.75 persons per 10,000 residents; provinces (autonomous regions and municipalities) of more than 500,000 square kilometers with population density fewer than 25 persons per square kilometer can set the proportion at up to 3 persons per 10,000 residents. The provincial-level CDCs exercise overall control and arrangements and dynamic adjustment of staff quotas. In the personnel structure, professional and technical personnel account for not less than 85 percent of the total, and health technical personnel for not less than 70 percent. Comprehensive management work should be done, if possible, by the professional and technical personnel, and logistics services will be gradually socialized.

(Table continued next page)

TABLE 7A.5   **Headcount quota formulation standards for Chinese health institutions**   *Continued*

Scope of application	Issue date	Policy directives	Standards
Sanitation inspection institutions	2010	Advice on Implementing Supervising Responsibilities and Strengthening Food Safety and Sanitary Inspection	In accordance with the principle of consistent responsibilities, accountability, and appropriate personnel to perform duties and safeguard work implementation, and considering the factors of population, workload, service scope, and economic level, 1–1.5 health supervisors should be allocated per area with 10,000 residents.
Maternal and child care stations	1986	Quota Standards for Maternal and Child Care Stations (trial)	The staff quota in MCH institutions at or above the county level should be set at 1 per 10,000 total population. In regions with vast land area and fewer people as well as inconvenient transport, as well as in large cities, the ratio is 1 per 5,000; for provinces with dense populations, it is 1 per 15,000. Medical technical personnel should account for 75–80 percent of the total personnel in MCH hospitals and 80–85 percent in MCH centers. Managerial positions can be set according to the actual situation and scale: above the prefecture level, at 2–4 for MCH hospitals and 1–3 for MCH centers.
Village clinics	2014	Management Guidelines on Village Clinics (trial)	According to the target population, rural health services status, expected demand, and geographical conditions, in principle at least 1 village doctor per 1,000 population should be provided. Specific standards will be formulated by the provincial health administrative departments.

Note: CDCs = centers for disease control and prevention; GP = general practitioner; MCH = maternal and child care institution; TCM = traditional Chinese medicine.

Notes

1. "Guidance of the National Health and Family Planning Commission and Seven Other Departments on the Establishment of a Standardized Residency Training System," NHFPC (*Guowei kejia fa* 2013, No. 56).
2. "Guiding Opinions of the State Council on the Establishment of a General Practitioner System in China, July 2, 2011," State Council (2011).
3. This reflects a broader picture of the health workforce in China: only 28.6 percent have a university or higher degree (more than five years' medical education), and 38.8 percent have three years' junior college or even less education.
4. Compensation data from "National Health Financial Annual Report 2012," NHFPC, Beijing.
5. Survey data from "Survey of China's Highest-Scoring Students in National University Entrance Exam, 2013," Ai Rui Shen Research Institute, affiliated with the Ai Rui Shen China University Alumni Alliance Network (cuaa.net).
6. There were 17,243 incidents of violence against medical staff in 2010 (Hou and others 2014).
7. The headcount quota system was created in 1956 after the Working Committee on Headcount of the State Council and the Ministry of Health issued a joint policy directive, "Principles of Headcount Management for Hospitals and Outpatient Clinics." Under the quota system, the Chinese government establishes the management system for all public institutions and defines employee-headcount standards for various PSUs (including hospitals, THCs, CHCs, centers for disease control and prevention, sanitary inspection stations, and so forth). Based on these national standards, provinces formulate provincial standards, taking local conditions into consideration.
8. "Guideline on General Hospital Organization Quota Formulation (78)," Ministry of Health (No. 1689).
9. "Provisional Regulations for Professional Certificate System," Ministry of Personnel (1995).
10. "Notification on Pilot of Physicians' Dual Practice," Ministry of Health (2009, No. 86).

11. "Deepening Personnel Reform in Public Medical Service Units" (2000).
12. "Personnel Management Regulations for Public Service Units," State Council (2014).
13. The executive order improved "Guideline on Strengthening Health Professional Titles Evaluation," Ministry of Personnel and MoH (2000), which is further described in annex 7A, table 7A.4.
14. Compensation data from "National Health Financial Annual Report 2012," NHFPC, Beijing.
15. "2013 National Physicians Survey" (data set) of the College of Family Physicians of Canada, the Canadian Medical Association, and the Royal College of Physicians and Surgeons of Canada (accessed July 19, 2018), http://nationalphysiciansurvey.ca/surveys/2013-survey/.

References

Aran, Meltem, and Claudia Rokx, eds. 2014. "Turkey on the Way of Universal Health Coverage Through the Health Transformation Program (2003–2013)." Health, Nutrition, and Population Discussion Paper No. 91326, World Bank, Washington, DC.

Boyle, Seán. 2011. "United Kingdom (England): Health System Review 2011." *Health Systems in Transition* 13 (1): 1–486. European Health Observatory on Health Systems and Policies, World Health Organization Regional Office for Europe, Copenhagen.

Buchan, J. 2015. "Health Sector Wages in Context." Background report commissioned by the World Bank, Washington, DC.

Buchan, J., A. Kumar, and M. Schoenstein. 2014. "Wage Setting in the Hospital Sector." Health Working Paper No. 77, Organisation for Economic Co-operation and Development (OECD), Paris.

Cashin, Cheryl, Y-Ling Chi, Peter Smith, Michael Borowitz, and Sarah Thomson, eds. 2014. *Paying for Performance in Health Care: Implications for Health System Performance and Accountability.* Berkshire, U.K.: World Health Organization (acting as the host organization for, and secretariat of, the European Observatory on Health Systems and Policies).

Daermmich, A. 2013. "The Political Economy of Healthcare Reform in China: Negotiating Public and Private." *SpringerPlus* 2 (1): 448.

DH (Department of Health). 2010. *Equity and Excellence: Liberating the NHS.* London: HMSO.

Doran, Tim, and Martin Roland. 2010. "Lessons from Major Initiatives to Improve Primary Care in the United Kingdom." *Health Affairs* 29 (5): 1023–29. doi:10.1377/hlthaff.2010.0069.

Freund, Tobias, Christine Everett, Peter Griffiths, Catherine Hudon, Lucio Naccarella, Miranda Laurant, and Lincoln Chen. 2015. "Skill Mix, Roles and Remuneration in the Primary Care Workforce: Who Are the Healthcare Professionals in the Primary Care Teams Across the World?" *International Journal of Nursing Studies* 52 (3): 727–43.

Gragnolati, M., M. Lindelow, and B. Couttolenc. 2013. *Twenty Years of Health System Reform in Brazil: An Assessment of the Sistema Único de Saúde.* Directions in Development Series. Washington, DC: World Bank.

Gregory, R. G., and J. Borland. 1999. "Recent Developments in Public Sector Labor Markets." In *Handbook of Labor Economics,* vol. 3, edited by Orley Ashenfelter and David Card, 3573–3630. Amsterdam: Elsevier.

Hou, Jianlin, Catherine Michaud, Li Zhihui, Zhe Dong, Baozhi Sun, Junhua Zhang, Depin Cao, and others. 2014. "Transformation of the Education of Health Professionals in China: Progress and Challenges." *The Lancet* 384 (9945): 819–27.

Johnson, C. D., J. Noyes, A. Haines, K. Thomas, C. Stockport, and A. N. Ribas. 2013. "Learning from the Brazilian Community Health Worker Model in North Wales." *Globalization and Health* 9 (1): 25.

Kringos, Dionne, Wienke Boerma, Yann Bourgueil, Thomas Cartier, Toni Dedeu, Toralf Hasvold, Allen Hutchinson, and others. 2013. "The Strength of Primary Care in Europe: An International Comparative Study." *British Journal of General Practice* 63 (616): e742–50.

Kroneman, Madelon, Pascal Meeus, Dionne Sofia Kringos, Wim Groot, and Jouke van der Zee. 2013. "International Developments in Revenues and Incomes of General Practitioners from 2000 to 2010." *BMC Health Services Research* 13 (1): 436.

Liu, X. 2015. "Health Worker Labor Market Situation Analysis in China." Background report commissioned by the World Bank, Washington, DC.

Marchildon, Gregory. 2013. "Canada: Health System Review." *Health Systems in Transition* 15 (1): 1–179.

McPake, Barbara, and others. 2015. "Wage Setting in Hospital and Primary Care: Case Studies of Five OECD Countries." Unpublished background report commissioned by the World Bank, Washington, DC.

NHDRC (National Health Development Research Center). 2014a. "Establishing in Public Hospitals the Compensation System which Aligns with the Sector Features." Study report, NHDRC, National Health and Family Planning Commission, Beijing.

———. 2014b. "Monitoring and Evaluation Report on Talent Planning, 2013–14." Report, NHDRC, National Health and Family Planning Commission, Beijing.

NHFPC (National Health and Family Planning Commission). 2004. *China Health and Family Planning Statistical Yearbook 2004*. Bejing: Peking Union Medical College Press

———. 2014. *China Health and Family Planning Statistical Yearbook 2014*. Beijing: Peking Union Medical College Press.

———. 2015. "Report on the Development of Standardized Residency Training in China (2014)." Report, NHFPC, Beijing.

Paris, V., M. Devaux, and L. Wei. 2010. "Health Systems Institutional Characteristics: A Survey of 29 OECD Countries." Health Working Paper No. 50, OECD, Paris.

Qin, X., L. Li, and C. R. Hsieh. 2013. "Too Few Doctors or Too Low Wages? Labor Supply of Health Care Professionals in China." *China Economic Review* 24 (1): 150–64.

Roland, M., B. Guthrie, and D. Thomé. 2012. "Primary Medical Care in the United Kingdom." *Journal of the American Board of Family Medicine* 25 (1): S6–S11. doi:10.3122/jabfm.2012.02.110200.

Waldmeir, P. 2013. "China's Doctors Not Part of Society's Elite." *Financial Times*, October 6.

Woodhead, M. 2014. "How Much Does the Average Chinese Doctor Earn?" *China Medical News*, March 31.

Wranik, D. W., and M. Durier-Copp. 2010. "Physician Remuneration Methods for Family Physicians in Canada: Expected Outcomes and Lessons Learned." *Health Care Analysis* 18 (1): 35–59.

Ying, Yachen. 2014. "Achieve Win-Win-Win Situation by Jointly Reforming the Drug Sector, Health Service Sector and Health Insurance Sector: Field Study Report on Public Hospital Reform in Sanming." August. Unpublished case study. Beijing: Health Development Research Center (NHFOC).

Yip, W. C., W. Hsiao, Q. Meng, W. Chen, and X. Sun. 2010. "Realignment of Incentives for Health-Care Providers in China." *The Lancet* 375 (9720): 1120–30.

8

Lever 7: Strengthening Private Sector Engagement in Health Service Delivery

Introduction

The health care system in China has moved from an exclusively state-run system to one that is decentralized and open to private sector investment and service provision. The foundations for private participation in the production, financing, and delivery of health goods and services were laid during the early days of liberalization of the economy in the 1970s. Over time, the government has relaxed the rules for private investment in health care and explored ways to nudge it closer to the emerging vision of the future of health care in China. Reforms since 2000—and especially in the 12th Five-Year Plan (State Council 2011) and the State Council policy directives issued in 2015[1]—affirmed the role of private capital in developing China's health care system and of further encouraging private participation in the health sector.

The rapid rise of the private sector in health care poses many opportunities and challenges for the government, investors, and people of China. There are now more than 10,000 private hospitals in China, constituting 52.6 percent of all hospitals in the country. Most are small (with fewer than 100 beds), and together they accounted for 19.4 percent of all hospital beds, 14.7 percent of admissions, and 12 percent of outpatient visits in 2015. The number of private primary care facilities also has grown considerably recently, and is about equal to the number of public primary care facilities.

Limited in size but rapidly growing in market share, private investment is set to transform the health market in China. On the one hand, the private sector offers alternatives. On the other hand, the development of a health care delivery system in which providers, whether public or private, have strong incentives to generate revenues and operating surpluses is raising ethical, legal, economic, and political issues. Despite central policies pushing for a greater role for the private sector in health care, many local governments continue to focus their service planning and public financing on public service providers. Whether guided by prospects of more and better health care or by concerns related to high levels of profit making, the continuing development of private health care enterprise in China is being watched closely by all stakeholders.

This chapter examines the private health sector in China and proposes a way forward to strengthen private engagement in health care delivery as it relates to the government's objectives of reforming health service delivery and improving value for money.

The rest of the chapter is organized as follows:

- *"Evolution of Policies on the Private Health Sector"* briefly reviews the changes in government policy toward the private sector's engagement and investment in the Chinese health care system.
- *"Scope and Growth of China's Private Health Sector"* describes the private sector's current size, scope, and recent growth.
- *"Key Challenges"* discusses the challenges China faces in dealing with private enterprise in health care.
- *"Recommendations for Strengthening Private Sector Engagement"* draws upon experiences from within China and Organisation for Economic Co-operation and Development (OECD) countries to offer a series of actionable recommendations for strengthening private sector participation and engagement in health care.

Evolution of Policies on the Private Health Sector

Policies related to the development of the private sector in health care in China have evolved over time, and can be categorized into five phases, as discussed in detail below (table 8.1).

Phase 1: Socialization of Medicine, 1949–78

Before the People's Republic of China (PRC) was founded, health services were delivered primarily by the private sector. During this period, China moved to socialized medicine, and in 1963, private practice became illegal.

Over the next three decades, the government developed the largest public health institutional network and health workforce in the world (Huang and others 2009). The number of health facilities in the public sector grew 20 times and manpower 5 times compared with 1949 levels (Liu 1994).

Phase 2: Opening of Health to the Private Sector, 1979–92

Remarkable economic growth and rising standards of living after 1978 spurred increased demand for health care, which outpaced the government's ability to expand health services. To alleviate the increasing shortages in health services, the government decided to relegalize private medical practice in 1980. This laid the foundation for the conversion of state- and collective-owned medical institutions to private ownership.

By 1985, private investment in health care was legally allowed. During this period, the Cooperative Medical System collapsed, and many "barefoot doctors" started private practice with fee-for-service payment (Liu and others 2006; Ramesh, Wu, and He 2014).[2]

Phase 3: Experimentation in the Private Sector, 1993–99

As economic reforms took hold in the 1990s and pressures to deliver more and better health care intensified, the State Council and Ministry of Health published several policies, rules, and laws encouraging cautious development of nonstate health organizations to supplement the government system. New ownership categories were created for health institutions, including state, collective, private, and Chinese-foreign joint ownership.

By the end of the 1990s, almost all rural ambulatory care was delivered by private providers, either in private practice or contracted by the village health post (Liu and others 2006). Some regions set up small and medium-size private hospitals, but the policy and planning environment still did not encourage large-scale or organized growth of private hospitals (Gu and Zhang 2006).

Phase 4: Gradual Growth, 2000–08

During the 2000s, a series of important policies opened up the health sector to

TABLE 8.1   Evolution of policies on the private health sector in China, 1949–present

Phase	Policies, opinions, regulations	Impact on private sector
Phase 1: Socialization of medicine, 1949–78	• 1951 MoH Policy adjusting relationships between public and private health sectors • 1951 MoH Policy implementing cooperatives between public and private sectors • 1963 MoH interim management measures for medical practitioners	• Rationalized health services and practices between sectors during 1950s • Eventually closed all private practice by mid-1960s
Phase 2: Opening up to the private sector, 1979–92	• 1978 3rd Plenary Session of 11th Central Committee • 1980 MoH regulations permitting individual private practice • 1985 State Council and MoH circular on policy issues in health care reform • 1989 MoH/MoFTEC rules on establishing international hospitals and clinics in China and on governing	• Opening up of Chinese economy including the health sector to private enterprises • Policies lay foundation for private practice, private ownership of state- or collective-owned medical institutions, and foreign investment in health • Reforms stress improving efficiency and quality of health services through public-private competition
Phase 3: Experimentation in the private sector, 1993–99	• 1992 South Inspection Speech of senior leader Deng Xiaoping and the 14th National Congress • 1994 State Council document regulating administration of health institutions • 1998 State Council creation of medical health insurance for urban workers • 1999 MoH guidance on regional health planning • 1999 MoH opinions on urban community health services	• Chinese leadership and 14th National Congress set the direction for market opening • State Council and MoH respond by cautiously opening up health sector to nonstate forms of ownerships • Other health policies reference nonstate medical institutions • However, government stresses dominance of the public sector in health, describing the private sector as "supplemental"
Phase 4: Gradual growth, 2000–08	• 2000 State Council guidance on health system reforms in cities and towns • Notice of health affairs planning in 11th Five-Year Plan and of issuing planning on medical and health affairs "12th Year"	• In early part of decade, many policy reforms further open up the health sector to nonstate actors, offering unprecedented opportunities • Private sector experiences some setbacks • Private sector growth is limited, less than expected
Phase 5: Renewed opportunities, 2009–15	• 2009 Central Committee and State Council publish opinions on deepening health system reform • 2010 MoH notice guiding pilot reforms of public hospitals • 2010 State Council opinions encouraging further development of private medical institutions • 2012 State Council document on planning medical and health sectors in 12th Five-Year Plan • 2013 State Council issues several opinions promoting development of health services industry • 2013 Opinions accelerating development of private ownership of health care • 2015 Main tasks of deepening medical reform	• 2008–09 reforms have significant impact on the private sector • Reforms reinforce dominance of public sector in all aspects of the health system but also allow for increased private sector role in financing and delivery of health services • In 2012, first targets for private sector set by the State Council: 20 percent of all beds and outpatient volume by 2015 • Article 40 envisions nonprofit institutions as the central component of a new, more diversified health system • Draft NHFPC Five-Year Plan specifies key areas for private sector growth beyond hospitals and opens the door for contracting the private sector to deliver services on behalf of the government • Private sector policies accelerate, laying the foundation to redirect private sector growth and explicitly reiterating "vigorous" support for a mixed ownership health system to achieve health for all

Note: MoFTEC = Ministry of Foreign Trade and Economic Co-operation; MoH = Ministry of Health; NHFPC = National Health and Family Planning Commission.

nonstate actors, offering unprecedented opportunities, including for Chinese-foreign jointly owned medical institutions. The private-for-profit (PFP) and private-not-for-profit (PNFP) categories came to be recognized, and all private health facilities were required to register as either of the two (Gu and Zhang 2006).

Several PFP and PNFP hospitals opened across China during this period, which also saw many hospitals converting from public to private ownership status. At the same time, some private hospitals that were too small to be economically viable converted to public ownership.

Phase 5: Renewed Opportunities for the Private Sector, 2009–15

To further promote the growth of the private sector in the health market, the 2009 health reforms and 2010 public hospital reforms created additional "space" for the private sector in the financing and delivery of health services. This encouragement has continued with a series of new policies, opinions, and regulations that have come out each year since, including the following:

- The 2010 State Council opinion was a landmark policy that prompted all provinces and metropolitan centers to publish supporting documents to grow the private health sector in ways that reflected their local conditions.
- In 2012, the State Council, in the Twelfth Five-Year Plan, enunciated a specific target for the share of the private sector in the health sector at 20 percent of all beds and outpatient service volume by 2015 (State Council 2011).
- In 2013, Article No. 40 reinforced health reform goals set in 2009 and encouraged additional future development of health service delivery through the private sector. It envisioned the development of nonprofit institutions as an important part of a more diversified health system, to be established with "social" capital and market-driven development.

- In 2014, the Ministry of Health (MoH) outlined specific areas for private sector growth, including premium services, niche services in rehabilitation and geriatrics, diagnostic and laboratory services, and pharmacy chains. It also supported expanding the number of joint ventures. This opened the door to the contracting of the private sector for delivery of publicly financed health services, and to the transfer of business and management skills to public facilities.

Recent policies related to the role of the private sector in health are more specific, designating subsectors in which private sector expansion is encouraged. For example, the "Planning Layout of National Medical and Health Services System (2015–2020)" explicitly notes that nonpublic hospitals could deliver basic medical services, compete with public hospitals, offer premium services to meet nonbasic needs, provide niche services on rehabilitation and geriatric nursing, and so on.[3] The guideline encourages the nonpublic sector to run health facilities, including specialized traditional Chinese medicine (TCM) hospitals; rehabilitation hospitals; nursing homes (stations); and medical facilities specializing in oral diseases, geriatrics, and noncommunicable diseases.

In 2015, the policy statement enshrined in the "Main Tasks of Deepening Medical Reform 2015" laid the foundation for redirecting private health sector growth and explicitly reiterated commitment to a mixed-ownership health system to achieve health for all.[4] This "vigorous" support called for a greater private sector role in areas beyond conventional medical service delivery, including fitness and prevention. The 2015 policy statement also moved away from national targets and envisioned a mixed health system in which "public medical institutions lead joint development with nonpublic medical institutions" and suggested a complementary role with "nonprofit medical institutions as the main body and for-profit medical institutions as the supplement." Key themes running through the 2015 policy statement include "creating a level playing field," "loosening restrictions over market access," "relaxing price control over medical services provided by nonpublic medical institutions," and strengthening "multi-site practice and markets for human resources and talent in health."

Scope and Growth of China's Private Health Sector

Government statistics show the current status and development of key segments of the private sector since 2005, when the "private" category was first established. To enable international comparisons, providers and facility ownership are reported using the three categories commonly used internationally: public (as reported in official Chinese statistics also), private not-for-profit, and private for-profit, as described in box 8.1.

Private Sector Activity in Hospital Services

The number of private sector hospitals in China, especially PNFP hospitals, has grown rapidly in recent years. Between 2005 and 2012, the total number of hospitals grew by 24 percent, from 18,644 to 23,170. During this period, the number of public sector hospitals fell by 14 percent; PFP hospitals increased by 116 percent (from 2,971 to 6,403); and PNFP hospitals increased

---

BOX 8.1   Hospital ownership categories in China: Public, PNFP, and PFP

Standard international reporting has three categories: public, private not-for-profit (PNFP), and private for-profit (PFP). "Not-for-profit organizations" are those established for purposes other than generating profit and in which none of the organization's income is distributed to owners or investors. Not-for-profits include private not-for-profit organizations as well as government-owned nonprofit organizations such as public hospitals and government-owned community health centers (CHCs).

Chinese statistics report two categories of registration status (按登记注册类型分):

- *Public* (公立) *government-owned providers:* public hospitals and other providers, including both state-owned (central and local governments) and collective-owned providers
- *Private providers:* "people-run" (minying 民营) or nongovernment (feigongli 非公立), including joint ventures, cooperatives, purely private providers, and hospitals funded from sources in Hong Kong SAR, China; Macao SAR, China; Taiwan, China; or foreign countries.

Statistics also report a separate category of profit status or "management form" (按分类管理分): for-profit (yinglixing 营利性) and not-for-profit (fei yinglixing 非营利性), which may be either government-owned or private.

To enable comparisons using the three ownership categories commonly used internationally, we used the Chinese statistics to create a category of PNFP (minying feiyinglixing) by removing government-owned not-for-profits from all not-for-profits (fei yinglixing 非营利性); and a category of PFP (minying yinglixing) by removing the PNFPs from the official statistics on nonstate providers. The assumption is that public providers such as public hospitals are registered as not-for-profit organizations according to management form—that is, there are a negligible number of public for-profits, regardless of whether public hospitals may behave similarly to for-profit organizations.

The three-way ownership definition used in this book is consistent with China's own definition of public hospital (our "public" category exactly matches the official statistics of gongli) and with international standards differentiating not-for-profits from for-profits within the private category (fei gongli). It is difficult to develop a comprehensive picture of China's overall health sector beyond hospitals, in part because grassroots providers (jiceng yiliao jigou), including village clinics, do not have consistently reported statistics on ownership or management. Even in 2009, the profit status for many grassroots providers was listed as "unknown."

China also usually reports statistics (for example, for hospitals or ambulatory clinics) using a different

(Box continued next page)

> **BOX 8.1   Hospital ownership categories in China: Public, PNFP, and PFP** (continued)
>
> three-way ownership categorization, by "management work unit" (zhuban danwei 主办单位):
>
> - Government-managed (zhengfu ban 政府办)
> - Managed by society (shehui ban 社会办)
> - Managed by individuals (siren ban 私人办).
>
> Although these categories provide additional information about management form, they are not legal definitions of ownership, residual control rights, or legal authority. Providers managed by "society" (or by individuals) may be for-profit or not-for-profit. The statistics on the "government-managed" category include substantially fewer facilities than the numbers registered as public; those managed by society or by individuals do not only include private providers. It is not known how consistently contracted-out facilities are categorized in different parts of China, that is, if a government-owned hospital is contracted out to be managed by a PFP firm, whether it is classified as government-managed (zhengfu ban 政府办) or managed by society (shehui ban 社会办). During fieldwork interviews, some localities reported that they did not
>
> collect data that allowed consistent categorization of private providers as PFP or PNFP.
>
> China may wish to retain China-specific categories that use the management work unit and registration to define "government-managed public" (政府办公立医疗机构), "society-managed public" (社会办公立医疗机构), and "society-managed private" (社会办民营医疗机构), which include provider organizations managed "by society" and "by individuals." But these ownership categories are not the international standard, and China could enable meaningful international comparisons by also reporting according to international standard categories, just as China reports and compares health expenditures internationally according to the World Health Organization (WHO) and Organisation for Economic Co-operation and Development (OECD) international standard categories (public financing and private financing) with their respective subcategories, while retaining China's own three categories of health financing (government, social health insurance, and out-of-pocket).
>
> *Sources:* Morris and others 2014; Rudd 2011; Turner and others 2016.

by 1,681 percent (from 190 to 3,383) (figure 8.1).[5] During the same period, the percentage of all hospitals that were in the public sector fell from 83 percent to 58 percent, and their share of inpatient admissions fell from 96 percent to 89 percent.

PFP hospitals increased from 16 percent to 28 percent of the total, and their share of admissions rose from 3 percent to 6 percent. PNFP hospitals increased from under 1 percent to 15 percent of the total, though their share of admissions grew from 1 percent to just 5 percent, reflecting their small size (figure 8.2). These trends make it unlikely that the target set by the government in 2012 of a 20 percent private sector share of hospital beds and outpatient services, with an emphasis on PNFP ownership, would have been met by 2015.[6]

Growth and shares of inpatient admissions are similar to outpatient visits (figure 8.3). By 2010, the private health sector had taken root firmly in China, even though

9 out of 10 outpatient and inpatient visits to hospitals still took place in the public sector.

Private hospitals are generally smaller than public hospitals in China, as is reflected in their shares of hospital beds. In 2012, 86 percent of all hospitals beds were in the public sector, with the private sector accounting for the remaining 14 percent (figure 8.4).

Almost all private hospitals (96 percent) have fewer than 100 beds, while only 60 percent of public hospitals are that small (figure 8.5). Because capital investment and management requirements are less demanding in small and medium-size hospitals, the private sector expands more easily in that size facility (Hou and Coyne 2008). Almost all hospitals of more than 500 beds are operated by the public sector.

About 30 percent of private sector hospitals are specialty hospitals, where higher margins for advanced technologies produce huge profits, compared with only 13 percent of public sector hospitals (Hou and Coyne 2008;

FIGURE 8.1   **Number of Chinese hospitals, by ownership type, 2005–12**

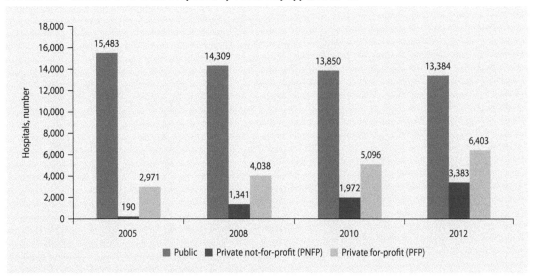

Source: World Bank analysis of data from *China Health Statistical Yearbook 2013*, Ministry of Health, Beijing.
Note: For complete definition of the PNFP and PFP categories, see box 8.1 of the chapter text.

Tang and others 2014). Almost all new private hospitals are specialty hospitals because it is easier for a specialty hospital to become eligible for insurance reimbursements than for a general hospital (Yip and Hsiao 2014).

Much of the private sector expansion has been in urban private hospitals that deliver high-end services, such as cosmetic surgery, VIP services,[7] and "checkups" that are not integrated with chronic disease case management (Yip and Hsiao 2014). Key informant interviews indicated that difficult market conditions and regulatory policies have driven investment and growth in nonessential service areas where fewer obstacles exist. At the same time, there are also important cases of private companies providing specialty or essential services (not elective services) to the general public under the social health insurance schemes. Indeed, although systematic data are lacking, existing studies do not support the common perception that private providers only serve the wealthiest patients in China. Liu and others (2006) report that there is nothing in the literature, nor in any data, that supports the notion that the private sector serves primarily the better-off people; in fact, the available data suggest that the private sector extensively serves low- to middle-income groups as well.

FIGURE 8.2   **Market share of inpatient admissions in China, by hospital ownership type, 2005 and 2012**

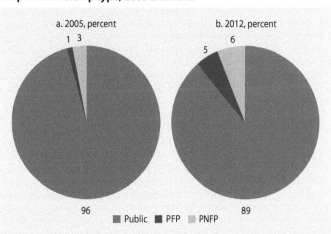

Source: World Bank analysis of data from China Health Statistical Yearbook 2013, Ministry of Health, Beijing.
Note: PFP = public for-profit; PNFP = public not-for-profit. For complete definition of the PNFP and PFP categories, see box 8.1 of the chapter text.

Nationally, a disproportionate percentage of private hospitals—41.5 percent—are in eastern China (table 8.2). This is also true of other types of hospitals. Western China has the next largest share (32.5 percent) of private hospitals, and Middle China has the least (26 percent).

There is no correlation between level of economic development in provinces, measured by income per capita, and the size of

FIGURE 8.3   **Trends in hospital use in China, by ownership type, 2005–12**

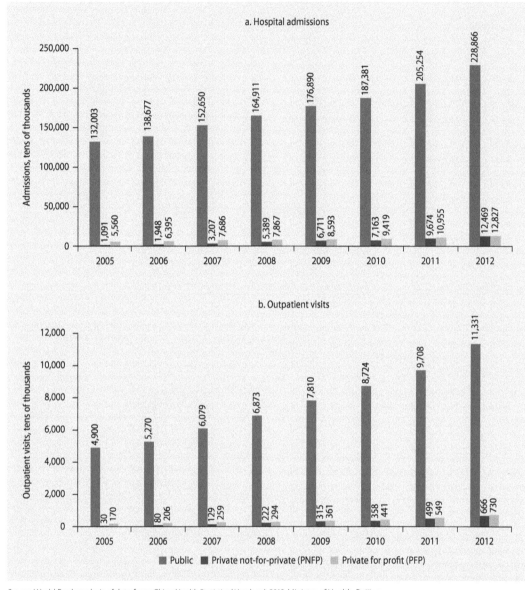

Source: World Bank analysis of data from *China Health Statistical Yearbook 2013*, Ministry of Health, Beijing.
Note: For complete definition of the PNFP and PFP categories, see box 8.1 of the chapter text.

the private health sector, measured by percentage of outpatient visits (figure 8.6).[8] The share of private visits is low (6 percent) in the rich provinces (such as Shanghai) and in poor provinces (such as Gansu) alike; it is also equally high in the well-off province of Jiangsu (19 percent) as well as in the low-income province of Guizhou.

Private Sector Activity in Primary Health Care Services

The number of primary health care (PHC) facilities in the private sector—using the Chinese definition of grassroots providers (jiceng yiliao jigou), which includes all non-hospital facilities such as village clinics;

FIGURE 8.4   **Number of beds in Chinese hospitals, by ownership type, 2005–12**

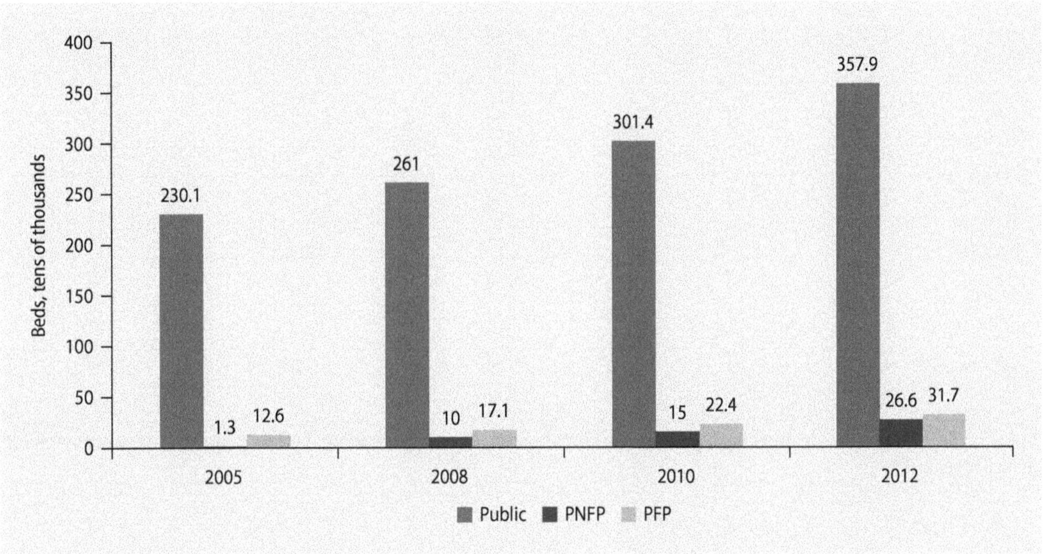

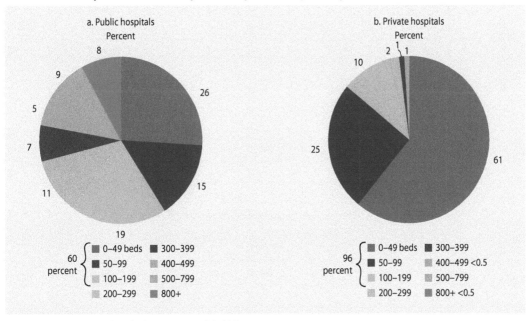

Source: World Bank analysis of data from *China Health Statistical Yearbook 2013*, Ministry of Health, Beijing.
Note: PFP = public for-profit; PNFP = public not-for-profit. For complete definition of the PNFP and PFP categories, see box 8.1 of the chapter text.

FIGURE 8.5   **Composition of Chinese public and private hospitals, by number of beds, 2012**

Source: China Health Statistical Yearbook 2013, Ministry of Health Beijing.

township health centers (THCs); clinics (zhen-suo, menzhenbu, yiwushi); community health stations; and community health centers—has also grown. The number of PNFP PHC facilities increased the most, from 15,204 in 2008 to 216,614 in 2012 (figure 8.7). The number

of PFP PHC facilities increased by only 9 percent, from 202,537 in 2008 to 220,642 in 2012.

By 2012, PFP and PNFP facilities each accounted for 24 percent of PHC facilities, and the combined private sector share

TABLE 8.2   Regional distribution of private hospitals in China, 2012

Hospital type	Total number	Regional share (%)		
		East	Middle	West
General hospital	6,047	39.8	22.4	37.7
TCM hospital	571	48.0	32.4	19.6
Combination	187	40.1	26.7	33.2
Ethnic	23	8.7	30.4	60.0
Specialty	2,905	43.1	32.4	24.8
Nursing	53	90.6	3.8	5.7
Total	9,786	41.5	26.0	32.5

Source: Ministry of Health service statistics.
Note: TCM = traditional Chinese medicine.

FIGURE 8.6   Correlation between private hospital share of outpatient visits and per capita income across provinces, 2012

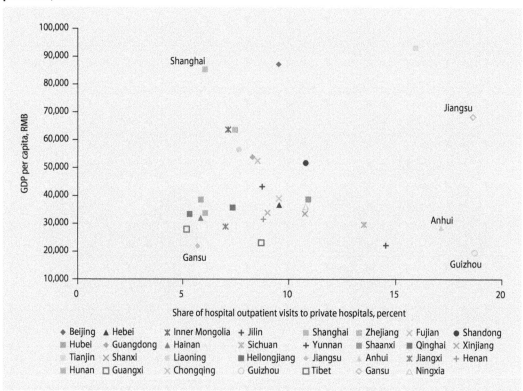

Sources: China Health Statistical Yearbook 2013, table 5-2-3, Ministry of Health, Beijing.

(48 percent) approached the public sector share (52 percent) in number of facilities but not in share of outpatient visits, which is not consistently reported.

Recategorization reduced the percentages of PFP and public PHC facilities from 32 percent and 66 percent, respectively, in 2008 to 24 percent and 52 percent in 2012. Key informants in China noted that the private sector share of the supply chain has grown for other goods and services, such as diagnostics, drug supplies, medical equipment, and dentistry services.[9]

The private sector employs a greater percentage of all health workers in China than its 10–11 percent share of admissions and

FIGURE 8.7   Growth in Chinese PHC facilities, by ownership type, 2005–12

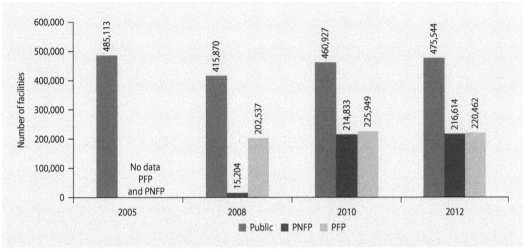

Source: World Bank analysis of data from *China Health Statistical Yearbook 2013*, Ministry of Health, Beijing.
Note: PHC = primary health care; PFP = private for-profit; PNFP = private not-for-profit. For complete definition of the PNFP and PFP categories, see box 8.1 of the chapter text.

beds (table 8.3). Of the 9.1 million health personnel in China in 2012, 18 percent worked in the private sector and 82 percent in the public sector (table 8.4). The percentage is similar for all cadres from physicians to administrative staff, except that 37 percent of village physicians are in the private sector.

Key Challenges

Even though laws and regulations in China encourage private capital investment in the health sector, private providers still face many challenges entering the health market at the local level. Despite the acceleration in recent years in the pace and scope of policies promoting private health care production and delivery, the country still lacks a unified vision for the role of private providers in improving service delivery or contributing to national health objectives. And no consensus has yet formed across government agencies on whether the private sector should be complementary, supplementary, or integral to the public delivery system. Quantity targets have spurred private sector growth in ways not consistent with national health objectives.

Private sector expansion needs to be strengthened to address key health sector priorities—such as greater access to health care in poorer regions—or to complement government efforts in priority areas like rehabilitation, elderly care, and integrated management of noncommunicable diseases. Provinces seek to attract private capital to remote rural areas or new peri-urban areas not already well served by government providers, whereas private capital demonstrates an inclination to stay in cities where medical resources are already plentiful. This section discusses these issues in detail.

Difficulty in Developing a Shared Vision of the Private Sector Role

The central government has enacted a rich set of national policies related to private sector engagement, but the accelerated pace of policy development has added to uncertainty and wide variability in interpretation and action by provinces (Brixi and others 2013). Some provinces and municipalities have hesitated, while others have taken decisive steps. (Annex 8A, table 8A.1, summarizes major relevant national polices, grouped by 14 topics, showing examples of the regional

TABLE 8.3   **Health employees in China, by sector, 2010–12**
Tens of thousands

Year	Hospitals			Primary health care[a]		
	Public	Private	Private (%)	Public	Private	Private (%)
2010	377.0	45.8	10.8	235.0	93.2	28.4
2011	398.1	54.6	12.1	241.8	95.7	28.4
2012	428.2	65.5	13.3	248.3	95.4	27.8

Source: Ha 2014.
a. "Primary health care" comprises grassroots providers using the Chinese definition (jiceng yiliao jigou), which includes all nonhospital facilities such as village clinics; township health centers; clinics (zhensuo, menzhenbu, yiwushi); community health stations; and community health centers.

TABLE 8.4   **Health employees in China, by type and sector, 2012**

Health cadre	Total number (tens of thousands)	Sector	
		Public (%)	Private (%)
Physician	261.6	81.5	18.5
Nurse	249.7	86.3	13.7
Pharmacist	37.7	86.4	13.6
Technician	36.4	88.2	11.8
Other	81.5	88.0	12.0
Village physician	109.4	62.7	37.3
Other technicians	31.9	88.4	11.7
Administrative	37.3	85.1	15.0
Logistics	65.4	84.6	15.4
Total	9.1 million	82.2	17.8

Source: Ha 2014.

differences in their interpretation and implementation.) The inconsistency is a challenge but also an opportunity to learn from varied experiences across China.

National policies support private investments in the health sector in China. For example, the "Opinions of the State Council on Comprehensively Scaling up Reform of County-Level Public Hospitals" calls for local authorities to "implement policies that support and guide nongovernment investment in hospitals."[10]

However, not all provincial governments follow up with the same sense of urgency or scale. One example of differences across provinces is in their implementation of the target of a 20 percent private sector share of hospital beds and inpatient admissions by 2015. Some provinces, such as Yunnan, have

adopted the national goal, while some others, like Hunan, have set even more ambitious targets by suggesting that by 2020, the two indicators should exceed 25 percent of the total.[11] Changsha went further, aiming to exceed 30 percent by 2020. Likewise, Shenzhen also aims for the two indicators to exceed 30 percent by 2015 and to have two to three private medical institutions that meet the standards for tertiary hospitals.

Overall, about two-thirds of provinces and municipalities encourage private sector hospitals, and more than half especially encourage "high-end" (that is, modern and high-tech) and specialty hospitals. Many refer to "hospitals with certain scale and level" and a few, such as Hubei, set targets for the number of beds by type of hospital.

One approach to increasing the private sector share in hospitals has been to convert ownership of public hospitals. For example, the Zhejiang provincial government adopted mixed state-private ownership as a transition stage to promote private investment ("social capital") while exploring ways to assure service quality and to handle state assets. However, some provinces proceeded with ownership conversions without strong mechanisms in place to prevent loss of state assets. One example is Kunming Children's Hospital, for which the city intended to build a new campus with joint contributions from the hospital and the government. The hospital was taken over by CR Pharmaceutical, which, despite state ownership, is publicly listed, creating the risk of state assets being transferred to private investors.

There is much less policy clarity about the role of the private sector in primary care and community services, which reflects differing interpretations of whether the private sector should be an integral part of the health sector or have a more limited supplementary role. Almost all provinces encourage the private sector to set up medical services in geographic areas with inadequate public services, especially new towns, rural and remote areas, and peri-urban areas. However, private (and public) providers prefer to stay in urban areas where medical resources are already abundant.

Many provinces encourage private investment in specific medical areas where existing health care resources are lacking or weak, such as rehabilitation, nursing, geriatrics, and chronic disease management. A few provinces encourage private sector delivery of basic services at CHCs and THCs. A few stress traditional Chinese medicine or Hui and Tibetan medicine. Anhui province stands out in having a comprehensive vision for the private health sector role that follows practices in OECD countries. Anhui encourages the private sector to provide basic medical services in rural areas and to establish high-end specialty medical institutions in urban areas.

The overall result is that a lot of private sector development has been in services that are not well aligned with people-centered integrated care (PCIC) and that do not complement government efforts. The incentives created by the current fee-for-service payment system have driven both private and public provider investment into nonessential areas that generate revenue (such as VIP services, overprescribing, cosmetic surgery, and "checkups" not integrated with chronic disease management) rather than into areas that improve health and strengthen PCIC.

Special private sector incentives and constraints differ considerably across health authorities. For example, Yunnan set up a special fund of RMB 20 million annually in 2010 (increased to RMB 40 million per year in 2014) to encourage private sector expansion and to develop exemplary institutions. Yunnan offers special support to private firms, including medical institutions, to attract talent, such as an RMB 150,000–300,000 housing subsidy for key personnel. Some provinces and municipalities limit development of public hospitals to facilitate entry by nongovernmental institutions. For example, Shaanxi province regulations do not allow new public medical institutions, and they seek to shut down VIP medical services in public hospitals and leave this market segment for private medical institutions. Chongqing's health administration strictly controls VIP medical services allowed in its public hospitals. Shenzhen in Guangdong province spends its own budget to directly subsidize PFP medical institutions.

Stakeholders have been wary of policy changes that would shift the political context of private sector engagement and reverse previous policies. Many local initiatives were designed to be able to reverse course without much difficultly, so markets and investors could not be confident of long-term support that would make important complementary investments profitable, such as investing in human resource training. Policy uncertainty has encouraged a short-term investment focus, which fueled suspicion that private engagement pursued short-run profits and was ill-suited to long-term development goals in the health sector.

Shortcomings in the Regulatory Framework Overseeing Private Sector Development

To grow, the private sector requires a well-functioning governmental stewardship mechanism—one that has the capacity of monitoring (and shutting down, as necessary) facilities seen to be endangering patient safety or defrauding social health insurance. Regulatory frameworks for accountability and quality assurance, however, exhibit wide local variations and are not uniformly strong. It is widely believed that private providers are more likely than their public counterparts to engage in false advertising, overtreatment, or fraudulent billing practices, and unsurprisingly, the private health sector in China does not have a good reputation with health consumers. Even though some private sector providers have overcome this perception and established a reputation of higher quality of services than public hospitals (for example, United Family Hospital in Beijing and Shanghai), and some have achieved high operational efficiency (such as the Aier Eye Hospital Group and Wuhan Asia Heart Hospital),[12] this general impression is unlikely to change soon, given limited government capacity to monitor and sanction low-quality or unqualified providers.

Qinghai is an example of the serious difficulties that localities with limited resources and experience face in monitoring health services. Qinghai has only two quality supervision staff to monitor approximately 300,000 medical personnel, and information systems are incomplete. The province relies on borrowed personnel from the health and family planning commission and other related organizations in the area to carry out special checks. Even in relatively rich Fujian and Zhejiang provinces, regulatory frameworks for accountability and quality assurance are not sufficient and have wide local variation. Localities that aggressively promote private sector development, such as Suqian city in Jiangsu, have recognized the need for rigorous regulatory policies to ensure that interests of patients are protected (Chen 2015; Liu 2015; Zhou 2015).

Compliance with regulations is much more likely, and hence enforcement much easier and more feasible, if those being regulated agree that the regulations serve a useful and desirable purpose. The modern and more successful approach to regulation is to approach it in a collaborative way rather than in a coercive way. However, there is limited capacity in China to engage the private sector in policy discussions, and there are almost no direct interactions between policy makers and the private health sector.

Difficult Market Entry

Public and private sector stakeholders interviewed in 2014 and early 2015 agreed that market conditions have been a significant barrier to private sector growth in the health sector. The "Measures to Promote the Growth of Nonpublic Medical Institutions" include detailed policies to relax entry barriers, expand financing channels, promote resource flows, and improve the regulatory environment for private sector development.[13] However, private health sector growth still faces constraints, especially relative to other sectors.

It is not easy to open a private health facility. There are multiple agencies to deal with, several reports to file, and many payments to make (Zhang 2006). If foreign investors are involved, a new facility requires approvals from the local health authority, the National Health and Family Planning Commission (NHFPC), the Ministry of Commerce, the National Development and Reform Commission, and environmental protection agencies; a business license from the State General Bureau of Industry and Commerce; and registration with the State General Bureau of Tax (Glucksman and Lipson 2010). The process can take more than a year.

Another barrier to expansion is the prohibition against consolidating finances across affiliates that allow the private business to offset tax liability. Each municipality wants its share of taxes, and so each subsidiary is considered a separate, individual cost center.

In addition, the numbers and types of medical equipment are highly regulated by local and provincial authorities in their annual capital plans. Consistent implementation of the "Measures to Promote the Growth of Nonpublic Medical Institutions" and the "Planning Layout of National Medical and Health Services System (2015–2020)"[14] could ease these barriers to expansion of qualified private providers.

Uneven Implementation of Reforms Allowing Doctors to Practice at Multiple Facilities

Government policies and practices tend to put the private health care industry at a disadvantage relative to the public sector and affect its ability to compete fairly in the marketplace. One huge problem until recently was access to human resources, with physicians responding to the requirement of registering and working in only one facility by opting to work in public hospitals, which offered them a known and stable career track. Professional recognition, career development, salary compensation, and pension benefits were all linked to the physician's employment contract with a specific (usually public) health facility.

Some hospitals have devised successful human resources strategies to counteract these disincentives. One PNFP 1,000-bed tumor tertiary specialty hospital with a joint-stock ownership system has explored reforms to attract and retain talent, including a retirement compensation fund to match the compensation levels of public hospitals as well as a special fund for managers and physicians to study and practice in other hospitals. A large tertiary general hospital in Zhejiang that achieved a top 10 national ranking after merging two public hospitals and converting to PNFP status retained authorized staff-quota status for more than 90 percent of the hospital employees. Its employees take the same bureau examination as public hospital employees, which has aided recruitment and retention of physicians.

The latest reforms allow doctors to practice at multiple facilities, including private

hospitals, and are making the best doctors more mobile and easier to recruit (as further discussed in chapter 7). Provincial governments have begun to experiment with multisite license policies, but implementation varies widely. Guangdong and Fujian, for example, have adopted a pioneering set of reforms, while Qinghai (a poorer province in western China with low population density and shortages of health personnel) has yet to implement the new multisite practice policy, and its private health care industry continues to face human resource shortages.

In practice, the multiple-institute—or "dual practice"— policy has not been enough to create a functioning labor market for health workers and is not working well for either the private or the public sector. It has not freed up as many staff as the private sector had hoped. Although the policy allows doctors to work in multiple institutes without approval, in practice public hospital administrators make it difficult. As an owner of one private hospital in Beijing noted, "Dual practice is an interim step, but it is not revolutionary. Doctors are still tied to public hospitals." A public hospital administrator explained the administrative challenge that dual practice creates for the public sector: "It is difficult to plan when a percentage of your most experienced staff are off-site each week." This is a particularly intractable policy reform to implement.

Out-of-date professional and malpractice liability also constrains labor movement between the sectors. Few private insurance companies offer limited liability insurance. Physicians and other health workers are reluctant to move the private sector where there is no safety net against malpractice.

Uneven Implementation of Reforms Restricting Social Health Insurance Reimbursement to Private Hospitals

Private hospitals face reimbursement restrictions from social health insurance (SHI), which gives preferential treatment to public facilities (Liu, Guan, and Gao 2013). In cities where private enterprises are eligible, limited insurance funds are first directed toward public facilities; they go to private enterprises only if there is money left over. The latest reforms are changing this, with more and more private hospitals being considered for inclusion in public health insurance networks on the same terms as public hospitals. Private facilities that are approved for SHI reimbursement report dramatic patient increases, including patients traveling from afar for specialized health care. More than any other policy initiative, SHI reimbursement reform is creating pressure on public hospitals and has started to enable the private sector to compete successfully for patients.

Even so, private sector representatives have complained that SHI reimbursement levels are too low. In principle, approval for SHI "dingdian" provider status is supposed to be ownership-neutral, but effective differences remain. For example, Yunnan's reimbursement rate is tied to the class of a medical institution as rated by the local social security department, which can be lower than the rating by the local health department, resulting in lower reimbursements to some private providers. (See box 8.2 for a discussion of Yunnan Kidney Hospital, an example of the difficult market conditions that even a PNFP medical institution catering to an underserved population has faced.)

The increasing adoption of budget caps or global budgeting experiments also implicitly favors incumbent market participants, usually public hospitals, over newer entrants. The global budgets are usually negotiated directly between local health insurance management offices and individual hospitals,

---

BOX 8.2   Difficult market conditions for Yunnan Kidney Disease Hospital

Founded in 1997, Yunnan Kidney Disease Hospital is a nonprofit specialty hospital in Kunming, the capital city of Yunnan province. At the end of 2014, the hospital had 140 employees, including 42 physicians. With 160 beds and about 100 hemodialysis machines, the hospital provides care for more than 400 renal patients who need long-term treatment. A new campus built in 2015 added 600 beds, a kidney medical center, cardiology center, and women and children medical center. The hospital often admits patients with severe complications who are declined by public hospitals. It sometimes reduces or waives fees for the poor who cannot afford to pay.

The chairperson explained the hospital's difficulties with finance, tax, staffing, and insurance as follows:

- *Finance:* The Guarantee Law of 1995 states that medical facilities belonging to a nonprofit hospital that operates for public objectives shall not be used as guaranties or collateral. This makes it very difficult to get bank mortgage loans. Private nonprofit hospitals have to turn to private equity (PE) or venture capital (VC) firms for funding to expand. However, once PE or VC firms control nonprofit medical institutions, they will no longer be considered nonprofit.

- *Tax burden:* The local government charges enterprise income tax at a rate of 25 percent of any retained earnings from all medical institutions (including nonprofit ones). This is not conventional practice in most other provinces.

- *Staffing:* The hospital recruited more than 100 doctors over the years, but only 32 chose to stay. Most, especially young doctors, left for public hospitals after acquiring professional credentials. The hospital has been able to attract doctors from public hospitals because it gives substantial authority to doctors, including the authority to reduce and even waive medical charges for low-income patients.

- *Insurance reimbursement:* In Yunnan, the reimbursement rate is tied to a medical institution's grading by the local social security department, which may differ from the rating system used by the local health department. For example, some hospitals rated Grade-3 by the local health department are only rated Grade-2 by the local social security department and are reimbursed at a higher rate. Regular delays in insurance payments adds to the hospital's financial pressure.

Sources: Morris and others 2014; Rudd 2011; Turner and others 2016.

based on average hospital revenue in several previous years. This policy is not supportive of private hospitals with their short history of development, especially recent entrants with limited hospital revenue in the start-up phase.

The current price structure gives incentives to both public and private providers to overtreat and overprescribe. This underscores the importance of changing payment and purchasing arrangements to promote social value from both public and private providers, as highlighted in recent policies reinforcing calls to "stop the mechanism of subsidizing health facilities with income from medicines" (county hospital reform) and instructions to "reduce prices for examination, treatment, and tests with large medical equipment" but set reasonable price increases for medical services to "reflect the technical value of the staff, particularly treatment, surgery, nursing, beds, TCM, and other services; and establish a dynamic price adjustment mechanism based on changes of cost and revenue composition." These proposed changes to the price structure will enhance the role of SHI in channeling both private sector growth and existing public sector providers toward providing better social value in health.

Some private investors have entered into public-private partnership (PPP) with public hospitals as a strategy to work around market difficulties, especially to gain access to qualified physicians and specialists and to market their services to high- and middle-income consumers. In exchange for an annual service fee to the public hospital and direct payment to public doctors, a private hospital can use the public hospital's name and staff. In a few cases, the public hospital is a minority shareholder in the newly created private facility.

There are opposing views on whether both partners benefit from these PPP arrangements. Almost no evaluation has been done of the impact on patients' well-being or on efficiency and costs. There are numerous anecdotes about private parties not fulfilling contractual agreements and necessitating government repurchase. Instead of being broadly beneficial partnerships that promote

quality and efficiency, these arrangements of convenience can undermine potential gains to society from fair competition, especially if they promote market power and even monopolies. This highlights the importance of developing institutions in China to promote and regulate well-functioning health markets that promote coordination and integration.

Recommendations for Strengthening Private Sector Engagement

China has taken important steps to formulate policies that enable the private sector to deepen and expand its role in the health system. However, much remains to be done to nudge private sector entities to deliver high-quality, effective health services that improve the lives and health of China's population. The experiences of OECD countries in their struggles to reconcile expectations, policies, ideologies, and actions may also be useful to China's own reform process.

Three core action areas and corresponding implementation strategies include the following (as summarized in table 8.5):

1. A clear, shared vision of the private sector's potential contribution to health system goals
2. Regulatory and enforcement capacity to steer health services production and delivery toward social goals
3. A level playing field across public and private providers to promote active private sector engagement.

Core Action Area 1: A Clear, Shared Vision of the Private Sector's Contribution to Health System Goals

Strategy 1: Identify how the private sector can contribute most effectively to China's vision for health sector development, and publicly endorse and articulate this shared vision
A clear articulation of the role of private enterprise in China's health care system is important to send an unambiguous message to the industry and to allay any ethical or

TABLE 8.5   **Three core action areas and implementation strategies to strengthen private sector engagement in health service delivery**

Core action areas	Implementation strategies
1: A clear, shared vision on private sector's contribution to health system goals	• Identify areas where the private sector can contribute most effectively to China's broad vision for the health sector's development; endorse the shared vision and articulate it publicly and communicate it widely • Move away from quantity targets for private sector market share and instead use a combination of supportive policies and regulatory structures to align private sector entities with health system goals • Formalize the engagement process by drafting guidelines for provincial leadership groups to implement according to local conditions
2: Regulatory and enforcement capacity to steer health service delivery toward social goals	• Conduct a systematic review of existing regulations to harmonize and eliminate out-of-date and inconsistent regulations • Review the current institutional framework and empower it with skills and resources needed to govern a mixed health system with both public and private participants • Adopt policies and regulatory measures to guide private sector engagement and minimize risks associated with growth of poor-quality private providers • Implement guidelines for key regulatory functions • Strengthen regulatory capacity at different levels of the government by training provincial and municipal governments in indirect management of mixed (public and private) health systems, tools of government, and the new regulations and implementation guidelines • Allocate sufficient resources for enforcement
3: Level playing field across public and private providers	• Issue clear guidance on private sector planning, entry requirements, surplus use, and community service requirements • Identify and remove access barriers related to health professionals, land use, equipment purchasing, and professional title appraisal • Introduce equal contracting standards and payment principles for public and private providers

ideological concerns that may be lingering in any sections of the government or society. This vision should be widely communicated to all stakeholders and publicly endorsed. Central to this articulation are clear statements on

• Whether the private sector is seen as becoming an integral part of China's health system;
• Which forms of organization are preferred (for-profit versus not-for-profit); and
• Which areas private participation is most sought in (such as outpatient or inpatient care, specialist tertiary care, VIP services, pharmacies, rehabilitation therapies, eldercare, diagnostics and laboratory services, and prevention).

In most OECD countries, the government plays a much larger role in health care

financing (averaging 75 percent) than in service delivery (averaging 35 percent as measured by the share of inpatient beds and of licensed medical professionals in 15 OECD countries) (Rothgang and others 2010). Private ownership is usually highest in primary care and smallest in hospital services, with outpatient specialist services tending to fall in between (table 8.6). Private sector service delivery is often done by independently licensed physicians who contract with the government or the social insurance system.

Self-employed doctors or private organizations under contract with public or social insurance organizations deliver primary care in most OECD countries; the general practitioners (GPs) in the United Kingdom are a well-known example. As table 8.6 shows, only 10 OECD countries—Chile, Finland, Hungary, Iceland, Israel, Mexico, Portugal, Slovenia, Spain, and

TABLE 8.6   Shares of predominant mode of service provision in OECD countries, by subsector, early 2010s

Country	Primary care		Outpatient specialist		Hospital acute care	
	Predominant form	Share (%)	Predominant form	Share (%)	Predominant form	Share (%)
Australia	Private	89	Private		Public	70
Austria	Private	80+	Private		Public	73
Belgium	Private	75	Private	80	NFP	66
Canada	Private	52	Public		Public	100
Chile	Public	30	Public	40	Public	
Czech Republic	Private	90	Private	60	Public	91
Denmark	Private		Public		Public	97
Estonia	Private	77	Public	84	Public	
Finland	Public	88	Public	90	Public	89
France	Private	65	Private	90	Public	66
Germany	Private	76	Private	76	Public	49
Greece	Private	60	Private	60	Public	69
Hungary	Public	100	Public	61	—	
Iceland	Public	95	Private	60	Public	100
Ireland	Private		Public		Public	88
Israel	Public		Public		—	
Italy	Private	65	Public		Public	82
Japan[a]	Private		Private		NFP	74
Korea, Rep.	Private		Private		NFP	65
Luxembourg	Private		Private		Public	68
Mexico	Public	78	Public		Public	65
Netherlands	Private	54	Private	50	NFP	100
New Zealand	Private	52	Public		Public	81
Norway	Private		Public	70	Public	99
Poland	Private	76	Private		Public	95
Portugal	Public	100	Public		Public	86
Slovak Republic	Private	98	Private		Public	60
Slovenia	Public	67	Public	65	—	
Spain	Public	97	Public	88	Public	74
Sweden	Public		Public	17	Public	98
Switzerland	Private		Private	60	Public	83
Turkey	Public		Public		Public	90
United Kingdom	Private	100	Public	95	Public	96
United States	Private		Private	30–50	NFP	60

Sources: Hospital acute care data from Paris, Devaux, and Wei 2010. Primary care and outpatient specialist service data (as of April 2014) from Question 27, OECD Health System Characteristics (HSC) survey 2012 (http://www.oecd.org/els/health-systems/characteristics.htm) and Secretariat estimates.
Note: — = not available; NFP = not-for-profit; OECD = Organisation for Economic Co-operation and Development. Shading of table cells designates the following: <gray> = private; <light blue> = public; and <dark blue> = not-for-profit.
a. Japan "private clinic" data from the OECD HSC 2008 questionnaire.

Turkey—provide primary care mainly through public clinics and salaried health personnel.[15] Any private primary care provision is segmented: that is, it takes place outside the core network and is paid for privately, often out-of-pocket.

OECD countries offer many examples of different relative sizes of for-profit and not-for-profit private enterprises in the health sector (figure 8.8). Denmark, Iceland, and New Zealand limit the core hospital network to government-owned hospitals.[16] Most countries have relatively little private ownership of hospitals. Canada and the Netherlands permit only not-for-profit hospitals in the private sector. In the few countries with relatively large private hospital sectors, not-for-profit hospitals dominate in Belgium, Japan, the Republic of Korea, and the United States; the private for-profit sector plays an important role only in Germany, Greece, France, Mexico, and the Slovak Republic.

Strategy 2: Move away from quantity targets, instead combining policies and regulatory structures to align private sector entities with health system goals
No OECD country has used quantitative targets to expand the private sector. Policy initiatives that expand private activity in OECD countries always involve considerable effort to build and strengthen policies, processes, and regulatory structures for "indirectly" governing health care service provision.

Likewise, OECD countries also offer many examples that can inform the preferred subsector concentration of private health service providers. In most OECD countries, private service provision plays a strong role in health care delivery—more so in certain subsectors such as primary care than in others such as hospital services. Private providers deliver a large share of services in outpatient care, where services are delivered by independently licensed physicians who contract with the government or the social insurance system. This subsector (and others such as retail pharmacies, laboratory services, and so on) is characterized by well-established quality criteria, which makes it readily contractible and open to competition.

These characteristics do not apply to all inpatient services, and, accordingly, the share of private provision is comparatively lower in the hospital subsector in OECD countries. Outpatient specialist services tend to fall in between, with more public ownership than in primary care services and with policies deployed that constrain operation more than in primary care but less than in hospitals.

FIGURE 8.8   Composition of hospital beds in OECD countries, by ownership type, 2012 or latest data

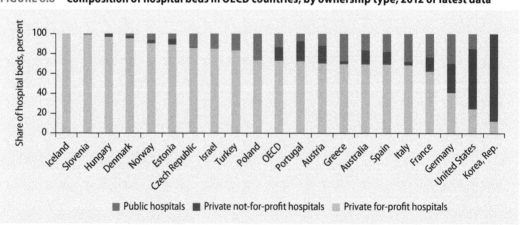

Source: OECD Health Statistics 2013 database 2013.
Note: OECD = Organisation for Economic Co-operation and Development.

Differing historical trajectories are one reason for the different shares of not-for-profit and for-profit hospitals. The other reason is the perceived policy trade-off between mobilizing capital (easiest with corporate for-profit entry) and aligning incentives, because corporate for-profit entities may be more predisposed to opportunistic behavior to increase profits unless a rigorous regulation framework is in place and enforced (Deber 2002). Unlike in primary care where private provision is well accepted, profit-oriented hospitals are viewed with concern—perhaps because hospital services are inherently harder to measure and therefore harder to purchase wisely and regulate (Preker, Harding, and Travis 2000).[17]

Strategy 3: Formalize the engagement process by drafting guidelines for provincial leadership groups
An expanded and integrated private sector role will need sound regulations to ensure patient safety, assure quality, and promote efficiency to align private sector development with social value in health. As noted earlier, regulations are easier to enforce if they are well accepted by those being regulated. Acceptance is more likely if the private sector is consulted and input solicited and if regulations are informed by a good understanding of the perspective of nonstate actors. Dialogue that enables the government and private sector to understand and appreciate each other's perspectives can build trust and foster collaboration.

The State Council might consider drafting guidelines for dialogue between provincial leadership groups and the private health sector. The guidelines could explain the rationale for dialogue and engagement; engagement principles (such as mutual respect, accountability, and results reporting); and mechanisms (forums, meetings, and workshops) that could be implemented according to local conditions, including the range of relevant stakeholders.

It is important that China decide and state its preferences for select forms and subsectors in the health sector where it would like

private enterprise to focus. This clarity will help the capital markets as well as subnational governments, both of which can then develop appropriate supervisory and regulatory mechanisms to guide the private sector in ways that best complement the existing public system of health production and delivery.

Core Action Area 2: Regulatory and Enforcement Capacity to Steer Health Service Delivery Toward Social Goals

The private sector can potentially make a strong contribution to helping achieve national health goals, but this requires a conducive policy and regulatory environment. Indeed, regulations and incentives have a powerful influence on all health providers, whether public or private.

Strategy 1: Conduct a systematic review to harmonize and eliminate outdated and inconsistent regulations
Private provision is widespread in OECD health systems, but providers do not operate in totally free markets. Expanded private activity in OECD countries has invariably come with considerable effort to build and strengthen policies and processes for "indirectly" governing health care service provision.

Governments use several kinds of policy tools to manage mixed health systems by influencing service providers to achieve health care goals of access, financial protection, efficiency, and cost containment (table 8.7). China can draw on considerable international experience in designing and implementing effective regulatory mechanisms to oversee and guide the provision of health services, whether delivered by the public sector or by private enterprises.

Strategy 2: Review the institutional framework and empower it with the skills to govern a mixed health system with both public and private participants
In New South Wales, Australia, the Ministry of Health is the regulatory authority for

TABLE 8.7   Tools of health care governance or indirect policy

Tool	Description	Health sector example
Social regulation	Rules to influence individual and organizational behavior, with an administrative apparatus to sanction noncompliance	All medical doctors must belong to a professional association, and follow its guidelines for high-quality care.
Economic regulation	Rules on prices, output, or entry and exit of firms into markets, with laws and judicial processes to implement and enforce them	Medical insurance reimbursement rates are set for specific services, with maximum markup margins for pharmaceuticals.
Public information	Information to a target audience to influence knowledge and positively alter behavior	Websites give public access to data on hospital quality measures.
Contracting	Enlistment of private organizations to deliver services on behalf of government agency to an identified group via a formal agreement	Government contracts with a private provider for diagnostic services in a defined geographical area.
Accreditation	A recognition of quality and other characteristics, based on well-specified criteria—usually required for social funding eligibility	Health facilities that meet a set of clearly specified criteria (for staffing, quality standards, services, size, opening hours, and so on) receive accreditation, which is reviewed periodically.
Taxation	Tax laws that encourage or discourage certain behaviors by individuals or organizations by diminishing or increasing tax obligations and affecting costs	NFP hospitals are exempt from certain taxes if a percentage of their patients are of low socioeconomic status. Import duties or sales taxes are waived or reduced on items with strong social benefits (such as vaccines).

Source: Adapted from Salamon 2002.
Note: NFP = not-for-profit; OECD = Organisation for Economic Co-operation and Development.

privately owned and operated private health facilities across the state. Guided by the Private Health Facilities Act of 2007, regulation focuses on maintaining appropriate and consistent standards of health care and professional practice in private health facilities as well as on planning for and providing comprehensive, balanced, and coordinated health services throughout the state. The legislation also sets requirements for licensing, including minimum standards for safe, appropriate, and high-quality health care for patients in private health facilities.

Regulating hospital services poses a quite different set of challenges than regulating outpatient services. There are two different approaches to managing mixed hospital networks: an "integrated" approach where all hospitals operate under the same regulations, and a "segmented" approach in which different regulations apply depending on ownership or whether organizations operate for-profit or not-for-profit. Different ownership and organizational structures in OECD countries and their regulatory systems offer useful illustrations for China to consider.

Canada and the Netherlands take a "segmented" approach, in which the core hospital provider network includes only public and private nonprofit hospitals. There is an assumed degree of alignment between national health goals and those of managers of public and nonprofit hospitals who are not under pressure to generate surplus revenues. The policy tools used to guide core networks like these are sometimes referred to as a form of trust-based governance, and they are likely to be ill suited to for-profit organizations (Costain 2000; Deber, Topp, and Zakas 2004). For-profit private hospitals are not eligible for social insurance reimbursement in Canada and the Netherlands. They are lightly regulated and exempt from regulations that seek to ensure equal access and financial sustainability, because they do not have contractual relationships with funding bodies (Busse and others 2002).

In France, Germany, and Switzerland, the core provider network takes an "integrated" approach, consisting of public, nonprofit, and for-profit hospitals that all operate under the same governance regime. Hospitals are relatively independent, and corporate (for-profit) hospitals deliver a substantial share of services. These countries use mechanisms for managing capacity expansion (services and infrastructure) that work with providers of all ownership types (Ettelt and others 2008). This approach allows health agencies to ensure adequate and equitable access, and it gives private hospitals a degree of certainty about expected volume of demand.

These integrated systems have well-established institutional contracting processes that specify providers' obligations and constitute the main mechanism for resolving compliance issues. Contracts typically include both case-based reimbursement rates and agreed minimum and maximum service volumes.[18] Rates and volumes are agreed upon and updated in negotiations between representatives of the purchaser organizations and the hospitals (Busse and others 2002, 136–41), supported by agencies capable of sophisticated cost analyses of case-based reimbursement levels.[19] Box 8.3 describes the indirect policy tools used in Germany's fully integrated mixed hospital market. This governance regime was developed and refined over many years.

BOX 8.3   Use of indirect policy tools in Germany's hospital market

Germany has around 2,000 general hospitals, with about equal numbers of private for-profit, private not-for-profit (owned by churches or other charitable bodies), and public (owned by the subnational governments). Even public hospitals are largely autonomous of government in their day-to-day operations.

Hospitals get most of their funding from (non-profit) social health insurance organizations and are paid per case. (There is also a small private insurance sector.) Providers are reimbursed at agreed-upon rates, which are set to reflect the costs of treatment. Social health insurance organizations' representative body and an association representing all participating hospitals meet periodically to review reimbursement rates and permitted extra charges (such as copayments; supplements for superior accommodation) as well as to negotiate changes. Patients choose hospitals; funds follow those choices.

Prices are fixed, so hospitals compete on quality. Those with reputations for higher-quality health care are likely to be more successful at attracting patients and thus earn more income. However, patients typically have little information or expertise to assess quality. So, even strong competition for patients does not ensure high-quality services. This problem is offset (to some degree) by the use of social regulation policy tools including

- Extensive and effective professional self-regulation and a requirement that all physicians be members of their professional association;

- Mandatory quality reporting to the Federal Quality Assurance Agency; and
- Social insurance reimbursement contracts that require providers to have quality management systems in place and to collect and submit standardized quality information.

Hospitals are accredited by the Cooperation for Transparency and Quality in Healthcare (established by the Association of Social Health Insurers), the Chamber of Physicians, the Hospital Federation, and the Nursing Council. Accreditation is voluntary, but hospitals have strong incentives to earn accreditation because patients and referring physicians can choose among hospitals.

Policy makers also use economic regulations. The Federal Cartel Office, a key economic regulatory agency, reviews proposed mergers and sales of hospitals and is responsible for curbing potential monopoly power and excessive prices. Regional hospital planning bodies also estimate demand for hospital services and approve new hospital facilities or extensions, irrespective of ownership, for inclusion in the socially funded network.

The outcomes from the governance regime are not perfect. Prices are higher than in some other markets in the region. There is a tendency for providers to oversupply well-reimbursed services. But overall, the system supplies a sufficient quantity of mostly high-quality medical services for an overall cost that the public is, on average, willing to pay.

Source: Busse and Blümel 2014.

Strategy 3: Adopt policies and regulatory measures to guide private sector engagement and minimize risks associated with growth of poor-quality private providers

China's early initiatives experimenting with hospital ownership conversions had some successes, but many joint ventures and conversions to full private ownership had such disappointing results that the government repurchased them or reasserted strong oversight (Chen and Zhang 2015). These experiences underline the importance of (a) payment incentives that nudge private providers to national goals, and (b) contractual and other institutional arrangements to regulate and monitor quality as well as to ensure accountability. There are also cautionary examples of potential conflicts of interest when supplier firms invest in hospital ownership.

The famous (or infamous) ownership transformations that took place in Suqian city in Jiangsu after 2000 have provoked sharply conflicting opinions.[20] Opponents of market-oriented approaches cite negative aspects: anecdotal evidence of supplier-induced demand, overtreatment, higher medical cost increases, and compromised medical quality due to profit-driven behavior. Proponents of market-oriented approaches argue that the privatizations brought vitality and increased supply and diversity of health services through market competition.

There has been no rigorous evaluation of the outcomes of Suqian's reforms, and indeed few facts are available for many of the hundreds of ownership conversion cases and other early private sector engagement efforts in China. This is a missed opportunity for valuable learning. Systematic and transparent study of the results of new policies are essential to be able to expand and replicate successes as well as to understand and redirect or stop reforms that fail to achieve their intended goals or that have unacceptable, unexpected negative effects.

Strategy 4: Implement guidelines for key regulatory functions

Denmark is a good example of how rigorous and transparent data collection is a core part of the policy tools used to regulate private providers and ensure good performance (box 8.4). These illustrate the methods most frequently used to regulate and manage primary care delivery in the OECD countries.

Primary care practitioners in Denmark must obtain a license to practice from the Health and Medicines Authority, which is part of the Ministry of Health. They operate under contract with the regional governments that manage capacity and quality by regulating a list of approved practitioners who can receive public reimbursement. A new practitioner cannot obtain authorization for public reimbursement unless a regional government determines it needs an additional practice; otherwise, the practitioner can buy a retiring doctor's practice (and reimbursement authorization). Contracts are nationally standardized and define services to be provided, opening hours, required postgraduate education, and payments, which are a combination of capitation and fee-for-service. A set of social regulations also influence how professionals practice.

All practitioners must follow practice guidelines and quality standards, which are set and continuously updated by their professional associations. They must also allow the national Quality Unit of General Practice to collect quality data and standardized user survey responses from their patients (electronic records automate this). The Quality Unit provides reports to each practice that track and compare their prescribing, use of tests, consistency with treatment guidelines, and patient outcomes with aggregated data for other doctors in the area. This has enabled improved quality of care and patient outcomes, less hospitalization, and lower total costs (Schroll and others 2012).

China's own experience includes examples of effective and successful contracting for primary care services (box 8.5). A study by Hou and others (2012) of more than 5,000 community health stations in 28 cities in 2008 found that government-owned and private stations provided similar basic medical services, and private stations provided public health services (such as

BOX 8.4 Use of indirect policy tools in primary care in Denmark

Primary care and hospital services in Denmark are free of charge as part of the universal, tax-funded health system. Primary care practitioners play a gatekeeping role: patients must be referred by a primary care unit to obtain care from a specialist or hospital. Practitioners are private and self-employed, and most work solo or in small group practices. Patients can choose among nearby practices, and most patients register with a practitioner. Primary care practitioners are contracted by regional authorities, using a nationally agreed-upon contract that is negotiated every two years between the General Practitioners' Association and the payers' association (Health Service Bargaining Committee). This kind of "institutional contracting" is common in health care.

Primary care reimbursement is sufficiently high that the average incomes of primary care practitioners are higher than those of many doctors working in hospitals. The regional government pays a capitation for each registered patient, which provides about one-third of income; the rest comes from fee-for-service reimbursement. Patients can switch registration to a different practice after three months. The "money follows the patient," so practitioners' incomes depend on their success in attracting and keeping patients. Because reimbursement rates are administratively determined, and primary care is free of charge to patients (except for small copayments for pharmaceuticals), the only way practitioners can compete for patients is to offer better care.

There are also social regulations that influence practice. All practitioners belong to the General Practitioners' Association, which, along with the College of General Practice, continuously develops and updates guidelines and distributes them to all primary care practitioners. The Quality Unit of General Practice, a joint body between the Association of Regions and the General Practitioners' Association, coordinates quality development activities and establishes practice quality standards, which members must follow. Patient and practice data are submitted to the Quality Unit as well as patients' responses to standardized user surveys about the care they receive. The Quality Unit uses these data to identify unusual patterns of prescribing, diagnostic tests, and noncompliance with guidelines and also to benchmark patient health outcomes, all with the goal of identifying opportunities to improve quality of care and patient outcomes.

A review of 31 European countries exploring the strength of various features of primary care found Denmark to be particularly strong (Kringos and others 2013). Danes are satisfied with primary care services: 91 percent of Danish respondents to a Eurobarometer survey rated the quality of family doctors as "good," compared with the European Union average of 84 percent (EC 2007). Of course, no system is perfect; a 2013 OECD review concluded that primary health care in Denmark faces challenges related to increasing public and political expectations around the continuity of care (OECD 2013), and the balance between capitation and fee-for-service is contentious. But overall, Denmark's governance regime for primary care appears to work well and align private actors with social goals.

Source: Pedersen, Andersen, and Søndergaard 2012 if not otherwise indicated.

establishing resident health records and distributing health education materials) when paid adequately to do so.

This finding supports those of numerous studies and reviews in other countries that ownership or organizational form has far less effect on results than regulatory oversight, contractual management, quality monitoring, and effective incentives or disincentives. Effective harnessing of private entrepreneurship will be more scalable once China strengthens its regulatory frameworks for governance and accountability, including financial reporting, internal and external audits, and quality assurance mechanisms.

OECD countries have encountered many challenges in developing effective policy and regulatory structures to govern mixed-ownership health service delivery systems. It is a long-term process that requires constant monitoring and improvement, and adjustments in response to evolving conditions. China can avoid many of the pitfalls encountered in other countries as they opened up the health sector.

BOX 8.5   Chinese experiences in purchasing community services from private and public providers

Shandong province has experimented with purchasing community services since 2008 and has established a new model of community health service characterized by government leadership, social responsibility, market mechanisms, and purchasing of services from public and private providers. In Weifang city, for example, the system involves public bidding and competitive awarding of contracts to public and private community health centers (CHCs).

The coverage areas of CHCs and community health stations (CHSs) were defined scientifically at the city level. Community health service centers are set up in places with high concentrations of population without existing centers. Medical institutions in the defined areas can bid to operate these centers. Large hospitals, enterprise hospitals, private medical institutions, and other health resources are guided to run community health care services by the municipal finance bureau and health bureau. In the Municipal Government Procurement Center open tender, bids were won by 16 CHCs (of which 4 were private) and 64 CHSs (of which 38 were private). Public community health service organizations are run by public hospitals or the Chinese Center for Disease Control and Prevention (China CDC); private community health service institutions are either purely private or were transferred from enterprise hospitals.

To ensure a reasonable and data-based fee schedule, a third-party professional organization estimated the costs of labor and transportation, communication, basic supplies, and public health services in accordance with the relevant standards. The payment and purchasing mechanisms were designed to be simple yet achieve accountability for the multiple government objectives. The third-party

assessment mechanism links provider performance to government subsidies and involves accounting firms, experts in community health care, local officials, and community representatives. Payment includes an element of pay-for-performance in that the criteria for CHS performance scores include multiple dimensions of basic care, chronic disease management, community outreach, and community resident satisfaction. Organizations with poor performance receive informed criticism (and no performance rewards). Organizations with two consecutive low rankings can be removed from the social health insurance (SHI) community services network.

A case study assessing Weifang's experience in contracting with private providers for urban primary and preventive health services used data from administrative records; a household survey of more than 1,600 community residents in Weifang and in comparator City Y; and a provider survey of more than 1,000 staff at CHSs in Weifang and City Y, supplemented by interviews with key informants (Wang and others 2013). All CHSs in both cities are nonprofit (public or private-not-for-profit [PNFP]). Analysis revealed that government and private CHSs in Weifang did not differ statistically in their performance on contracted dimensions, after controlling for size and other CHS characteristics. In contrast, comparison City Y had lower performance and a large gap between public and private providers. This was not because the public providers served a more vulnerable mix of patients. In fact, residents in the communities served by private CHSs were of lower socioeconomic status (more likely to be uninsured and to report poor health) than residents in communities served by a government-owned CHS.

Source: Wang and others 2013.

Achieving a regulatory environment that offers similar, predictable, and consistent conditions for public, PFP, and PNFP service providers will be greatly helped by a systematic review of the implementation of the "Measures to Promote the Growth of Nonpublic Medical Institutions"[21] and other recent policies to harmonize and eliminate

out-of-date or inconsistent regulations. The research for this study found examples of underregulation in some areas and overregulation in others as well as inconsistent interpretations and implementation of regulations on PNFPs. Making both public and private health service organizations subject to a "scientific performance evaluation system"[22] will enhance accountability across the health system. Indeed, many of the issues discussed in earlier chapters that need to be resolved to enable China to develop a world-class health care system also undermine China's ability to harness the private sector to help meet social goals in health.

Many observers allege with considerable justification that public and private hospitals in China, regardless of profit status, act very much like for-profit hospitals. Under the current circumstances, public nonprofit and private not-for-profit hospitals might be considered illustrations of what Weisbrod (1988) referred to as "for-profits in disguise." If China wishes to foster nonprofit-oriented behavior among public and PNFP providers, as stated in official policy documents, then incentive, policy, and regulatory structures need to support that goal. OECD country regulations on ownership category (PFP versus PNFP); market size and antitrust enforcement (preventing market dominance and/or monopolies under the pretense of integration and coordination); and conflict of interest (avoiding financial incentives for improper behavior) could be useful examples.

Strategy 5: Strengthen regulatory capacity by training provincial and municipal governments in indirect management of mixed (public and private) health systems, tools of government, and the new regulations and implementation guidelines

In addition to regulations that apply to providers, regulations also need to enable and support provincial governments to use indirect policy tools. A comprehensive review could identify gaps, duplication, and inconsistencies in these regulations. It is also likely that some new or additional institutions, skills, and resources will be needed to govern a mixed health system.

Reforms in Sweden (box 8.6) provide a good example of how governing a mixed health system involved new tasks for existing government agencies and the need for new central agencies. (Similar reforms were made in Finland, Norway, and several East European countries: the Czech Republic,

Estonia, Latvia, Lithuania, Poland, and Romania.)

Strategy 6: Allocate sufficient resources for enforcement

New tasks may require learning new skills. Provincial governments will need training to build capacity to monitor and improve quality of all health care providers, using quality standards that are ownership-neutral. Eligibility for SHI reimbursement is a strong incentive to meet quality standards and can apply equally to public and private providers. It is likely that more resources will be needed by provincial and municipal governments to ensure the staff, transport, and training needed to monitor compliance and enforce regulations.

Researchers have tried to study whether competition has improved quality and reduced cost in China (Liu and others 2009; Pan and others 2015). Consistent with the international evidence, the available evidence from China shows that competition has the potential to improve quality and reduce cost for specific services or cases, but the evidence is mixed on broader systemwide effects (as discussed in box 8.7). This is partly because the institutional context (such as payment incentives and regulatory enforcement capacity) matters greatly when assessing the impact of competition and ownership, and these factors vary across China's provinces and over time.

Researchers and policy makers have been handicapped by the lack of systematic data on quality of care and the extent of essential services provision, as well as a lack of meaningful indicators of the case mix of patients served by different providers. For example, Pan and others (2015) use emergency room mortality as a hospital quality metric, but the hospital's case mix, and mortality after patients leave the hospital, would be important variables to include in an actionable quality evaluation. Similarly, Pan and others (2015) use outpatient waiting times as a measure of outpatient care "quality," because no systematic data are available yet (or released for third-party assessment) in China to

BOX 8.6   Sweden's "Choice" reforms: From government direct delivery to indirect governance of the primary care market

Historically, Sweden's primary care sector of publicly owned health centers employing a multidisciplinary workforce was not as strong as the hospital sector. General practitioner (GP) visits per capita and proportions of GPs to total physicians were low compared with Organisation for Economic Co-operation and Development (OECD) peers. As in China, decision making in Sweden is decentralized; 21 counties operate most hospitals and primary care facilities. Thus, the "Choice" health care reforms—begun in 2007 to improve access, responsiveness, and quality of care while strengthening primary care overall—had to consider the political ideologies of national and county governments.

It was left to counties to decide on the relative importance of the different reform goals and to vary the reform design for the county accordingly. For instance, Stockholm county emphasized increasing access to care and therefore based a large share of provider payments (approximately 40 percent of reimbursement) on the number of GP visits per capita. This was less important in all other counties, where 80 percent or more of reimbursement was through fixed capitation payments based on the number of people listed at each clinic.

The Choice reforms started as a local initiative in one county in 2007; two other counties voluntarily implemented the reform later. Based on these experiences, in 2010 the central government issued a new law requiring all counties to give "freedom of establishment" to private primary care providers that fulfilled local market entry requirements, and provide public payment to people's chosen providers. It was up to county councils to develop the details of the reform based on their context and objectives. Counties decided on eligibility criteria for market entry, levels of public financing, whether patients would register with a clinic actively or passively, and reimbursement models. The national government set the direction but did not provide specific guidance to county councils for developing their individual reform models. Many county councils wanted to learn from the pioneers' experience, and learning exchanges were facilitated.

New functions were established at the central level, and various existing agencies were given new tasks:

- *The Swedish Competition Authority* would evaluate the competitive conditions of the primary care market, to ensure that public and private providers faced the same market conditions.
- *The Legal, Financial and Administrative Services Agency (Kammarkollegiet)* became responsible for providing procurement support to the 21 county councils and developing a national website for tender documents to ensure transparent public procurement.
- *The National Board of Health and Welfare* continued its previous role of supervising and monitoring the quality of care and operations of all counties.
- *The Swedish Association of Local Authorities and Regions* (an employer-interest organization) offered legal advice, provided process support, and organized conferences for county councils implementing the reforms.
- *The Swedish Agency for Health and Care Services Analysis (Vårdanalys)*, was established to strengthen the position of patients and users by analyzing health care and social care services from the perspective of patients and citizens.

These central-level functions were key to providing the framework within which the locally developed reforms operated.

Evaluation of the Choice reforms shows that access to primary care has improved. The number of primary care providers increased 20 percent, contacts with GPs and other primary care providers per capita increased, and providers expanded their phone and visit availability. Evaluations find no systemic differences between public and private providers in quality and efficiency of care. Most counties (except Stockholm) used capitation as the main basis for reimbursement, so the cost of the reform was predictable and cost neutral. Counties that decided to strengthen primary care shifted spending from inpatient care to primary care. There has been heated debate, however, on whether the reform affected equality in health care. Continuity of care does not seem to have improved in most counties. Comparisons of performance of counties is complicated by varying definitions of primary care tasks and compensation requirements.

(Box continued next page)

BOX 8.6   Sweden's "Choice" reforms: From government direct delivery to indirect governance of the primary care market (continued)

County councils continue to tinker with and improve the Choice reforms. In Stockholm county, for instance, the development department has considered how to strengthen coordination of primary care, which reimbursement mechanisms have yielded best results, how to strengthen procedures for banning nonperforming providers from the market, how to improve quality of care for patients with multiple and chronic diseases, and whether competitive neutrality is being sustained. A 2015 report shows that the prerequisites for quality competition are met in all counties; however, in areas with very low population density, the choice of providers is limited by geographical distances. The report also found that some counties have allowed public providers (owned by the counties) to operate with a net loss, which was reprimanded since it threatens competitive neutrality. The report recommends that county councils closely monitor the financial situation of private providers to anticipate and prevent adverse impacts on patients of possible provider bankruptcy.

Sources: Anell 2015; KKV 2014; Swedish NAO 2015; and interviews with Prof. Anders Anell and staff from the Stockholm county council in Stockholm, March 2015.

BOX 8.7   Health care quality assurance and the role of fair competition

Private sector advocates sometimes argue that another layer of bureaucracy for quality assurance is counterproductive because it deters innovation and stifles entrepreneurial experimentation. Fair competition with public hospitals, they suggest, will automatically raise quality standards. But this is not consistent with evidence from China and internationally.

Although public-private competition may bring China benefits in innovation, years of rigorous impact evaluations in Organisation for Economic Co-operation and Development (OECD) countries show that competition does not always improve efficiency and quality. Several studies in the United Kingdom and the United States have found that competition improves quality (Bloom and others 2015; Cooper and others 2011; Gaynor, Moreno-Serra, and Propper 2013; Kessler and McClellan 2000; Propper, Burgess, and Green 2004). Yet other equally rigorous studies have found that competition can lead to quality problems (Capps 2005; Gowrisankaran and Town 2003; Ho and Hamilton 2000; Propper, Burgess, and Gossage 2008).

Competition with appropriate payment incentives (to control spending and reward quality without underservicing) can contribute to social value, whereas competition under fee-for-service can lead to a wasteful "medical arms race." A key challenge is establishing purchasing and payment mechanisms that align entrepreneurship with the goals of people-centered integrated care (PCIC) and social value.

---

evaluate ambulatory care quality in terms of process and outcomes of both private and public providers. Systematic evaluations will be extremely important to know whether reforms are having their intended effect, including whether private providers are helping improve health outcomes.

There are many useful examples of quality assurance measures. One of the most rigorous is that of the Helios hospital group in Germany (box 8.8), which has been adapted by Switzerland as a national system.

Core Action Area 3: Level Playing Field across Public and Private Providers

Leveling the playing field across public and private providers of health services promotes

---

BOX 8.8   Hospital quality measures at Germany's Helios group

Many health care providers in Europe use benchmarking and related management tools to improve the level and consistency of care. The Helios group systematically compares its performance with results for other German hospitals, monitoring 30 diseases and procedures using 142 indicators related to complications, death rates, and so on. All quality data are posted on the company intranet and provided to the health insurance organizations (Krankenkassen), which maintain quality management statistics and publish most of the data regularly. The Helios managers have noted that close

examination of the hospital's results promotes better performance, and they treat quality data for each clinic or department with the maximum degree of transparency.

Helios also ensures that medical protocols are appropriate and regularly updated. At monthly internal conferences, doctors from a selected specialty present difficult cases they have encountered recently, and care protocols are reviewed in the light of specific cases four times a year. Twice each year, the heads of specialty departments meet in groups of 25 to review the medical protocols.

Source: Busse and Blümel 2014.

---

active private sector engagement by helping to create a competitive environment for cost-effective service delivery.

Strategy 1: Issue clear guidance on private sector planning, entry requirements, surplus use, and community service requirements

Licensing a private health facility in China remains variable and costly compared with public facilities. China may consider providing clearer guidance to provincial governments on private sector planning, entry requirements, surplus use, and other community service requirements as well as strictly monitoring enforcement. Periodic reviews and reforms of policies and regulations may be needed to ensure similar treatment of the private sector and public institutions.

Strategy 2: Identify and remove access barriers related to health professionals

China may consider lifting the remaining restrictions, in policy and practice, on allowing doctors to practice at multiple facilities so

that they are mobile and the labor market works. Many examples from within China could be elaborated, especially from provinces such as Guangdong and Fujian, which have been pioneers in this field.

Additionally, China may like to continuously implement policies and regulations to ensure the private sector of treatment similar to public institutions in such aspects as land use, equipment purchasing, and professional title appraisal.

Strategy 3: Introduce equal contracting standards and payment principles

Finally, China may wish to ensure fair and even implementation across all regions of the recent reforms, lifting restrictions on reimbursing private facilities from SHI so that patients have access to more providers. Equal contracting standards and payment principles for both public and private providers are necessary to establish a level playing field, one in which both public and private sector health providers can grow.

Annex 8A   Supplementary Tables

TABLE 8A.1   Overview and comparison of Chinese national and provincial private sector policies in health care service delivery

Policy category	National policy	Regional interpretation and implementation
Market entry		
Vision	• There is lack of clarity in the national government's vision of the private sector role in health.	• Without a shared vision, there is "space" for provincial governments to develop their own vision.
Ownership types	• Private sector policy focuses on the 20 percent target for hospital beds and outpatient service volume. • The PFP and PNFP categories are established in business licensing and tax registration. • PNFPs are established and operated for the public's benefit rather than institutional profits. Any balance or surplus in revenue after expenditures can only be spent on developing the organization to improve quality, introduce advanced technology, expand services, and so on. • PFP health care organizations are those whose earnings are an economic return for investors. • Nongovernment services of a certain quality and scale are encouraged, with emphasis on shifting from small to large medical groups and hospitals with high quality and advanced technology. • PNFPs are preferred because they are more aligned with the public interest.	• Interpretation of ownership types—particularly PNFP—varies by province. • Provincial interpretation of the private sector role falls into three categories: (a) deliver services in rural, peri-urban areas where there are weak public services; (b) establish high-end, large specialty hospitals; and (c) invest in specific medical areas—rehabilitation, nursing, geriatrics, chronic diseases—where the public sector is weak. Few mentioned basic medical services at community and township levels. • Anhui province's vision is comprehensive: encourage the private sector to provide basic medical services in rural areas and to establish high-end specialty medical institutions in urban areas. • To facilitate nongovernmental medical institutions, some provinces limit the number of public hospitals and VIP services offered in public hospitals.
Public hospital conversion	• Policies propose reducing the number of public hospitals by encouraging private entities to assume ownership of public hospitals in a variety of ways. • Initially, the government will pilot reforms of public hospitals in specific regions and in some hospitals run by state-owned enterprises (SOEs). • Hospital conversions should prioritize prevention of national property loss and safeguarding of employee resettlement.	• Provinces want to convert underperforming public and state-owned hospitals. • The reform process focuses on (a) evaluation and disposition of the property of the public hospitals, and (b) resettlement of personnel. • Government is concerned that national property ownership will contract and the workforce will lose stability. • All local governments published regulations governing hospital conversions. • Experience has been mixed, with examples of both failure and success.
Foreign capital	• Foreign business actors can establish medical institutions in China through joint ventures or co-ownership with Chinese counterparts. • The percentage of foreign-owned capital is expected to decline over time. • Qualified foreign capital can eventually establish wholly owned medical institutions in China. • Disagreement remains on allowing WOFIs at the national level. • Overseas investors are allowed to sponsor both PNFP and PFP health care institutions in China. • Overseas investors are encouraged to establish health care institutions in the central and western regions of China. • Investors in Hong Kong SAR, China; Macao SAR, China; and Taiwan, China, receive preferential access in establishing foreign institutions according to relevant rules.	• Many provinces are gradually relaxing limitations on overseas investments. Some are experimenting with wholly owned foreign investments (WOFIs). • At present, most encourage overseas capital to establish high-end facilities and/or services in areas where public resources are relatively weaker. • There are many gaps in policies related to foreign investment.

(Table continued next page)

TABLE 8A.1 Overview and comparison of Chinese national and provincial private sector policies in health care service delivery *Continued*

Policy category	National policy	Regional interpretation and implementation
Land policy	• Relevant departments are responsible for allocating land use for nonpublic medical institutions and should align demand with the urban land plan. • PFP and PNFP medical institutions are subject to land policies and must be qualified licensed operations. • Private medical institutions are not allowed to change the use of land without authorization.	• Most provinces follow similar land use practices in the private health sector. • PNFP medical institutions cannot change the use of land, but can access land through transfers and approved sales or leases. • PFP medical institutions can purchase land. • Private medical institutions receive preferential treatment in Jiangsu if land is used for specific health services (such as nursing, geriatrics, and so on), and in Shaanxi if land is used for hospitals with 500 or more beds.
Approval and licensing	• Regional health planning departments are responsible for authorizing and licensing new PNFP institutions. • Health departments are responsible for verifying that facility types, clinical specialties, bed volume, and so on are appropriate for service capacity. • Priority is given to private medical institutions that conform to local health priorities and plans. • Once entry requirements are met, approval should be timely. • There are no restrictions on nonpublic practice scope. • Foreign investors—through Chinese-foreign joint ventures or cooperation—seek approval from provincial health and commerce departments. • Wholly foreign-owned medical institutions seek approval from the MoH and Ministry of Commerce.	• No two provinces issue licenses alike. There are still many unnecessary procedures and multiple "fees." • Multiple departments within health are involved, depending on the type of activity and size. Approvals are required from multiple public agencies (Commerce, Trade, Fire, and so on). • Key regulations governing market entry are out of date, including the Regulations on Administration of Medical Institutions (State Council and MoH) and the Basic Standard of Medical Institutions (Trail). • Most provinces are trying to simplify the approval process. For example, some provinces assign approval rights to different levels of authority according to the investment scale or number of beds. Others delegate approval right to the county and municipal levels. Some set time limits to encourage faster turnaround.
Operations		
Taxes	• PNFP medical institutions are entitled to the preferential tax policy according to national rules.	• Policies and regulations governing taxes for private medical institutions are generous. • In many provinces, PNFP are exempt from value added tax (VAT) and other taxes (for example, land tax, building tax, and so on). • "Self-made" and "self-used" preparations are exempted from VAT, building tax, land use tax, and car and vessel tax. • In most provinces, PFP medical institutions engaged in improving medical conditions are exempted from the building tax and land use tax for the first three years of business. Some provinces extend this tax holiday beyond three years.

(Table continued next page)

TABLE 8A.1   Overview and comparison of Chinese national and provincial private sector policies in health care service delivery   *Continued*

Policy category	National policy	Regional interpretation and implementation
Price	• The prices of health services and medicine provided by PNFP medical institutions must comply with government pricing schemes. • PFP medical institutions can set their prices of medical services independently.	• Policies governing PNFP medical institutions, health services, and medicine prices are consistent across all the provinces because they must conform to centrally set public health prices. • PNFP and public medical institutions are charged the same cost for electricity, water, and gas. • PFP medical institutions are free to set prices for health services and drugs. Most provinces require PFPs to offer open public access to pricing schemes. • Some provinces set price ceilings—Tianjin for specialty services and technologies, and Hunan for medicines.
Medical Insurance	• Eligible nonpublic medical institutions should be incorporated into the designated hospital lists for the Urban Basic Medical Insurance Scheme for Employees, Retirees and Residents; the New Rural Cooperative Medical Scheme (NRCMS); medical assistance; employment injury insurance; and maternity insurance. • Reimbursement policies for eligible nonpublic medical institutions should be the same as for public institutions. • Local government authorities are prohibited from providing preferential approval of participation with insurance providers based on ownership.	• From the policy review, almost all local governments do not limit social health insurance (SHI) provision to public facilities. The only exception is Shanghai. • However, key informant interviews reveal this is not the actual practice.
Large equipment	• Nonpublic medical institutions are allowed to equip facilities reasonably for practice scope, size, and target population. • Health departments approve the allocation of large medical equipment based on the regional or local large medical equipment allocation plan. • Nonpublic medical institutions' equipment needs should be given full consideration and integrated into the formulation and adjustment of the large medical equipment allocation plan. • Approval of large medical equipment is simultaneous with institutional and services license approval. • The health authority cannot limit the allocation of large medical equipment for qualified institutions that meet allocation quota.	• Similar to facility and business licensing, approval for large medical equipment is implemented in different ways across provinces. • Although most provinces have relaxed the quotas for large medical equipment for nonpublic medical institutions on paper, in practice, provincial and local governments continue to limit the number of approvals.

(Table continued next page)

TABLE 8A.1   Overview and comparison of Chinese national and provincial private sector policies in health care service delivery   *Continued*

Policy category	National policy	Regional interpretation and implementation
Government purchasing	• Health authorities are encouraged to contract eligible nonpublic medical institutions to provide health services on behalf of public health or government authorities. • Priorities for contracting include supporting health services in rural and remote areas. • Nonpublic medical institutions, especially community-level medical service centers and clinics, are encouraged to play an active role in the basic medical service system. • Nonpublic medical institutions shall receive compensation from the government in accordance with relevant regulations. • Nonpublic medical institutions should complement government initiatives during public health emergencies.	See chapter 6 (Realigning Purchasing and Provider Incentives)
Switching legal status	• PNFP medical institutions are not allowed to change to PFP status in principle unless there is approval by the original administrative authorities. • PFP medical institutions can apply to change to PNFP status by following procedures outlined in the law. After conversion, the institution must comply with applicable national price policy and tax policy.	All provinces, except for Jiangsu province, implement the policies consistently according to terms outlined in State Council policies.
Personnel	• Medical personnel sign labor contracts with nonpublic medical institutions according to the law and should be enrolled in social insurance.	• All provinces now encourage the "free flow" of health personnel between public and private health facilities.
Multisite practice	• The National Health and Family Planning Commission (NHFPC), the National Development and Reform Commission (NDRC), the Ministry of Human Resources and Social Security (MoHRSS), the State Administration of Traditional Chinese Medicine, and the China Insurance Regulatory Commission issued the policy opinions on doctor multisite licensed practice in January 2014, encouraging flow of medical personnel between public and nonpublic medical institutions.	• Several provinces have policies prohibiting public health facilities from preventing multisite practice. • Most provinces are moving to liberalize restrictions on multisite practice such as no longer requiring public hospital administrators' approval. • Beijing is a pioneer in promoting multisite practice. • However, in practice many provincial public hospitals restrict labor movement. See chapter 7 (Strengthening the Health Workforce) for more details.
Professional status	• Academic status, title evaluation, vocational skill evaluation, or professional and vocational skill training of medical personnel should not be influenced by place of employment. • MoHRSS authority should include nonpublic institutions in professional training and other regular guidance according to their grade.	

(Table continued next page)

TABLE 8A.1 **Overview and comparison of Chinese national and provincial private sector policies in health care service delivery** *Continued*

Policy category	National policy	Regional interpretation and implementation
Supervision of medical institutions	• Nonpublic medical institutions are subject to State Council and MoH regulations on administration of medical institutions. • Health authorities should include nonpublic medical institutions in the medical quality control evaluation system. • Practice conditions of nonpublic medical institutions and associated personnel should be checked, evaluated, and verified through daily supervision and management, site visits, and physician assessments. • Illegal medical practice and medical fraud is punishable by law. • Medical advertisements of nonpublic medical institutions are regulated, and false and illegal medical advertisements are forbidden.	• All provinces stress the need to bring nonpublic medical institutions into the quality system. • Provincial regulations emphasize quality and client satisfaction as well as the importance of accurate and regular reporting. • However, many provincial government officials interviewed explained that they do not have sufficient staff or capacity to effectively monitor and supervise the growing number of nonpublic medical providers.

Note: MoH = Ministry of Health; MoHRSS = Ministry of Human Resources and Social Security; PFP = private for-profit; PNFP = private not-for-profit; WOFIs = wholly owned foreign investments.

TABLE 8A.2 Summary of policies on the social capital sponsoring medical institutions, by region

Regions	Access policies						Human resource policies			Medical insurance	Price policies	Tax policies	Supervision policies
	Encouraged in high-tech and characteristic regions	Encouraged in remote/developing regions	Encouraged in urban center districts	Encouraging public hospital ownership conversión	Permitting overseas capital	Simplifying and regulating the approval procedures	Introducing high-end talent	Hiring retired staff	Doctor multisite licensed practice	Incorporating into the designated hospital lists	Non-profit hospital: government guidance price / profit-hospital: market adjusted price	For-profit medical institution: exempt from business tax	Establishing supervision mechanism
Beijing	✓	✓		✓	✓	✓	✓		✓	✓	✓	✓	✓
Tianjin	✓	✓		✓	✓	✓			✓	✓	✓	✓	
Hebei	✓	✓		✓	✓	✓			✓	✓	✓	✓	✓
Shanxi	✓	✓		✓	✓	✓			✓	✓	✓	✓	✓
Inner Mongolia	✓	✓		✓	✓	✓		✓	✓	✓	✓	✓	✓
Liaoning	✓	✓		✓	✓	✓			✓	✓	✓	✓	✓
Jilin	✓	✓		✓	✓	✓			✓	✓	✓	✓	✓
Heilongjiang						✓			✓				✓
Shanghai	✓	✓		✓	✓	✓	✓		✓	✓	✓	✓	✓
Jiangsu	✓	✓		✓	✓	✓		✓	✓	✓	✓	✓	✓
Zhejiang	✓	✓	✓	✓	✓	✓		✓	✓	✓	✓	✓	✓
Anhui	✓	✓		✓	✓	✓		✓	✓	✓	✓	✓	✓
Fujian	✓	✓		✓	✓	✓	✓	✓	✓	✓	✓	✓	✓
Jiangxi	✓	✓		✓	✓	✓		✓	✓	✓	✓	✓	✓
Shandong	✓	✓		✓	✓	✓		✓	✓	✓	✓	✓	✓
Henan		✓	✓	✓	✓	✓	✓	✓	✓	✓	✓	✓	✓
Hubei	✓	✓		✓	✓	✓		✓	✓	✓	✓	✓	✓

Notes

1. "Planning Layout of National Medical and Health Services System (2015–2020)"; "Opinions of the State Council on Comprehensively Scaling up Reform of County-Level Public Hospitals"; and "Measures to Promote the Growth of Nonpublic Medical Institutions," General Office of the State Council (*Guo Ban Fa* 2015, Nos. 14, 33, 45).

2. Barefoot doctors are "farmers who received a short medical and paramedical training, to offer primary medical services in their rural villages" (Yang and Wang 2017).

3. "Planning Layout of National Medical and Health Services System (2015–2020)," General Office of the State Council (*Guo Ban Fa* 2015, No. 14).

4. "Main Tasks of Deepening Medical Reform," General Office of the State Council (*Guo Ban Fa* 2015, No. 34).

5. Hospital numbers and ownership data in the tables and graphs are from the *Chinese Health Statistical Year Book 2013* (published through 2013 by the Ministry of Health) unless otherwise indicated. The team analyzed the data using standard international definitions (as explained in box 8.1) to determine the number of PFP and PNFP hospitals.

6. Statistics for 2015 were not yet available at the time of writing.

7. "VIP service" refers to enhanced patient access to services for an extra charge.

8. The correlation coefficient between per capita income and private share is near zero (0.06) and becomes negative when outliers Tianjin or Jiangsu are excluded.

9. The review focused on private health services only.

10. "Opinions of the State Council on Comprehensively Scaling up Reform of County-Level Public Hospitals," State Council (*Guo Ban Ga* 2015, No. 33a).

11. "Opinions on Promoting the Development of Health Services Industry," Hunan Provincial People's Government (*Hunan Provincial Governmental Announcement* 2012, No. 30).

12. For a more detailed discussion of the Aier Eye Hospital Group and Wuhan Asia Heart Hospital, see chapter 5.

13. "Measures to Promote the Growth of Nonpublic Medical Institutions," State Council General Office (*Guo Ban Fa* 2015, No. 45).

14. "Planning Layout of National Medical and Health Services System (2015–2020)," General Office of the State Council (*Guo Ban Fa* 2015, No. 14)

15. Budget allocations to public clinics are typically based on the number of residents served in a defined geographical area or catchment area.

16. OECD country hospital network data from the OECD Health System Characteristics Survey 2012, http://www.oecd.org/els/health-systems/characteristics.htm.

17. "Measurability" refers to the precision with which health care service inputs, processes, outputs, and outcomes can be specified and measured (Preker, Harding, and Travis 2000, 782).

18. In "cost and volume contracts" (widely used in the United Kingdom also), hospitals receive an agreed-upon sum for a specified baseline level of activity (number of cases, treatments), and beyond that level, funding is per case, at a specified rate per case. The baseline helps hospitals plan, and the maximum volume helps authorities control expenditure (see Duran and others 2005).

19. For an overview of these mechanisms and processes, see the introduction to Busse and others 2011.

20. Suqian—a large city in Jiangsu, with very limited government health assets and resources to expand health services—from 2000, tried three different models to convert ownership of all township hospitals and most urban hospitals: a transfer of net assets and auction of intangible assets; a joint-stock cooperative system; and a merger and mandatory administration. Among many changes, the reformed hospitals gained decision rights (including inputs, outputs, outcomes, and process/management) and became residual claimants to hospital net revenues for all hospital operations, competing on the market for patients. Hospitals undertook some social functions without government compensation (Chen 2015; Liu 2015; Zhou 2015).

21. "Measures to Promote the Growth of Nonpublic Medical Institutions," State Council General Office (*Guo Ban Fa* 2015, No. 45).

22. As called for in the "Opinions on County Public Hospitals," State Council General Office (*Guo Ban Fa* 2015, No. 33).

References

Anell, Anders. 2015. "The Public-Private Pendulum—Patient Choice and Equity in Sweden." *New England Journal of Medicine* 372 (1): 1–4.

Bloom, Nicholas, Carol Propper, Stephan Seiler, and John Van Reenen. 2015. "The Impact Of Competition on Management Quality: Evidence from Public Hospitals." *Review of Economic Studies* 82 (2): 457–89.

Brixi, H., Y. Mu, B. Targa, and D. Hipgrave. 2013. "Engaging Sub-national Governments in Addressing Health Equities: Challenges and Opportunities in China's Health System Reform." *Health Policy and Planning* 28 (8): 809–24.

Busse, Reinhard, and Miriam Blümel. 2014. "Germany: Health System Review." *Health Systems in Transition* 16 (2): 1–296.

Busse, Reinhard, Alexander Geissler, Wilm Quentin, and Miriam M. Wiley, eds. 2011. *Diagnosis-Related Groups in Europe: Moving towards Transparency, Efficiency and Quality in Hospitals*. Berkshire, U.K.: Open University Press, McGraw-Hill International, for the World Health Organization on behalf of the European Observatory on Health Systems and Policies.

Busse, Reinhard, Tom van der Grinten, and Per-Gunnar Svensson. 2002. "Regulating Entrepreneurial Behaviour in Hospitals: Theory and Practice." In *Regulating Entrepreneurial Behaviour in European Health-Care Systems*, edited by Richard B. Saltman, Reinhard Busse, and Elias Mossialos, 126–45. Buckingham, U.K.: Open University Press for the World Health Organization.

Capps, Cory Stephen. 2005. "The Quality Effects of Hospital Mergers." Economic Analysis Group Discussion Paper 05-6, Antitrust Division, U.S. Department of Justice.

Chen, Qiulin, and Wei Zhang. 2015. "To Privatize or Not to Privatize: The Political Economy of Hospital Ownership Conversion in China." Working paper, Renmin University of China and Chinese Academy of Social Sciences.

Chen, X. J. 2015. "Chen Xingjie: Falling Qiu He Did the Right Thing to Wipe Out All Public Hospitals in Suqian." Caijing.com article.

Cooper, Zack, Stephen Gibbons, Simon Jones, and Alistair McGuire. 2011. "Does Hospital Competition Save Lives? Evidence from the English NHS Patient Choice Reforms." *The Economic Journal* 121 (554): F228–F260.

Costain, D. 2000. "Regulating Quality & Price in Private UK Health Markets." Oxford Policy Institute (OPI) Seminar Series "Issues in Health Sector Regulation," Oxford, U.K.

Deber, R. 2002. "Delivering Health Care Services: Public, Not-for-Profit, or Private." Discussion Paper No. 17, Commission on the Future of Health Care in Canada (Romanow Commission).

Deber, R., A. Topp, and D. Zakas. 2004. "Private Delivery and Public Goals: Mechanisms for Ensuring that Hospitals Meet Public Objectives." Unpublished background paper for the World Bank, Washington, DC.

Duran, Antonio, Igor Sheiman, Markus Scheider, and John Øvretveit. 2005. "Purchasers, Providers, and Contracts." In *Purchasing to Improve Health Systems Performance*, edited by Josep Figueras, Ray Robinson, and Elke Jakubowski, 187–214. London: European Observatory on Health Care Systems and Policies.

EC (European Commission). 2007. "Health and Long-Term Care in the European Union." Special Eurobarometer Report No. 283, EC, Brussels.

Ettelt, Stefanie, Ellen Nolte, Sarah Thomson, and Nicholas Mays. 2008. "Capacity Planning in Health Care: A Review of the International Experience." Policy brief, World Health Organization on behalf of the European Observatory on Health Systems and Policies, Copenhagen.

Gaynor, Martin, Rodrigo Moreno-Serra, and Carol Propper. 2013. "Death by Market Power: Reform, Competition, and Patient Outcomes in the National Health Service." *American Economic Journal: Economic Policy* 5 (4): 134–66.

Glucksman, James, and Roberta Lipson. 2010. "Private Healthcare: A Tough Market to Crack." *China Business Review* 37 (1): 30–34.

Gowrisankaran, Gautam, and Robert J. Town. 2003. "Competition, Payers, and Hospital Quality." *Health Services Research* 38 (6 Pt 1): 1403–22.

Gu, Edward, and Jianjun Zhang. 2006. "Health Care Regime Change in Urban China: Unmanaged Marketization and Reluctant Privatization." *Pacific Affairs* 79 (1): 49–71.

Ho, Vivian, and Barton H. Hamilton. 2000. "Hospital Mergers and Acquisitions: Does Market Consolidation Harm Patients?" *Journal of Health Economics* 19 (5): 767–91.

Hou, Wanli, Hong Fan, Jing Xu, Fang Wang, Yun Chai, Hancheng Xu, Yongbin Li, Liqun Liu, Bin Wang, and Zuxun Lu. 2012. "Service Functions of Private Community Health Stations in China: A Comparison Analysis with Government-Sponsored Community Health Stations." *Journal of Huazhong University of Science and Technology* 32 (2): 159–66.

Hou, X., and J. Coyne. 2008. "The Emergence of Proprietary Medical Facilities in China." *Health Policy* 88 (1): 141–51.

Huang, Cunrui, Haocai Liang, Cordia Chu, Shannon Rutherford, and Qingshan Geng. 2009. "The Emerging Role of Private Health Care Provision in China: A Critical Analysis of the Current Health System." Asia Health Policy Program Working Paper No. 10, Stanford University, Stanford, CA.

Kessler, Daniel P., and Mark B. McClellan. 2000. "Is Hospital Competition Socially Wasteful?" *Quarterly Journal of Economics* 115 (2): 577–615.

KKV (Konkurrensverket [Swedish Competition Authority]). 2014. "Etablering och konkurrens bland vårdcentraler – om kvalitetsdriven konkurrens och ekonomiska villkor" [Establishment and Competition among Health Centers: About Quality-Driven Competition and Economic Conditions]. Report No. 2014:2, KKV, Stockholm.

Kringos, D., W. Boerma, Y. Bourgueil, T. Cartier, T. Dedeu, T. Hasvold, A. Hutchinson, and others. 2013. "The Strength of Primary Care in Europe: An International Comparative Study." *British Journal of General Practice* 63 (616): e742–50.

Liu, G. L. 1994. "Privatization of the Medical Market in Socialist China: A Historical Approach." *Health Policy* 27 (2): 157–74.

Liu, G., H. Guan, and C. Gao. 2013. "Analysis on Status Quo of Private Care in China." *China Journal of Health Policy* 6 (9): 41–46.

Liu, Gordon G., Lin Li, Xiaohui Hou, Judy Xu, and Daniel Hyslop. 2009. "The Role of For-Profit Hospitals in Medical Expenditures: Evidence from Aggregate Data in China." *China Economic Review* 20 (4): 625–33.

Liu, W. 2015. "Why Did Suqian Rebuild the Public Hospital Ten Years after Selling It?" Southern Weekend, infzm.com, March 5. http://www.infzm.com/content/108036.

Liu, Yuanli, Peter Berman, Winnie Yip, Haocai Liang, Qingyue Meng, Jiangbin Qu, and Zhonghe Li. 2006. "Health Care in China: The Role of Nongovernment Providers." *Health Policy* 77 (2): 212–20.

OECD (Organisation for Economic Co-operation and Development). 2013. *OECD Reviews of Health Care Quality: Denmark 2013. Raising Standards*. Paris: OECD.

Pan, Jay, Xuezheng Qin, Qian Li, Joseph P. Messina, and Paul L. Delamater. 2015. "Does Hospital Competition Improve Health Care Delivery in China?" *China Economic Review* 33 (C): 179–99.

Paris, V., M. Devaux, and L. Wei. 2010. "Health Systems Institutional Characteristics: A Survey of 29 OECD Countries." Organisation for Economic Co-operation and Development Health Working Paper No. 50, OECD, Paris. doi:10.1787/5kmfxfq9qbnr-en.

Pedersen Kjeld Møller, John Sahl Andersen, and Jens Søndergaard. 2012. "General Practice and Primary Health Care in Denmark." *Journal of the American Board of Family Medicine*. 25 (Suppl 1): S34–S38. doi:10.3122/jabfm.2012.02.110216J.

Preker, A. S., A. Harding, and P. Travis. 2000. "'Make or buy' Decisions in the Production of Health Care Goods and Services: New Insights from Institutional Economics and Organizational Theory." *Bulletin of the World Health Organization* 78 (6): 779–90.

Propper, Carol, Simon Burgess, and Denise Gossage. 2008. "Competition and Quality: Evidence from the NHS Internal Market 1991–9." *The Economic Journal* 118 (525): 138–70.

Propper, Carol, Simon Burgess, and Katherine Green. 2004. "Does Competition between Hospitals Improve the Quality of Care? Hospital Death Rates and the NHS Internal Market." *Journal of Public Economics* 88 (7): 1247–72.

Ramesh, M., Xun Wu, and Alex Jingwei He. 2014. "Health Governance and Healthcare Reforms in China." *Health Policy and Planning* 29 (6): 663–72. doi:10.1093/heapol/czs109.

Rothgang, H., M. Cacace, L. Frisina, S. Grimmeisen, A. Schmid, and C. Wendt. 2010. *The State and Health Care: Comparing OECD Countries*. Basingstoke, U.K.: Palgrave Macmillan.

Salamon, Lester M., ed. 2002. *The Tools of Government: A Guide to the New Governance*. New York: Oxford University Press.

Schroll, Henrik, René dePont Christensen, Janus Laust Thomsen, Morten Andersen, Søren Friborg, and Jens Søndergaard. 2012. "The Danish Model for Improvement of Diabetes Care in General Practice: Impact of Automated Collection and Feedback of Patient Data." *International Journal of Family Medicine* 2012: Article ID 208123. doi:10.1155/2012/208123.

State Council. 2011. "The 12th Five-Year Plan for Economic and Social Development of the People's Republic of China (2011–2015)." Translated by the Compilation and Translation Bureau, Central Committee of the Communist Party of China. Beijing: Central Compilation & Translation Press.

Swedish NAO (National Audit Office [Riksrevisionen]). 2015. "Primärvårdens styrning – efter behov eller efterfrågan?" [Primary Care Management: As Needed or Demand?]. Review Report No. 2014:22, Swedish NAO, Stockholm.

Tang, C., Y. Zhang, L. Chen, and Y. Lin. 2014. "The Growth of Private Hospitals and Their Health Workforce In China: A Comparison with Public Hospitals." *Health Policy and Planning* 29 (1): 30–41.

Wang, Yan, Karen Eggleston, Zhenjie Yu, and Qiong Zhang. 2013. "Contracting with Private Providers for Primary Care Services: Evidence from Urban China." *Health Economics Review* 3: 1–20. doi:10.1186 /2191-1991-3-1.

Weisbrod, B. 1988. *The Nonprofit Economy.* Cambridge, MA: Harvard University Press.

Yang, Le, and Hongman Wang. 2017. "Medical Education: What about the Barefoot Doctors?" *The Lancet* 390 (10104): 1736.

Yip, Winnie, and William Hsiao. 2014. "Harnessing the Privatization of China's Fragmented Health-Care Delivery." *The Lancet* 384 (9945): 805–818. doi:10.1016/ S0140-6736(14)61120-X.

Zhang, Mengzhong. 2006. "The Development of Private-Owned Hospitals in China: Can Health Policies be Transferred from Other Countries in China?" Network of Asia-Pacific Schools and Institutes of Public Administration and Governance, New Delhi.

Zhou, Qiren. 2015. "Zhou Qiren Talks about Suqian Health-Care Reform." 22ccom.net article.

Lever 8: Modernizing Health Service Planning to Guide Investment

Introduction

To promote people-centered integrated care (PCIC) and ensure that the health system places more emphasis on people's needs, capital investment decisions must reinforce the strengthening of primary health care (PHC) so that the population can obtain access to affordable health care at the right place and at the right time. This implies shifting the focus of capital investments from tertiary to primary health care and, within tertiary care, to deepening the delivery system rather than expanding it further. This is at the fundamental basis of service planning, which is the substance of this chapter.

More than half of all first contacts with the health care delivery system in China for an illness occur in hospitals, which account for 54 percent of the country's health spending, according to the *China Health Statistical Yearbook 2013*. The number of inpatient discharges has grown at a rate of 12 percent per year, and in keeping with this trend, hospital revenue has grown at an annual rate of 23.6 percent (2011–13) and is expected to exceed RMB 4 trillion by 2017. Fueling this growth are the huge capital investments in the hospital sector, which have made the

system increasingly top-heavy and have contributed to further escalating costs.

As mentioned in chapter 1, patients tend to go directly to hospitals even for outpatient care, and there is no gatekeeping at lower levels. Since 2005, bed-per-population ratios have increased by 56 percent and admission rates have more than doubled, reaching levels higher than in most middle-income countries and approaching Organisation for Economic Co-operation and Development (OECD) averages.

The health sector in China is growing rapidly. Industry analysts predict it will exceed US$1 trillion and constitute over 7 percent of the country's gross domestic product (GDP) by 2020, which would triple 2010 levels and make it the second largest health care market in the world, behind the United States (EIU 2015; Le Deu and others 2012). Annual capital investment in the health sector will potentially reach US$50 billion within the same time frame. The question of value for money with these resources—important even at existing levels—will become fundamental, especially as the country progresses toward its commitment of affordable, equitable, and effective health care for all by 2020.

This chapter examines capital planning strategies in China and in selected OECD countries, and proposes a framework to introduce modern service planning techniques in the capital investment planning process. The next section examines the challenges in China's current capital investment planning practices. Later the chapter draws upon experiences from within China and OECD countries to offer a series of actionable recommendations for aligning capital investments with the service needs of the population served by the health system.

Capital Investment Challenges in China's Health Sector

Capital investment refers to the acquisition of capital assets or fixed assets such as land, clinics, hospitals, or equipment that is expected to be productive over many years. Two key challenges characterize China's current capital investment planning (CIP) model: (a) a lack of investment planning, which contributes to super scaling of investments, particularly at the hospital level; and (b) a focus on construction to expand network capacity rather than to deepen the existing infrastructure's capacity to better meet the population's health needs. With disproportionate expansion of hospital infrastructure in urban areas, the net result is a hospital-centric system characterized by large, well-endowed urban hospitals and relatively few or poorly endowed rural ambulatory facilities.

A Call for People-Centered Capital Investment Planning

Capital spending in the health sector among provinces in China accounts for 5–10 percent of total public spending on health. In comparison, the average capital spending in OECD countries is 7 percent of total public spending on health,[1] while among European countries, capital spending varies between 2 percent and 6 percent of total public health spending (Rechel and others 2010).[2]

However, each yuan invested in capital also determines future recurrent expenditure

allocations, as a result of which more than 54 percent of total public health spending is directed to hospitals. In comparison, levels in OECD countries are predominantly below 50 percent (and averaging 38 percent). Furthermore, the ratio of beds to population in most provinces has already exceeded the average among OECD countries.

In the past decade, the number of hospitals increased by 50 percent. During this period, the number of public hospitals has decreased, while the number of private hospitals has increased, and the number of beds nationwide has doubled. Although these levels of investments in hospitals may have been necessary to satisfy unmet demand and growing population needs, continued expansion can have serious fiscal implications for the health sector in the near future.

Addressing these problems calls for a shift in how capital investment is planned in China's health sector. The traditional input-based planning system—in which decisions are not based on actual demand but are driven by high-level macro standards—has to give way to an approach that considers the changing epidemiological and demographic profiles and emphasizes effective regionalization and integration of care with new technologies (box 9.1). This people-centered service planning approach—in which production and delivery of services are based on population needs—prioritizes public investments according to the burden of disease, where people live, the kind of daily care people need, wellness, and so on.

Under this people-centered approach, CIP identifies and exploits all funding opportunities (including insurance and direct public budgetary funding) to guide the development of facilities of the future and ensure that excess capacity is not created that further exacerbates inefficiency and capital misallocation. It offers the opportunity to remake the health provider network—its design, culture, and practices—to better meet the needs of patients and families and the aspirations of those that provide them with health care. Consideration of the private sector's role in meeting the population's service needs is also

---

BOX 9.1   **Distinguishing features of an effective health service planning approach**

- Needs-based planning linked to specific health challenges
- Long-term perspective by using demographic, epidemiological, and urban development plans
- Balance in real demand and supply
- Integrated networks that deliver services required by catchment populations
- Capital expenditure (CAPEX) allocations to provinces that correct for equity and level of deprivation

- Increased proportion of outpatient care, including primary health care, day surgeries, and day hospitals
- Increase in general hospitals with fewer mono-profile facilities
- Use of spatial analysis with geographic information system (GIS) to ensure access
- Integrated perspectives in terms of buildings, people, and technology
- Use of private sector as partner in reaching health goals.

---

critical to reducing the public sector's capital requirements and optimizing utilization of existing capacity.

The need to develop a CIP model driven by service planning based on population needs is well understood in China, and several efforts have already been undertaken to improve resource allocation and investment planning. Since the 1990s, regional health planning has been conducted as part of health policy reforms to improve performance of the health sector. In 1997, the National Development and Reform Commission (NDRC), Ministry of Health, and Ministry of Finance jointly issued "Guidance of Implementation of Regional Health Planning," which provided details on the concepts, contents, methods, procedures, and implementation of regional health planning, and demonstrated recognition of the need for capital planning to be driven by population health needs. Local governments were expected to plan and project health care delivery according to these guidelines.

However, despite the efforts of the national government agencies, regional and local health planning has still not adopted an efficient and integrated service approach, and capital planning strategies continue to favor larger hospitals. A significant share of all hospital investments is funded from debt financing, off-balance sheet operations, or land swaps, which also compromise the

government's efforts to reduce the pressure on prices. Further, the high level of fragmentation and lack of transparency and accountability limit the effectiveness of these subsidies as policy instruments. Public subsidies for capital investments are not being fully used as a top-down mechanism to develop a rational, patient-centered network capable of responding to the population's changing health needs while delivering value for money.

A key challenge, therefore, relates to coordination and compliance with the national guidelines and standards at the provincial level to ensure that capital investments are used to shape a people-centered provider network that delivers the right care, at the right place, and at the right time. Although the National Health and Family Planning Commission (NHFPC)[3] leads on setting broad planning goals, and the NDRC examines and approves the project, much of the investment is based on bottom-up goals from the provinces and cities without consideration of the service needs or the existing installed (public and private) capacity before approvals are issued.

An initial step in the right direction was the 2015 issuance of policy guidelines that aim to rationalize capital investments— specifying functions and roles of health facilities, staffing standards, vertical integration across tiers, and horizontal integration across types of care and aim to rationalize capital investments.[4] However, capital investment needs to be further integrated into regional service planning and ensure that private sector capacity is considered within the targets for 2020.

Health Investment Planning Challenges: A Survey of Three Provinces

An analysis of capital investment decisions in three provincial administrative regions—Sichuan province, Hubei province, and the Tianjin municipality, which vary across demographic, economic development, public resources, and health indicators—reveals many fundamental challenges in the investment models being employed in the health sector in China.

Sichuan province. The main challenges for the western province of Sichuan include control of hospital expansion and an uneven distribution of health personnel. Figure 9.1 depicts the results of hospital-centric CIP in Sichuan. Although hospital growth reached a plateau in 2010–12, the average annual

growth rate (10 percent) over the four-year period remained significantly higher than that of other types of health facilities, while the average annual growth rates of other facility types, including PHC facilities, became negative over time.

From 2012 to 2014, the local government spent RMB 1.01 billion on capital investment projects related to prefecture-level facilities, while only spending RMB 369.96 million on capital investment projects related to major disease prevention and control. Furthermore, in 2012, Sichuan hospitals (including general or comprehensive, traditional Chinese medicine, and special and national hospitals) represented RMB 40.79 billion of fixed assets, whereas health care institutions at the basic level (including hospitals, township hospitals, community health centers, and outpatient departments) represented RMB 9.6 billion in fixed assets.

Figure 9.2 shows the heavy capital investment expenditures on hospitals in Sichuan province relative to other types of health facilities over a four-year period: 2009–12.

The distribution of health care personnel in Sichuan is likewise unbalanced: there are roughly twice as many health personnel per 1,000 residents in city or urban settings than in county and rural settings (table 9.1). To provide higher-quality care, officials in Sichuan province must assess how to encourage a more even distribution of health professionals according to service need.

Hubei province. The tendency to favor larger hospitals is also apparent in the eastern province of Hubei. Figure 9.3 shows the growth rate of health facilities from 2008 to 2013. Hospitals were the only facility type to maintain a steady increase after 2009. If these trends continue, capital investment in Hubei will remain hospital-centric, and the health system will inadvertently attract patients who should otherwise be seeking care at primary facilities.

Tianjin municipality. In the northeastern municipality of Tianjin, health expenditure consistently increased from 2000 to 2013, and far more money went to city hospitals

FIGURE 9.1   Growth rates of health facilities, Sichuan province, 2008–09 to 2011–12

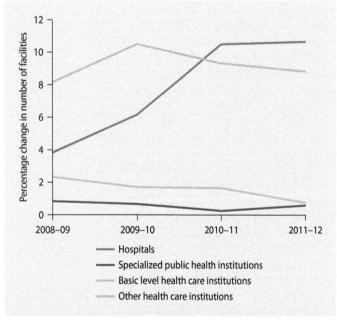

Source: Sanigest Internacional.
Note: "Hospitals" include general or comprehensive, traditional Chinese medicine, and special and national hospitals. "Basic-level health care institutions" include hospitals, township hospitals, community health centers, and outpatient departments.

FIGURE 9.2 **Distribution of total capital expenditures in health, Sichuan province, 2009–12**

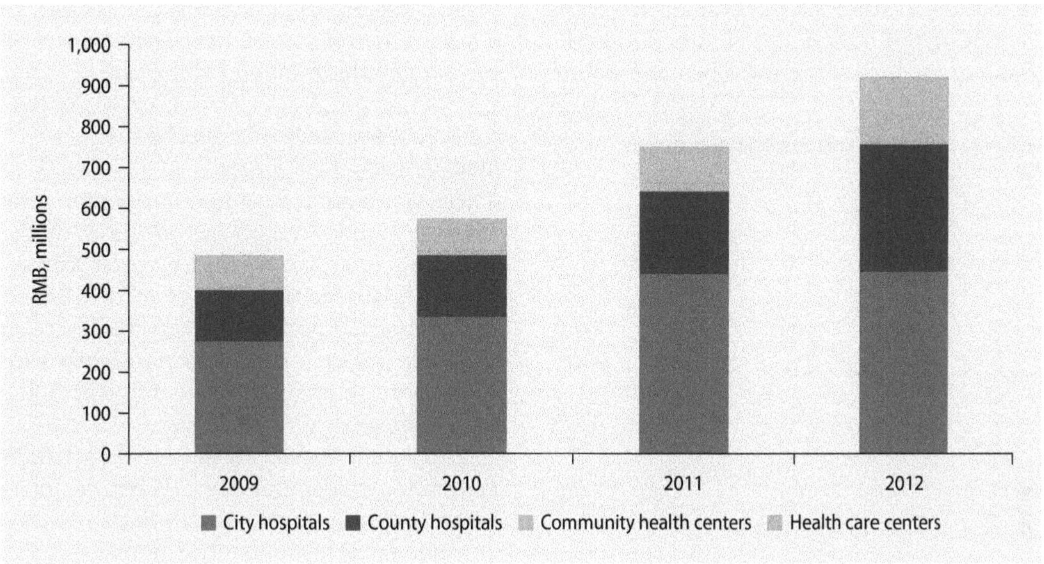

Source: Sanigest Internacional.

TABLE 9.1 **Distribution of health personnel, Sichuan province, by location type, 2008–12**
Workers per 1,000 residents

Personnel type	2008	2009	2010	2011	2012
Licensed (assistant) doctors					
City	2.18	2.31	2.44	2.60	2.73
County	1.06	1.09	1.11	1.17	1.23
Health technical personnel					
City	4.85	5.32	5.78	6.29	6.82
County	2.08	2.22	2.30	2.49	2.74
Licensed (assistant) doctors					
Urban	2.02	2.15	2.32	2.45	2.58
Rural	1.13	1.32	1.35	1.43	1.50
Health technical personnel					
Urban	4.79	5.29	5.79	6.26	6.82
Rural	2.51	2.68	2.80	3.05	3.33

Source: Sichuan Health Yearbook 2012, Sichuan Bureau of Health, Chengdu.

than to any other type of health facility (figure 9.4).

Survey methodology. A standardized questionnaire was prepared to evaluate the CIP process in the three provinces, benchmarking existing practices against best practice for a service-led planning model. Interviews using a structured questionnaire were completed with government officials in charge of health care CIP in each of the three provinces. These government officials represented the most relevant government departments: the Health and Family Planning Commission (HFPC), the Development and Reform Commission, the Finance Department, the Human Resources and Social Security Department, and the Construction Department. Hospital administrators were also interviewed by employing the same questionnaire during site visits to medical facilities. The case studies addressed the following key components: knowledge of CIP, financing CIP (ability to assess value for money of investments), and project identification and evaluation.

Limited knowledge of capital investment and planning techniques

There was significant unanimity among the three provinces' responses to many of the interview questions regarding their knowledge of CIP. Decision makers acknowledged the importance and necessity of needs-driven CIP. The HFPC officials explained that all infrastructure projects were developed in line with strategic health objectives.

Population health care needs were stated as the main consideration for CIP, but the interviewed officials gave different measures. For example, in Sichuan province, population size and providers' service radius were given as the primary measure to define health care needs. In the Tianjin municipality, disease pattern and incidence and services utilization (for example, number of visits, types of services, medical expenses, and so on) were stated as the main measures of health care needs.

In each of the three CIP components examined, the respondents stated that rates

FIGURE 9.3   Growth rate of health facilities, Hubei province, 2008–09 to 2012–13

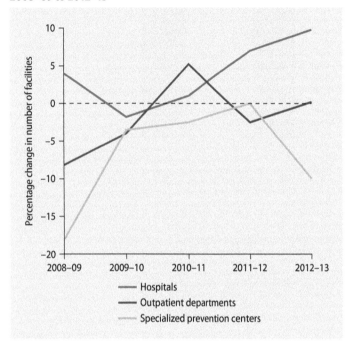

Source: Sanigest Internacional.

FIGURE 9.4   Distribution of health capital expenditures, Tianjin municipality, 2000–13

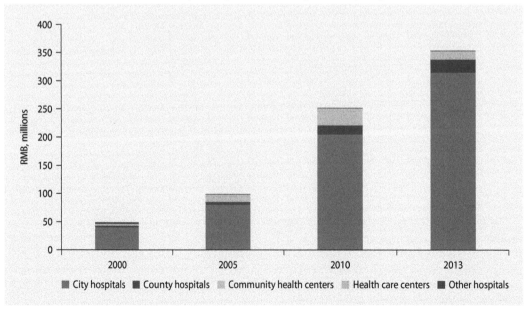

Source: Sanigest Internacional.

of service utilization and disease prevalence were the primary factors behind CIP by Health Bureau planners. Furthermore, only the respondents from Tianjin stated that health objectives have a "very high" influence on capital investment decisions; in Hubei, the influence was stated to be "medium" and in Sichuan, "high." In either case, however, only population density is documented as the key factor of consideration for capital investments, and beds per population are used as the key indicator for configuring health sources (table 9.2). Both of these are the traditional standards for CIP and bear little or no relation to service needs.

The data also indicate that in the three provinces surveyed, the practical configuration of health resources has been driven by medical facilities rather than by population needs. For example, in a feasibility study report of a county-level hospital in Renshou that applied for relocation and expansion, the number of beds, construction planning, and selection of location were initiated according to facility needs (table 9.3). There is no indication that the CIP considered the optimal location(s) for the population to be served.

Facility-based planning is not unique to Renshou; regional or local facilities often deviate from national standards. This indicates

TABLE 9.2 **Capital investment planning for health facilities, beds, and health personnel in studied Chinese provinces**

Province	Health facilities (population: health facility)	Beds	Personnel (per 1,000 residents)
Sichuan	• 30,000–100,000 pop.: 1 community health center • 300,000–500,000 pop.: 1 county-level hospital and 1 county-level traditional Chinese medicine hospital • County with population over 500,000: permissible to increase number of public hospitals, which should achieve 2nd-level standards • County with population over 800,000: hospitals should achieve 3rd-level standards • 1–2 million pop.: 1–2 city hospitals (2nd level); service radius of each should reach 50 kilometers	Per 1,000 residents: • Hospitals: 4.8 (of which public hospitals should be more than 3.3) • Grassroots health facilities: 1.2	• Health technical personnel: 7 • Licensed (assistant) doctors: 2.5 • Nurses: more than 2.8 • GPs: 2.5
Tianjin	• 2,000–3,000 pop.: 1 community health station (village clinics) with service radius of 1.5 kilometers • 15,000–25,000 pop.: 1 community health station (city) • 50,000 pop.: 1 community health center • 300,000–500,000 pop.: 1 city-level hospital (2nd level)	For comprehensive or general hospitals: • 3rd-level hospitals: 1,000–1,500 • 2rd-level hospitals: 500–800 For traditional Chinese medicine hospitals: • 3rd-level hospitals: 800–1,500 • 2nd-level hospitals: 500–800 Grassroots medical facilities (per 100,000 residents): • Community health centers or township hospitals: 15–30 (maximum should be lower than 50)	—
Hubei	• More than 3,000 pop.: 2 village clinics • 5,000–10,000 pop.: 1 community health station • 30,000–100,000 pop.: 1 community health center in urban area • More than 100,000 pop.: 2 community health centers • More than 800,000 pop.: 1–2 county hospitals in rural areas	Per 1,000 residents: • In general: 4.0–4.5 (Wuhan city: 7.0–7.5) • Township hospitals: 0.6–1.2 • Grassroots health facilities: 0.3–0.6 Taking residents as standard for county-level hospitals: • Below 100,000 population: 100–150 • 100,000–300,000 population: 200–300 • 300,000–500,000 population: 300–500 • 500,000–800,000 population: 400–600 • 800,000–1 million population: 500–800 • More than 1 million population: 800–1,000	In general, for licensed doctors: 1.95–2.15

Sources: Adapted from Configuration Standards of Health Resources in Sichuan 2008–20 and Sichuan Health Care Service Planning 2015–20; Tianjin Medical Facilities Layout Planning 2014–20; and Configuration Standards of Health Resources in Hubei 2011–15.
Note: — = not available; GP = general practitioner.

TABLE 9.3   Feasibility study results on relocation and expansion of Renshou County People's Hospital, 2009

Reasons for relocation and expansion	Project planning	Financing estimation (RMB, tens of thousands)
• Increased outpatient and inpatient needs by population (estimated by rate of utilization) • Acute shortage of beds • Department scattered in different places • Vulnerability of some buildings to weather-related risks (earthquakes) • Shortage of land for hospital expansion • Department setting restricted by limited space	• *Total number of beds needed:* 2–4 beds per 1,000 pop. × total population • *Bed gap:* total number of beds needed—existing number of beds • *Planned number of beds for the hospital:* current number of beds (498) + bed gap × 30%) • *Bed dimensions:* 88 square meters per bed (following national guideline) • *Construction area:* 800 (number of beds) × 88 = 70,400 square meters (following national guideline) • *Selection of location (factors considered):* convenient transportation, safety, nice environment	• Total investment: 16,451 • Infrastructure investment (three years): 16,451 • Floating fund: 0 • Capital sources: 16,451 • Funds for postdisaster reconstruction: 8,111 • Asset replacement: 4,650 *2,417.64 [1st year] + 2,232.36 [2nd year] + 0 [3rd year]* • Loans (financial discount guaranteed by government): 3,690

Source: Adapted from feasibility study report of Renshou County People's Hospital 2009.

that CIP in China is often driven by medical facility demand rather than population health care needs.

Absence of clear procedures to assess value for money of investments

Financing is a crucial part of capital investment planning. Without proper financial management and planning, capital investment projects tend to lack direction and have a high probability of failure. All three provinces studied demonstrated an absence of clear management and economic principles to assess the potential profitability and sustainability of long-term investments or to determine the value for money of competing investment projects. Although the government is moving to establish three-year budgeting, the NDRC investment approval process does not yet evaluate the sustainability of the investments based on projected cash flow and operating expenditure or value for money in terms of efficiency and affordability.

Responses from each province indicate that all three levels contributed to the capital costs of health care, yet it was not specified which carried a greater burden of the cost for each province. Each official indicated that each facility bore the brunt of long-term costs. It was not specified how much of a burden these costs are on facilities or whether they are deterrents to investing in capital improvement projects.

Project identification and evaluation

Project identification and evaluation are important components of the CIP process. As in the other components of the survey, the results were remarkably similar across the three provinces. In each case, investments are prioritized based upon criteria set by government policy and feasibility. Each official stated that existing infrastructure is always examined in each province before approving new projects, but there was no mention as to how this was done. It is interesting to note that each province indicated there does not exist a means to monitor, evaluate, and report on infrastructure effectiveness, efficiency, and sustainability. The respondents also indicated that an information management system is not in place to support monitoring and evaluation, nor are any cost-accounting tools and norms used in CIP decision processes. Furthermore, each respondent indicated there is no risk management process in place for capital investment projects.

A lack of these components is cause for concern. Although management and evaluation processes exist, if they do not employ the best, most up-to-date tools, they may not be reliable. It is reasonable to suggest that efficiency issues in China's health care capital investment may be alleviated with the proper use of management and evaluation tools.

Mismatch in procedures for administrative reporting and planning clearances

In China, the principle of administrative-affiliated management is employed in the planning process, and hospitals (including those at the provincial, city, community, and county levels) are administratively linked with their corresponding level of government. Each level of the government develops its own capital investment plan, while the provincial government makes the final decision in the overall planning. For example, Tianjin Medical University General Hospital is directly affiliated with the Ministry of Education instead of with the Tianjin municipal government; however, this Level 3 hospital develops its capital investment plan under the administration of the Development and Reform Commission of Tianjin. This creates confusion, especially because common information is not shared across different types and levels of governments involved, and project identification and evaluation suffer in this process.

Excessive capital investment in hospitals, particularly in urban areas, continues in Sichuan, Hubei, and Tianjin. Unless there are principles to guide the development of facilities of the future, there is a real danger that capital investment planning will simply perpetuate the status quo, or worse yet, create excess capacity that will exacerbate the existing inefficiencies and capital misallocations. Planning clearances should consider the private sector's capacity and planned investments in each province to ensure that the overall targets are achieved based on service planning needs and population-based needs.

Recommendations to Modernize Service Planning

China is not alone in its efforts to modify its capital investment strategy from one driven by macro standards to one determined by service planning based on real population needs. OECD countries, although diverse, face a number of common challenges when it comes to capital investment for health: demographic and epidemiological transitions associated with an aging population, advances in medical technologies and pharmaceuticals, rising public expectations, persistent health inequalities, and so on. The challenge for these countries, as well as for China, is to reconcile health needs and expectations with available resources. Several OECD countries have made or are making this transition, and their experiences offer important lessons for China.

Another major challenge that China needs to keep in mind concerns the lengthy time periods involved in planning, financing, construction, and operation of new health facilities. The interval between concept and commissioning of major hospitals can range from 5 to 10 years, while several more years are needed to construct the hospital (Rechel, Erskine, and others 2009). This has implications both for hospital sustainability and for responsiveness of health care delivery to population needs. The long time period from commissioning to operation can mean that many hospitals, when beginning to operate, do not meet the current (or future) health needs of their population.

Meanwhile, population needs are constantly shifting. Health care demand is highly sensitive to variations in the hospital's catchment population, including demographic changes and migration. The dynamic context of hospitals makes demand difficult to predict, both in terms of quantity and type of use. Furthermore, medical technologies have advanced rapidly since the 1970s, with a far-reaching impact on demand for clinical services (Rechel, Erskine, and others 2009). Ensuring that hospitals created today can retain their relevance and value in the future is a profound challenge. Although providing health care goes beyond the physical asset, it is the starting point in the delivery of sustainable and high-quality clinical services at the right place and the right time. This means that the design of hospitals should be sufficiently flexible to meet new requirements.

The following sections—each discussing a core action area for modernizing CIP for health service delivery—provide illustrative case studies from OECD countries from which lessons can be drawn for China. The case studies provide a variety of perspectives on how the challenges outlined above are being met in various contexts. They also demonstrate a variety of different approaches to adopting a service-based capital investment strategy—from needs-based planning for care of the elderly, persons with disabilities, and stroke patients to reform of regional capital planning.

Although the case studies are diverse, common themes can be identified on the response of health services to population needs. For example, there is a clear trend toward using systematized "care pathways" as a means of characterizing the provision of health care services, including their links and integration with capital investment. Care pathways aim to describe health care services for specified disease syndromes and, ideally, encapsulate measurable inputs and outcomes. They provide a possible basis for translating demographic and epidemiological trends into concepts that can be used for planning health capital investment. Furthermore, they offer a means of engaging with clinicians while

simultaneously providing levers for economic control. Care pathways are likely to have greatest impact on health capital investment when (a) they are applied across care settings, not only to hospitals, and (b) they are backed by appropriate systems of resource allocation (Hindle, Dowdeswell, and Yasbeck 2004).

In addition, the case studies highlight the need for comprehensive systems of capacity planning and for the use of new measures of hospital capacity that go beyond bed numbers. Bed numbers to measure hospital capacity, although obsolete, are still used by many countries (both OECD and non-OECD). Other countries are seeking measurements derived from systemized care pathways, or at least more closely linked to actual capacity rather than bed numbers. However, this is a methodology that is still in its infancy, and more work is needed to develop a reliable and robust characterization of hospital capacity other than that based on bed numbers. Figure 9.5 shows how best practice in OECD countries is linking the service planning with the estimated investment cost requirements.

The OECD case studies demonstrate the need for linking the operation of hospitals

FIGURE 9.5   Translating health services to costs in OECD countries

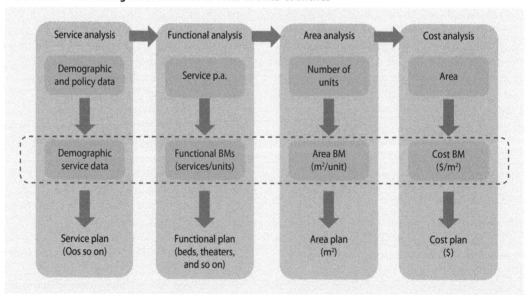

Source: Interpretation of OECD 2008; Rechel, Erskine, and others 2009; Rechel, Wright, and others 2009.
Note: BM = benchmark; m² = square meters; OECD = Organisation for Economic Co-operation and Development.

with flexible financing models. The time periods for renewing medical technologies and buildings are becoming shorter, and issues of the life-cycle effectiveness and economic sustainability of hospitals are being recognized as more important. Those hospital projects that have sought to design more adaptable buildings and services have also tended to turn to more adaptable capital financing models.

Five core action areas and corresponding implementation strategies that can strengthen capital investments in the health sector in support of PCIC include the following (as summarized in table 9.4):

1. A shift from the traditional input-based planning toward people-centered planning of capital investments based upon region-specific epidemiological and demographic profiles
2. Engagement with all relevant stakeholders and local communities in the planning process
3. Empowerment and enabling of regions and provinces to develop their own capital investment plans
4. Introduction of a Certificate of Need program to evaluate and approve new capital investments in the health sector
5. Prioritization of community health projects.

TABLE 9.4   Five core action areas and implementation strategies to strengthen capital investments

Core action area	Implementation strategies
1: Shift from traditional input-based planning toward people-centered planning	• Develop a regulatory framework in which capital investment in health is focused on improvement and value • Adopt the service planning approach to capital investments, and require all future investments to be guided by an assessment of population needs • Develop a capacity planning tool that estimates financial and physical resource needs for the country's hospital system by province, medical specialty, and level • Prepare province-level strategic plans that include 5–10 year perspectives on investment needs for infrastructure, equipment, technology, and human resource development • Integrate capital planning into a medium-term expenditure framework, and bring together planning and budgeting including consideration of private sector capacity • Create an enabling legal framework to support the new planning and governance arrangements, and support enforcement and compliance arrangements to ensure execution
2: Engagement with all relevant stakeholders and local communities in the planning process	• Identify different stakeholder groups and prominent community and private sector leaders, and formulate an engagement strategy for each stakeholder type • Conduct consultation sessions according to the strategy • Require rigorous evaluation and public disclosure of all capital projects, including self-funded capital projects, financed through philanthropy or other in-kind contributions • Publish benchmark spending per bed by level of care and average bed size across provinces to ensure that standards are met
3: Empowerment and enabling of regions and provinces to develop their own capital investment plans	• Establish provincial commissions on health investment and capital development • Prepare province-level strategic plans (master plans) that include 5–10 year perspectives on investment needs for infrastructure, equipment, technology, and human resource development to ensure consistency with the population's evolving health needs • Include private capital investment in the establishment of regional health accounts that include total capital expenditures
4: Introduction of a Certificate of Need program to evaluate and approve new capital investments	• Require feasibility studies for all capital investments to be based on population health needs • Require feasibility studies to demonstrate that the proposed capital investment is necessary to meet the identified and targeted need, considering the public and private supply in each region • Require all applications for new capital investments to be supported by a Certificate of Need as developed in the feasibility study
5: Prioritization of community health projects	• Earmark a percentage of provincial and city capital budgets for community projects • Identify high-priority communities, and formulate multiyear community capital investment plans within the context of the new budgetary frameworks

Core Action Area 1: Shift from Traditional Input-Based Planning Toward People-Centered Planning

China is a very large country and has a diverse demographic and epidemiological profile. An investment planning method that is based on region-specific population needs instead of country-level averages will better meet the health objectives of the population.

Several specific strategies will help reverse the current planning logic and allow population needs to determine service planning.

The needs-based Horizon method used to plan capital investment for care of the elderly in the Netherlands is an example of CIP focused on meeting the health needs of the population while simultaneously carefully planning long-term capital investments (box 9.2).

Comparisons between the Horizon needs-based approach and the old demand-based approach reveal interesting differences. For example, the needs-based model predicted a slightly increased bed capacity for the Netherlands as a whole in 2009, because of the demographic of elderly citizens in the country. Because it takes into account the unequal demographic distribution of people in the municipalities, it is more accurate than the demand-based, linear approach.

A good example of CIP using the Horizon approach is in The Hague. In 2009, the needs-based model predicted that 4.3 beds (per 1,000 population) would be needed for care profiles 4 and 5, whereas the demand-based model predicted 3.5 beds (Nauta, Perenboom, and Galindo Garre 2009). The needs-based model took into account the differences between The Hague and the national population and calculated the need for the different care profiles, giving The Hague a more accurate representation of capital needs for elderly care.

BOX 9.2   Horizon's three-step CIP model for eldercare in the Netherlands

Like many countries, the Netherlands is faced with the problems associated with an aging population. To better plan for infrastructure for the elderly, Dutch health officials transitioned from linear, demand-based estimations to the needs-based Horizon method, which has given more accurate estimations of the population, allowing for more efficient capital investment planning (CIP) centered on population health needs.

CIP for eldercare in the Netherlands has traditionally used a demand-based method, which calculates demand using the percentage of citizens above the age of 75. By 1998, it had become obvious that the approach was proving to be insufficient, and the Netherlands moved to a needs-based approach. Called Horizon, this three-step approach uses measures of actual physical and mental disabilities to help plan capital investment projects (Nauta, Perenboom, and Galindo Garre 2009).

In Step 1, questionnaires and surveys are issued to capture personal health status, physical abilities, well-being, and ability to cope with daily routines. Information about care issues is gathered from multiple sources, and patterns are distinguished using latent class analysis. Care profiles developed from the analyses indicate prevalent health concerns for the elderly. A random population survey is then carried out to check whether the profile is reflective of the entire population. This survey is carried out yearly, ensuring that the data are updated and reflect the most current health needs of the elderly population. The number of persons belonging to a certain profile for a set geographical area is predicted using demographics and predictions about future demographic trends.

Step 2 in the process is to determine the care needed for each profile, as each care profile states a general condition of a surveyed group. This step is relatively short, because the profiles are broken down and precategorized.

Step 3 involves ascertaining the most appropriate setting of care, given the type of care needed. This step assesses the needs of each profile and examines the best option for the setting of care. The analysis conducted in this step is crucial for CIP because it informs the plan of the care needs of the elderly population.

Source: Nauta, Perenboom, and Galindo Garre 2009.

The needs-based Horizon model is flexible and allows for greater long-term predictions. For example, the linear approach of the demand-based model suggests that the number of beds in The Hague be raised to around 4.0 beds for 2019. The needs-based model, however, predicts that the need for beds will decrease to 3.9 by 2019. The needs-based model allows for future-friendly capital investments, and it can be translated to different sectors of health care.

Horizon has proven to be a good model in the Netherlands for long-term, needs-based capital investments for care of the elderly. It shows that making needs-based projections is possible and, in fact, may give more accurate estimations for capital investment projects.

China is faced with an aging population, so such an approach could be used to help direct CIP toward meeting the needs of the elderly population in China. A planning method such as Horizon would allow Chinese health officials to plan capital investments based upon a location's unique demographics instead of generalizing health needs across the vast country. This will allow for personalized health capital investments designed to meet specific health needs; as a result, the health needs of each unique region will be met more readily by the capital, a step in the right direction toward improving population health.

Core Action Area 2: Engagement with All Relevant Stakeholders and Local Communities in the Planning Process

Involving all relevant stakeholders in the planning process, especially the target population and the private sector, allows for capital investment decisions to be made in ways that simultaneously meet health needs as well as policy requirements. Key action steps include the following:

- Identify different stakeholder groups and prominent community and private sector leaders, and formulate an engagement strategy for each stakeholder type

- Conduct consultation sessions according to the strategy.
- Require rigorous evaluation and public disclosure of all capital projects, including self-funded capital projects, financed through philanthropy or other in-kind contributions.
- Publish benchmark spending per bed by level of care and average bed size across provinces to ensure that standards are met.

New South Wales (NSW), a state on the east coast of Australia, has begun to implement a new capital investment method to better meet the needs of its population of people with disabilities. Known as the Sector Planning Framework, its flexible approach can be modified to fit any population subgroup. Among its key features, it places local communities, including people with disabilities, their families, and caretakers at the center of the planning process and as joint parties in the planning process. It also helps the state deliver on its commitments to local communities in ways that best suit each community. It recognizes that each community has unique health needs and that capital investments cannot be made in a "one size fits all" manner if they are to meet all the disparate health needs.

NSW is currently transitioning to this new approach (figure 9.6). Previously, capital planning for disability services was a centrally driven, program-based planning method that focused on service outputs and defined service models, driven by agency-based priorities (NSW Government 2011).

This new Sector Planning Framework approach will contribute to a service system that does the following;

- Is people-centered, with the population of people with disabilities, their families, and caretakers being the focus of decision making and allowing them to provide input about the support they receive, who provides the support, and how and when they receive it
- Is based on a lifespan approach that empowers people with disabilities to be

FIGURE 9.6   Delivering a new approach to health sector planning in New South Wales, Australia

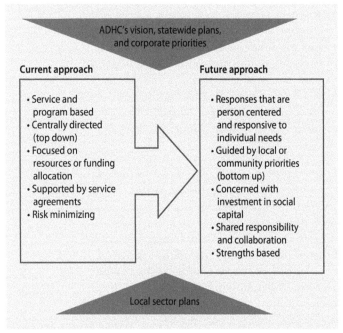

Source: NSW Government 2011.
Note: ADHC = Ageing, Disability, and Home Care.

actively involved in planning and designing their own support arrangements
• Focuses on maximizing the experiences and opportunities of people with disabilities;
• Promotes economic participation and employment opportunities
• Actively develops the capacity and social capital of the nongovernmental organization (NGO) sector and local communities.

In terms of logistics, the Sector Planning Framework will focus on long-term investments of 5-10 years. It will involve planning based upon robust evidence, research, and data. This will help better meet the population's needs while also embedding benefits realization into the planning cycle. It will integrate planning at various levels: statewide, regional or local, and organizational. This will allow for a tailored approach for each community that still communicates well with NSW's overall goals. It will strengthen planning at the organizational level as well, providing tools to support planning at the local level with the help of organizations.

Further, it will feed into the broader Family and Consumer Services (FACS) planning framework and ensure that locally based strategies are reflected in the wider FACS and in the NSW government's plans to support the population of people with disabilities (NSW Government 2011).

This approach allows for open dialogue among all different levels of planning. Robust research and strong community involvement allow for investment plans to incorporate projects that best fit the health needs of any given population. Further, it helps tailor capital investments to the unique needs of individual communities, contributing to the development of service-based investment decisions. NSW has recognized that this method of planning is not limited to capital planning only for people with disabilities; it is an approach that can be modified for any given population.

NSW's Sector Planning Framework offers many attractive options for China. It offers a way for China to incorporate each planning level into the investment planning process, allowing for capital investment decisions that meet health needs and policy requirements. The Sector Planning Framework is designed to achieve coordination and alignment in the priorities among governments, agencies, providers, and communities, and it builds cross-agency and public-private partnerships to enable easy integration into future systems. China may wish to employ the flexibility of this approach to address a variety of different health concerns, while not having to reinvent the process every time.

Core Action Area 3: Empowerment and Enabling of Regions and Provinces to Develop their Own Capital Investment Plans

Empowering subnational levels in China to develop their own capital investment plans require several key actions. The "Planning Layout of National Medical and Health Services System (2015–2020)" provides an incipient framework for this planning and ensures its implementation will be a step in the right direction.[5] China may wish to further study.

One such example is the capital investment framework in France, where the health sector investment planning is based on population needs and is executed through Regional Strategic Health Plans (Schéma Régional d'Organisation Sanitaire, or SROSs). SROSs set the overall strategic goals for health care delivery; define priorities, objectives, and targets; and determine quantitative targets and the distribution of health care facilities within a region. SROSs are developed by regional health agencies in consultation with stakeholders, including the Ministry of Health, health insurance funds, hospital federations, health care professionals, and patient representatives (EOHSP, n.d.; Ettelt and others 2008). The Ministry of Health plays a coordinating role and generates a catalogue of health services based on an assessment of national needs and priorities, which the regions incorporate in their own plans (Ettelt and others 2008).

The regional health agencies are generally responsible for planning services and for authorizing hospitals to deliver services within the social health insurance system. They also oversee changes to the existing hospital infrastructure, including restructuring and mergers. The only exceptions are new hospital developments (both private and public) and comprehensive emergency centers, which have to be authorized by the Ministry of Health. Strategic planning requires regional agencies to assess population health care needs on the basis of regional health care utilization data and relevant demographic data (such as on mortality and morbidity). Data for each region are analyzed and compared with those for other regions to identify demand and supply. Expert estimates of future trends in demand and technological change—largely based on epidemiological data and trends observed in other countries (mainly the United States)—are taken into consideration for these assessments (Ettelt and others 2008).

The SROS is the most important tool in France's regional capital investment and health care delivery planning. It focuses on hospital planning and on expensive treatment and technology provided in hospital settings. Since its implementation in 2003, the SROS in each region has replaced the "national medical map," which was the quantitative planning tool used by the Ministry of Health to divide each region into health care sectors and defined norms for bed-population ratios for major disciplines within a geographical area (EOHSP, n.d.; Ettelt and others 2008). In contrast to previous national planning practices, the purpose of the SROS is to better tailor health care delivery to the needs of the local population.

Related to capital investment planning, SROSs determine capacity by specifying the number of facilities in each region and subregion for each area of care (including general medicine, surgery, maternity care, accident and emergency care, neonatal care, radiotherapy, cardiologic intensive care, and psychiatric care, as well as expensive technical equipment such as magnetic resonance imaging scanners). They also define the volumes for certain types of service and benchmark them for comparison. "Service volumes" refer to units such as numbers of patients, sites, days (length of stay), procedures performed, and admissions, and they are expressed in numbers of services or rates and show changes relative to previous volumes. The objective of planning on the basis of service volumes rather than on bed-population ratios is to limit oversupply, which is a persistent problem in some cities (Paris) and regions (south of France) (Ettelt and others 2008).

Since the reform of national health planning in 2003, trends in the French health care system have moved toward increased efficiency. For example, the percentage of outpatient care has risen from 48 percent in 2001 to 53.4 percent in 2006, mostly through an increase of day cases in acute care (from 30.9 percent to 39.2 percent) and in the follow-up and rehabilitation sectors (60.3 percent to 67.4 percent). The average length of stay in acute care decreased from 5.7 days in 2001 to 5.4 days in 2006. However, the utilization rate in the acute care sector (73.4 percent in 2005) is relatively low compared with that of neighboring countries, indicating continued overcapacity (EOHSP, n.d.).

The French experience—and in particular how the SROSs are developed—offer lessons to China on how to involve all relevant stakeholders in the planning process. More important, however, are the lessons the French experience offers in how to transition away from a bed-population ratio method of determining health service configuration. As discussed earlier in the Chinese case studies, CIP is still largely based upon population projections and bed numbers. The same was true in France before the reforms in 2003; this method often led to oversupply of health services, especially in urban centers like Paris and in southern France. China could learn from France by adopting the service volume method, whereby health service configuration and capacity are calculated based upon volumes of service (that is, type of service, numbers of patients, sites, lengths of stay, procedures performed, and admissions), which are then benchmarked with current levels.

Core Action Area 4: Introduction of a Certificate of Need Program to Evaluate and Approve New Capital Investments in the Health Sector

China already has a system of requiring feasibility reports for all capital investments. However, these feasibility reports use norms set according to macro standards governing the size and scope of the intended service.

Feasibility studies are essential for governments to evaluate and approve new capital investment projects. The earlier discussion of a feasibility study for possible relocation and expansion of the Renshou County People's Hospital noted that the construction planning and selection of location were determined according to facility needs rather than population needs. The Certificate of Need (CON) program presents a possible solution.

The Certificate of Need (CON) program is used extensively in the United States to evaluate and approve new capital investment projects. In 1974, the federal Health Planning Resources Development Act mandated that all 50 states evaluate CONs before allowing the continuation of any health capital investment projects, such as building expansions, and ordering new high-technology devices. The goal was to restrain facility costs and allow for a more coordinated planning of health services and construction. Many states established CON programs to receive federal funding. Even though the Health Planning Resources Development Act, along with its funding, was cut in 1987, 36 states still maintain some form of a CON program, and the remaining 14 states that do not have CON programs have other mechanisms in place to regulate costs and duplication of services.

Maine CON program

Each state in the United States has developed its own unique approach to the program. Many states have recognized the importance of population health needs in CIP and rely on the analysis of population health needs to implement capital investment projects. For example, in 2002, Maine passed a Certificate of Need Act in an attempt to decrease unnecessary construction and modification of health facilities and duplication of health services and hence to decrease costs and provide higher-quality health care.

The core principles of Maine's CON program are as follows (Ashcroft and Maine State Legislature 2011):

- Supporting effective health planning
- Supporting the provision of quality health care in a manner that ensures access to cost-effective services
- Supporting reasonable choice in health care services while avoiding excessive duplication
- Ensuring that state funds are used prudently in the provision of health care services
- Ensuring public participation in the process of determining the array, distribution,

quantity, quality, and cost of these health care services
- Improving the availability of health care services throughout the state
- Supporting the development and availability of health care services regardless of the consumer's ability to pay
- Seeking a balance, to the extent a balance assists in achieving the purposes of this law, between competition and regulation in the provision of health care
- Promoting the development of primary and secondary preventive health services

The Certificate of Need Unit (CONU) is composed of a manager, three financial analysts, and administrative support. To distribute the workload throughout the year, the CONU processes applications for different projects on a staggered timeline. For a project to be considered, a CON application must be submitted to the CONU. After receiving the application, a public information meeting is scheduled, and a public notice is issued. This part of the process is essential for the CON program's success. It allows for open feedback from the public regarding projects, allowing for citizens to express their needs and concerns. Any Maine citizen has the opportunity to provide a public testimony about a potential health capital investment project (Ashcroft and Maine State Legislature 2011).

The CONU considers the public testimonies, along with input from organizations such as the Maine Quality Forum, the Maine Center for Disease Control & Prevention (CDC), and the Bureau of Insurance. By consulting with the Maine CDC, the CONU can make informed decisions based upon population health needs. Throughout this process, several important factors are considered in CON determinations (Ashcroft and Maine State Legislature 2011):

- The applicant is fit, willing, and able to provide the proposed services at the proper standard of care.
- The proposed services are economically feasible.

- There is a public need for the proposed services.
- The proposed services are consistent with the orderly and economic development of health facilities and health resources for the state.
- The proposed services are consistent with the State Health Plan.
- The proposed services ensure high-quality outcomes and do not negatively affect the quality of care delivered by existing service providers.
- The proposed initiative does not result in inappropriate increases in service utilization.
- The proposed project can be funded within the capital investment fund (CIF).

Notably, the Maine CON program requires the existence of public hearings for a proposed service before a capital investment project can begin. Applicants must prove their proposed capital investment is geared toward meeting some public need. Furthermore, for each application, the CONU solicits comments on the impact of each project on the health of Maine citizens from both the Maine Quality Forum and the Maine CDC (figure 9.7).

Maine's CON program requires in-depth evidence of the potential worth of a capital investment project. Population health is considered to be of crucial importance, and because of the CON process, no capital investment project can be approved without detailed consideration of population health needs from the applicant, the CDC, and the Maine Quality Forum. This thorough examination is less likely to favor larger hospitals in a disproportionate way, allowing for efficient CIP to occur at all levels of health care to best meet population health needs (Ashcroft and Maine State Legislature 2011).

Similarly, China can consider the Maine example in designing a CON program to approve CIP that is based on population health and public need.

Kentucky CON program

The state of Kentucky has also used the CON program to incentivize development of a full

FIGURE 9.7   Certificate of Need application and approval process in Maine, United States

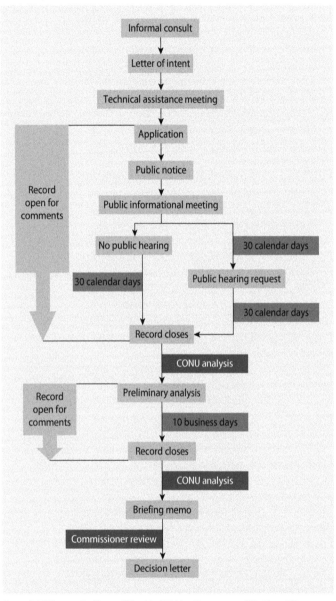

Source: "2010 Report, Certificate of Need Act."©Maine Department of Health and Human Services (Maine DHHS). Reproduced, with permission, from Maine DHHS; further permission required for reuse.
Note: CONU = Certificate of Need Unit.

continuum of care. The program works to promote and support providers and facilities that seek to develop a robust continuum of care alone or in partnership with others, in part owing to the evolving payment structures and the ever-changing environment of the health care sector in the United States.

The program also incentivizes the attainment of robust quality indicators. This is especially important, given that Kentucky currently has a poor health profile. Health officials wish to incentivize greater access to care for Medicaid members, the newly insured, and any remaining uninsured citizens—a particularly important priority for poor rural communities, where chronic diseases are rampant and the rates of uninsured high.

The CON program will also focus on achieving greater price transparency, especially as health care in the United States transitions from a fee-for-service model to a value-based purchasing framework. In addition, to modernize the health systems in Kentucky, CON will favor the adoption of new health technologies geared toward the prevention and treatment of chronic diseases. Finally, the program encourages further modernization by being more reflective of modern health care trends and population health needs. All the aforementioned points were brought forth in October 2014 as core principles for CON modernization.[6]

Michigan CON program
Another example from the United States that may be relevant for China is from Michigan. The CON program in for Michigan's health sector has evolved over the years to include more services and to move away from a hospital-centric system. Michigan also introduced requirements to ensure that capital projects comply with standards, which has proved to be a challenge in China.

Initially, Michigan's CON program was based solely on the costs of capital investment projects; as a result, primary attention was given to hospitals, because they accounted for most health spending. The program initially only covered hospital capital investment projects. However, as time passed, health policy officials realized that a CON program based solely on costs could have a distorting effect on health care, adversely affecting both quality and access. For example, the least costly location in which to start a new service might not be one that improves access or might not have enough of the health professionals needed to meet demand. The Michigan CON program evolved accordingly into a more patient-centric, needs-based process, although considerable attention is still paid to bed numbers (CRC of Michigan 2005).

Michigan's Act 256 of 1972 states a hospital facility shall not be constructed, converted, added to, or modernized without first obtaining a CON that documents a demonstrated need for the proposed project. This need-based component has remained a part of the CON program. This act also placed the responsibility for CON on the Department of Public Health, and a commission was established to oversee the program. This helps to protect the state's health-related CIP from any biased political agendas. According to this act, a capital investment proposal must contain the following (CRC of Michigan 2005)—good examples of the potential criteria for capital investment projects in China:

- The patterns and level of utilization, availability, and adequacy of existing facilities, institutions, programs, and services in the immediate community and region
- The degree to which residents and physicians in a community are provided access to the hospital applying for the Certificate of Need
- The availability and adequacy of services such as preadmission, ambulatory, or home care services that may serve as alternatives to hospital care
- The economies and service improvements that could be achieved from consolidation of highly specialized services or from shared central services such as laboratory, radiology, and the like
- The economies and service improvements that could be achieved from affiliation or contractual arrangements between hospitals and others
- The availability of personnel to fulfill the services to be offered
- Proof that the hospital does not discriminate in activities including employment, room assignment, and training

- Proof that consumers make up the majority of a nonprofit hospital's governing body
- Proof that the hospital has the financial capacity to both fund the construction and operate the facility following completion
- Proof that the project complies with local and regional rules, regulations, and standards
- Other factors that contribute to the orderly development of quality health care.

Public Act 368 of 1978 further amended Michigan's CON program, extending its coverage to nonhospital facilities (including nursing homes) and to certain clinical services. This allowed Michigan to further consider population health needs in its CIP as it moved away from the hospital-centric model.

Ten years later, Public Acts 331 and 332 extended the CON program to include more clinical services and defined seven covered medical equipment categories in state law. It also continued authorizations for regional health planning agencies under state law. Act 332 allowed the Department of Public Health to require the submission of data and statistics as a part of a CON application, and it established in law the obligation to monitor CON projects after approval to confirm alignment with the approved project and with population health needs (CRC of Michigan 2005).

Michigan's CON program is notably more complicated than Maine's, which highlights the diversity of the CON programs in the United States. Each program is designed to fit the state's unique health policy procedures and allows each state to create a program that best suits its health population needs and governmental processes. A proposed project in Michigan must meet the following six requirements (CRC of Michigan 2005):

- Meet an unmet need.
- Include alternatives that have been considered and the reasons why the proposed particular approach is best (if there are no alternatives, the application must state why).

- Show that the proposed service is the least costly.
- Be delivered in compliance with operating standards and quality assurance standards; include a description of how the proposed project will assure appropriate utilization; indicate how project effectiveness will be measured; and show that the applicant has complied, both currently and historically, with federal and state licensing and certification requirements.
- Demonstrate, if the project relates to a facility, that the facility where the proposed service will be delivered is viable by meeting one of six requirements.
- If a nonprofit applicant, show that consumers make up a majority of the board.

Such requirements could prove useful for China, especially for provinces that have not fully complied with federal mandates. These requirements help base CIP on realistic health needs and ensure that capital investment projects contribute to the betterment of population health.

Michigan's CON program is an example of how such a program can evolve over time and show that CON programs that are not hospital centric are the most successful at providing capital investment guidance that is aimed at improving the entire health sector. Michigan's CON program is another example of how to orchestrate a CON program to better plan capital investment structures around existing and unmet needs.

U.S. Certificate of Need programs as a model for China

The CON programs as practiced in the United States hold a lot of promise for China, where facility needs are often paramount in determining hospital expansion. A close look at the feasibility study of possible relocation and expansion of the Renshou County People's Hospital in Meishan city, Sichuan province, for instance, reveals that construction planning and selection of location for the Renshou hospital were determined according to facility needs rather than population needs.

A program akin to the CON program presents a possible solution to this.

Each state's CON program in the United States holds important lessons for China:

- *In Kentucky,* the state recognized the dire state of its population health and sought to refocus its CON program on developing capital focused on the health needs. China can consider doing the same by developing CON program-like processes to respond to health needs. By focusing on the health needs of a population, capital investment projects can help provide the best, most accessible care, improving overall population health. Kentucky has a long way to go in terms of improving its population health, but it is starting by redirecting its CIP, providing a positive example of the importance of service-based CIP.
- *In Maine,* applicants for capital investment projects must prove that their proposed capital investment is geared toward meeting some public need. This is important, because it helps reduce duplicated services and helps direct capital investment to areas of the state that need it most. Also, public hearings are important features of the CON program process. In these hearings, citizens can voice their needs and opinions regarding potential capital investments. This increases communication with health officials and the public and further provides for a people-centered CIP. Like Maine, China could develop a CON program-like process that relies heavily on actual population health data to make informed decisions on capital investment.
- *In Michigan,* the state realized that a CON program based solely on costs could have a distorting effect on health care, adversely affecting both quality and access—an important lesson for China. The CON program evolved over the years to include more services and move away from hospital-centric CIP. Several requirements also ensure that capital projects comply with standards; China has experienced difficulty with compliance, so

such requirements could help its practices to better reflect actual policy. Michigan's CON program shows how CON programs that are not hospital-centric are the most successful at providing capital investment guidance aimed at improving the entire health sector. Michigan's CON program is another example of how to orchestrate a CON program to better plan capital investment structures around existing and unmet needs.

Core Action Area 5: Prioritization of Community Health Projects

As in China, capital investment in Northern Ireland was once hospital centric and was largely focused on the acute sector. Beginning in 2007, Northern Ireland started to redirect its capital investments toward community-level facilities. The new model sought to create an integrated continuum of facilities—from home care to primary, community, subacute (step-down), and acute facilities—all supported by structured networks.

The underlying strategy had two main components: enhanced services within the community and concentration of complex services. Regarding the first component, Northern Ireland carried out a comprehensive regionwide planning exercise and decided to develop 42 new community health

centers at population centers throughout the country (box 9.3).

Meeting the second component (concentration of complex services) required greater centralization—from local general hospitals to acute centers or to regional centers of excellence—of those services that, because of their complexity, required specialized skills and expertise that could not easily or affordably be replicated in local hospitals. A key criterion in the process of determining the final locations of those hospitals being designated as "acute" was that patients should have a maximum travel time of one hour from anywhere in Northern Ireland to an acute facility offering full accident and emergency services.

A primary objective of this new model of care is to improve accessibility of the public to high-quality, timely services. The specific location of individual facilities was determined by a number of key factors, including the core principles within the regional health strategy, urban or rural setting, size of the local population, epidemiology, travel times and distances, critical mass for staff, critical mass for specialist equipment, state and location of current facilities, improved accessibility, reduced waiting times and reduced hospital admissions, and affordability.

Additionally, Northern Ireland has attempted to incorporate flexible design principles into its new configuration (figure 9.8).

BOX 9.3   **Physical redesign of Northern Ireland's health system model**

Five elements defined the physical redesign of the health system in Northern Ireland:

1. Reduction of the number of Health and Social Care Trusts (service provider organizations) from 17 to 5, according to geographic need, each providing a full continuum of health and social care services to its local population
2. Designation or development of regional centers as the sole providers of a range of tertiary services that will benefit from centralization

3. Reduction in the number of general hospitals providing the full range of acute services from 18 to 10
4. Redevelopment of seven of the remaining nine hospitals as new nonacute step-down facilities with a focus on their local communities and the ability to provide a wider range of intermediate care services
5. Creation of 42 new, one-stop community health centers (without bed accommodation) with the key objective of preventing unnecessary hospitalization.

Source: Rechel, Erskine, and others 2009.

FIGURE 9.8   **The integrated health services model in Northern Ireland**

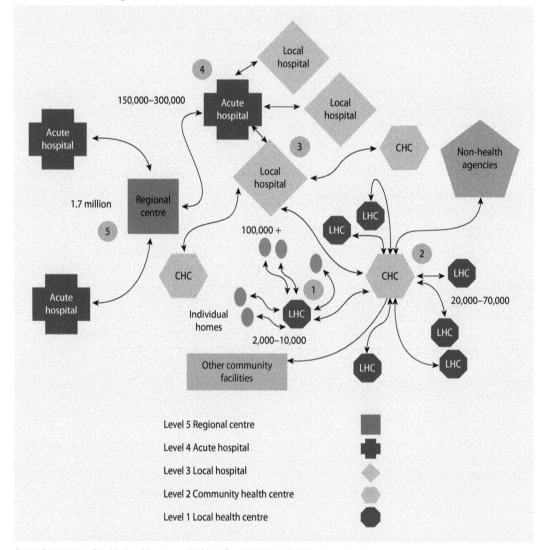

Source: Department of Health, Social Services and Public Safety (DHSSPS), Belfast, Northern Ireland.
Note: CHC = community health center; LHC = local health center.

These principles included phased construction to transition from existing to new facilities; insertion of "soft" spaces (for example, office space or educational accommodation that can be relatively easily relocated) beside complex areas (such as those for critical care or imaging) that are likely to expand in the future and would be very expensive to move; and standardization (Rechel, Erskine, and others 2009).

The colocation of Level 1 and Level 2 facilities has been encouraged within the model, particularly in areas of high population density, where travel distances are more likely to be acceptable for access to general practitioners. Where sites for Level 3 or Level 4 facilities are already located at natural population centers with good access to public transport, there are potential benefits in colocating Level 1 and Level 2 facilities while ensuring the retention of their separate identities and organizational structures. Where such colocation is proposed, the resultant arrangement has come to be referred to as "a health village." The typical range of services intended to be provided at each level is outlined in table 9.5.

The example of Northern Ireland shows that it is possible for a health system to undergo such a physical transition and move away from a hospital-centric system. Citizens of Northern Ireland now have greater access to both community facilities and acute facilities, both of which have been designed to improve population health.

The focus on specific geographic needs offers an important lesson for China, which could greatly benefit from investing more

TABLE 9.5 Services under Northern Ireland's integrated health services model, by level

Level	Services
Level 1: Local health centers • Construction cost range: £1–5 million • Level 1 facilities frequently incorporated into Level 2 facilities	• General practices • Noncomplex diagnostic testing • Basic treatments and nursing care • A limited range of therapies
Level 2: Community health centers • Construction cost range: £5–15 million	• After-hours GP service • Outpatient clinics • Minor procedures • Noncomplex imaging and diagnostics • Children's services • Physiotherapy • Speech therapy • Podiatry • Dental services • Social services • Mental health services • Multidisciplinary outreach teams • Voluntary sector • Community facilities • Pharmacy
Level 3: Local hospitals • Construction cost range: £40–70 million	• Urgent care center (as opposed to full accident and emergency care) • Ambulatory care center • Full diagnostics including radiological services • Day procedures or day surgery unit (Level 3 facilities can be designated to act as "protected elective centers") • Step-down, rehabilitation, and GP beds • Mental health unit • Support services
Level 4: Acute hospitals • Construction cost range: £200–300 million	Full range of standard acute hospital services, including the following: • Specialist-led accident and emergency care • Critical care department • Acute medical and surgical departments • Pediatrics • Outpatient department • Radiology
Level 5: Regional centers of excellence • Construction cost varies • Generally, but not always, colocated with a Level 4 acute hospital	Specialized care, including the following: • Cancer treatment services • Orthopedic services • Cardiac surgery • Neurosurgery

Source: Adapted from Rechel, Erskine, and others 2009.
Note: GP = general practitioner.

in community health capital projects and increasing access to quality care. Recognizing the unique health and capital investment needs at the community level, Northern Ireland is focusing its capital investment on community-level facilities, transitioning away from hospital-centric models. Further, Northern Ireland has dedicated some capital investment toward creating flexible facilities, which increases efficiency in the long term and enables the health system to better respond to future population health needs without needing to invest in new capital or completely redesign facilities to meet unforeseen needs. China may wish to explore this flexible design.

Notes

1. OECD health spending data are from the 2015 OECD.Stat Health Statistics Database, https://stats.oecd.org/index .aspx?DataSetCode=HEALTH_STAT.
2. National accounts data provide an idea of the type of assets and capital spending. Although capital spending can fluctuate from year to year, in OECD countries overall, there is an even split between spending on construction (that is, building of hospitals and other health care facilities) and spending on equipment (medical machinery, ambulances, and information and communication technology [ICT] equipment). Together they account for 85 percent of capital expenditure. The remaining 15 percent is accounted for by intellectual property products—the result of research, development, or innovation.
3. The NHFPC was created in 2013 from the former Ministry of Health and National Population and Family Planning Commission. In March 2018, however, its functions were integrated into a new agency called the National Health Commission ("China to Set Up National Health Commission," *Xinhua*, March 13, http://www.xinhuanet.com /english/2018-03/13/c_137035722.htm).
4. "Planning Layout of National Medical and Health Services System (2015–2020)" (*Guo Ban Fa* 2015, No. 14).
5. "Planning Layout of National Medical and Health Services System (2015–2020)" (*Guo Ban Fa* 2015, No. 14).

6. For more information on Kentucky's CON program, see the Cabinet for Health and Family Services of Kentucky website: https:// chfs.ky.gov/agencies/os/oig/dcn/Pages/cn.aspx.

References

Ashcroft, Beth, and Maine State Legislature. 2011. "Certificate of Need: Process Appears Clear, Consistent and Transparent, 2011." Paper 26, Office of Program Evaluation and Government Accountability, Augusta, ME.

CRC of Michigan (Citizens Research Council of Michigan). 2005. "The Michigan Certificate of Need Program." Report 338, CRC of Michigan, Livonia, MI.

EIU (Economist Intelligence Unit). 2015. "China Healthcare Industry Report." http://www.eiu .com (requires subscription).

EOHSP (European Observatory on Health Systems and Policies). n.d. "Health Systems in Transition (HiT) Profile of France." Country health system report, EOHSP, World Health Organization (WHO) European Centre for Health Policy, Brussels.

Ettelt, Stefanie, Ellen Nolte, Sarah Thomson, and Nicholas Mays. 2008. "Capacity Planning in Health Care: A Review of International Experience." Policy brief, World Health Organization on behalf of the European Observatory on Health Systems and Policies, Copenhagen.

Hindle, D., B. Dowdeswell, and A.-M. Yasbeck. 2004. "Report of a Survey of Clinical Pathways and Strategic Asset Planning in 17 EU Countries." Report, Netherlands Board for Hospital Facilities, Utrecht.

Le Deu, Franck, Rajesh Parekh, Fangning Zhang, Gaobo Zhou. 2012. "Healthcare in China: Entering Uncharted Waters." McKinsey Insights compendium, McKinsey & Co., Shanghai.

Nauta, J., R. Perenboom, and F. Galindo Garre. 2009. "A New Horizon for Planning Services and Health Care Infrastructure for the Elderly." Proceedings, HaCIRIC (Health and Care Infrastructure Research and Innovation Centre) International Conference 2009: 44–53.

NSW Government (New South Wales Government). 2011. "Sector Planning Framework: Policy Statement [Version 1.0]." Ageing, Disability, and Home Care (ADHC) policy document, NSW Department of Family and Community Services (FACS), Sydney.

OECD (Organisation for Economic Co-operation and Development). 2008. "OECD Annual Report 2008." OECD, Paris.

Rechel, B., J. Erskine, B. Dowdeswell, S. Wright, and M. McKee. 2009. *Capital Investment for Health: Case Studies from Europe.* Observatory Studies Series No. 18. Copenhagen: World Health Organization, on behalf of the European Conservatory on Health Systems and Policies.

Rechel, B., S. Wright, B. Dowdeswell, and M. McKee. 2010. "Even in Tough Times: Investing in Hospitals of the Future." *Euro Observer* 12 (1): 1–3.

Rechel, Bernd, Stephen Wright, Nigel Edwards, Barrie Dowdeswell, and Martin McKee. 2009. *Investing in Hospitals of the Future.* Observatory Studies Series No. 16. Copenhagen: World Health Organization, on behalf of the European Conservatory on Health Systems and Policies.

10

Strengthening the Implementation of Health Service Delivery Reform

Introduction

The next phase of China's health care system development will center on comprehensive improvement in the value of care across all levels of the system. Previous chapters have discussed the details of what must be changed in each of the eight reform levers. Drawing on lessons from national and international cases, they have also provided specific strategies to guide the implementation of each core action area. This chapter addresses the central challenge of how to implement these important changes and focus on creating an enabling organizational environment; it also discusses the tools needed to operationalize and sustain the core action areas and implementation strategies suggested in the previous chapters. Putting this environment in place is a precondition for effective implementation and thus a critical first step. Without it, progress may be elusive.

The rest of the chapter is organized as follows:

- *"Implementation Challenges"* reviews barriers to implementation in China's institutional and organizational environment and discusses specifics of an implementation model for spreading and scaling up the recommended reforms described in earlier chapters.
- *"A Four-Part Actionable Implementation Framework"* presents an operational implementation framework that focuses on four implementation systems: (a) macro implementation and influence, (b) coordination and support, (c) service delivery and learning, and (d) monitoring and evaluation.
- *"Moving Forward: Effective, Sustainable Local Implementation"* proposes, for each of the four implementation systems listed above, strategies that are specific and relevant to China. The organizational platforms for frontline service delivery improvement and learning are particularly important. For example, it is unlikely that changes in payment incentives will be enough to enable low-performing organizations to transform themselves (Cutler 2014); improvement will also require a support system that builds capacity and creates a facilitative climate to foster organizational (and individual) change.[1]
- *"Toward a Sequential Plan for Full-Scale Reform Implementation in China"* contains recommendations on sequencing and reaching full-scale health service delivery reform.

Implementation Challenges

There is consensus that China has sufficiently robust policies in place for health sector reform, but most observers acknowledge that the country has had difficulty translating these policies into scalable and sustained actions that improve service delivery. Typical of its development strategy in other sectors, China has promoted health reform implementation mainly through pilot projects. Experimenting with small-scale pilots operated by local governments has been effective in promoting and expanding economic reforms (Heilmann 2008), but it needs to make further progress in expanding health reforms.[2] This need has become particularly evident in efforts to address deep-rooted and complex issues related to provider incentives, private sector engagement, public hospital reform, and rebalancing service delivery.

Part of the problem is the difficulty of shifting away from direct facility management by government agencies to an arm's-length or indirect approach to governance, in which government agencies steer the health system through a combination of incentives, regulation, and other checks and balances (Meessen and Bloom 2007). Institutional fragmentation, diffuse leadership, and vested interests make this transition even more challenging. Under these conditions, even effective pilots cannot be maintained or scaled up.

Moving forward to implement the recommendations related to the eight reform levers will depend on careful management of implementation impediments at three levels of the system: central government, provincial and local governments, and frontline service providers. The impediments at each of these levels is taken up in turn.

Central Government: Dispersed Oversight and Monitoring of Reform Implementation

Typical of China's governance style, central government policy directives consist of principles and general guidelines to stimulate local innovation, while allowing flexibility in applying the principles to local conditions. Innovations are usually tried through pilot activities, which tend to be sanctioned by the central government. As observed in a number of case studies reviewed in this report, successful innovations have indeed occurred, but few have been scaled up.

Some policy makers suggest that innovations and reform implementation tend to be "personalized," responding to the preferences of local leaders, and therefore are difficult to replicate. This may relate to the lack of evidence-based analysis and feedback on reform progress and problems. Few innovations have been evaluated using rigorous methods, especially since all pilots were implemented under local contexts, and the background of different localities nationwide varies greatly.

The State Council's Health Reform Leading Group is responsible for policy formation and oversight, but various central government agencies monitor how these policies are implemented, with each agency focusing on specific aspects of reform (such as pricing, insurance, drug standards, human resources, medical services) aligned with their respective mandates. Supervisory reports tend to be based on short fact-gathering site visits, which are often conducted separately by representatives of different agencies. In addition, the independence of any assessment can be questioned because central-level departments are not totally separate from their decentralized counterparts in provincial and local governments. China has yet to systematically put in place independent mechanisms for gathering information and evaluating reforms. These conditions suggest that the central government may need to provide implementation-oriented guidance, consolidate and strengthen implementation oversight, and introduce systems to scrupulously monitor and validate progress and assess implementation from a more systemic, "big picture" perspective.

Provincial and Local Governments: Fragmented Coordination and Leadership

Given the dispersion of roles over many institutions, health reform has not been prioritized at some local levels. Resilient mechanisms for holding local government leaders accountable for health reform implementation have yet to be put in place. Incentives for local officials to plan and implement health reforms are generally weak compared with, for example, the incentives to promote economic growth and development (Huang 2009; Ramesh, Wu, and He 2013). Local leaders' performance and promotion are not determined by the progress on health reform. Under these conditions, local officials are justifiably reluctant to take on complex issues such as the profit-making interests of public hospitals.

Putting in place new models of health service delivery will require the strengthening of broad system coordination, particularly to overcome institutional fragmentation—both horizontal (across many government departments) and vertical (across the municipal, county, and district levels of government). Sustainable and scalable reform implementation is compromised under the current situation in which each department and agency tends to act to defend its own interests. Decisions on complex issues are often made through interagency bargaining, which weakens reform implementation (Huang 2009; Qian 2015). Patchwork administrative actions negotiated among diverse government departments (with divergent interests) to address elements of the reform may be effective in the short term but are not sustainable unless the government builds and institutionalizes its coordination capacity and creates the organizational arrangements to make them operational (He 2011). In sum, effective, scalable, and sustainable implementation will require putting in place incentives and accountability mechanisms that will drive local leaders and government departments to coordinate and enforce health reforms.

Frontline Service Providers: Weak Organizational Mechanisms for Providers to Lead and Share Learning about Health Care System Reform and Improvement

Health care improvement occurs on the front lines: in households, village clinics, community and township health centers, and hospital wards. Transformational value is seldom created by a single clinician or facility; it is more often generated by a group of providers who cooperate with each other and are collectively responsible for patient care. Reliable implementation of policy reform at the facility level does not happen by accident or by chance: deliberate and focused plans to ensure implementation must be created and then executed. This has been amply demonstrated internationally: good examples include the United Kingdom's Primary Care Collaborative (described in annex 10A), the U.S. Veterans Health Administration's Patient Aligned Care Teams (discussed in chapter 2), and the U.S. Centers for Medicare and Medicaid's recent Partnership for Patients (discussed in chapter 3).

International experience demonstrates that the proposed shift in organizational goals from treatment delivery to outcomes improvement requires fundamental changes in organizational culture. "Naming and blaming" denunciations to motivate changes in provider practices are insufficient to encourage creation of a value-oriented delivery system. Instead, the evidence supports the use of health-systems improvement methods, including performance reporting, data transparency, and, perhaps most importantly, systematic application of specific learning models that allow institutions to make changes and learn from their impact (Garside 1998; Greene, Reid, and Larson 2012; Schouten and others 2008). Facilitated collaborative approaches that allow peer institutions to learn from one another's successes and failures in a fear-free environment can rapidly accelerate implementation of policy reforms.

A Four-Part Actionable Implementation Framework

Implementation consists of the set of activities, processes, and interventions used to put policies, reforms, and evidence into practice. High-quality implementation is associated with obtaining desired impacts (Aarons and others 2009; Durlak and DuPré 2008; Meyers and others 2012; Wilson, Lipsey, and Derzon 2003). For example, in a review of 483 studies in five meta-analyses and 59 additional studies, Durlak and DuPré (2008) found a significant association between the level of implementation and the achievement of program outcomes. High-quality implementation increases the statistical probability of better program performance and can lead to better benefits for program participants.

There is a well-recognized gap between the health gains that could be achieved and those that are actually being realized around the world (WHO 2007). Part of this gap results from shortcomings in implementation and putting knowledge into practice. In other words, evidence-based health technologies and service models are not reliably implemented in many contexts. As the editors of the journal *Implementation Science* wrote in their inaugural issue, "Uneven uptake of research findings—and thus inappropriate care—occurs across settings, specialties, and countries" (Eccles and Mittman 2006, 1).

Drawing on a large body of literature, the science supporting implementation has advanced considerably during the past two decades. A number of actionable frameworks have emerged to assist planners, implementers, and communities in their implementation efforts (Aarons, Hurlburt, and Horwitz 2011; Damschroder and others 2009; Durlak and DuPré 2008; Fixsen and others 2005; Meyers, Durlak, and Wandersman 2012; Meyers and others 2012; Peters, Tran, and Adam 2013; Wandersman, Chien, and Katz 2012; Wandersman and others 2008). These frameworks provide evidence-based guidance on the critical phases, action steps, and components that contribute to effective

implementation, and ultimately to sustained institutionalization of successful practices.

Despite the strong evidence base supporting these frameworks, some caution is warranted. Some components have stronger empirical support than others. Also, implementation is inherently intertwined with the contexts where it occurs: general, "one size fits all" solutions do not exist, and adaptations tailored to local contexts will invariably take place. The implementation steps and organizational platforms proposed below, and their sequencing and timing, will vary according to local capacity, the supporting environment, and other starting conditions.

Bridging the gap between policies and practice requires capacity, resources, accountability, and a commitment to collaboration, evaluation, and learning. Drawing on the literature on implementation guidelines, the discussion below proposes a simplified but actionable implementation framework consisting of four systems adapted broadly to the Chinese context. It is important to note that these systems overlap and that further adaptations probably will be required for specific situations.

The Macro Implementation and Influence System

This system involves establishing the external "influence factors" that would create a climate that facilitates effective and sustained implementation (Fixsen and others 2005, 59). Implementation does not occur in a vacuum; it occurs within an institutional, political, and financial environment that establishes leadership and advocacy (for a focus on implementation practices), sets goals and performance targets, and scrutinizes the quality of implementation practices and their impacts. This enabling environment is essential for successful implementation of transformative reforms, which entail a need for new models and learning to overcome well-established routines and embedded interests. Research shows that a facilitating macro environment is associated with better outcomes and with *fidelity* of implementation—that is, the degree to which implementation is aligned with intended expectations, design, and plans (Fixsen and others 2005; Meyers, Durlak, and Wandersman 2012; Meyers and others 2012).

Greater attention to and scrutiny of implementation practices by senior policy makers and leaders is critical to the process of service delivery reform. Specific considerations include the following:

- Creating clear accountabilities for implementation performance
- Demonstrating leaders' commitment to the implementation process
- Specifying expected implementation milestones and outcomes
- Building a monitoring and feedback system to learn from implementation experiences and adjust policies and guidelines
- Mobilizing resources to support implementation processes
- Arranging independent evaluations.

One strategy for fostering an enabling environment (as further described below) is to strengthen the central government's oversight and monitoring role in reform implementation.

The Coordination and Support System

The coordination and support system aims to create the capacity and an enabling environment for effective implementation of frontline reform. Key functions of the coordination and support system include the following:

- Coordinating and ensuring the commitment of key local stakeholders
- Arranging training and technical assistance
- Developing and adapting implementation plans and timelines
- Communicating reform activities and expectations to communities, health care organizations, and health workers
- Making frontline providers accountable for implementation progress and results

- Ensuring that reform has adequate administrative support
- Conducting on-site monitoring of implementation activities, including documenting adaptations of original plans and designs.

The coordination and support system requires an organizational structure near the frontline implementation to carry out these functions and oversee the implementation process. Some countries have set up special implementation task forces to encourage the involvement and commitment of key stakeholders, monitor and control institutional and political pressures, and guide frontline providers through the complex change processes (Dewan and others 2003). As described below, China may consider establishing a fully empowered "leading group" or steering committee at the provincial or local governmental levels to perform these functions.

The Delivery and Learning System

The delivery and learning system is the main locus of implementation and where many service delivery reforms and care improvement solutions are designed and executed. It is at the front lines of service delivery: health care organizations (for example, hospitals, township health centers, and community health centers); networked groups of health care organizations; and communities. It involves individual behavioral and broader organizational change but also making the "culture of the organization" open to change (Garside 1998, S8). This system is where evidence is put into practice and where implementers learn from their own experience and customize and tailor experience from elsewhere to their own situation.

Operationally, it involves creating organizational arrangements for problem solving, practitioner-to-practitioner coaching and collaboration, and shared and continuous learning. Transformation Learning Collaboratives (TLCs) are proposed as the organizational building blocks for a delivery and learning system in China, as described later in this chapter.

A learning system includes a set of methods including observation, experimentation, and feedback that is applied to build knowledge and enable the achievement of a patient-centered result. In the United States, the National Science Foundation has supported multidisciplinary, cross-sector workshops to explore the potential for a new "science of learning systems" (Etheredge 2014; Friedman and others 2014). A variety of technical models for generating new insights (innovation), developing supporting evidence (research), and ensuring reliable implementation of impactful findings (dissemination and implementation) have been described (IHI 2003; Rogers 2010). Recognizing the need and importance for a health care system to be able to learn rapidly from its own efforts to improve patient care, the U.S. Institute of Medicine established a Committee on the Learning Health Care System in America (Yong, Olsen, and McGinnis 2010).[3]

The Monitoring and Evaluation System

Monitoring and evaluating the effectiveness of implementation and the impact of reform is a critical but often overlooked component of the implementation process. Evidence needs to be gathered to learn from implementation and contribute to evidence-based adjustments and future policy making. Careful monitoring can detect whether implementation is aligned with stated objectives, whether it is on track (or going off track), and whether the implemented reforms match those that were intended.

To that end, it requires careful measurement, which in turn must respond to the information needs of the various stakeholders. Good measurement will require prioritizing the establishment and strengthening of high-quality national and subnational information platforms. Previous attempts to improve the quality of common data repositories for health care improvement have established a basis on which primary care data can be captured and analyzed for the purposes of making ongoing improvements. For these data to become operationally

useful for frontline practitioners to make system-level improvements, the information will need to be returned to the front line for those practitioners' interpretation and use. Systems may already be in place to aggregate local data, create distribution tables, and benchmark values that can be fed back to service delivery units for their reflection. Guidance on how to improve the accuracy, completeness, and timeliness of data submission, processing, and feedback can be found in the international literature (Mate and others 2009).

In addition, it is highly recommended that implementation be accompanied by a combination of effective health services research (HSR) and impact evaluations to allow rigorous measurement of intended and unintended effects and outcomes. Though these activities are more methodologically demanding than monitoring, HSR and impact evaluations can provide valuable information for understanding a reform's effects and can provide practical guidance to key stakeholders, including policy makers, about the progress of reform implementation. One additional focus—combining both monitoring and impact evaluation—is understanding *why* implementation was successful or not (Berwick, Nolan, and Whittington 2008). In China, putting in place a robust monitoring and evaluation system to accompany reform implementation will require the close attention of the central government in coordination with provincial and local governments.

Moving Forward: Effective, Sustainable Local Implementation

Numerous experiments are under way in China to operationalize the health reform policies, but for the reforms to be successful and brought to scale, they need to be deep, comprehensive, and implemented in a coordinated and deliberate manner. In building a better health care delivery system for China, a major challenge is reaching full scale: being able to test and spread reforms to health care delivery systems in every municipality, county, township, and village.

Following the four-part implementation framework presented in the previous section, this section suggests strategies and corresponding actions that China can consider to facilitate robust reform implementation and scaling-up. These strategies are the critical elements for planning, prioritizing, and sequencing interventions necessary to build a 21st-century health system. All will need strong, persistent central government support to make them work. The main strategies for each system are the following (as further outlined in table 10.1):

- *Macro implementation and influence system*: Establish strong central government oversight linked to national policy implementation and monitoring guidelines
- *Coordination and support system*: Establish fully empowered coordination

TABLE 10.1 Responsibility levels, strategies, and actions to scale up health service delivery reform, by implementation system type

| Actionable implementation systems | | |
System and level of responsibility	Main strategies and responsibilities	Actions
Macro implementation and influence system (central level)	Establish the external "influence factors" that would create a facilitative climate for effective and sustained implementation Focus greater attention and scrutiny on implementation practices by senior policy makers and leaders	Establish strong central government oversight, linked to national policy implementation and monitoring guidelines, responsible for the following activities: • Create clear accountabilities for implementation performance, demonstrating leaders' commitment to the implementation process, by specifying expected implementation milestones and outcomes • Build a monitoring and feedback system to learn from implementation experiences to adjust policies and guidelines • Mobilize resources to support implementation processes • Arrange for independent evaluations
Coordination and support system (provincial and local levels)	Create capacity and an enabling environment for effective reform implementation by resolving overlapping accountabilities and interagency complexities	Institute coordination and leadership mechanisms at the provincial and local governmental levels (such as "leading groups" or steering committees) that build capacity and foster accountability for effective reform implementation as follows: • Coordinate and ensure buy-in of key local stakeholders • Arrange training and technical assistance • Develop and adapt implementation plans and timelines • Communicate reform activities and expectations • Conduct on-site monitoring of implementation activities, including documenting adaptations to original plans and designs
Delivery and learning system (frontline providers)	Set up a robust learning system—a set of methods including observation, experimentation, and feedback—that frontline workers can use as they implement service delivery reforms and help design and execute care improvement solutions, enabling them to build and share knowledge during implementation	• Develop local Transformation Learning Collaborative models to foster frontline reform implementation and care improvement • Create an organizational arrangement for problem solving, practitioner-to-practitioner collaboration and coaching, and shared and continuous learning
Monitoring and evaluation system (central level in partnership with provincial level)	Monitor and evaluate the effectiveness of reform implementation and impact—a critical but often overlooked component of the implementation process	• Ensure strong and independent monitoring with robust data feedback to the front line where care decisions are made • Conduct rigorous impact evaluations to understand progress against overall health reform objectives

and leadership mechanisms at the provincial and local governmental levels that build capacity and foster accountability for effective reform implementation

- *Delivery and learning system:* Create local Transformation Learning Collaboratives at the network and facility levels that foster frontline reform implementation and care improvement
- *Monitoring and evaluation system:* Ensure strong and independent monitoring and impact evaluation.

Macro Implementation and Influence System: Establish Strong Central Government Oversight

The central government might consider taking a more hands-on lead in guiding and monitoring the implementation of the reforms, including the eight levers. China could consider assigning this mandate to the State Council, which would mean expanding the authority, roles, and functions of the State Council Health Reform Leading Group currently responsible for health-reform policy making (figure 10.1).

Guidelines for policy implementation and monitoring could be prepared to orient reform planning and execution by provincial and local governments. Drawing on the core action areas presented in chapters 2–9, many activities could be covered by such guidelines (table 10.2). The guidelines could describe verifiable (and measurable) tasks or intermediate outcomes related to reform implementation, and thus foster greater integrity of reform implementation at local levels. They would not constitute an implementation plan or a generalized blueprint but would need to be operational in nature, specifying categorically "what to do." In turn, provincial and local governments would need to have full authority to decide on "how to do it" — developing, executing, and sequencing implementation plans based on local conditions.

Given the large number of government institutions involved in the health sector, the decentralized nature of implementation, and the well-known difficulties in aligning institutional positions, China may want to consider assigning an official with a rank higher than Minister to head the State Council Health Reform Office (SCHRO). While controversial, an appointment with this very high rank may be needed to influence institutional stakeholders and provincial governors. China might also consider granting SCHRO

FIGURE 10.1 Proposed oversight, coordination, and management for implementation and scaling up of health service delivery reform

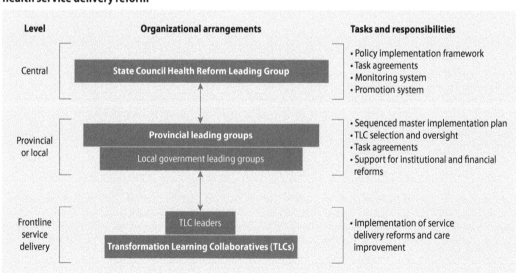

TABLE 10.2   Sample monitoring guidelines for implementation of China's value-driven future health system

Reform component	Key elements, selected core action areas
Service delivery system	
A tiered health care delivery system based on people-centered integrated care (Lever 1)	1. *Strengthened primary care is the first point of contact* and the gatekeeper for patients' use of the health care delivery system, and is responsible for providing continuous and comprehensive care. (Primary care includes m-health outreach to communities, social services, and homes through use of community health workers virtually connected to general practitioners and specialists.) 2. *Within each care network, well-organized multidisciplinary teams* of clinical and nonclinical personnel provide full cycle of care to patients. (People enroll with care teams and are stratified by risks and conditions. Teams assume joint accountability for treatment, prevention, and patient engagement.) 3. *Vertical integration of care* is provided at hospitals, primary care facilities, and communities by establishing multidisciplinary teams, evidence-based integrated clinical pathways and referral systems (such as for postdischarge care), and individualized care plans for patients with chronic conditions. 4. *Horizontal integration of individual preventive and curative care* services takes place at the primary care level. (Centers for disease control emphasize public health; individual preventive care is transferred to primary care.) 5. *Information and communication technologies* support provider-to-provider integration and empower frontline health workers. 6. A Transformation Learning Collaborative leadership team (separate from hospital management) forms and operates networks.
Quality of care and patient engagement (Levers 2, 3)	1. *National authority* assesses, regulates, and oversees quality of care in all institutions. 2. *Evidence-based health literacy campaigns* are used to encourage healthy behaviors. 3. *Patients' self-management* of chronic conditions is part of care plans. 4. *Information on provider quality* is publicly disclosed.
Hospital reform and service integration (Levers 1, 4)	1. *Public hospitals are granted more autonomy* in management but within a strong regulatory and accountability framework that ensures accountability for supporting care integration, reducing costs and unnecessary care, and shifting low-complexity care to lower levels. 2. *Managerial capacity building* is supported by putting a professionalization plan in place for hospital management. 3. *Tertiary hospitals provide highly complex care* while supporting secondary hospitals and primary care facilities with technical assistance, research, and workforce development. 4. *Secondary hospitals provide essential specialty care* and are closely linked to primary care, providing technical support, supervision, and training. Professional medical staff are shared with primary care through formation of multidisciplinary care teams.
Financial and institutional environment	
Incentives in purchasing and provider payments (Lever 5)	1. *Strategic purchasing of health services* is based on quality and efficiency criteria. 2. *Health providers' income* is delinked from service volume. 3. *Provider payment systems* gradually shift from paying individual facilities to paying integrated care networks (for example, using capitation) and to paying for a package of services (for example, bundled payments for treating groups of patients with certain conditions).
Strengthening of human resources (Lever 6)	1. *Standardized scientific professional development and education* is in place for all health care professionals, including physicians, nurses, and pharmacists. 2. *Professional standing and sufficient income* for primary health care providers are ensured to keep the health profession attractive. 3. *Physician compensation and hospital-based quota systems* are reformed to enable a more flexible labor market and efficient workforce management. 4. *New and alternative cadres of workers* are produced and integrated into the health workforce to strengthen primary health care delivery.
Private sector engagement (Lever 7)	1. *Regulations support a level playing field* whereby high-quality private providers can deliver cost-effective services and compete on the same terms as the public sector. 2. *Social health insurers purchase from private providers* the services for which they are licensed and that meet quality standards.
Service and capital planning (Lever 8)	1. *A new, people-centered planning model* is based on province-specific population health needs and demographic profiles. 2. *Capital investment planning* integrates all public financial resources. 3. *An integrated capital planning process* incorporates private provider participation and capacity.

sufficient authority and institutional independence to influence how resources are allocated and how provincial and local leaders are assessed in terms of reform implementation. SCHRO staffing would need to be strengthened to perform this proposed expanded role. SCHRO should also consider establishing strong accountability mechanisms to enforce reform implementation at the provincial and local levels, such as "task agreements" with provincial and local governments (as further discussed below).

Coordination and Support System: Establish Coordination and Organizational Mechanisms for Provincial and Local Accountability and Frontline Reform Implementation

Strengthening of accountability arrangements, particularly at the provincial and local levels, is another essential ingredient to facilitate effective implementation of reforms. Any accountability arrangement should be sufficiently powerful to align institutional interests and leverage government priorities when dealing with providers and vested interests.

One solution would be to form empowered leading groups or steering committees at the provincial level, led by high-level leaders (governors or party chiefs). Leading groups could also be formed at local government levels (county, municipality, and prefecture), depending on the context. Such groups already exist in China and could be enabled to oversee reform implementation and support frontline execution. The leading groups would need strong, active leadership by high-level officials, broad political support, and full empowerment (and accountability) to implement reform within their jurisdictions. The proposed leading groups could consist of representatives from the various government agencies involved in the health sector, but they should also include private sector representatives and community leaders.

An advantage of the proposed leading-group arrangement is that it is a well-known mechanism for interagency coordination and has been applied successfully within China's

current institutional framework. It could be considered an interim organizational arrangement, in part to mitigate the potential adverse effects of institutional fragmentation on reform implementation—it would not institutionalize interagency coordination. A longer-term solution would involve institutional consolidation as part of a much broader reform to streamline the government's administration systems and organizational structures (box 10.1).

In Sanming (as mentioned in chapter 5), concerted and coordinated actions led by a leading group at the prefecture level and buttressed by exceptionally strong political support enabled a successful series of deep reforms. The Sanming experience suggests that the leading-group arrangement can effectively coordinate decision making across multiple government departments for planning and implementing complex reforms, at least in the short term. Reformers have yet to put in place an institutionalized platform for coordinating stakeholders that would formalize accountability mechanisms and incentives for sustained reform implementation.

As it considers the organizational structures, distribution of responsibilities, and coordination of functions across agencies for health system governance, China may wish to review the experiences in Organisation for Economic Co-operation and Development (OECD) countries. Both international and Chinese experience suggest that implementing health reform is a long-term endeavor, is technically and politically complex, and requires numerous adjustments while it is in progress. Desired outcomes may take time to materialize because of many intervening factors, and unintended negative consequences can occur. In a country as large as China, flexibility is also required to allow for the wide variation in starting conditions and local contexts.

The leading-group arrangement can be strengthened to support longer-term implementation in several ways:

- The proposed provincial leading groups could be made accountable to central government through intergovernmental

BOX 10.1   Government administrative reforms and international experience

Organizational restructuring has been a major feature of China's administrative reforms for several decades (Saich 2015; Xue and Liou 2012). Policies have called for streamlining administrative functions to promote coordination and reduce the overlapping of authorities and responsibilities. More recently, these reforms are seen as part of a broader process to transform government functions to enable deepening of economic, social, and other sectoral reforms; strengthen regulations; and delegate government power (Li 2015). Making government agencies more effective through streamlining functions and "building a unified supervision platform" (Li 2015) is also considered critical to improving reform oversight and implementation. Whether these reforms will lead to institutional consolidation or creation of an institutionalized platform for an interagency coordination in the health sector remains an open question.

China may consider examining organizational structures, distribution of responsibilities, and coordination of functions across agencies for health system governance among the Organisation for Economic Co-operation and Development (OECD) countries. Most OECD countries have an array of agencies—including central line ministries, self-governing bodies, professional associations, affiliated institutes, independent commissions, and regional health authorities—that constitute the governance configurations of the health sector.[a] Institutional configurations depend on the following (Jakubowski and Saltman 2013; Mossialos and others 2015):

- The type of system (that is, a tax-financed national health system or social insurance system)
- The extent of decentralization
- The degree of state involvement in three core health system functions: regulation, financing, and service delivery.

Over the past two decades, China has been migrating from a tax-funded national health service in which the state plays a dominant role in regulation, financing, and service delivery to a social insurance system in which the state retains regulatory functions but delegates financing to social insurance agencies and service delivery to public and (increasingly) private providers. China may want to explore the institutional governance arrangements of health systems based on social insurance financing such as in Austria, Germany, the Republic of Korea, and the Netherlands.

In the OECD, all agencies involved in health system governance are generally under the jurisdiction of a single governing institution responsible for policy making, strategies, and regulations. Over the past two decades, OECD countries have enacted governance reforms that have added national agencies (that is, for quality oversight, assessment, and improvement as well as for performance and regulatory monitoring) while at the same time consolidating overlapping functions and responsibilities across different levels of government, including the consolidation of social insurance funds (Jakubowski and Saltman 2013). These reforms aimed to exert greater central influence. Similarly, in part to address coordination, cost containment, and equity concerns, national governments have strengthened their decision-making power along with that of the corresponding lead health organization, inducing the recentralization of functions. These centralizing trends have been noted in different systems, including those based on the tax-funded National Health Service in the United Kingdom and the social insurance system in Germany.

However, in countries with strongly decentralized systems, greater central-level authority does not always result in greater policy or policy implementation integrity. Moreover, international experience suggests that stronger government authority should not mean, for example, government interference in operating social insurance systems. Clear division of roles and authorities between government health institutions and social insurance agencies combined with well-defined accountability to align the latter with government health policies and priorities are critical to coherent decision-making structures (Savedoff and Gottret 2008).

a. For more details about the institutional configurations of the health sectors in OECD countries, see Mossialos and others 2015 and the Health in Transition (HiT) Series of the World Health Organization's (WHO) European Observatory on Health Systems and Policies: http://www.euro.who.int/en/about-us/partners/observatory/publications/health-system-reviews-hits/. For similar information about Asian countries, see the online resources of the Asia Pacific Observatory on Health Systems and Policies: http://www.wpro.who.int/asia_pacific_observatory/hits/series/chn/en/.

performance contracts or task agreements, signed with SCHRO, that specify implementation benchmarks, anticipated results of the reforms, and, ultimately, population-health indicators. These agreements could be assessed and revised annually or twice a year. SCHRO could consider rewards and sanctions related to performance.

- A subset of these implementation-performance measures should be incorporated into the career-promotion system as yardsticks to measure provincial and local government performance in reform implementation.

- As suggested above, performance in implementing agreed-upon reforms should be vigorously monitored by SCHRO and independently verified by SCHRO in partnership with academic institutions. National and regional workshops could be held to review and compare performance across provinces. These reviews would identify some higher performers, whose efforts could be more carefully examined to learn the contextually relevant ingredients for success that may be replicable by others.

Delivery and Learning System: Create Transformation Learning Collaboratives to Implement, Sustain, and Scale Up Frontline Reforms

The shift to focus on improving outcomes rather than just delivering treatments—that is, on value rather than procedures—will require fundamental changes in organizational culture. Health care organizations (whether networks, hospitals, community health centers, or township health centers) would greatly benefit from adopting continuous learning and problem-solving approaches to hasten the successful implementation of reforms. The service delivery reforms recommended in earlier chapters include a number of important changes at care facilities throughout China: using evidence-based care protocols, extending e-health innovations, integrating care, following clear guidelines for referral to specialists and hospitals, measuring and tracking outcomes, and more. Although these changes can and should be driven by national and provincial leadership, implementing them at local sites will require assistance for local learning, problem solving, and adaptation.

To achieve better outcomes at lower costs, providers in China need to learn new ways to deliver care. To support this learning process, public and private providers can come together to form associations committed to implementing the people-centered integrated approach and the corresponding financial and institutional reforms. If these associations are properly organized and led, participating providers will benefit from not having to reinvent their care alone and separately; they can learn together and help each other. Associations or groups of providers can be organized in either urban or rural settings and be made accountable for on-the-ground implementation of reforms, under the oversight of the provincial leading group and aligned with the policy implementation framework to be developed by the State Council Health Reform Leading Group. These associations could help move the care systems more quickly toward a new culture of coordinated, cooperative, outcome-oriented care.

Drawing from international experience, we propose that Transformation Learning Collaboratives—partnerships of groups of facilities within a county, district, or municipality—should be established to implement, manage, and sustain reforms on the front line.[4] The driving vision behind the TLC concept is to assist and guide local care facilities such as village clinics, township health centers, community health centers, and county and district hospitals to implement and scale up the reformed service delivery model and close the gap between "knowing" and "doing." Provincial (and local) leading groups can select the facility alliances or networks, hospitals, and primary care facilities to participate in TLCs.

This approach for shared joint learning among all parties in a geographic area has been tried and tested all over the world, including in Brazil, Chile, Germany, Portugal,

---

BOX 10.2   **Evidence supporting the use of TLC methodology**

The Transformation Learning Collaborative (TLC) methodology has led to impressive results in several large health care systems in a number of countries, and it has been adopted and locally improved by many organizations. These sample results are representative of hundreds more like them:

- *The U.S. Veterans Health Administration* (VHA) used a collaborative learning approach to reduce waiting times in primary care clinics by 53 percent, from 60 days to 28 days. As the largest integrated delivery system in the United States, caring for more than 6 million patients, the VHA continued to work to spread its "advanced access" model[a] to health services across its entire system. From July 2002 to October 2003, the total number of veterans waiting decreased from more than 300,000 to fewer than 50,000 (IHI 2004; Schall and others 2004).
- *The United Kingdom's National Health Service (NHS)* launched its National Primary Care Collaborative in 2000. The Collaborative is now perhaps the world's largest health care improvement project. Encompassing nearly 2,000 practices nationwide and covering almost 18.2 million patients, it has helped to reduce the waiting time for an appointment with a general practitioner by an average of 60 percent (Oldham 2004).
- *The United Kingdom's NHS Modernization Agency* formed the Cancer Services Collaborative in 1999 to improve access and care for cancer

patients. Project teams tested 4,400 changes between September 1999 and August 2000, involving about 1,000 patients. Sixty-five percent of the projects showed at least a 50 percent reduction in the time to first treatment (Griffith and Turner 2004).
- *The Boston-based nonprofit Partners in Health (PIH)* adapted the "Breakthrough Series" model to improve care for people in low- and middle-income nations. In Peru, where 9 out of 10 people with tuberculosis die, PIH's patients have an 80 percent cure rate. The program's success persuaded the World Health Organization (WHO) to add medicines for this disease to the WHO list of essential drugs (Shin and others 2004).
- *Nash Health Care Systems* in North Carolina in the United States reduced the average number of days on a ventilator by 34 percent and the average length of stay by 25 percent for ventilator patients. Cases of ventilator-associated pneumonia dropped by more than 50 percent during the collaborative. Patients in the protocol group averaged more than US$35,000 savings in hospital charges, compared with patients in the baseline group (IHI 2003).
- *The Singapore Healthcare Improvement Network (SHINe)* has used collaborative methods to improve patient safety in all acute-care medical institutions in the country, including hospitals that serve the behavioral health and long-term care needs of the population.[b]

a. The "advanced access" model is also known as open access or same-day scheduling, in which a sizable share of the day's appointments are reserved for patients desiring a same-day appointment (IOM 2015).
b. For more information, see the SHINe website: http://shine.com.sg/.

Singapore, Sweden, the United Kingdom, and the United States. Box 10.2 summarizes some of these experiences and their impact. Annex 10A describes how the TLC methodology has been used in Scotland to improve patient safety and more broadly in the United Kingdom to strengthen primary care.

The rest of this subsection discusses how China might structure and operationalize TLCs, including (a) the basic principles, structure, and managerial philosophy underlying TLCs; (b) the tiered management system to support TLCs; (c) processes that TLCs

use to help their members make improvements; and (d) proposed sequencing of interventions within a TLC.

Principles, structures, and managerial philosophy of TLCs

A TLC is a structure that supports shared learning and rapid change among a group of providers or organizations. Instead of trying to achieve results alone and separately, participants in a TLC have the opportunity to learn together, exchange ideas and lessons learned, and share information on measurements and results to encourage that exchange. A TLC capitalizes on the idea that "two heads are better than one" and that "many heads are better than a few."

The approach moves away from defining performance indicators, identifying under-performers, and public "naming and sham-ing." Naming and shaming can generate a culture of fear—a situation that often leads to incomplete and distorted data, corrodes the spirit of innovation, and undermines the will to improve. In the TLC model, continu-ous improvement for everyone is the goal, and everyone (even the best performers) is recognized as having the capacity to improve. Facility-level teams are encouraged to test and improve new systems without fear of failure. Data are scrutinized, not to identify underperformers but rather to high-light, celebrate, and learn from those who have outperformed the rest. Recognition and celebration of performance, not the instillation of fear, is the currency of the TLCs and drives all parties to higher levels of performance.

The TLC model is a structure for rapidly disseminating better practices to all facilities in a geographic region, whether in a rural county or an urban municipality. At the start of service delivery reform implementation, each participating province would select the most natural administrative level for the TLC: county, district, municipal, or prefec-ture. TLCs would be formed and rolled out over time, and all health care organizations (public or private) within the province would be expected to join a TLC at some point.

In most provinces, some combination of TLC types would be needed. For example, in a rural setting, a TLC could consist of a county hospital, township health centers, vil-lage clinics, and private providers. Urban TLCs could consist of tertiary hospitals, dis-trict hospitals, community health centers, community health stations, and private pro-viders. Other combinations of facilities are also possible. Figure 10.2 displays three pos-sible examples of TLC partnering arrange-ments: at the county or rural level, at the municipal or urban level, and at the prefec-tural rural and urban level.

The TLC management system

Depending on local conditions, TLCs can be formed and overseen by provincial leading groups (PLGs) or by local leading groups

FIGURE 10.2   The TLC model in three different arrangements

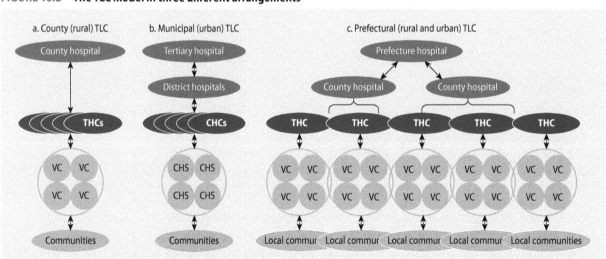

Source: ©World Bank. Permission required for reuse.
Note: CHC = community health center; CHSs = community health services; THC = township health center; TLC = Transformation Learning Collaborative; VC = village clinic.

(LLGs). The PLG or LLG would define the number of participating facilities and the geographical scope of the TLC, appoint leaders, invite facilities and teams to participate, and host its activities. It would appoint a TLC management team consisting of trusted local hospital and clinic leaders, assisted by a systems improvement adviser and program management staff from the participating hospitals.

Given the operational nature of TLCs, PLGs should consider making TLC management separate from government administrative leadership. Strong communication and continuous data flow between the TLCs and PLGs would strengthen the PLGs' governance and stewardship roles while allowing the TLCs sufficient room to innovate. The PLGs should also ensure the active participation of multiple providers and avoid hospital capture of TLC leadership. The leading groups could sign task agreements with the TLC's leadership.

It would be important that the PLGs work on the more macrolevel changes and improvements in the institutional and financial environment across the multiple TLCs (that is, those at the provincial level) to remove specific barriers that impede progress within several TLCs operating in a province. For example, as TLC participants seek to spread the changes that are needed to produce better care at lower cost, they will encounter barriers that make the reforms difficult. Removing those barriers would require actions by senior leaders and leading groups above the level of the TLC participants. For example, the TLCs probably would need the PLGs' support to deal with issues relating to changes in human resources policies, supply-chain problems, reorientation of incentives, capital planning and investment, and promoting engagement with the private sector. International experience demonstrates that a critical function of senior leadership (in this case, provincial leadership) is to remain in touch with the TLC members and focus on solving upstream problems to allow the TLCs to progress.

Establishing the appropriate managerial capacities to guide, support, and operate TLC activities is critical for the success of any individual TLC. This set of tasks would include building the capability and technical skills of TLC members in how to manage scientific improvement of systems. To acquire these skills, TLCs should consider forming technical partnerships with leading Chinese academic institutions that would contribute technical know-how and confer some of their reputational strength on the TLCs. International partners and technical assistance could also be provided through the Chinese academic institutions as needed.

TLC processes to make improvements

Each TLC would be organized as a time-delimited (18- to 24-month) learning system. Before launching the TLC, the PLGs or LLGs would agree on the specific set of reform initiatives to be implemented and on a set of measures to track the implementation progress of all the participating facilities and institutions. For example, one reform initiative could involve the transition to team-based care, which would facilitate care for chronic diseases such as diabetes. All the participating facilities could track their progress using agreed-upon "process measures" (such as the proportion of frontline staff on the clinical care teams, the proportion of patients assigned to a clinical care team, the numbers of annual visits by patients assigned to a care team, or the numbers of medicines prescribed) and "outcome measures" (such as the percentage of diabetic patients with glycosylated hemoglobin levels of less than 8 percent).

Figure 10.3 illustrates how a collaborative could work—from formation of facility-level teams to attend the TLC learning sessions to action periods between meetings, all supported by various knowledge-sharing activities.

Formation of facility-level teams. Organizations participating in the TLC would send facility-level teams to the TLC meetings. The facility-level teams would consist of three to five people from each facility, including operational leadership and key clinical staff.

FIGURE 10.3   **Design of a Transformation Learning Collaborative**

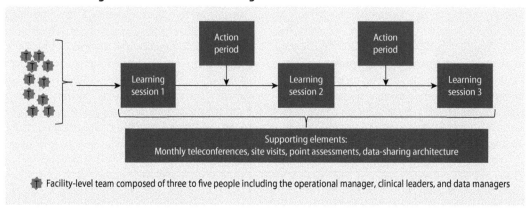

Source: ©World Bank. Permission required for reuse.

Learning sessions. TLC teams from all participating facilities would meet face-to-face in learning sessions every four to six months to discuss successes, barriers, and challenges; share better practices; and describe lessons learned as they collectively seek to implement the reforms in primary health care. Learning sessions are a mixture of collective will-building; didactic training on specific improvement skills and technical issues that might be pertinent to the health reform; and sharing of lessons and ideas by participating teams to overcome specific implementation barriers.

Learning sessions conclude with each team establishing a plan for implementation during the action period that follows each learning session. For example, in a recent learning session of a collaborative that focused on improving access to primary care, participants spent one quarter of the time learning technical skills in a plenary format, one quarter working in their teams to plan future actions, and the rest of the time exchanging practical tips and tools with other participating teams.

Action periods. Between the face-to-face TLC learning session meetings, there would be action periods when the facility-based teams would test and implement interventions in their local settings and collect and report data to measure the interventions' impact.

Supporting activities. Teams would submit monthly progress reports and be supported by conference calls, peer site visits, and web-based discussions to enable them to share information and learn from national experts and other health care organizations. The aim is to build collaboration and support member organizations as they try out new ideas, even at a distance.

Throughout the process, teams would use a methodology known as the Plan-Do-Study-Act (PDSA) cycle to iteratively test ideas for improving system performance (as further described in annex 10B).[5] During an action period, for example, teams would test different ways of implementing team-based care. Teams might try different approaches to structuring their teams or different communication strategies, such as a daily morning meeting to review all assigned patients. Scheduling might take various forms. Teams might test an innovative technology for grouping patients according to various characteristics and conditions to perceive patterns. Teams would use a web-based data collection portal to submit monthly progress reports on the agreed-upon measures. To continue the example mentioned above, such measures might include the percentage of diabetic patients with glycosylated hemoglobin of less than 8 percent or with blood pressure under control. These data would be available to the entire TLC community for all to see and review.

Reform sequencing and measurement within a TLC

As TLCs begin to be rolled out in the selected reform provinces, it would be important to think about the sequence of implementation. (For an example of an implementation pathway and guidelines, see annex 10C.) TLCs might focus on one or more of the eight reform areas. It would be difficult to predict which reforms each TLC would select, because the details of their circumstances would likely determine which reforms are most important to the TLC leaders. A full menu of the reforms should be made available to the TLC leaders at the outset, and as soon as a team starts work, its leaders should devise a master "reform pathway" in consultation with representatives from the participating health care facilities.

Monitoring and Evaluation System: Ensure Strong and Independent Monitoring and Impact Evaluation

The State Council may consider establishing a strong monitoring and evaluation system capable of independently assessing and verifying implementation progress and reform impacts. This could be achieved in partnership with academic institutions. Based on the proposed implementation guidelines and existing monitoring systems, SCHRO could develop implementation benchmarks and other metrics to track reform implementation. Table 10.3 contains examples of value-oriented indicators categorized by the three overarching goals of the reform effort: better care, better health, and lower cost.

Regardless of the specific pathway taken through the available reform priorities, each reform would need a clear, universal measurement framework to help guide TLC leaders and the provincial leadership groups to understand the progress being made on the front lines. As a particular reform matures within facilities, progress would need to be measured and understood so that TLC leaders and PLGs can encourage the TLCs to move on to new areas of reform.

More operationally, the PLGs could track the TLCs' progress and, together with the central government, monitor data on selected indicators of utilization, cost, quality, and outcome (table 10.4). The tracking of progress should be complemented by impact

TABLE 10.3 Sample indicators for monitoring health reform implementation, by reform goal

Reform goal	Indicators
Goal 1: Achieve better care for individuals	• Admission rates for complications for diabetes, hypertension, and chronic lung disease in secondary and tertiary hospitals: aim for 20 percent reduction in two years • Number of patients whose first contact for an illness episode occurs in primary care: aim for a 20 percent increase in two years • Antibiotics prescriptions at primary care facilities and outpatient clinics: aim for a 25 percent reduction in two years
Goal 2: Achieve better health for populations	• Percentage of population ages 18–75 years with hypertension and whose blood pressure was adequately controlled (below 140/90): aim for 20 percent improvement in two years • Percentage of patients with diabetes with hemoglobin A1c below 8 percent: aim of 20 percent improvement in two years • Percentage of women ages 16–64 years who received one or more Pap tests to screen for cervical cancer: aim of 20 percent improvement in two years
Goal 3: Achieve affordable costs	• Inpatient admissions per 1,000 population: aim of 15 percent reduction in two years • Length of stay: aim of 20 percent reduction in stays at secondary and tertiary hospitals in two years • Total spending per insured: aim of health cost inflation similar to consumer price inflation, as indicated by quarterly reports of social insurance agencies

TABLE 10.4   Scoring system for Transformation Learning Collaboratives

TLC stage	Indicators
1. Formation	• TLC has been formed.
	• Aim for implementation has been set, and baseline measurement has begun.
2. Activity	• TLC is meeting regularly.
	• Participating teams are beginning local implementation activities.
3. Testing	• Changes are being tested, but no improvements are seen yet.
	• Data on measures are being reported consistently.
4. Process improvement	• Improvements have been recorded in processes identified as critical to achieving collaborative aim.
5. Outcome improvement	• Improvements have been recorded in outcomes related to the collaborative aim.

Note: TLC = Transformation Learning Collaborative. Each TLC is graded 1–5 on this scale based on how the TLC is progressing. These data can be averaged at the desired level of aggregation for performance review by provincial and national authorities.

FIGURE 10.4   Sequential plan for scaling up reform implementation

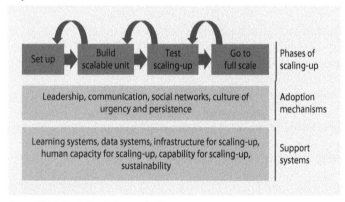

Source: ©World Bank. Permission required for reuse.

evaluations that use rigorous methodologies to measure impact and allow comparison across sites that are implementing similar reforms.

Toward a Sequential Plan for Full-Scale Reform Implementation in China

The province is the recommended unit of focus for implementing health reform in China over the next five to seven years. A well-designed and detailed plan is needed for scaling-up across a province—that is, for ensuring that all facilities in a province participate in a TLC and implement the reforms.

This section describes a "waved" sequence that could be used to achieve provincewide spread of the eight reform levers (Barker, Reid, and Schall 2016).

TLCs could be rolled out gradually in phases to all counties and districts. Depending on the local context and starting conditions, there might be more than one TLC per jurisdiction (such as a large municipality or county). Four phases would be required to spread TLCs throughout a province:[6]

- *Phase 1:* Set up the TLC, including the provincial and local preparatory steps for implementation of reforms
- *Phase 2:* Develop the scalable unit—a prototyping phase.
- *Phase 3:* Test scaling-up—a phase that expands the core knowledge in a variety of settings that are likely to represent different contexts that will be encountered at full scale
- *Phase 4:* Go to full scale—a phase that unfolds rapidly to enable a larger number of sites or divisions to adopt or replicate the intervention.

Figure 10.4 illustrates this sequential implementation and also shows a series of adoption mechanisms and support systems that facilitate the implementation sequence. "Adoption mechanisms" are the system elements needed to facilitate the implementation

TABLE 10.5   TLC sequential implementation plan, by phase, time interval, and jurisdiction

Phase	Time interval	TLC rollout in counties and districts
1. Set up	Month 0	0 counties
2. Develop scalable unit	Month 3	1–2 "initial" C&Ds
3. Test of scaling-up	Month 12	Wave 1: 10 C&Ds
4. Full-scale rollout	Month 24	Wave 2: 10 additional C&Ds
	Month 36	Wave 3: 10 additional C&Ds
	Month 48	Wave 4: 10 additional C&Ds
	Month 60	Wave 5: 10 additional C&Ds
	Month 72	Wave 6: 10 additional C&Ds

Note: C&Ds = counties and districts; TLC = Transformation Learning Collaborative.

of change: leadership, communication, social networks, and a culture of urgency and persistence. "Support systems" are the health-system building blocks that must be strengthened to enable implementation: learning systems, data systems, infrastructure, human resources, and technical capability.

Table 10.5 shows a sample sequence for the rollout of TLC across counties and districts in a hypothetical province with about 60 counties and districts.

Phase 1: Set Up the TLCs

In the set-up period, provincial leaders would begin to build the "how" of implementation, first examining the province's administrative structures to identify where the TLCs ought to be created. Decisions would need to be made on how many urban and rural TLCs would be needed, which specific facilities would join specific TLCs, and which TLCs would be launched first and which in subsequent years. PLGs or LLGs would be set up, and the TLC management teams would be established to begin developing the province's first TLC. Governance arrangements, measurement frameworks, task agreements, and pathways would be agreed upon between national, provincial, and local management teams.

Provincial leaders would also examine the full menu of reforms and SCHRO's implementation guidelines to derive a master reform pathway particular to their local circumstances. Such a master pathway would outline the key change concepts, goals, and

core action areas to design a series of more-specific reform interventions (as shown in the example in box 10.3). It is essentially a guide that identifies, sequences, and, to the extent possible, synchronizes the reform actions, adapting them to the local setting. It would focus on the core actions presented in chapters 2–9 but would be carefully sequenced, taking into account key elements of hospital reform, the PCIC model, and quality improvement, as well as structural changes to payment mechanisms, purchasing arrangements, team configurations, and workforce development that would need to precede certain changes in clinical processes. No master pathway will be perfect, and therefore its components should be flexible and iterative, allowing provincial leaders to work with TLC leaders to amend the master reform pathway over time. This phase could be accomplished quickly, within three months.

More in-depth implementation pathways, derived from specific core action areas of the master pathway, would provide more detailed specifications for what needs to be done. Annex 10A presents an example of such an implementation pathway to guide and sequence activities for implementing specific components of the proposed PCIC model. Implementation pathways provide clear objectives, overall milestones, measurable outputs, and specific activities to achieve them. Based on contextual requirements, each province would choose its own implementation pathways.

BOX 10.3   Example of a master reform pathway: primary care enhancement for patients with complex needs

This master pathway is designed to help primary care teams redesign care to meet the needs of patients living with complex needs. It illustrates a master pathway that includes ideas that teams can test and implement; tips and guidance culled from the experience of expert faculty and primary care teams from around the world; resources to support teams' progress; and examples of care models.

Several key change concepts are necessary to improve the health and cost outcomes of patients with complex needs (figure B10.3.1). Teams with existing care models and those just beginning to develop programs for the complex-needs population are encouraged to work through this design process to refine and focus care interventions.

Choose your BHLC (Better Health at Lower Cost) population and learn about its assets and needs includes the following tasks:

- Identify your overall population.
- Identify population segments and select the focus population for intervention.

Identify individuals who are good candidates for your enhanced care design includes these tasks:

- Identify individuals through a combination of approaches.
- Use real-time identification.

Revolutionize patient engagement includes these tasks:

- Develop processes to recruit people into care.
- Adopt patient engagement strategies that are tailored to and informed by your focus population.

Develop an enhanced care model to fit the needs and assets of the focus population includes these tasks:

- Co-create individualized care plans to learn about and prepare for care redesign.
- Develop your transformed care model through iterative testing.
- Develop work processes to ensure consistent care delivery.

FIGURE B10.3.1   Sample "Better Health at Lower Cost" reform pathway

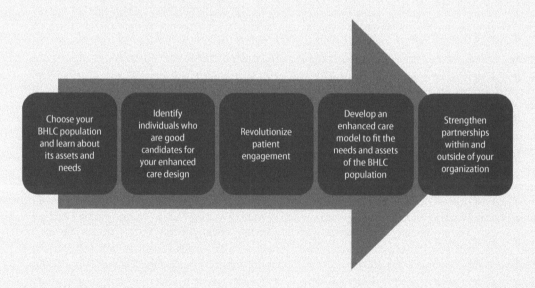

Source: ©World Bank. Permission required for reuse.
Note: BHLC = Better Health at Lower Cost.

(Box continued next page)

Example of a master reform pathway: primary care enhancement for patients with complex needs (continued)

Strengthen partnerships within and outside of your organization includes these tasks:

- Strengthen community partnerships to meet the needs and enhance the strengths of the focus population.
- Cultivate a healthy team in your enhanced care design.

Finally, the data must be used effectively. Even the best models will fail if implementation is poorly accomplished. To help teams use data efficiently

and effectively and to work at scale, execute these strategies:

- Understand the data and how to use them
- Cultivate ongoing investment to build a sustainable program
- Develop a learning system
- Work at scale
- Scale up services to all individuals in the target population.

Phase 2: Develop the Scalable Unit

The "scalable unit" is the smallest representative unit of the system targeted for full-scale implementation. The county, district, or municipality would be the ideal scalable unit within the province. This is where the action happens for implementation and where the TLC would be operationalized.

In each geographical area that is targeted in a province, at least one and preferably more than one initial TLC would be set up in the first year. The purpose of these initial TLCs is to intensively test local ideas for best-practice implementation. An important outcome of this work would be a set of well-documented, context-sensitive strategies to aid implementation of specific reforms that could be further tested and refined.[7]

The choice of facilities to participate in this initial phase of implementation is of the utmost importance. Research on change management and the diffusion of innovation suggests it is good practice to identify front-runner innovators who have the will and motivation to make a change. Further, experience in China and internationally has shown that strong political commitment is needed to overcome entrenched interests in the health sector, make the difficult choices involved, and bring about the relentless focus on execution that is needed to achieve results. This phase will last approximately nine months.

Phase 3: Test of Scaling-Up

This phase involves testing the set of interventions to be taken to scale. The successful strategies that aided implementation in the initial TLCs would need to be tested in a broader range of settings before going to full scale. International experience suggests that testing should take place in 10 additional TLCs in each of the selected reform provinces starting in Year 2 of the reform period.

During this phase, all necessary infrastructure required to support full-scale implementation should be documented, understood, and adjusted as needed, including workforce development (for example, leadership, managerial, and frontline capacity); information systems management; and the supply chain. This phase is an important opportunity to build the confidence and will of leaders and frontline staff to support the changes. As the work proceeds, new insights from the reform implementation will lead to a more nuanced and mature set of context-specific strategies and ideas for change that can be used for full-scale implementation throughout the province. This phase would last one year.

Phase 4: Go to Full Scale

This is a rapid deployment phase in which a tested set of reforms within each province, now supported by a reliable data feedback system, can be rapidly adopted by frontline staff throughout the province. While some adaptation of the intervention to local environments may still be required, there would be less emphasis on contextual adaptation during this phase. Significant will, knowledge, experience, and infrastructural support and capacity need to be in place before moving to this phase of scaling-up.

At this point, a series of waves of TLCs would be launched within each of the provinces selected for reform (as shown in table 10.5). Each wave of scaling-up would be informed by the knowledge gained from the previous wave. The best-performing TLC participants from early waves may coach new TLC teams in subsequent waves. This developmental step needs to be explicitly described

and supported in the early stages so that TLCs can be prepared to take on the role of mentoring subsequent TLC participants. In this way, successes are multiplied across the province and transformation is greatly accelerated.

As shown earlier (in table 10.3), the suggested plan for achieving provincewide implementation is to spread the reforms in successive annual waves of 10 counties and districts until the full province is covered. After the first year (in which one or two initial TLCs are established in each province), the second year would see TLCs launched in the next wave of jurisdictions (counties, districts, and municipalities) as a test of scaling-up. A year after that, the next round of 10 counties and districts would be launched, and so on until the full province is covered.

Annex 10A   Case Examples of Transformation Learning Collaboratives (TLCs)

Case 1: The Scottish Patient Safety Programme

Background

Since 1999, Scotland has had its own National Health Service, NHS Scotland, independent from the NHS in the rest of the United Kingdom. Scotland has 36 acute-care hospitals, supervised by 14 local health boards. NHS Scotland has a long history of focusing on value, safety, and innovation. In 2004, it participated in the United Kingdom's Safer Patients Initiative, a large-scale improvement program that tested organizationwide ways to improve patient safety within hospitals. Through this program, one hospital, Ninewells Hospital, reduced patient harm by more than 60 percent in three years.

Inspired by that success, in 2007 Scotland launched the Scottish Patient Safety Programme (SPSP)—a Transformation Learning Collaborative (TLC) to improve patient safety in all of the country's hospitals. This collaborative proved so successful that it has now been replicated by NHS Scotland in primary care, long-term care, mental health, and maternity care.[8]

Goals

The initial aim of the SPSP collaborative was to reduce in-hospital mortality by 15 percent over five years. To achieve this larger mortality objective, the collaborative's leadership set specific goals, such as to reduce "crash calls" by 30 percent and reduce *Staphylococcus aureus bacteraemia* infections by 30 percent. An additional goal was to field-test the collaborative methodology in the NHS for the first time. If the test proved successful, the plan was to apply this methodology to primary care and postacute care as well.

Implementation

The model for collaborative learning was introduced in four clinical areas: general clinical wards, critical care units, perioperative theatres, and stewardship and use of medications. To spread successful changes and share learning, teams at different hospitals came together to participate in face-to-face learning sessions where they learned from their peers' successes and challenges in trying to implement the same changes.

In preparation for this collaborative work, Scotland engaged extensively in building motivation and knowledge at the leadership level and established crucial organizational infrastructure for improvement. The national leadership set the policy framework, and local health boards developed focused implementation plans and communicated them to the hospital staffs. Safety was deemed a priority, as reiterated by leaders at all levels of the system in discussions at health board meetings and safety walk-arounds in hospitals (during which leaders discuss safety issues with frontline staff).

The local health boards were also asked to appoint a program manager for patient safety, and later an executive leader, for each of the four clinical areas. A leadership team (including leaders from the Scottish government and Scottish nongovernmental organizations [NGOs]) was formed specifically for the program. The Scottish government also set up the National Advisory Board, chaired by the chief medical officer, to oversee the program, with representatives from the NHS, government, and patient groups.

To develop capability for implementation and improvement, more than 200 clinicians across the 36 hospitals received extensive instruction in the science of implementation and improvement. Board members and leaders also received instruction in providing appropriate leadership to steward these efforts effectively.

The structure of the SPSP included biannual nationwide meetings (learning sessions), during which the leadership team and the local health board teams from the four clinical areas met to share their experiences in overcoming obstacles and solving problems. Importantly, prominent national leaders such as the chief executive of NHS Scotland attended these sessions, sending the message that the collaborative was a national priority and that teams would be held accountable. In addition, regular events were held to convene 50–300 clinicians for one or two days to build skills in measurement, testing changes, and spreading innovation.

Between the in-person events were the action periods when teams returned to their hospitals to test and implement changes. During these times, clinicians from each of the four clinical areas participated in monthly calls, reporting progress and setbacks and discussing them with other teams. There were also regional facilitators who became well acquainted with the hospitals in their region, conducted site visits, and provided support. Frequent informal discussion also took place throughout the collaborative. Leaders reached out to chief executives, board chairs, medical directors, nurse directors, and patient groups to discuss planning and progress, and teams spoke frequently to other teams when they had questions or encountered challenges.

Clinical teams were asked to select a series of improvements from the SPSP collaborative's toolkits, but implementation was decidedly a local activity with local teams encouraged to make changes to the interventions as needed to tailor them to their own environments and experiences. For example, for one intervention procedure, one organization set up a cart to transport supplies to the bedside, while another developed a procedure pack containing all the necessary supplies for one patient. What mattered was that each team decided on an approach to implementation that worked for them, and adhered to it rigorously.

Data management was another key element. Clinicians were required to enter all patient-care data into a web-based data portal that was developed expressly for the SPSP. To minimize the workload, data already collected by other programs—such as on infection rates—were integrated automatically.

After an initial focus on acute care, the initiative gradually expanded to incorporate mental health, primary care, and pediatric and maternal care. Each clinical community has its own collaborative learning structure. In November 2014, delegates from all four communities came together to share learning at a national conference.

Outcomes

Through late 2012 and early 2013, SPSP achieved its aim of reducing hospital mortality by 15 percent. Other specific outcomes include (a) a 66 percent reduction in ventilator-acquired pneumonia; (b) a 70 percent reduction in the central-line bloodstream infection rate; (c) a 79 percent reduction in *Clostridium difficile* (commonly called "*C. diff*") infections in patients 65 and older; (d) a 15 percent decrease in the crash call rate; and (e) at least a 21 percent increase in medication reconciliation.

Case 2: The Primary Care Collaborative, United Kingdom (Prepared in Collaboration with Sir John Oldham)

Background

In 1997, a new government was elected in the United Kingdom on a promise to improve public services, in particular the NHS. The National Primary Care Development Team (NPDT), a small national leadership group, was formed. The NPDT was charged with improving primary care throughout the country by reducing waiting times and improving the effectiveness of service delivery. To spread change, the team used the collaborative methodology described in this chapter through a project called the Primary Care Collaborative. In late 2000, the government launched the NHS Plan, a policy framework for reforming the health service and, along with it, the Primary Care Collaborative as its "effector" or implementation plan. This policy framework envisaged primary care redesigned around the patient; "seamless" service; and a focus on patient experience and outcomes (Oldham 2004).

In the United Kingdom at the time, primary care doctors typically worked together in small group practices of three to four physicians. These small group practices were organized into primary care groups (PCGs) that were reorganized later into primary care trusts (PCTs). At the start of the collaborative, there were 310 PCGs or PCTs, each containing about 20–25 physician group practices. These PCGs or PCTs were the scalable units that joined the Primary Care Collaborative.

Goals

The goals of the NPDT were to create measurable improvement in access to primary care; improve the management of patients with established coronary heart disease; and build capacity- and demand-management systems between primary and secondary care. All primary care practices participating in the collaborative were asked to work on all three areas at the same time.

The broader goal was to develop a team that would create capacity and capability for improvement in primary care group clinical practice. Government leaders were committed to sustainable, long-term change.

Implementation

The initial collaborative structure began with 20 PCGs or PCTs and was closely managed by the NPDT. Each PCG or PCT was invited to select five group practices to participate. Thus, about 100 primary care group practices participated in the first "wave" of the collaborative.

At the individual clinic level, each primary care practice would choose a full-time project manager, employed by the site but trained by and accountable to the national collaborative management team. The project managers' responsibilities were to coach the core practices, ensure that data were submitted, generate local awareness, and recruit new PCGs or PCTs. They received bimonthly training in coaching and group skills, process flow and redesign, data management, communication and spread techniques, and improvement science. They also created a community among themselves, sharing challenges and solutions. They had a dedicated area on the Primary Care Collaborative website to facilitate information sharing in this community.

To expand the national learning collaborative, the initial five participating practices would coach the remaining 15–20 colleague practices within each PCG or PCT. This led to faster spread of better practice ideas for policy implementation: there was an almost palpable unleashing of the power of peer-to-peer coaching and knowledge building. The five initial participating practices linked the remaining 15–20 practices within the same PCG or PCT to the collaborative formally, through their coaching and mentoring. Typically, the collaborative effort would run for two years. In Year 1, the initial five sites would focus on learning and on making changes to their own practices; in Year 2, they would seek out their colleagues and coach them on the better practices and implementation ideas that they had learned.

To expand this further, the NPDT launched a series of four subsequent "waves," each of which was its own collaborative of 20 PCG or PCTs of 100 primary care practices. Each proceeded along similar lines to the initial collaborative. Year 1 focused on changes within the initial participating sites. Year 2 focused on coaching the remaining practices to adapt and adopt the reforms. The launch of the waves was staggered with four to five months between the start of each wave. Each collaborative wave was chaired by a knowledgeable and experienced clinician who had credibility with participants. The main role of the chairpersons was to lead the in-person learning sessions, chair meetings during and between the learning sessions, and represent the collaborative to a wider audience.

Throughout the two years of a wave, the core practices, and the spread practices as they joined, supplied monthly data. By the end of 2001, some 1,500 practices covering 1 million patients were engaged in this national transformative initiative, and there was strong momentum for change.

This was good progress, but how to reach the remaining 3,000 practices covering 30 million additional patients?

Here the NPDT needed a different solution. It created regional nodes: small semiautonomous administrative units that were typically headquartered at the site of one of the best performers from the nationally led collaborative. These nodes were called NPDT centers and were tasked by the NPDT to coordinate regional collaborative waves that essentially duplicated the formula used for the national collaborative implementation just described.

Outcomes

What was achieved by all this implementation activity? Within three years, 4,900 practices were engaged in the nationwide initiative, covering 31 million people. By January 2004, the collaborative had achieved a 72 percent improvement in access to primary care doctors (that is, reduced waiting time) and a fourfold reduction in mortality due to cardiovascular disease in the participating collaborative sites compared with the rest of the United Kingdom. Most importantly, it had established a robust, sustainable infrastructure for improvement and spread.

Annex 10B   Plan-Do-Study-Act Cycles of Change

The Plan-Do-Study-Act (PDSA) cycle guides individuals and organizations to test ideas for change systematically to determine whether the change can generate viable improvement. PDSA cycles have emerged from a long tradition of hypothesis testing and change management in both science and industry. Originally expressed by statistician Walter Shewhart as the Plan-Do-Check-Act cycle, it was later refined by W. Edwards Deming to its current Plan-Do-Study-Act form (Kiran 2016). This simple four-step process has been used in a variety of health care and non-health care settings to guide the conduct of small-scale tests to improve system performance.

The PDSA Cycle

A PDSA cycle includes four key steps, as further outlined below. *Plan* refers to a specific planning phase. *Do* is a phase for trying the change and observing what happens. *Study* is the phase for analyzing the results of the trial. *Act* is the phase for devising next steps based on the analysis (keep the change, adjust the change, or discard the change and try something else).

Step 1: Plan—Plan the test or observation, including a plan for collecting data

- State the objective of the test.
- State the questions you want to answer, and make predictions about what will happen and why.
- Develop a plan to test the change. (Who? What? When? Where? What data need to be collected?)

Step 2: Do—Try out the test on a small scale

- Carry out the test.
- Document problems and unexpected observations.
- Begin analysis of the data.

Step 3: Study—Set aside time to analyze the data and study the results

- Complete the analysis of the data.
- Compare the data to your predictions.
- Summarize and reflect on what was learned.

Step 4: Act—Refine the change, based on what was learned from the test

- Determine what modifications should be made.
- Prepare a plan for the next PDSA cycle.

Methods for PDSA Implementation

The PDSA cycle can be implemented in any organization and by any team by using these methods:

- *Forming the team:* Including the right people on an implementation team is critical to a successful improvement effort. Teams vary in size and composition. They might include some combination of primary care physicians, specialists, nurses, and other health care workers. Each organization builds teams to suit its own needs and the improvement goal at hand.

- *Setting aims for improvement:* The aim should be time-specific and measurable; it should also define the specific population of patients or other system that will be affected. Examples of an aim would be that all diabetic patients receive optimal care according to World Health Organization (WHO) guidelines within the next year, or that all identified tuberculosis patients are managed according to WHO's Integrated Management of Adolescent and Adult Illness (IMAI) guidelines in the next 18 months.
- *Establishing measures:* Teams use quantitative measures to determine whether a specific change actually leads to an improvement. For the aims cited above, measures might include the percentage of diabetic patients with glycosylated hemoglobin of less than 8 percent or the percentage of identified tuberculosis patients who convert to sputum- or culture-negativity.
- *Selecting changes:* Ideas for change may come from the insights of people who work in the system, whether from change concepts or other creative thinking techniques or by borrowing from the experience of others who have successfully improved.
- *Testing changes:* The PDSA cycle is shorthand for testing a change in the real work setting—by planning it, trying it, observing the results, and acting on what is learned. This is the scientific method adapted for action-oriented learning.
- *Implementing changes:* After testing a change on a small scale, learning from each test, and refining the change through several PDSA cycles, the team may implement the change on a broader scale—for example, for an entire pilot population or on an entire unit.
- *Spreading changes:* After successful implementation of a change or package of changes for a pilot population or an entire unit, the team can spread the changes to other parts of the organization or in other organizations.

Annex 10C   Example of a Detailed Implementation Pathway

Lever 1: Shaping Tiered Health Care Delivery System with People-Centered Integrated Care

The core action areas of Lever 1 selected for the sample implementation pathway include the following (further detailed in chapter 2):

- *Core Action Area 1:* Primary care as the first point of contact (Pathway 1.1, as shown in table 10C.1), using population empanelment and risk stratification (Pathway 1.2 [table 10C.2] and Pathway 1.3 [table 10C.3])
- *Core Action Area 2:* Functional multidisciplinary teams (Pathway 1.3, as shown in table 10C.3)
- *Core Action Area 7:* Measurement, standards, and feedback (Pathway 1.4 [table 10C.4] and Pathway 1.5 [table 10C.5])

TABLE 10C.1   Pathway 1.1: Increase the use of primary care as first point of contact

Pathway 1.1 rationale: Having primary health care perform gatekeeping functions limits specialty care access and can help systems reduce overuse of inappropriate care and move toward providing the right care at the right place at the right time.

Milestone	Outputs	Activities
Milestone 1: Protocol for community-concordant gatekeeping is developed that encourages individuals to make their primary care provider the entry point into the health system when they need care, while also maintaining elements of patient choice that promote trust. *Timeline:* Years 1–2	*Output 1:* Means of concordant gatekeeping is determined.	*Activity 1:* Assess community and provider perceptions of gatekeeping functions, including severity of concerns about restricted choice.
		Activity 2: Determine package of incentives and consequences for gatekeeping in concert with providers and insurance mechanism. Get input from a variety of local and provincial stakeholders, especially regarding successful and problematic gatekeeping efforts in the past.
		Activity 3: Determine options for financial incentives to encourage PHC utilization and discourage patients from bypassing to specialist care.
	Output 2: Patient education about primary health care and services is provided to increase community trust in the health care system.	*Activity 1:* Provide physicians with the knowledge necessary to build strong, long-lasting relationships with their patients.
		Activity 2: Reach out to local patient groups and the public around a campaign to encourage utilization of PHC services first.
Milestone 2: Pilot program to test whether agreed-upon gatekeeping scheme is under way. *Timeline:* Years 1–2	*Output 1:* Begin institutionalizing incentives and processes devised under Milestone 1.	*Activity 1:* Depending on results of community input above (during Milestone 1 activities), develop metrics and measure capture systems to monitor Output 2.
	Output 2: Measure uptake of gatekeeping.	*Activity 1:* Set indicators such as visit rates at PHC facilities, bypass rates for a set of conditions that could be treated at PHC facilities, and patient and provider experience with the system. *Activity 2:* Set monitoring systems to measure indicators (see Pathway 1.5 [table 10C.5]).
	Output 3: Use continuous learning, and feedback from providers and clients, to inform future iterations of the model.	*Activity 1:* Establish feedback system for providers and patients to assess their perspectives on strong and weak points of the gatekeeping model (see Pathway 1.5 [table 10C.5]).
Milestone 3: Increase accessibility of primary care services to patients using existing facilities for care delivery. *Timeline:* Years 1–2	*Output 1:* Increase the hours that primary care services are available.	*Activity 1:* Pilot offering weekend and evening hours at PHC facilities on a limited basis.
		Activity 2: Publicize campaign about after-hours care as an alternative to long wait times and high out-of-pocket costs for specialist or hospital visits.
		Activity 3: Provide financial incentives to PHC providers to offer more available times for patient visits.
		Activity 4: Measure the effect of these access policies on visit rates and use of specialist services in affiliated network providers.
	Output 2: Offer same-day visits to patients with acute needs.	*Activity 1:* Work with PHC providers in two counties to save at least 30 percent of visit slots each day for acute or urgent walk-in patients.
		Activity 2: Measure the effect of this open-access plan on the volume of visits and nearby hospital utilization.

Note: PHC = primary health care.

TABLE 10C.2   Pathway 1.2: Stratify panels based on risk for poor outcomes and high utilization, and develop care plans for most at-risk population

Pathway 1.2 rationale: Proactively targeting individuals at risk for poor outcomes and high utilization of health services enables provision of higher-intensity, coordinated care in a PHC setting.

Milestone	Outputs	Activities
Milestone 1: Empaneled populations are stratified by risk. *Timeline:* Years 1–2	*Output 1:* Algorithm(s) for risk stratification are developed.	*Activity 1:* Determine goals for risk stratification (such as to improve health or reduce costs).
		Activity 2: Determine which algorithm for risk stratification fits best with local needs, including disease burden, stated goals, and available resources. Potential algorithms used elsewhere include Adjusted Clinical Groups, Hierarchical Condition Categories, Elder Risk Assessment, Chronic Comorbidity Count, Charlson Comorbidity Index, and Minnesota Health Care Home Tiering.
		Activity 3: Pilot the algorithm(s) using historical data and determine the threshold for designation as "high-risk."
	Output 2: Risk stratification of patients is initiated.	*Activity 1:* Beginning with populations already empaneled to MDTs, use the algorithm(s) to identify "high-risk" patients per panel.
		Activity 2: Determine how often to update the list(s) of "high-risk" empaneled patients (for example, every three months or six months).
		Activity 3: Assign high-risk patients for longitudinal care management by one member of the MDT.
Milestone 2: Individualized care plans for high-risk patients are developed. *Timeline:* Years 1–2	*Output 1:* Care pathways for the highest-burden diseases are developed.	*Activity 1:* Select the highest-burden and/or highest-cost diseases for targeting.
		Activity 2: Assemble MDTs of experts from across care levels (primary care and hospitals) for consultation.
		Activity 3: Review literature to determine the best evidence-based practices for treatment.
		Activity 4: Develop standardized care pathways that clarify team members' roles and responsibilities at each level of care, establish explicit referral criteria, and establish postdischarge follow-up procedures.
	Output 2: Care pathways for a small number of selected diseases are piloted.	*Activity 1:* Establish a monitoring framework for assessing care pathway processes and associated health outcomes (see Pathway 1.5 [table 10C.5]).
		Activity 2: Begin applying care pathways for selected disease(s).
		Activity 3: Institute regular review meetings with MDTs across care levels to assess bottlenecks to implementation, propose solutions, and set new coverage and completeness targets.

Note: MDT = multidisciplinary team; PHC = primary health care.

TABLE 10C.3   Pathway 1.3: Form multidisciplinary teams and empanel population

Rationale: Multidisciplinary team (MDT) formation and population empanelment promote the accountability of primary health care system and providers for population health outcomes; shift care from hospital-centric to people-centered integrated care; improve patient-provider relationships and trust; and alleviate the consequences of acute shortages of human resources for health by maximizing reach and efficacy through multidisciplinary teams.

Milestones	Outputs	Activities
Milestone 1: Care provision is reorganized into multidisciplinary teams *Timeline:* Years 1–2	*Output 1*: Location-specific optimal composition of MDTs is determined.	*Activity 1:* Assess the disease burden, demographic profile, and preferences of the local population.
		Activity 2: Assess available human resources, including physicians, registered nurses, nurse practitioners, community health workers, and other health personnel such as mental health experts, pharmacists, nutritionists, and social workers. (Work to harmonize these efforts with the human resource reforms recommended in chapter 7.)
		Activity 3: Conduct a rapid inventory of skills and technical areas for which staff at lower-facility levels need support.
		Activity 4: Delineate each team member's roles and responsibilities and designate a team leader.
		Activity 5: Develop technical assistance support plans that are appropriate for the local setting and meet the needs of lower-level staff. Plans should include details on the frequency of assistance provision, the topics to be covered, and the roles and responsibilities of staff at all levels. Potential activities include on-site mentoring at primary care facilities by higher-level staff (including outpatient services, inpatient rounds, case discussions, and lectures) or embedding primary care staff at higher-level facilities for extended training opportunities.
	Output 2: MDTs are formed and providing services. A culture of cooperation is fostered.	*Activity 1:* Conduct outreach events (seminars, roundtable discussions, and so on) with health care providers to explain the rationale for transitioning to team-based care, answer questions, and address concerns.
		Activity 2: Group the care providers according to the criteria established in Output 1.
		Activity 3: Provide opportunity for teams to review their roles and responsibilities and adapt to local and team needs.
		Activity 4: Designate a care coordinator on each team. The exact training and professional status of this person can vary across regions; what is important is that the care coordinator fulfills a standardized function of tracking high-risk patients across care settings and proactively reaching out to them.
		Activity 5: Roll out the MDTs in a small pilot setting.
		Activity 6: Plan and implement regular team-based trainings to promote a collaborative culture with supportive supervision.
Milestone 2 (concurrently with Milestone 1): The population is empaneled to MDTs. *Timeline:* Years 1–2	*Output 1*: The guidelines and protocol for choosing and implementing different empanelment strategies are prepared.	*Activity 1:* Weigh the options for empanelment, based on community feedback and available technical capacity. Options include purely geographic empanelment, empanelment based on patient choice, or a combination of the two. Empanelment based on patient choice and the combination approach require the technical capacity and real-time communication to track patients if (or as) they switch between providers to ensure that gaps in care are minimized.
		Activity 2: Test different empanelment approaches in a small sample of diverse geographic areas.
		Activity 3: Develop patient registries and the information technology (IT) and human resource capacities needed to maintain and use them.
		Activity 4: Define the panel type and size based on these protocols.
	Output 2: Provider and community buy-in for empanelment is generated. Empanelment is initiated.	*Activity 1:* Conduct training events for multidisciplinary provider teams to explain the rationale for empanelment and to clarify provider roles in the new system.
		Activity 2: Conduct community outreach events to provide information on the goals of empanelment and to explain what these changes mean for how patients access care.
		Activity 3: Register people in the panels and assign them to MDTs.

Note: MDT = multidisciplinary team.

TABLE 10C.4   Pathway 1.4: Review pilot and scale up

Rationale: A systematic review of the progress made on pilots facilitates scaling-up.

Milestone	Outputs	Activities
Milestone 1: Spread the rollout of risk stratification and care pathways. *Timeline:* Years 3–4	*Output 1:* Develop the algorithm(s) for risk stratification based on the needs and goals of the new locale.	*Activity 1:* Determine the goals for risk stratification (for example, to improve health or to reduce costs) within the new geographic area.
		Activity 2: Determine which algorithm for risk stratification fits best with local needs (including the disease burden) and available resources.
		Activity 3: Pilot the algorithm using historical data and determine the threshold for designation as "high-risk."
	Output 2: The expanded pool of patients is risk stratified.	*Activity 1:* Within new geographic areas, use the algorithm to identify "high-risk" patients per panel.
		Activity 2: Determine how often to update list of "high-risk" empaneled patients (for example, every three months or six months).
		Activity 3: Assign high-risk patients for longitudinal care management by one member of the MDT.
	Output 3: Care pathways are applied to newly risk-stratified patient panels.	*Activity 1:* Establish a monitoring framework for assessing the care pathway processes and associated health outcomes (see Pathway 1.5 [table 10C.5]).
		Activity 2: Begin applying the care pathways for selected disease(s).
		Activity 3: Institute regular review meetings with MDTs across care levels to assess bottlenecks to implementation, propose solutions, and set new coverage and completeness targets.
	Output 4: Care pathways are revised based on the technical capacity of local providers and the population burden of disease.	*Activity 1:* Assemble local MDTs of experts from across care levels (primary care and hospitals) for consultation.
		Activity 2: Update the care pathways based on new feedback from local experts.
Milestone 2: Clinical pathways are developed for new diseases. *Timeline:* Years 3–4	*Output 1:* The highest-burden or highest-cost diseases not already covered by clinical pathways are identified.	*Activity 1:* Assemble MDTs of experts from across care levels (both primary care and hospitals) for consultation.
		Activity 2: Review literature to determine the best evidence-based practices for treatment.
		Activity 3: Develop standardized care pathways that clarify the roles and responsibilities of team members at each level of care, establish explicit referral criteria, and establish postdischarge follow-up procedures.
Milestone 3: Establish process for regular review of pathways. *Timeline:* Years 3–4	*Output 1:* Each clinical pathway is assessed at least once every two years.	*Activity 1:* Conduct listening sessions with local providers to determine bottlenecks to implementation, technical problems with clinical pathways, or other perceived needs for change.
		Activity 2: Review new literature to ensure fidelity of disease-specific clinical pathways to the most recent evidence base.
		Activity 3: Make necessary updates to the pathway based on Activities 1 and 2.
		Activity 4: Review revised pathway(s) with local stakeholders from multidisciplinary care teams across care levels.

(Table continued next page)

TABLE 10C.4   Pathway 1.4: Review pilot and scale up   *Continued*

Milestone	Outputs	Activities
Milestone 4: MDT capacity is spread and deepened through technical assistance between upper- and lower-level facilities. *Timeline:* Years 3–4	*Output 1:* Use of MDTs is expanded beyond pilot sites, following the process described in Milestone 1.	*Activity 1:* Determine location-specific optimal composition of the MDTs. *Activity 2:* Facilitate formation of teams and a culture of cooperation; continuous training is essential.
	Output 2: Health workers staffing community and township health centers (THCs) receive technical assistance from specialists in county and district hospitals.	*Activity 1:* Identify appropriate facilities for scaling-up within the tiered care system, including county hospitals, THCs, and village clinics *Activity 2:* Conduct an inventory of skills and technical areas for which staff at lower-facility levels need support. *Activity 3:* Develop technical assistance support plans that are appropriate for the local setting and meet needs of lower-level staff. Plans should include details on frequency of assistance provision, topics to be covered, and roles and responsibilities of staff at all levels. Potential activities include on-site mentoring at primary care facilities by higher-level staff (including outpatient services, inpatient rounds, case discussions, and/or lectures) or embedding primary care staff at higher-level facilities for extended training opportunities. *Activity 4:* Implement technical assistance activities within defined groups of care teams. *Activity 5:* Continually assess patient perspectives, provider perspectives and knowledge, and health outcomes (see Pathway 1.5 [table 10C.5]).
Milestone 5: Empanelment of populations to multidisciplinary teams is scaled up to additional localities. *Timeline:* Years 3–4	*Output 1:* Guidelines and protocols are developed or fine-tuned for choosing and implementing empanelment strategies for new locales.	*Activity 1:* Assess available options, local technical capacity, and community needs. *Activity 2:* Test different empanelment approaches. *Activity 3:* Develop patient registries. *Activity 4:* Define panel type and size based on protocols. *Activity 5:* Register the panels to MDTs.
	Output 2: Provider and community buy-in for empanelment is achieved.	*Activity 1:* Conduct a training event for multidisciplinary provider teams to explain the rationale for empanelment and clarify provider roles in the new system. *Activity 2:* Conduct community outreach events to provide information on the goals of empanelment and to explain what these changes mean for how patients access care.

Note: MDT = multidisciplinary care team; THC = township health center.

TABLE 10C.5   Pathway 1.5: Implement a continuous M&E plan to track reform progress and inform iterative improvements

Rationale: Continuous monitoring and evaluation, implemented as an integral part of the reforms from the start, is critical to the success of reforms. Ongoing measurement helps to ensure that reforms are undertaken with fidelity to the planned process; enables the collection of feedback from critical reform stakeholders (providers, clients, and communities); allows for early detection and correction of unintended negative consequences; and provides up-to-date data with which to track outcomes.

Milestones	Outputs	Activities
Milestone 1: Conduct continuous M&E of multidisciplinary team rollout. *Timeline (continuous with Pathway 1.1):* Years 1–4	*Output 1:* The measurement system is prepared.	*Activity 1:* Design an M&E framework and identify key processes, intermediate outputs, and outcomes to track, including critical PCIC functions such as care continuity and coordination, patient feedback, and provider perspectives. *Activity 2:* Assess the available data sources for tracking key indicators identified in the M&E plan. *Activity 3:* Develop new data collection tools to track indicators not captured by existing data sources, as needed.

(Table continued next page)

TABLE 10C.5   Pathway 1.5: Implement a continuous M&E plan to track reform progress and inform iterative improvements *Continued*

Milestones	Outputs	Activities
	Output 2: Ongoing M&E and quality improvement are conducted.	*Activity 1:* Implement continuous monitoring of the identified indicators
		Activity 2: Iterate within the pilot site to address any identified problems or improvement opportunities.
		Activity 3: Continue the measurement and improvement cycle for expanded rollout of MDTs in Years 3–4.
Milestone 2: Conduct continuous M&E of empanelment rollout. *Timeline (continuous with Pathway 1.1):* Years 1–4	*Output 1:* The measurement system is prepared.	*Activity 1:* Design an M&E framework and identify key processes, intermediate outputs, and outcomes to track, including critical measures of key PCIC functions such as care continuity and coordination, patient feedback, and provider perspectives. Key indicators to track include the following: Are the panel sizes within the guidelines and manageable for teams? Do the MDTs know the patients and communities they are responsible for?
		Activity 2: Assess the available data sources for tracking key indicators identified in the M&E plan.
		Activity 3: Develop new data collection tools to track indicators not captured by existing data sources, as needed.
	Output 2: Ongoing M&E and quality improvement is conducted.	*Activity 1:* Implement continuous monitoring of the identified indicators.
		Activity 2: Iterate to address any identified problems or improvement opportunities.
		Activity 3: Continue the measurement and improvement cycle for expanded rollout of empanelment in Years 3–4.
Milestone 3: Conduct continuous M&E of risk stratification and clinical pathway rollout. *Timeline (continuous with Pathway 1.2):* Years 1–4	*Output 1:* Assess appropriateness of risk stratification strategy.	*Activity 1:* Based on the criteria used to select a risk stratification algorithm, identify key indicators to track to determine whether most at-risk patients are being identified. For example, if high risk for cardiovascular outcomes is a criterion for risk stratification, indicators to track might include CHADS$_2$ scores, the ACC-AHA CVD risk calculator, and others.
		Activity 2: At regularly scheduled intervals, compare populations identified as high-risk with those not designated as high-risk on selected outcome measures such as admissions for MI, CVA, COPD, and PAD.
		Activity 3: If the risk stratification algorithm is not adequately capturing high-risk patients, change as needed.
	Output 2: The measurement system is prepared.	*Activity 1:* Design an M&E framework, including identifying key processes, intermediate outputs, and outcomes to track.
		Activity 2: Assess available data sources for tracking key indicators identified in the M&E plan.
		Activity 3: Develop new data collection tools to track indicators not captured by existing data sources, as needed.
	Output 3: Ongoing M&E and quality improvement is conducted.	*Activity 1:* Building on the scheduled pathway review meetings, implement continuous M&E of the pilot, including measures of key PCIC functions such as care continuity and coordination, patient feedback, and provider perspectives.
		Activity 2: Iterate within the pilot site to address any identified problems or improvement opportunities.

Note: ACC-AHA CVD = the American College of Cardiology and American Heart Association cardiovascular disease risk prediction algorithm; CHADS$_2$ = stroke risk assessment score in atrial fibrillation (standing for congestive heart failure, hypertension, age ≥ 75, diabetes mellitus, stroke); COPD = chronic obstructive pulmonary disease; CVA = cerebrovascular accident; MDT = multidisciplinary team; M&E = monitoring and evaluation; MI = myocardial infarction; PAD = peripheral artery disease; PCIC = people-centered integrated care; PHC = primary health care.

Notes

1. Such an environment will also be needed for effective and sustained implementation and scaling-up.
2. "Guidance on Comprehensively Scaling-Up Reform of County-Level Public Hospitals," State Council General Office (*Guo Ban Fa* 2015, No. 33); "Guidance of the General Office of the State Council on Promoting Multi-level Diagnosis and Treatment System," State Council General Office (*Guo Ban Fa* 2015, No. 70).
3. For more information, see the Institute of Medicine website on the Roundtable on Value & Science-Driven Health Care: http://iom .nationalacademies.org/Activities/Quality /VSRT.aspx.
4. This subsection draws on the following sources for evidence: Brush and others 2009; Franco and Marquez 2011; Hulscher, Schouten, and Grol 2009; IHI 2003; Jones and Piterman 2008; Kritchevsky and others 2008; and Schouten and others 2008.
5. The Plan-Do-Study-Act (PDSA) cycle guides individuals and organizations to test ideas for change systematically to determine whether the change can generate a viable improvement. PDSA cycles have emerged from a long tradition of hypothesis testing and change management in both science and industry. Briefly, the cycle works as follows: Teams thoroughly *plan* to test the change, taking into account cultural and organizational characteristics. They *do* the work to make the change in their standard procedures, tracking their progress using quantitative measures. They closely *study* the results of their work for insight on how to do better. They then *act* to make the successful changes permanent or to adjust the changes that need more work. This process continues iteratively over time, and refinement is added with each cycle. For a more detailed description, see annex 10B.
6. Similar efforts to scale reforms using the same approach have been used in the United Kingdom, for example, with great success, leading to major improvements in waiting times, cardiovascular care, and patient satisfaction.
7. For example, in a project seeking to reduce cesarean sections in Brazil, teams tested various approaches to reduce financial incentives to perform this procedure. Ultimately, one of the most successful approaches was to pay physicians a salary instead of paying them based on the volume of procedures performed. This had an immediate impact on C-section rates and became a key strategy that other organizations implemented also.
8. For more information about the Scottish Patient Safety Programme, see https://ihub .scot/spsp/about-us/.

References

Aarons, G. A., M. Hurlburt, and S. M. Horwitz. 2011. "Advancing a Conceptual Model of Evidence-Based Practice Implementation in Public Service Sectors." *Administration and Policy in Mental Health and Mental Health Service Research* 38 (1): 4–23.

Aarons, G. A., D. Summerfield, D. B. Hecht, J. F. Silovsky, and M. J. Chaffin. 2009. "The Impact of Evidence-Based Practice Implementation and Fidelity Monitoring on Staff Turnover: Evidence for a Protective Effect." *Journal of Consulting and Clinical Psychology* 77 (2): 270–80.

Barker, Pierre M., Amy Reid, and Marie W. Schall. 2016. "A Framework for Scaling Up Health Interventions: Lessons from Large-Scale Improvement Initiatives in Africa." *Implementation Science* 11 (1): 1–11.

Berwick, Donald M., Thomas W. Nolan, and John Whittington. 2008. "The Triple Aim: Care, Health, and Cost." *Health Affairs* 27 (3): 759–69.

Brush, John E. Jr., Edna Rensing, Frank Song, Sallie Cook, Janet Lynch, Leroy Thacker, Sarat Gurram, Robert O. Bonow, Joani Brough, and C. Michael Valentine. 2009. "A Statewide Collaborative Initiative to Improve the Quality of Care for Patients with Acute Myocardial Infarction and Heart Failure." *Circulation* 119 (12): 1609–15.

Cutler, David. 2014. *The Quality Cure: How Focusing on Health Care Quality Can Save Your Life and Lower Spending Too.* Berkeley and Los Angeles, CA: University of California Press.

Damschroder, Laura J., David C. Aron, Rosalind E. Keith, Susan R. Kirsh, Jeffery A. Alexander, and Julie C. Lowery. 2009. "Fostering Implementation of Health Services Research Findings into Practice: A Consolidated Framework for Advancing Implementation Science." *Implementation Science* 4 (1): 50.

Dewan, N. A., D. Conley, D. Svendsen, S. P. Chon, J. R. Staup, and A. L. Miller. 2003. "A Quality Improvement Process for Implementing the Texas Algorithm for Schizophrenia in Ohio." *Psychiatric Services* 54 (12): 1646–49.

Durlak, J. A., and E. P. DuPré. 2008. "Implementation Matters: A Review of Research on the Influence of Implementation on Program Outcomes and the Factors Affecting Implementation." *American Journal of Community Psychology* 41 (3–4): 327–50. doi:10.1007/s10464-008-9165-0.

Eccles, Martin P., and Brian S. Mittman. 2006. "Welcome to *Implementation Science*." *Implementation Science* 1 (1): 1.

Etheredge, L. M. 2014. "Rapid Learning: A Breakthrough Agenda." *Health Affairs* (Millwood) 33 (9): 1155–62.

Fixsen, Dean L., Sandra F. Naoom, Karen A. Blasé, Robert M. Friedman, and Frances Wallace. 2005. "Implementation Research: A Synthesis of the Literature." Monograph, National Implementation Research Network at the Louis de la Parte Florida Mental Health Institute, University of South Florida, Tampa.

Franco, L. M., and L. Marquez. 2011. "Effectiveness of Collaborative Improvement: Evidence from 27 Applications in 12 Less-Developed and Middle-Income Countries." *BMJ Quality & Safety* 20 (8): 658–65.

Friedman, C., J. Rubin, J. Brown, M. Buntin, M. Corn, L. Etheredge, C. Gunter, and others. 2014. "Toward a Science of Learning Systems: A Research Agenda for the High-Functioning Learning Health System." *Journal of American Medical Informatics Association* 22 (1): 43–50. doi:10.1136/amiajnl-2014-002977.

Garside, Pam. 1998. "Organisational Context for Quality: Lessons from the Fields of Organisational Development and Change Management." *Quality in Health Care* 7 (suppl): S8–S15.

Greene, S. M., R. J. Reid, and E. B. Larson. 2012. "Implementing the Learning Health System: From Concept to Action." *Annals of Internal Medicine* 157 (3): 207–10. doi:10.7326/0003-4819-157-3-201208070-00012.

Griffith, Clive, and Jill Turner. 2004. "United Kingdom National Health Service, Cancer Services Collaborative 'Improvement Partnership,' Redesign of Cancer Services: A National Approach." *European Journal of Surgical Oncology* 30 (Suppl 1): 1–86.

He, Jingwei Alex. 2011. "Combating Healthcare Cost Inflation with Concerted Administrative Actions in a Chinese Province." *Public Administration and Development* 31 (3): 214–28. doi:10.1002/pad.602.

Heilmann, Sebastian. 2008. "Policy Experimentation in China's Economic Rise." *Studies in Comparative International Developments* 43 (1): 1–26. doi:10.1007/s12116-007-9014-4.

Huang, Yanzhong. 2009. "An Institutional Analysis of China's Failed Healthcare Reform." In *Socialist China, Capitalist China: Social Tension and Political Adaptation under Economic Globalization*, edited by Guoguang Wu and Helen Landsowne, 75–86. New York: Routledge.

Hulscher, Marlies, Loes Schouten, and Richard Grol. 2009. *Collaboratives*. Quest for Quality and Improved Performance (QQUIP) Series. London: The Health Foundation.

IHI (Institute for Healthcare Improvement). 2003. "The Breakthrough Series: IHI's Collaborative Model for Achieving Breakthrough Improvement." Innovation Series white paper, IHI, Boston.

———. 2004. "The Courage to Act on 'What If . . .': 2004 Progress Report." IHI, Boston.

IOM (Institute of Medicine). 2015b. "Transforming Health Care Scheduling and Access: Getting to Now." Washington, DC: The National Academies Press.

Jakubowski, E., and R. B. Saltman, eds. 2013. *The Changing National Role in Health System Governance: A Case-Based Study of 11 European Countries and Australia*. Observatory Studies Series 29. Copenhagen: World Health Organization (acting as the host organization for, and secretariat of, the European Observatory on Health Systems and Policies).

Jones, Kay, and Leon Piterman. 2008. "The Effectiveness of the Breakthrough Series Methodology." *Australian Journal of Primary Health* 14 (1): 59–65.

Kiran, D. R. 2016. *Total Quality Management: Key Concepts and Case Studies*. Oxford, U.K., and Cambridge, MA: Butterworth-Heinemann. doi:10.1016/B978-0-12-811035-5.00003-9.

Kritchevsky, S. B., B. I. Braun, A. J. Bush, M. R. Bozikis, L. Kusek, J.-P. Burke, E. S. Wong, and others. 2008. "The Effect of a Quality Improvement Collaborative to Improve Antimicrobial Prophylaxis in Surgical

Patients: A Randomized Trial." *Annals of Internal Medicine* 149 (7): 472–80.

Li, Keqiang. 2015. "Streamline Administration, Delegate Power, Strengthen Regulation and Improve Services to Deepen Administrative Reforms and Transform Government Functions." National teleconference address, May 12, State Council, the People's Republic of China, Beijing. http://english.gov.cn /premier/speeches/2015/05/23/content_28147 5113213526.htm.

Mate, Kedar S., Brandon Bennett, Wendy Mphatswe, Pierre Barker, and Nigel Rollins. 2009. "Challenges for Routine Health System Data Management in a Large Public Programme to Prevent Mother-To-Child HIV Transmission in South Africa." *PloS One* 4 (5): e5483.

Meessen, Bruno, and Gerald Bloom. 2007. "Economic Transition, Institutional Changes and the Health System: Some Lessons from Rural China." *Journal of Economic Policy Reform* 10 (3): 209–31.

Meyers, Duncan C., Joseph A. Durlak, and Abraham Wandersman. 2012. "The Quality Implementation Framework: A Synthesis of Critical Steps in the Implementation Process." *American Journal of Community Psychology* 50 (3–4): 462–80. doi:10.1007/s10464-012-9522-x.

Meyers, Duncan C., Jason Katz, Victoria Chien, Abraham Wandersman, Jonathan P. Scaccia, and Annie Wright. 2012. "Practical Implementation Science: Developing and Piloting the Quality Implementation Tool." *American Journal of Community Psychology* 50 (3–4): 481–96.

Mossialos, Elias, Martin Wenzl, Robin Osborn, and Chloe Anderson, eds. 2015. "International Profiles of Health Care Systems, 2014: Australia, Canada, Denmark, England, France, Germany, Italy, Japan, The Netherlands, New Zealand, Norway, Singapore, Sweden, Switzerland, and the United States." Annual publication, The Commonwealth Fund, New York.

Oldham, John. 2004. *Sic Evenit Ratio Ut Componitur: The Small Book about Large System Change.* Chichester, U.K.: Kingsham Press.

Peters, David H., Nhan T. Tran, and Taghreed Adam. 2013. *Implementation Research in Health: A Practical Guide.* Geneva: Alliance for Health Policy and Systems Research, World Health Organization.

Qian, Jiwei. 2015. "Reallocating Authority in the Chinese Health System: An Institutional Perspective." *Journal of Asian Public Policy,* 8 (1): 19–35. doi:10.1080/17516234.2014. 1003454.

Ramesh, M., Xun Wu, and Alex Jingwei He. 2013. "Health Governance and Healthcare Reforms in China." *Health Policy and Planning* 29 (6): 663–72. doi:10.1093/heapol /czs109.

Rogers, E. M. 2010. *Diffusion of Innovations.* New York: Simon and Schuster.

Saich, Tony. 2015. *Governance and Politics of China.* 4th ed. London: Palgrave.

Savedoff, William D., and Pablo Gottret. 2008. *Governing Mandatory Health Insurance: Learning from Experience.* Washington, DC: World Bank. doi:10.1596/978-0-8213-7548-8.

Schall, Marie W., Terrence Duffy, Anil Krishnamurthy, Odette Levesque, Prashant Mehta, Mark Murray, Renee Parlier, Robert Petzel, and John Sanderson. 2004. "Improving Patient Access to the Veterans Health Administration's Primary Care and Specialty Clinics." *The Joint Commission Journal on Quality and Patient Safety* 30 (8): 415–23.

Schouten, Loes M. T., Marlies E. J. L. Hulscher, Jannes J. Evan Everdingen, Robbert Huijsman, and Richard P. T. M. Grol. 2008. "Evidence for the Impact of Quality Improvement Collaboratives: Systematic Review." *BMJ* 336 (7659): 1491–94.

Shin, Sonya, Jennifer Furin, Jaime Bayona, Kedar Mate, Jim Yong Kim, and Paul Farmer. 2004. "Community-Based Treatment of Multidrug-Resistant Tuberculosis in Lima, Peru: 7 Years of Experience." *Social Science & Medicine* 59 (7): 1529–39.

Wandersman, Abraham, Victoria H. Chien, and Jason Katz. 2012. "Toward an Evidence-Based System for Innovation Support: Tools, Training, Technical Assistance, Quality Assurance / Quality Improvement for Implementing Innovations with Quality to Achieve Desired Outcomes." *American Journal of Community Psychology* 50 (3–4): 445–59.

Wandersman, Abraham, Jennifer Louis Duffy, Paul D. Flaspohler, Rita Noonan, Keri Lubell, Lindsey Stillman, Morris Blachman, Richard Dunville, and Janet Saul. 2008. "Bridging the Gap between Prevention Research and Practice: The Interactive Systems Framework for Dissemination and Implementation."

American Journal of Community Psychology 41 (3–4): 171–81.

WHO (World Health Organization). 2007. *Everybody's Business: Strengthening Health Systems to Improve Health Outcomes: WHO's Framework for Action.* Geneva: WHO.

Wilson, S. J., M. W. Lipsey, and J. H. Derzon. 2003. "The Effects of School-Based Intervention Programs on Aggressive Behavior: A Meta-Analysis." *Journal of Consulting and Clinical Psychology* 71 (1): 136–49.

Xue, Lan, and Kuotsai Tom Liou. 2012. "Government Reform in China: Concepts and Reform Cases." *Review of Public Administration* 32 (2): 115–33. doi:10.1177/0734371X12438242.

Yong, Pierre L., LeighAnne Olsen, and J. Michael McGinnis. 2010. *Value in Health Care: Accounting for Cost, Quality, Safety, Outcomes, and Innovation: Workshop Summary.* Learning Healthcare System Series, Roundtable on Value & Science-Driven Health Care. Washington, DC: National Academies Press.

Supplementary Tables

TABLE A.1 Eight levers and recommended core actions for high-quality, value-based health service delivery in China

Levers (strategic directions)	Core action areas
Lever 1: Shaping tiered health care delivery system in accordance with people-centered integrated care (PCIC) model	1. Primary health care as the first point of contact
	2. Multidisciplinary teams
	3. Vertical integration, including new roles for hospitals
	4. Horizontal integration
	5. Advanced information and communication technology (e-health)
	6. Integrated clinical pathways and functional dual referral systems
	7. Measurement, standards, and feedback
	8. Accreditation and certification
Lever 2: Improving quality of care (QoC) in support of PCIC	1. Organizational structure to lead the creation of an information base and development of strategies for quality improvement
	2. Systematic QoC measurement and continuous use of resulting data to support quality improvements
	3. Transformation of management practice to improve QoC in health facilities
Lever 3: Engaging citizens in support of the PCIC model	1. Health literacy
	2. Self-management practices
	3. Shared decision making
	4. Supportive macro environment for citizen patient engagement in health promotion and improvement
Lever 4: Reforming public hospital governance and management	1. Strong accountability mechanisms for autonomous public hospitals to strengthen performance
	2. Incentives aligned with public objectives and accountabilities
	3. Sound organizational arrangements for public hospital governance
	4. Gradual delegation of decision rights to hospitals
	5. Managerial capacity building

(Table continued next page)

TABLE A.1 Eight levers and recommended core actions for high-quality, value-based health service delivery in China *Continued*

Levers (strategic directions)	Core action areas
Lever 5: Realigning incentives in purchasing and provider payment	1. Provider payment reforms in support of PCIC
	2. Coherent, consistent incentives and stronger integration of care
	3. Rational distribution of services by facility level
	4. Capacity building of insurance agencies to equip them to become strategic purchasers
Lever 6: Strengthening the health workforce	1. Strong enabling environment for development of primary health care (PHC) workforce to implement PCIC
	2. Balanced workforce composition and competency for PHC service delivery
	3. Compensation system with strong incentives for good performance
	4. Headcount quota system reform to enable a more flexible health labor market and efficient health workforce management
Lever 7: Strengthening private sector engagement in health service delivery	1. A clear, shared vision of the private sector's potential contribution to health system goals
	2. Regulatory and enforcement capacity to steer health service delivery toward social goals
	3. A level playing field across public and private providers
Lever 8: Modernizing health service planning to guide investment	1. Shift from traditional input-based planning toward people-centered planning
	2. Engagement with all relevant stakeholders and local communities in the planning process
	3. Empowerment and enabling of regions and provinces to develop their own capital investment plans
	4. Introduction of a Certificate of Need program to evaluate and approve new capital investments
	5. Prioritization of community health projects

TABLE A.2 Government policies in support of the eight levers for health service delivery reform in China

Levers	Government policy statements in support of each lever	References
Lever 1: Shaping tiered health care delivery system in accordance with people-centered integrated care (PCIC) model	• Adhere to the people-first principle, and attach primary importance to safeguarding the rights and interests of the people's health. • Adhere to the tenet of serving the people's health with health care undertakings; regard safeguarding the people's health as the center, and take the entitlement of basic health care services to everyone as the fundamental aim and outcome. • Emphasize the combination of prevention, treatment, and rehabilitation. Strengthen the prevention of chronic diseases. • Make community health the "gatekeeper." Strengthen the three-tiered health service net in rural areas. Improve the health service system based on the TCH. • Promote the construction of the health care information system. Take advantage of the network information technology to promote the cooperation between urban hospitals and community health service institutions. • Establish a coordinated service system, and on the basis of enhancing grassroots services, optimize allocation of resources with the application of legal, social, administrative, and market tools to improve the quality of medical care and guide reasonable medical treatment. • Establish the multilevel diagnosis and treatment model characterized by initial diagnosis by grassroots institutions, a two-way referral system, separate treatments for urgent and chronic disease, and close cooperation between hospitals at different levels. • Focusing on the cultivation of general practitioners, establish the system of basic medical and health personnel training.	• Opinions of the CPC Central Committee and the State Council on Deepening the Health Care System Reform (*Zhong Fa* 2009, No. 6) • The Notification on Health Sector "Twelfth Five-Year Plan" (*Guo Fa* 2012, No. 57) • Suggestions of the CPC Committee on the 13th Five-Year Plan for National Economic and Social Development • Guidance of the General Office of the State Council on Overall Pilot Reform of Urban Public Hospitals (*Guo Ban Fa* 2015, No. 38) • State Council General Office Opinions on the Full Implementation of Comprehensive Reform in the County Level Public Hospital (*Guo Ban Fa* 2015, No. 33) • Planning Layout of National Medical and Health Services System (2015–2020) (*Guo Ban Fa* 2015, No. 14) • Construction Planning of Grassroots Health Professionals Focusing on the General Practitioners (*Fa Gai She Hui* 2010, No. 561) • Guidance of the General Office of the State Council on Promoting Multi-Level Diagnosis and Treatment System (*Guo Ban Fa* 2015, No. 70) • Guiding Opinions on Further Regulating Community Health Service Management and Improving Health Service Quality (*Guo Wei Ji Ceng Fa* 2015, No. 93)
Lever 2: Improving quality of care (QoC) in support of PCIC	• Strengthen regulation of health care service behavior and quality, improve the health care service standards and quality evaluation system, regulate the management system and work flows, quicken the formulation of the treatment protocols, and complete the health care service quality surveillance networks. • Enhance the management and control of medical quality. Clinical examination, diagnosis, treatment, drug use, and the use of implant medical apparatus should be regulated.	• *Zhong Fa* 2009, No. 6 • *Guo Fa* 2012, No. 57 • *Guo Ban Fa* 2015, No. 38 • *Guo Ban Fa* 2015, No. 33 • Suggestions of the CPC Committee on the 13th Five-Year Plan for National Economic and Social Development
Lever 3: Engaging citizens in support of the PCIC model	• Strengthen health promotion and education. Carry out health education, strengthen the dissemination of medical and health knowledge, advocate a healthy and civilized lifestyle, promote rational nutrition among the public, and enhance the health awareness and self-care ability of the people. • Build sound and harmonious relations between health care workers and patients. • Investigate timely to irrational use of drugs, material, examination, and repetitive examinations for economic benefit. • Promote the transparency of hospital information and establish a regular display system, including financial situation, performance assessment, quality safety, price and inpatient cost, and so on.	• *Zhong Fa* 2009, No. 6 • *Guo Fa* 2012, No. 57 • *Guo Ban Fa* 2015, No. 38 • *Guo Ban Fa* 2015, No. 33 • *Guo Ban Fa* 2015, No. 14 • Suggestions of the CPC Committee on the 13th Five-Year Plan for National Economic and Social Development • *Guo Wei Ji Ceng Fa* 2015, No. 93

(Table continued next page)

TABLE A.2 Government policies in support of the eight levers for health service delivery reform in China *Continued*

Levers	Government policy statements in support of each lever	References
Lever 4: Reforming public hospital governance and management	• Transform government functions and promote separation of functions of government agencies and public institutions as well as separation of administration and business operations. • Perfect the management mechanism of public hospitals, and complete the corporate legal person management system. • Promote innovation in modern hospital management, promote the professional specialization of dean teams, and improve public hospital management. Implement the autonomous right of public hospitals, such as in personnel management, internal distribution, and operations management.	• *Zhong Fa* 2009, No. 6 • *Guo Fa* 2012, No. 57 • *Guo Ban Fa* 2015, No. 38 • Suggestions of the CPC Committee on the 13th Five-Year Plan for National Economic and Social Development
Lever 5: Realigning incentives in purchasing and provider payment	• Along with economic and social development, efforts should be made to uplift the fund-raising and pooling levels step by step, narrow the gap between different insurance schemes, and eventually achieve the fundamental unity of those schemes. • Explore the establishment of an integrated urban and rural health insurance scheme. • Implement the reform of the mode of health insurance payment. • Utilize the fundamental function of health insurance, strengthen the budget for revenues and expenditures of medical insurance fund, and establish various payment methods, in which payment according to the type of disease is the major form and other forms like payment by person and payment by service unit may also be used. Promote the diagnosis-related group (DRG) system. • Establish effective, open, and fair negotiation mechanisms and risk-sharing mechanisms between the insurance agencies and designated medical institutions. • Establish the restriction mechanism of medial expense growth; control the unreasonable growth. • Implement the basic health insurance settlement directly as well as cost accounting and control. The various health insurances should regulate, control, supervise, and restrict the behavior of medical services and medical prices, effectively control medical costs, and regulate the medical service behavior of the working staff.	• *Zhong Fa* 2009, No. 6 • *Guo Fa* 2012, No. 57 • *Guo Ban Fa* 2015, No. 38 • *Guo Ban Fa* 2015, No. 33 • Opinions on Implementing the Control of Total Medical Insurance Payment (*Ren She Bu Fa* 2012, No. 70) • Notification of Pilot of DRGs Reform (*Fa Gai Jia Ge* 2011, No. 674) • Opinions on Further Improving the Reform of Health Insurance Payment (*Ren She Bu Fa* 2011, No. 63) • *Guo Ban Fa* 2015, No. 70 • Suggestions of the CPC Committee on the 13th Five-Year Plan for National Economic and Social Development

(Table continued next page)

TABLE A.2 Government policies in support of the eight levers for health service delivery reform in China *Continued*

Levers	Government policy statements in support of each lever	References
Lever 6: Strengthening the health workforce	• Promote the medical talent system and innovation of mechanisms. • Establish the reasonable incentives of income distributions, and improve the treatment of medical staff. Establish a personnel system and salary system suitable for the medical industry. The salary of the medical staff should not be linked to profit. • Implement the system of comprehensive performance evaluation and post performance-based salary in line with service quality and workload, and effectively mobilize the initiatives of health care workers. • Deepen the reform of the headcount quota system. In terms of headcount setting, income distribution, professional title evaluation, management and deployment, and personnel inside or outside the authorized size should be considered as a whole, and the reform of endowment insurance system should be carried out according to national regulation. • Adopt the employment system and post management system, and establish a flexible employment mechanism. Ensure the autonomous right of public hospitals in recruiting people. • Promote registered physicians' multisited practice.	• *Zhong Fa* 2009, No. 6 • *Guo Fa* 2012, No. 57 • *Guo Ban Fa* 2015, No. 38 • *Guo Ban Fa* 2015, No. 33 • *Guo Ban Fa* 2015, No. 14 • Several Opinions on Promoting and Regulating Doctors' Multi-Sited Practice (*Guo Wei Yi Fa* 2014, No. 86) • *Guo Ban Fa* 2015, No. 70 • Suggestions of the CPC Committee on the 13th Five-Year Plan for National Economic and Social Development • *Guo Wei Ji Ceng Fa* 2015, No. 93
Lever 7: Strengthening private sector engagement in health service delivery	• Encourage and guide social capital to sponsor health care undertakings. • Promote the development of nonpublic health care institutions, and form a health care system with multiple categories of investors and diversified investment modes. Encourage social forces to invest in the medical industry through funding of new construction or participating in restructuring. • Encourage and promote the incentives of nonpublic hospitals. • Further ease entry requirements. • Carry out the tax policy of nonpublic hospitals. • Carry out the same policies with the public hospitals when the nonpublic hospitals are designated medical institutions. • Improve classification management of medical institutions, and introduce the regulation of nonprofit hospitals, such as the nature of business and the usage of surplus.	• *Zhong Fa* 2009, No. 6 • *Guo Fa* 2012, No. 57 • *Guo Ban Fa* 2015, No. 38 • *Guo Ban Fa* 2015, No. 33 • *Guo Ban Fa* 2015, No. 14 • Several Policy Measures to Accelerate the Development of Medical Institutions Sponsored by Social Force (*Guo Ban Fa* 2015, No. 45) • Notification on Launching the Pilot of Establishing Wholly Foreign-Owned Hospitals (*Guo Wei Yi Han* 2014, No. 244) • State Council General Office Opinions on Further Encouraging and Guiding the Social Capital to Hold a Medical Institution (*Guo Ban Fa* 2010, No. 58) • Suggestions of the CPC Committee on the 13th Five-Year Plan for National Economic and Social Development • *Guo Wei Ji Ceng Fa* 2015, No. 93

(Table continued next page)

TABLE A.2 **Government policies in support of the eight levers for health service delivery reform in China** *Continued*

Levers	Government policy statements in support of each lever	References
Lever 8: Modernizing health service planning to guide investment	• Strengthen regional health planning. • Optimize medical resources allocation. • Plan resources in a differentiated manner at different levels. At the city level and below, basic medical services and public health resources will be planned according to size of population and service radius; at the provincial level and above, resources will be planned according to needs and priorities in different regions. • Instruct the health facilities to procure equipment in a rational manner according to their functions, skill competency, disciplinary development, and the health needs of the general public and in the spirit of resource sharing. • The implementation condition of planning should be taken as the basis of the hospital construction, financial investment, performance assessment, medical insurance payment, personnel allocation, and beds arrangement. The constraint of planning should be enhanced, and the execution condition of the planning should be made public regularly.	• *Zhong Fa 2009, No.6* • *Guo Fa 2012, No. 57* • *Guo Ban Fa 2015, No. 38* • *Guo Ban Fa 2015, No. 33* • *Guo Ban Fa 2015, No. 45* • *Guo Ban Fa 2015, No. 14* • *Guo Ban Fa 2015, No. 70* • Suggestions of the CPC Committee on the 13th Five-Year Plan for National Economic and Social Development

TABLE A.3 New policy guidelines on tiered health service delivery and recommended core actions

Policy guideline	Levers supporting policy guideline	Core actions supporting policy guideline
1. First diagnosis at the grassroots	Shaping tiered health care delivery system in accordance with people-centered integrated care (PCIC) model (Lever 1)	Primary health care as the first point of contact
2. Dual referral	Shaping tiered health care delivery system in accordance with PCIC model (Lever 1)	Integrated clinical pathways and functional dual referral systems
3. Interaction between the upper and grassroots levels	Shaping tiered health care delivery system in accordance with the PCIC model (Lever 1)	Vertical integration, including new roles for hospitals
4. Specify diagnosis and treatment functions of medical institutions of different grades and categories	Shaping tiered health care delivery system in accordance with the PCIC model (Lever 1)	Vertical integration, including new roles for hospitals
5. Enhance capability building of the grassroots health care team	Strengthening the health care workforce (Lever 6)	Strong enabling environment for development of primary health care workforce to implement PCIC
		Compensation system with strong incentives for good performance
6. Enhance grassroots capability in health care	Shaping tiered health care delivery system in accordance with the PCIC model (Lever 1)	Vertical integration, including new roles for hospitals
	Realigning incentives in purchasing and provider payment (Lever 5)	Rational distribution of services by facility level
	Strengthening private sector engagement in health service delivery (Lever 7)	A clear shared vision on the private sector's potential contribution to health system goals
7. Consolidate sharing of regional medical resources	Realigning incentives in purchasing and provider payment (Lever 5)	Correct and realign incentives to reverse the current irrational distribution of service by level of facilities
8. Speed up health care informatization	Shaping tiered health care delivery system in accordance with the PCIC model (Lever 1)	Advanced information and communication technology (e-health)
9. Improve mechanism for reasonable allocation of medical resources	Shaping tiered health care delivery system in accordance with the PCIC model (Lever 1)	Vertical integration, including new roles for hospitals
	Realigning incentives in purchasing and provider payment (Lever 5)	Rational distribution of services by facility level
10. Improve medical insurance payment system reform	Realigning incentives in purchasing and provider payment (Lever 5)	Coherent, consistent incentives and stronger integration of care
		Rational distribution of services by facility level
11. Establish and improve the profit distribution mechanism	Realigning incentives in purchasing and provider payment (Lever 5)	Capacity building of insurance agencies to equip them to become strategic purchasers
12. Structure a division of labor and coordination mechanism for medical institutions	Shaping tiered health care delivery system in accordance with the PCIC model (Lever 1)	Vertical integration, including new roles for hospitals

Note: "New Policy Guidelines" refers to the "Guidance of the General Office of the State Council on Promoting Multi-Level Diagnosis and Treatment System" (*Guo Ban Fa* 2015, No. 70).

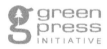